TISSUE MORPHOLOGY AND ANALYSIS

Dr. Greeshma Sharma

ALLIED
HEALTH
PRESS

Tissue Morphology and Analysis

Author: **Dr. Greeshma Sharma**

Allied Health Press
4164 Lakeshore Road
Burlington ON L7L 1A4
Canada
www.alliedhealthpress.com
Email: orders@arclereducation.com

ISBN: 978-1-77956-824-3

ABOUT THE AUTHOR

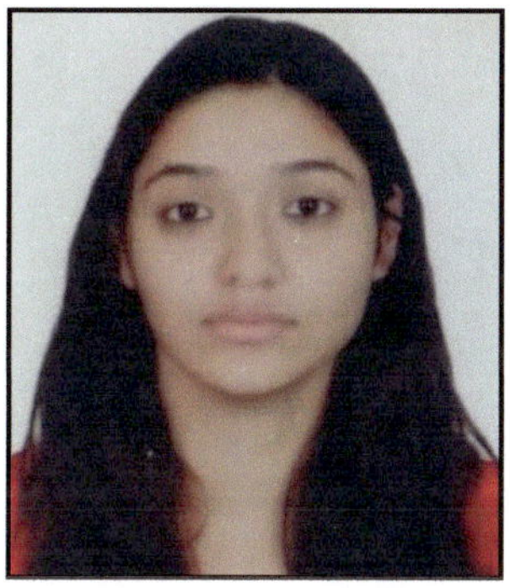

Dr. Greeshma Sharma, holds Ph.D. in Transfusion Medicine from PGIMER, Chandigarh, with a research focus on Neonatal Thrombocytopenia and Neonatal Alloimmune Thrombocytopenia (NAIT). She has completed her M.Sc. in Forensic Biotechnology from NFSU and a B.Sc. in Biological Sciences from Delhi University. She is currently working as a Project Research Scientist I under an ICMR-funded project on NAIT diagnosis and have previous experience as a Junior Research Fellow in DST-funded research. Some of her Publications include articles in Newborn Journal and Vox Sanguinis. She has qualified the UGC-NET (Forensic Science) and have received awards including the Harold Gunson Fellowship (ISBT 2020).

Brief Table of Contents

Detailed Table of Contents

CHAPTER 15

Digital Pathology and AI in Morphological Analysis 479

Index 513

LIST OF FIGURES

PREFACE

Understanding tissue structure is a foundation stone in a broad array of biomedical sciences. The tissue organization, shape, and cell-to-cell interactions of cells in tissues give us important clues about normal and disease function. From the early microscopy to molecular precision approaches of today, tissue study has remained at the focal point of research, diagnosis, and clinical decision-making. Not only does the investigation of cellular structure provide insight into the means whereby the body maintains homeostasis, but it also represents a useful window into the changes that accompany disease. A close familiarity with tissue morphology thus links basic biology and clinical medicine, bringing microscopic life together with the body's systemic response.

Improvements in tissue science have been driven by the continued development of laboratory techniques and imaging technology. Histological staining, immunolabeling strategies, and computational platforms have all contributed to improvements in tissue visualization and analysis. Furthermore, improvements in artificial intelligence and computational imaging now support high-throughput analysis, allowing both qualitative interpretation and quantitative measurement of tissue traits. Whether for identifying early cell change in cancer, quantifying organ biopsy fibrosis, or tracking developmental trends, the capacity to read tissue shape is more robust and specific than ever.

The text *Tissue Morphology and Analysis* has been planned as an encyclopedic work for students and scientists engaged in the disciplines of histology, pathology, and tissue-based research. It combines fundamental principles, general procedures, advanced techniques, and cutting-edge innovations into a cohesive book. Each chapter builds on the previous one, progressing from elementary topics to high-level applications, enabling the reader to develop a clear, sequential understanding of tissue morphology and its applications in scientific and clinical contexts. With proper emphasis on conventional histological concepts complemented by high-end computational algorithms, the book is approaching both conventional methods and newer cutting-edge methods that are changing the game for tissue analysis today.

Chapter 1 is an introduction to tissue morphology as a discipline, including the scope of its significance, historical development, and use in biomedical environments. It offers some key vocabulary, types of tissues, and the overall tissue examination process, setting the stage for the more technologically oriented discussions in later chapters.

Chapter 2 explains the fundamental principles of histological techniques. It is about tissue fixation, embedding, sectioning, and staining methods with emphasis on routine procedures carried out in laboratory settings. It explains how fixatives preserve tissue integrity and how staining differentiates structures within tissue.

Chapter 3 discusses the structural characteristics of epithelial tissues. In the chapter, epithelial types are categorized by layer and form, as well as the manner in which their structure relates to functions such as protection, absorption, and secretion. Diagnostic significance and clinical case examples are given.

Chapter 4 addresses connective tissues, defining components like collagen, elastin, and ground substance. It briefly addresses specialized connective tissues like cartilage, bone, and adipose tissue. The chapter relates structural diversity to functional functions in support, transport, and defense.

Chapter 5 explains muscle tissue morphology. It discriminates between skeletal, cardiac, and smooth muscle and mentions their different histological features and contraction modes. The chapter also provides visual criteria for the diagnosis of muscular disorders from tissue samples.

Chapter 6 covers nervous tissue morphology. This includes the morphology of the neuron and glial cells, synaptic morphology, and regional variations in the central and peripheral nervous systems. Histological methods in nervous tissue analysis are also covered.

Chapter 7 deals with the analysis of vascular and lymphatic tissue. It outlines the morphology of blood vessels, capillaries, and lymphatics, highlighting their structure in different organs. It also emphasizes the identification of vascular pathology and lymphatic involvement in disease processes.

Chapter 8 presents a detailed consideration of tissue preparation and sectioning. The technical considerations of trimming, orientation, and microtomy are discussed. Frequent artifacts and optimal tissue presentation are also troubleshooted.

Chapter 9 addresses histochemical and cytochemical techniques. It discusses the use of dyes and chemical reactions for the detection of tissue components, including carbohydrates, lipids, and enzymes. The practical utility of these techniques in research and diagnosis is illustrated by examples.

Chapter 10 introduces immunohistochemistry (IHC), focusing on antigen-antibody interaction, labeling protocols, and detection systems. The chapter explains how proteins are detected in tissue sections using IHC, with a focus on pathologic diagnostic markers.

Chapter 11 describes advanced imaging and analysis techniques such as confocal microscopy, multiphoton microscopy, and electron microscopy. The techniques are described in terms of resolution, sample requirements, and how they enhance tissue view depth.

Chapter 12 deals with *in situ* hybridization and molecular morphology. It describes techniques of nucleic acid sequence localization within tissues and how molecular probes may be employed to comprehend gene expression patterns.

Chapter 13 addresses morphometric analysis and quantification. It explains the structural tissue characteristics that are measured, analyzed, and statistically interpreted. The manual and automatic methods are contrasted, and the latter's role in diagnostic reporting and research is charted.

Chapter 14 covers pathological tissue morphology, with an emphasis on morphological alterations in diseases such as cancer, inflammation, and degenerative states. The chapter demonstrates the use of morphological characteristics in disease diagnosis and staging.

Chapter 15 considers the application of artificial intelligence and digital pathology in tissue analysis. It discusses image digitization, pattern recognition, tissue classification using algorithms, and integration of AI tools into diagnostic procedures.

This book may be adopted by undergraduate and postgraduate students of medical, dental, veterinary, and allied health sciences; laboratory technicians and technologists in pathology and research laboratories; academic researchers in histology and biomedical sciences; and clinicians seeking to learn about tissue structure for diagnostic or research purposes. It supports both independent learning and structured academic instruction through clear descriptions, visual reminders, and first-hand illustrations.

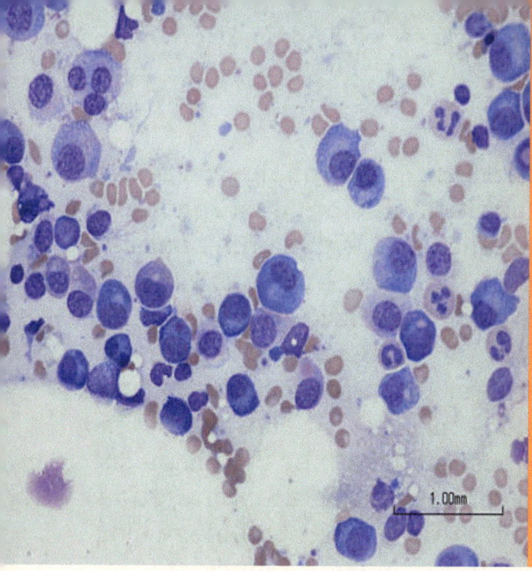

Chapter 1

INTRODUCTION TO TISSUE MORPHOLOGY

Contents

Introduction

Tissue morphology is the study of tissue form and organization at the cellular and extracellular levels. It seeks to understand how tissues develop, their organization, and how they work within biological systems and the implications of the interrelation between form and function. By techniques such as microscopy and histology, researchers are able to see and study the form of different tissues and therefore come to conclusions about their overall function. Tissue morphology is also important in numerous other fields, such as developmental biology and medicine, because it provides a foundation for how tissues respond to environmental changes, injury, and disease processes. Effectively, tissue morphology serves as an important doorway to understanding the complexities of biological systems, along with the mechanisms that determine organ development and tissue integrity. Tissue morphology also encompasses an appreciation of its evolutionary history, where variations in tissue structure may be traced along different species. Comparative anatomy is rich in information regarding adaptive processes that have come to fruition over millions of years. For instance, the morphological study of the marsupial mammal chondrocranium illustrates cryptic conservatism in cranial morphology, uncovering evolutionary constraints and adaptive functions. For instance, the wide lamina basalis and development of tactile sensory organs in neonatal marsupials illustrate how morphology contributes directly to survival adaptations. Also, the continuous modernization of imaging technology favors such studies, allowing for greater appreciation of morphological innovations in taxonomies. Such knowledge ultimately increases our understanding of evolutionary biology and highlights the intricate correlation between function and morphology in different ecosystems. In the medical context, comprehensive knowledge of tissue morphology is important for the diagnosis and treatment of disease. Abnormalities in the structure of tissues are generally a manifestation of inherent health disorders, so morphological analysis is a cornerstone of histopathology. For example, knowledge of the morphological changes associated with arrhythmias, as elucidated in studies of the atrioventricular conduction axis, is significant in uncovering mechanisms of cardiac dysfunction. The combination of morphological data with electrophysiological information enables a clearer view of disease processes, leading to improved diagnostic accuracy and therapeutic planning. Hence, tissue morphology not only informs normal biological processes but is also vital as an indispensable technology for the identification and treatment of complex diseases, underscoring its significance in both research and clinical practice (Figure 1.1).

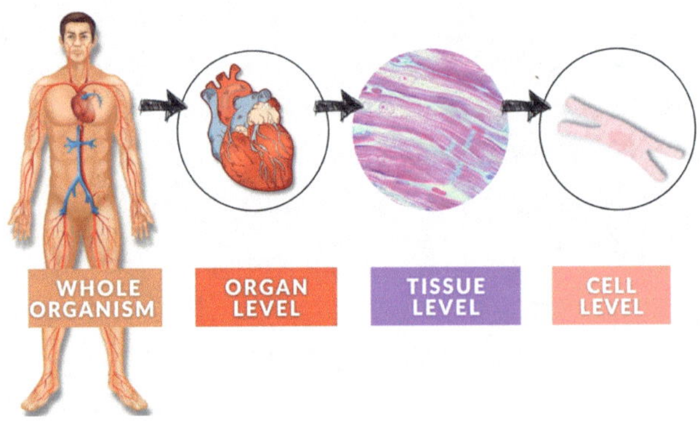

Figure 1.1. Definition of tissue morphology.

Source: https://www.biologyonline.com/wp-content/uploads/2019/10/types-or-levels-of-morphology.jpg.

Explanation of Tissue Morphology

Tissue morphology knowledge: Knowledge of tissue morphology is critical to the appreciation of biological system complexity because it examines the structure, organization, and function of cells in tissues. Tissue morphology comprises various levels of biological organization from cellular aggregations to extracellular matrices, which serve to support numerous physiological functions. For instance, the organization of epithelial tissues is key to forming protective barriers and facilitating selective permeability, while connective tissues supply structural support and anchorage. Cell types and their microenvironments interact reciprocally in intricate ways to decide the overall structure of the tissue, which is required for homeostasis and for the repair of tissues. Morphological tissue defects can lead to functional disturbances and are typically accompanied by disease pathology, underscoring the need for detailed investigation in both healthy and diseased states. Cell migration is one of the impressive aspects of tissue morphology, a dynamic process of behavior important in development, tissue repair, and disease. Studies have shown that migration behavior is characterized not only by biochemical signals but also by mechanical properties of the extracellular matrix and by neighboring cell structures. For example, in invasion from cancer, cells possess ameboid-like modes of migration depending on the rigidity and deformability of their surroundings. These mechanical interactions can also control cancer cell migratory phenotype and velocity in various environments, implying that tissue geometry can be particularly influential in disease phenomena. Emerging tools for modeling these phenomena, such as cellular Potts models to model cell behavior in confined spaces, offer insights into how structure in tissues influences cell migration and can thus be employed to develop drugs against malignancies and other diseases (Preziosi, L. & Scianna, M., 2013). Moreover, the morphology of organelles, including mitochondria, contributes additional context to tissue disease and function. Mitochondria play critical roles in energy generation, and dynamic morphology is linked with various cellular processes and disease states, e.g., cancer. Abnormalities in the shape and distribution of mitochondria can serve as markers of occult cellular stress or dysfunction, and these organelles' structural characteristics may reflect overall tissue health. High-resolution imaging techniques such as 2D confocal fluorescence and 3D electron micrograph reconstruction allow for thorough scrutiny of mitochondrial morphologies in real-time living cells. By measuring such morphological markers, researchers can gain insight into cellular responses to pharmacological challenges, thereby identifying potential biomarkers of disease progression and drug action (Achuthan et al., 2019). Hence, tissue morphology research transcends structural analysis to comprise more general knowledge of cellular dynamics and health.

Importance in Biological Sciences

The role of biological sciences in tissue morphology cannot be overemphasized. Understanding the intricate structures and mechanisms of tissues lies at the heart of knowing how organisms develop, maintain homeostasis, and respond to environmental stress. Tissue morphology provides a foundation for studying cell organization in tissues, providing insights into their functions. Utilizing sophisticated imaging modalities and histological methods, researchers can visualize the spatial relationships between cells, which are critical to the comprehension of physiological processes. This morphological information is crucial for identifying aberrations that lead to disease, demonstrating the intersection of cellular architecture and pathological states. These tests are not only essential to basic biological knowledge but also have practical applications in medical diagnosis and treatment therapies, demonstrating a practical application of tissue morphology within the biological sciences. Furthermore, tissue morphology is studied within the field of neuroscience as well, where an understanding of the structural design of neuronal tissue can enhance our knowledge of advanced brain functions. Brain morphology studies have revealed the intricate organization of neuronal circuits that form the basis of cognition and behavior. The striatal complexes' role in regulating motor activity is an excellent example of how tissue morphology bridges structural properties with functional implications in the nervous system. The integration of microscopic details into macroscopic representations, as suggested in Noori (2009), is another excellent example of how computational tools facilitate this understanding through simulation of brain compartment interactions. Such interdisciplinarity highlights the fundamental importance of tissue morphology in mediating organization and function, thereby providing insight into broader biological contexts, such as neurobiology. Of significance beyond its place within developmental biology and neuroscience, tissue morphology is central to the elucidation of mechanisms for many diseases, most particularly neurodegenerative disease. Investigation of molecular mechanisms involved in tissue and cellular integrity often has significant lessons for disease process. For instance, the role of p38 MAPK signaling in neuroinflammation and synaptic plasticity is interesting as it can potentially provide therapeutic target pathways for neurodegenerative diseases like Alzheimer's and Parkinson's, as discussed in Corrêa, S. A. L. & Eales, K. L. (2012). Knowing how molecular changes result in tissue-level morphological changes allows scientists to develop early diagnosis methods as well as targeted therapies. This association of tissue structure with disease makes it more applicable to biological sciences in general and underscores the need for a unified study of biological systems (Figure 1.2).

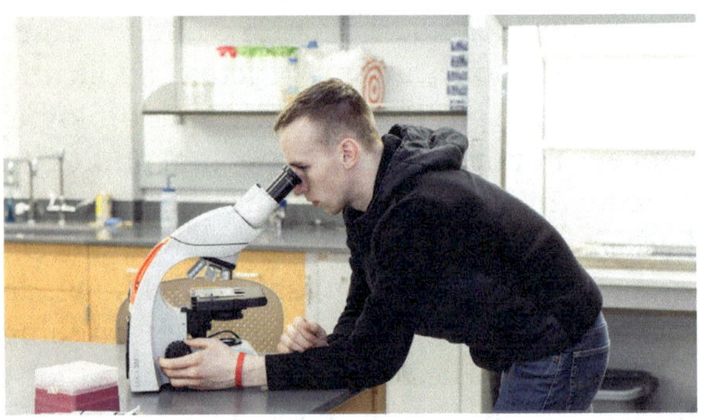

Figure 1.2. Importance in biological sciences.

Source: https://www.northcentralcollege.edu/sites/default/files/styles/full_image_large_2x/public/2021-11/biology-experiment-2.jpg?h=d0b5a34c&itok=fQE5BAKA.

Historical Context and Development

Tissue morphology possesses a rich and diverse history that underlies its modern meaning and uses. Early investigations of tissue structure were an immediate outgrowth of early research in histology, wherein scientists used rudimentary means to examine microscopic shapes within some organisms. Developments in histological techniques, particularly in the 19th century, led to discoveries about cell-based tissue architecture. Visionaries such as Rudolf Virchow pioneered the theory of cellular pathology and posited that pathological processes may be explained by examining tissue structure. This paradigm transformed the basis of correlating structure to function and highlighted the utility of tissue morphology in the broader biological sciences. Also, the interconnection of microscopy and histological investigation provided mounting levels of tissue organization that have persisted to the present era, further shaping contemporary disciplinary practice in the science of tissue morphology. As the discipline advanced, significant contributions were made through evolutionary developmental biology (evo-devo), which brought fresh insights into the interplay of tissue structure and evolution. One of the surprises to emerge from research in evolutionary developmental biology (evo-devo) is that increased diversity of body plans and morphology in animals among animal phyla is not paired with equally breathtaking alterations on the level of gene composition of their genomes. So, for instance, tissue-level simplicity frequently occurs alongside much genetic complexity. And also, in this conversation, it is suggested that rather than relying only on new adaptations of genes, evolutionary changes will happen more frequently due to variations in gene regulation and reorganization of existing genetic networks. All this is possible through rigorous adherence to the phylogeny and demographic history of the organisms, which, in turn, has implications for tissue morphology research at a broader level. During the past decades, the use of theories of urban morphology in studies of tissue morphology has introduced a new type of understanding into the nature of the development of complex biological systems. Although there are several excellent examples of the application of research into urban morphology to designing new developments of housing across Europe, it is very difficult to find examples relating to other types of land use and beyond Europe. The histological evolution of tissue organization is patterned after urban planning systems, where structure determines function and function determines structure. The comparative perspective allows tissues to see how they can transform over time according to varying pressures, just like urban centers transform according to socio-economic forces. Such interdisciplinarity not only enriches tissue morphological understanding but also propels progress in biomedicine by informing the design and implementation of regenerative therapies and tissue engineering according to a complete understanding of both structure and biological adaptation.

1.1. Types of Tissues

The multiclassification of tissues in biological organisms represents a general framework in tissue morphology studies. There are basically four types of tissues: epithelial, connective, muscle, and nervous tissues. All these tissue types possess characteristic structural features and functions. Epithelial tissue covers body surfaces and cavities and defends, absorbs, and secretes. Connective tissue, on the other hand, supports, binds, and protects other tissues and organs, often appearing as a loose arrangement of cells dispersed within an extracellular matrix. Muscle tissue, recognizable from its contractility, aids in locomotion and movement, while nervous tissue networks control body functions and processes via electrical impulses, highlighting complexity and specialization in tissue organization. As one further explores connective tissue, its various functions become known. It not only provides structural and physical support to the body but also plays a role in energy storage and immunity. Connective tissues fall under various subgroups, including loose connective tissue, dense connective tissue, adipose tissue, cartilage, bone, and blood. Each subtype possesses particular characteristics that are unique to its respective functions, such as adipose tissue for energy storage and body insulation, and bone providing support and firmness. The dynamic nature of connective tissues can be demonstrated by the discovery and definition of multipotent stem cells, such as dental neural crest-derived progenitor cells in the human third molar pad. These cells can differentiate into various types of tissues and thus mirror connective tissues' potential towards regenerative medicine (Degistirici et al., 2008).

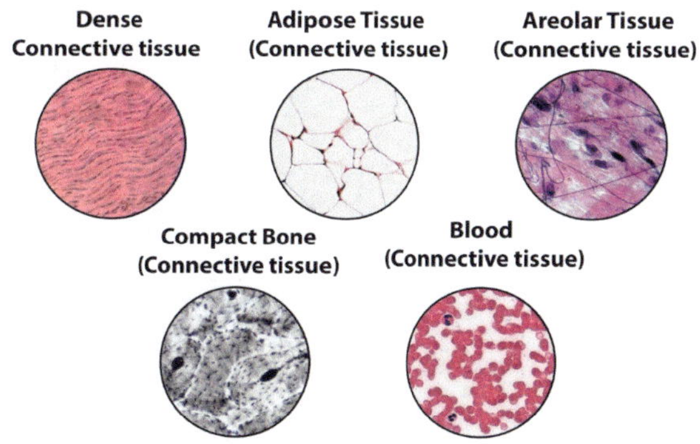

Figure 1.3. Types of tissues.

Source: https://www.vedantu.com/question-sets/04651295-3175-43d6-bad9-57b28f4cad533810317559862032324.png.

Muscle tissue, which is divided into three broad forms—skeletal, cardiac, and smooth—is essential in performing functions on behalf of the organism. Skeletal muscle, being striated and under voluntary control, plays a role in the movement process. In opposition to this, cardiac muscle, found solely in the heart, operates involuntarily and possesses a special organisation whereby it is able to contract perpetually. Smooth muscle, found within hollow organs such as intestines and blood vessels, also operates involuntarily but has an even more restrained appearance with no striations. The study of muscle tissue morphology provides information about its biomechanical function and capacity for regeneration. This understanding is critical in its use from injury repair to athletic performance, and here it is emphasized that well-defined types of muscle tissue are important in health as well as disease conditions (Figure 1.3).

1.1.1. Epithelial Tissue

Epithelial tissue is one of the four simple tissue types within the human body, characterized by its rigid cell structures that form protective coverings and scaffolds on various surfaces. Epithelial tissue is known for being continuous, typically in the form of slabs of tightly packed cells with minimal extracellular matrix between them. Functionally, epithelial tissue is critical in protection, secretion, and absorption functions that are crucial in homeostasis maintenance. Epithelial tissue can be classified by cell shape—squamous, cuboidal, or columnar—and by layer number—simple or stratified—which results in a large range of structures appropriate for specific functions in specific organs in the body. Its peculiar properties are borne out in its adaptability and responsiveness to a wide range of physiological stimuli.

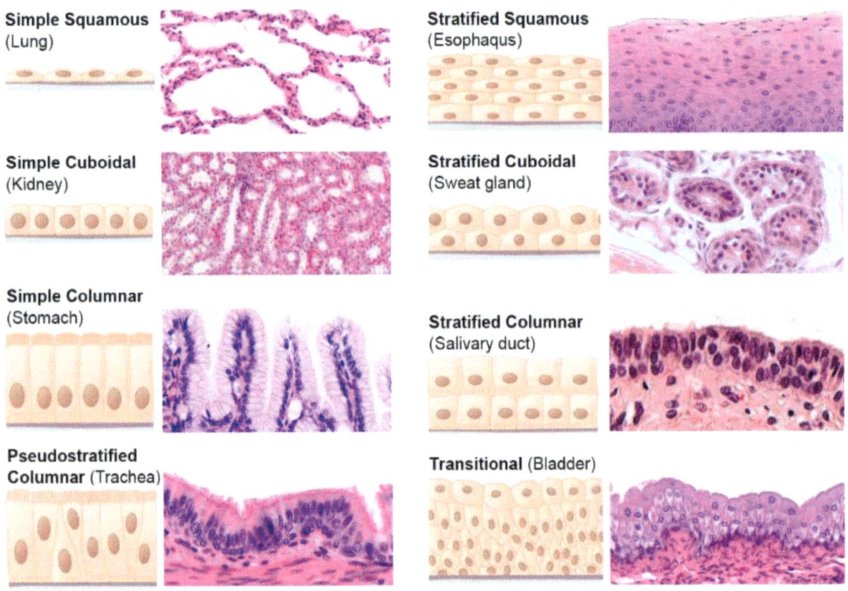

Figure 1.4. Epithelial tissue.

Source: https://medicinebtg.com/wp-content/uploads/2017/06/Epithelial-Tissues-In-Human-Body-tissue-is-classified-by-cell-shape-and-the-number-of-layers-it-therefore-found-1007x776.jpg.

Epithelial cells, for instance, possess the ability to regenerate themselves rapidly and self-repair, which is particularly relevant in areas subject to wear and tear, such as the skin and gastrointestinal tract. In addition, recent research has shown that certain proteins, such as TMIGD1, are essential in modulating cell morphology, adhesion, and survival in epithelial tissues. Knocking down TMIGD1 in cultured kidney epithelial cells increases cell death, underscoring the importance of this protein in maintaining epithelial cell integrity under stress. Thus, understanding the molecular mechanisms that govern epithelial tissue behavior not only explains normal physiological processes but also unravels potential therapeutic interventions in disease conditions such as kidney injury (Arafa, 2016). In addition to structural and barrier functions, epithelial tissue is critical in facilitating communication and interaction in multicellular environments. Recent advances in computational modeling have enabled a better understanding of cellular interactions within epithelial layers. An agent-based model, designed to simulate epithelial cell behavior, demonstrates how the dynamics of cell growth can be regulated by external conditions, such as calcium level in the growth medium.

The results of these simulations reveal qualitative agreement with experimentally observed patterns of growth of epithelial cells *in vitro*, emphasizing emergent properties that result from interactions among cells. These observations not only increment our understanding of tissue morphology but also highlight the complexity of cellular environments, paving the way for further work that can elucidate epithelial tissue response in health and disease (Hill et al., 2004) (Figure 1.4).

1.1.2. Connective Tissue

Connective tissue is a significant component in the overall structure of the body, differing from other tissues such as epithelial, muscular, and nervous tissue in function and structure. It is defined by a matrix that provides support, binding, and protection to various organs and structures. Noteworthy is that connective tissue is heterogeneous and consists of subtypes like loose connective tissue, dense connective tissue, adipose tissue, and specialized forms like bone and cartilage. This heterogeneity of each of these subtypes arises from variation in cell types and the extracellular matrix, which is rich in fibers, collagen, and elastin. This structural plasticity allows connective tissue to adapt to various mechanical stresses and facilitates physiological functions such as movement and nutrient delivery, and is critical for maintaining homeostasis and overall health. The sophistication of connective tissue extends beyond mere structural support; it is also an important part of physiological response. For instance, the mechanical characteristics of connective tissue control the plasticity of musculoskeletal structures to environmental conditions, such as in weightlessness during space travel. From research, the musculoskeletal system, which relies heavily on connective tissues, is plastic in the sense that it can support multiple mechanical loads. Prolonged periods of disuse, such as those endured by astronauts, lead to spectacular restructuring and changes in the function of such connective tissues, demonstrating their sensitivity to mechanical loads (N/A).

The understanding of this plasticity is essential in the development of countermeasures to minimize the adverse effects of microgravity on human health, depicting the complex interplay between connective tissue morphology and functional outcomes. Furthermore, specialized connective tissues such as bat wings show the intricate interrelationship between function and structure in the field of connective tissue morphology. The unique structure of bat wing membranes, which consist of specialized muscle fibers and elastin bundles, shows how connective tissues evolve to meet some functional requirements. They are thinner than typical mammalian skin and are well-organized to enable enhanced aerodynamics in flight. The structure of these connective components, like the presence of specialized types of muscles within the wing, enhances the ability of a bat to manage wing shape during flight (Fenton et al., 2017). These instances illustrate not only the variety of connective tissue but also its mandatory roles in specialized functions, which point to the importance of the morphology of connective tissue in informing the evolutionary adaptations of various organisms (Figure 1.5).

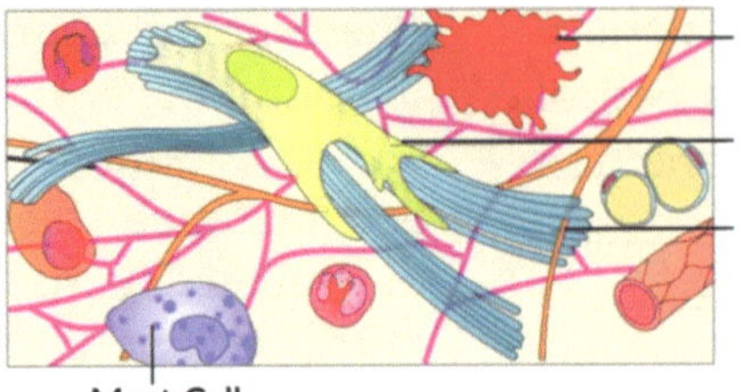

Figure 1.5. Connective tissue.

Source: https://st.adda247.com/https://www.careerpower.in/blog/wp-content/uploads/sites/2/2024/02/08172533/connective-tissues-1.png.

1.1.3. Muscle and Nervous Tissue

The intricate anatomy of muscle tissue plays a critical role in the effective operation of the human body. Muscle tissue is predominantly of three kinds: skeletal, cardiac, and smooth. Skeletal muscle is voluntary and striated and enjoys the support of the nervous system for precise movement. Cardiac muscle, while also striated, operates involuntarily to regulate heart rhythms, while smooth muscle is not striated and is found within the internal organ walls, and is employed to assist in involuntary movements such as peristalsis. It is significant to be aware of each muscle's morphological characteristics, as they significantly influence their own physiological functions. Moreover, the ability of muscle tissue to contract and generate force is not simply a result of cell composition but rather depends on the coordination of nervous tissue, illustrating the interdependence between the two tissue types in maintaining homeostasis and facilitating movement within an organism. Nervous tissue, tasked with mediating communication in the body, consists of neurons and glial cells, both of which have distinct but complementary roles. Neurons are adapted to transmit impulses, while glial cells provide support, nutrition, and protection to them. The complex morphology of neurons with dendrites, axons, and synapses allows for efficient transmission of the signal over large distances, facilitating responses to stimuli both internal and external. As discussed under evolutionary perspectives of neural elongations, such as those adopted by internal coordination models, was to enhance coordination between muscle contractions across multicellular bodies (de Wiljes et al., 2017). This relationship between nervous and muscle tissues illustrates how evolutionary adaptations have formed their anatomy in a way that enables them to create complex physiological systems needed for survival and responding to the surroundings. Furthermore, pathological changes that occur in contiguous tissues can reveal the functional relevance of muscle and nervous tissue. For instance, malfunctioning perivascular adipose tissue (PVAT) can influence vascular health with the engagement of both muscle and nervous responses in cardiovascular diseases (Guzik, T. J., & Nosalski, R., 2017). The inflammatory microenvironment resulting from aberrant cellular responses in PVAT can lead to systemic vascular impairment, suggesting the overall impact of tissue morphology on health. An appreciation of the interconnection of the function and structure of muscle and nervous tissues has the potential to create insights into certain diseases that detail new avenues for treatment. It is this interconnectivity that necessitates thorough studies in tissue morphology, ultimately leading us to understand how these tissues work together within biologically complex systems (Figure 1.6).

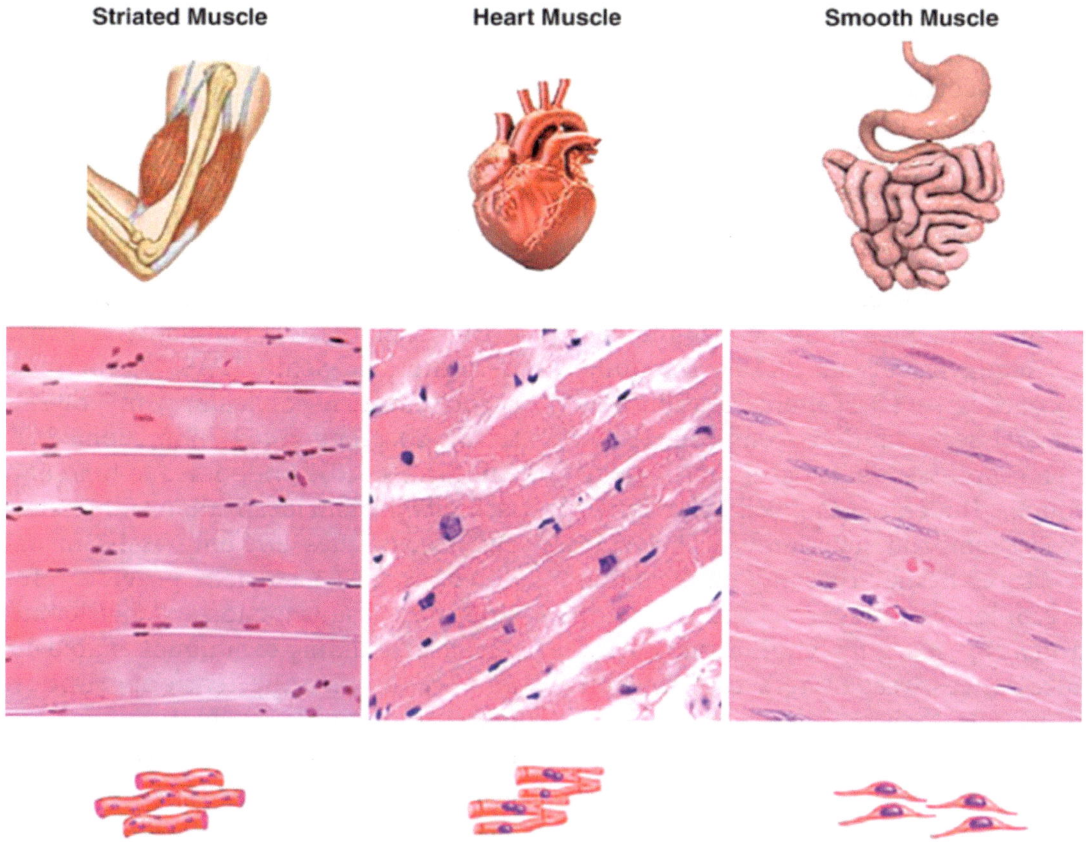

Figure 1.6 Muscle and nervous tissue.

Source: https://media.springernature.com/lw685/springer-static/image/chp%3A10.1007%2F978-3-031-33924-0_2/MediaObjects/532514_1_En_2_Fig2_HTML.png.

1.2. Techniques in Tissue Morphology

Tissue morphology investigation entails numerous techniques essential for understanding tissue structural organization and function. One significant approach is the use of three-dimensional (3D) scaffolding to enhance cell growth in a controlled environment. For instance, advances in the preparation of fibrous matrices have led to the creation of materials with an interbonded fiber structure with controlled pore size and porosity levels. These matrices not just maximized cell culture performance but also reproduced the natural extracellular matrix, leading to cellular behavior that is strikingly close to *in vivo* conditions. The efficiency of these scaffolds has been demonstrated by employing various cell lines, and this holds great potential in regenerative medicine and tissue engineering, which are critical characteristics of tissue morphology analysis (Kirkland et al., 2011). Another effective technique in the discipline of tissue morphology pertains to image analysis for the segmentation of nuclei in pathological analysis. Accurate measurement of nuclear characteristics in cancer tissues is essential to identify the degree and advancement of the disease. Traditional techniques, such as active contours, have been found to be insufficient for segmenting nuclei in images with heterogeneous staining. In order to solve these problems, studies have focused on fully automatic morphology-based approaches that further improve the segmentation accuracy. The novel approach offers the precise quantification of protein activity in histologically heterogeneous tissue sections and thus enhances the diagnostic capability of histological examinations. The ability to extract rich information from tissue images underscores the central role of advanced segmentation techniques in tissue morphology research (Acquaviva et al., 2010). Blending these approaches — 3D scaffold creation and advanced image segmentation — emphasizes the interdisciplinarity essential to tissue morphology breakthroughs. Understanding cell behavior in engineered systems and quantitatively analyzing tissue structures has far-reaching implications in both biomedical research and medical applications. By merging engineering with biological sciences, researchers can develop more efficacious therapeutic strategies and diagnostic reagents. With the development of tissue morphology techniques, the potential to move them into practical applications increases, holding out the promise of revolutionary advances in disease treatment, particularly for complex tissue structures. The fusion of engineering concepts with biological knowledge is a promising research and application in the field of tissue morphology.

1.2.1. Histological Staining Methods

Histological stains are an indispensable set of techniques in tissue morphology that allow scientists and clinicians to observe and differentiate cellular structures in biological specimens. Using specific dyes, these techniques provide tissue contrast, allowing pathological changes, cellular constituents, and tissue architecture to be readily identified. The most popularly employed stains, i.e., hematoxylin and eosin (H&E), provide good differentiation of nuclei and cytoplasmic material that is of most value in diagnostic pathology. As a main tool in the understanding of tissue structure and disease, staining methods may detect subtle aspects of cell morphology not seen in unstained specimens. The variety of histological stains also permits examination of specific cellular structures and elements, thus broadening the area of tissue study. Special stains specific to particular tissue types or cellular constituents are used to define structures such as collagen fibers, mucins, and other extracellular matrix components. For instance, periodic acid-Schiff (PAS) staining identifies carbohydrates, particularly in polysaccharide tissue. Correspondingly, immunohistochemistry employs specific antibodies to bind antigens to facilitate protein localization at the cellular level. Such techniques not only assist in pathologic detection but also help provide information regarding tissue function and development. Such advanced staining techniques enable diagnostic and research applications, underscoring the importance of histological protocols in contemporary biomedical research. The advancement in histological staining methods has also improved our ability to examine complex tissue structures. Techniques such as multiplexed staining can now observe multiple biomarkers simultaneously, improving diagnostic specificity and cell characterization precision. New techniques, such as the utilization of image analysis software, also enable better quantitation and comparison between staining results, providing a more data-driven understanding of tissue morphology. Current studies have explored the application of advanced staining techniques, showing their applicability in research contexts, such as analyzing engineered tissues. An example is the construction of organotypic models in regenerative medicine, which requires proper morphological analysis, as seen in the complex pathologies of the respiratory system, where histological analyses inform disease implications (Berry et al., 2017). Similarly, methods used in measuring chondrogenic differentiation give insights into the regeneration of articular cartilage, and this further illustrates the pivotal role staining techniques play in the demystification of complex biological processes (Asadian et al., 2020) (Figure 1.7).

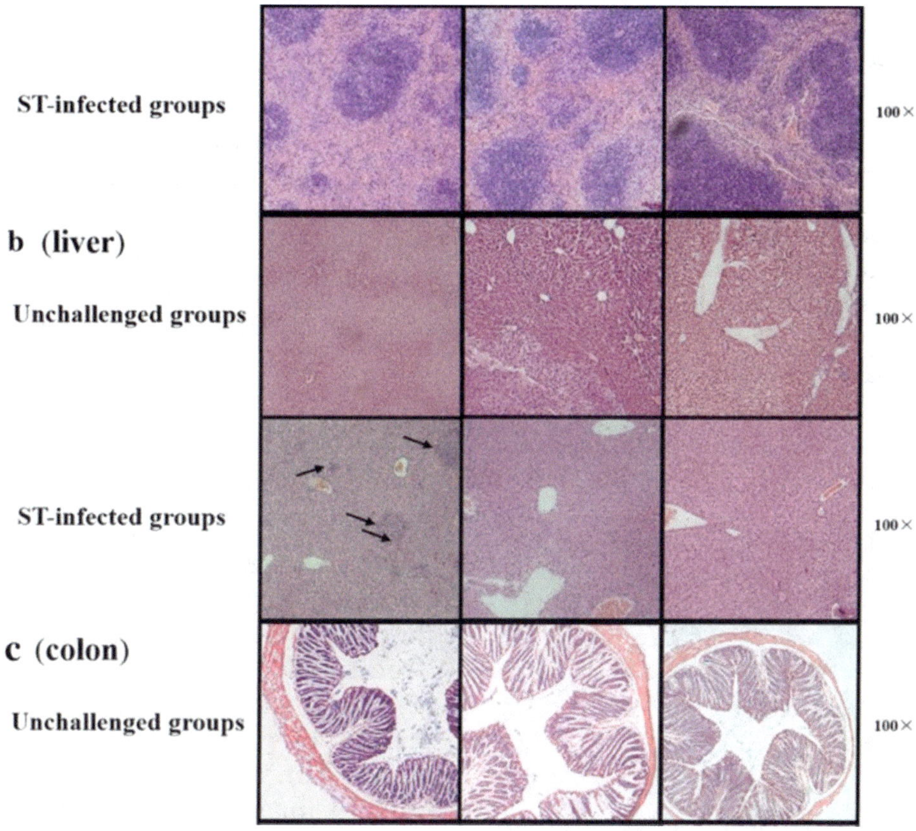

Figure 1.7. Histological staining methods.

Source: https://www.researchgate.net/publication/350738393/figure/fig1/AS:1010549110370333@1617945091313/Histological-morphology-was-determined-by-H-E-staining-a-Histological-morphology-of_Q640.jpg.

1.2.2. Microscopy Techniques

In tissue morphology research, various microscopy techniques are crucial in observing and analyzing the intricate structures of biological tissues. Light microscopy, for example, forms the foundation of histological analysis, which allows researchers to easily examine stained tissue sections. It enables researchers to determine cellular organization, tissue architecture, and morphological changes in pathological diseases. The ability to discriminate between different types of tissues and quantify cellular response to diverse stimuli is critical, particularly when investigating osseointegration of dental implants. For instance, studies show that microscopy at high resolution can potentially provide valuable information on the interfaces between bone and implant, an aspect that is critically relevant with respect to facilitating correct integration in the biological environment (Fujinaka, 2019). On the other hand, more recent microscopy techniques, such as multimodal nonlinear optical (NLO) microscopy, have been very promising in the research of cancer by identifying very fine changes in tissue morphology that are associated with malignancies. This new method employs several imaging modalities to enhance our understanding in morphological changes at the cellular and subcellular level. In cancer of the colon, NLO microscopy has been successful in revealing characteristic tissue microstructure patterns that are highly distinguishable in cancer and normal tissues. Through these advanced techniques, researchers can determine abnormalities in cell development and collagen architecture, which allows for the improvement of diagnostic and prognostic accuracy. This capability underscores the need to use multiple microscopy techniques to achieve a comprehensive understanding of disease and improve clinical outcomes (Adur et al., 2014).

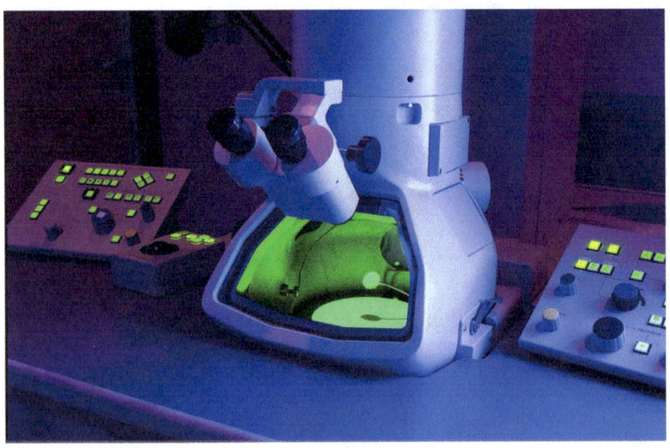

Figure 1.8. Microscopy techniques.

Source: https://scitechdaily.com/images/Electron-Microscope.jpg.

Besides, combining quantitative analysis with high-end imaging technologies offers overall tissue morphology a better insight. An example of the equipment used by researchers to facilitate quantitative measurements of structural properties such as bone volume and implant integration, thus providing a clearer definition of healing processes, is microcomputed tomography (μCT). In a recent comparative study of different implant configurations, μCT and histological analyses revealed extensive differences in osseointegration patterns, showing the advantage of piezoelectric surgery. These findings not only report the complex interactions between biomaterials and host tissue but also highlight the need for new imaging technologies to guide future development in tissue engineering and regenerative medicine. Ultimately, the continued advancement of microscopy techniques will go a long way toward advancing the science of tissue morphology, thereby providing greater understanding of tissue dynamics and disease across many fields of medicine (Fujinaka, 2019) (Figure 1.8).

1.2.3. Imaging Technologies in Tissue Analysis

The development of imaging techniques has transformed the field of tissue analysis by enhancing our understanding of tissue morphology and related pathological lesions. Traditional imaging techniques, such as histology, have been the core tools but are lacking in providing dynamic and detailed information about the architecture of tissues. Modern imaging devices, including Magnetic Resonance Imaging (MRI), Positron Emission Tomography (PET), and ultrasound, give three-dimensional images of tissue structure and function. All of these technologies have proven highly useful in clinical practice, particularly in detecting and staging diseases, as they allow non-invasive visualizations of the tissues without the requirement for bulky surgical interventions. Despite the advances, though, bridging phenotypic data generated by such imaging devices with genomic data is a gigantic problem, and this necessitates relentless innovation in imaging technology to bridge these critical gaps (Andrén et al., 2018). One of the most promising technologies in this direction is Imaging Mass Spectrometry (IMS), which is an innovative technique enabling the detection of molecular constituents in tissues. By comparing these molecular profiles and genomic characteristics, IMS can provide insights into gene expression patterns and detect potential mutations. This feature is particularly significant for decoding the complex biology of disease because it hastens the attribution of phenotypes observed with the molecular origins of such diseases. The spatial resolution offered by IMS allows the mapping of thousands of proteins and metabolites, thus revealing tissue structure and function's subtle details that could be lost using conventional imaging approaches. IMS is hence at the forefront of converting tissue analysis into a more holistic and comprehensive investigation of disease biology and promoting personalized medicine (Andrén et al., 2018). In addition, advanced optical technology, such as elastic light scattering spectroscopy, is playing an important role in non-invasive tissue analysis. Evidence has confirmed the use of advanced techniques such as the wavelet transform to produce measurable differences in elastic scattering distinguishable between dysplastic and normal tissues. These differences not only represent structural heterogeneity inherent in such tissue types but also represent increased complexity in dysplastic tissue in the form of multi-fractal behavior. Such observations further underscore the promise of optical probes for early cancer detection, enabling deconstruction of tissue morphological complexity with minimal invasiveness. As these technologies continue to advance, they hold the ability to create more efficient diagnostic platforms that enable us to gain a greater understanding of disease formation and improve patient outcomes through earlier treatment (Figure 1.9).

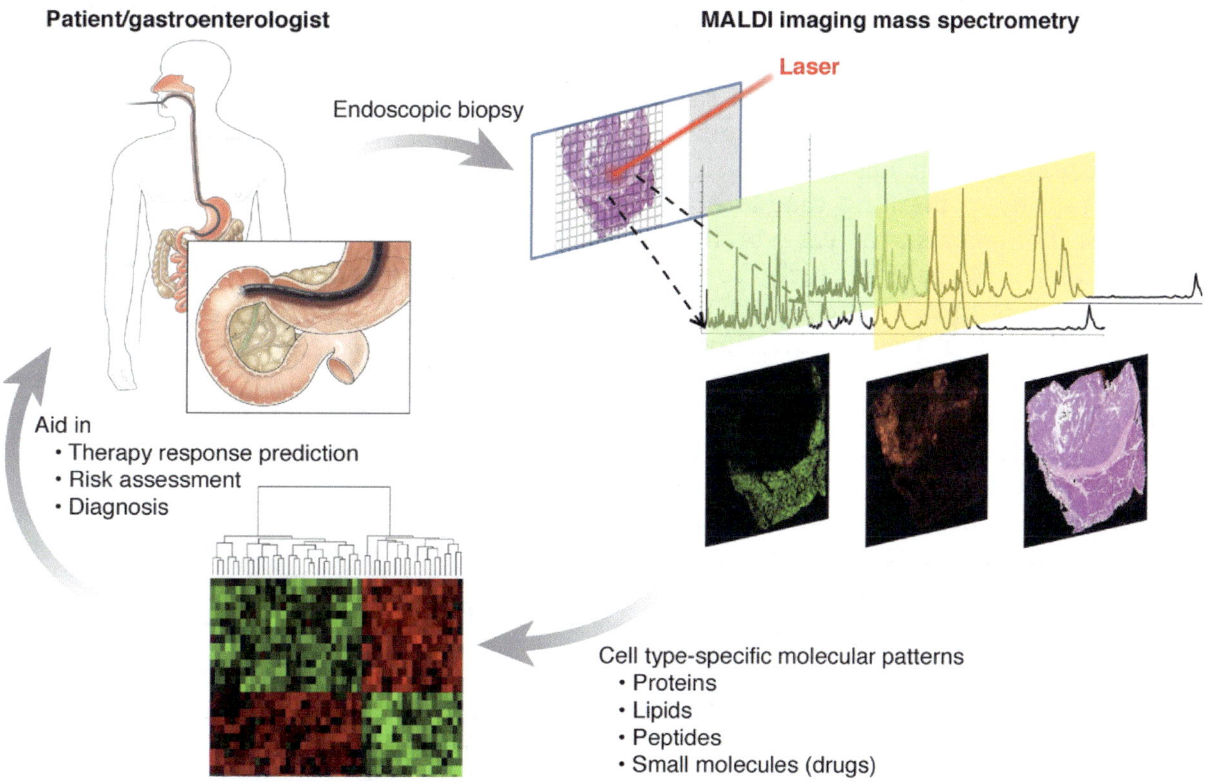

Figure 1.9. Imaging technologies in tissue analysis.

Source: https://els-jbs-prod-cdn.jbs.elsevierhealth.com/cms/attachment/a0957b52-ed4b-4afc-81f9-bcc6b1537880/gr1_lrg.jpg.

1.3. Epithelial Tissue Characteristics

Epithelial tissue, being a general component of numerous organ systems, is characterized by the packing density of its cells, their polarity, and their adhesion to the underlying basement membrane. Compared to the remaining tissues, epithelial cells are welded together, forming an uninterrupted sheet that possesses protective and functional roles in the body. It facilitates efficient absorption, secretion, and perception, demonstrating the diversity of epithelial tissue. Polarity, as differentiation of an apical from a basal surface, allows such cells to react differently to their environment, allowing them selective transport through their membranes. Adhesion to the basement membrane, a differentiated extracellular matrix, provides structural support and integrity and organization to epithelial layers and thus highlights their role in tissue morphology. One of the defining traits of epithelial tissue is that it has the capacity to regenerate rapidly, something that is highly essential for homeostasis in case of injury or disease. This is largely because the stem cells in the basal layer of epithelial structures undergo an ongoing process of dividing and differentiating into specialized cell types. For instance, computational modeling has been used to investigate the role played by calcium concentration in cell culture to analyze cellular behavior in interactions within epithelial tissues. The research implies that calcium oscillations can significantly influence cell growth behavior in monolayer cultures to mimic *in vivo*-like environments. These phenomena suggest the dynamic nature of epithelial cells, illustrating how the environment can play a key role in influencing physiology and morphology, something that is essential for both health and disease conditions (Hill et al., 2004). Furthermore, the diversity of types of epithelial tissue, such as simple, stratified, and transitional epithelium, highlights the adaptability of these tissues in a bid to carry out various physiological functions. Each type has unique structural features adapted to its specific function; for instance, simple epithelium facilitates efficient diffusion and absorption in places like the lung's alveoli, whereas stratified epithelium provides effective protection against abrasion in the skin. Such variations in form can be investigated using high-tech tools such as electron microscopy, providing deeper insight into cellular structure and function at the microscopic level. Recent cell culture experiments, particularly on adenoma cell cultures, have confirmed that such *in vitro* systems maintain key physiological characteristics, and hence established that epithelial tissues may be used as viable models for further study and also for therapeutic intervention (Bácsy et al., 2005) (Figure 1.10).

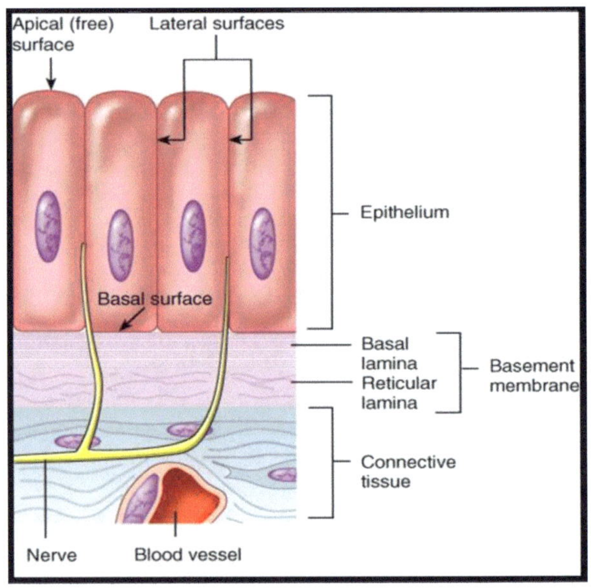

Figure 1.10. Epithelial tissue characteristics.

Source: https://blogger.googleusercontent.com/img/b/R29vZ2xl/AVvXsEj-WqNdL8Jkkz1BCiFB3a1_OdZ87Xm5c6YNzu77TOFKUJajD5YgHXXRj5aKzRAlnvyKqSp9WZd7Q6wTqDPIC0C-u2FnTrOtX-Ib9yfkxSsh0zoQozyT5TmHhuq3PyIBVUx9U2yc66x-YjI4/s1600/Picture1.jpg.

1.3.1. Structure and Function

The structural-functional correlation is a fundamental basis in tissue morphology studies, demonstrating the close relationship between tissues' physical characteristics and their functions within an organism. In many biological systems, cell and extracellular matrix organization control how tissues interact with their environment and fulfill some physiological requirements. For instance, muscle tissue shows a remarkable correspondence between its organized fiber arrangements and its capacity to move. Histological examinations of muscle tissue in model organisms such as Drosophila reveal how specialized anatomy is linked to function at the cellular level. The methods of prepping the muscle tissue sections, such as frozen samples and paraffin-embedded ones, disclose aspects of the tissue's functional anatomy. This is a process that is used to uncover morphological defects and map muscle-nervous system relationships, thus establishing the direct relationship between structure and functional use (Klepzig et al., 2010). Morphology of tissues is not merely about observing anatomy, but actually something that involves research into evolutionary adaptation that preconditions functional efficacy. Consider the diverse structural morphs of the patella across various animal groups; its anatomy presents a dramatic example of how evolution has molded biological structure to optimize the mechanics of function in locomotion. For palaeognathous birds, where there exists a range of patellar structure from none through to fusion with other elements of the skeleton, one can see how these various forms are evidence of adaptation to specific ecological niches. Detailed analyses exhibit how the patellar tendon, particularly in emus, has specific morphological structures that provide resistance to loads during movement. Structure-to-mechanical function interaction in the patellar anatomy demonstrates the evolutionary significance of form as a basis for further investigation into adaptations within bird locomotion (Alexander et al., 2014). The analysis of both vertebrate and invertebrate muscle tissues through the histological approach greatly improves our knowledge of structure-function relationships. In the study of *Drosophila musculature*, for instance, aside from unveiling the complexity of muscle fiber organization, it also informs us of the molecular processes associated with muscle function. The explanation of alterations in muscle form allows us to understand muscle degenerative diseases, thus creating a relationship between cellular structure and potential pathological conditions. In addition, recognition of varied structural characteristics in different species enhances our understanding of functional diversity within taxa. This convergence illuminates larger studies on how varied evolutionary forces shape tissue structure and function, proving the concept that morphological disparity is an indicator of ecological adaptation and functional differentiation of tissues. Such comprehensive studies emphasize the critical importance of integrating morphology, function, and evolutionary biology in tissue studies (Klepzig et al., 2010).

1.3.2. Types of Epithelial Tissue

Epithelial tissue is an elementary building material of the human body, which is categorized into various types based on structural and functional features. The broad categorization is simple and stratified epithelia. Simple epithelium consists of a single layer of cells, and its functions are absorption, secretion, and filtration because of its relatively thin composition. It is further divided into simple squamous, cuboidal, and columnar epithelia, which are modified to perform specific functions in various organs. Simple squamous epithelium, consisting of platelike cells, for instance, lines structures such as alveoli in the lungs to support gas exchange easily. Conversely, stratified epithelium consists of multiple layers, designed to protect underlying tissues from abrasion and chemical contact, such as keratinized stratified squamous epithelium of the skin, illustrating diverse functional adaptations of epithelial types in tissue structure. Cellular morphology in epithelia varies significantly, in keeping with specialized function. Transitional epithelium, for example, in the urinary bladder, is specially structured to accommodate fluctuations in volume. This specialized epithelium can extend when the bladder is distended, changing from many layers of cells when it is vacant to fewer layers when it is distended. Glandular epithelium, including endocrine and exocrine glands, also participates in secretion.

Endocrine glands secrete hormones into the circulatory system, whereas exocrine glands secrete their material by way of ducts to a specific location. It is critical to know these morphological variations to understand their physiological roles in the body, particularly where cell differentials are pathologic; e.g., cellular differences seen in reactive adenomas, as elucidated when interpreting morphology and secretion of hormone in pituitary adenoma cell cultures (Bácsy et al., 2005). The morphology of epithelial tissue extends beyond mere classification, such as the complex relationship between the structure and function of the cells. Recent work, such as evaluations of the tissue maceration method, has demonstrated the distinct characteristics of various epithelial cell types in organisms like hydra and interpreted them in terms of their diversity using phase contrast microscopy (David et al., 1973). This approach is important in the study of epithelial tissues as it discriminates between cell types depending on their morphology. Through the use of this and other sophisticated methods, scientists acquire information on how epithelial tissues react to physiological stress, how they respond to environmental change, and how they are involved in regeneration processes. Such understanding not only pushes the limits of tissue morphology but also paves the way to innovation in medical research, particularly in the creation of targeted therapies for diseases associated with epithelial dysfunction (Figure 1.11).

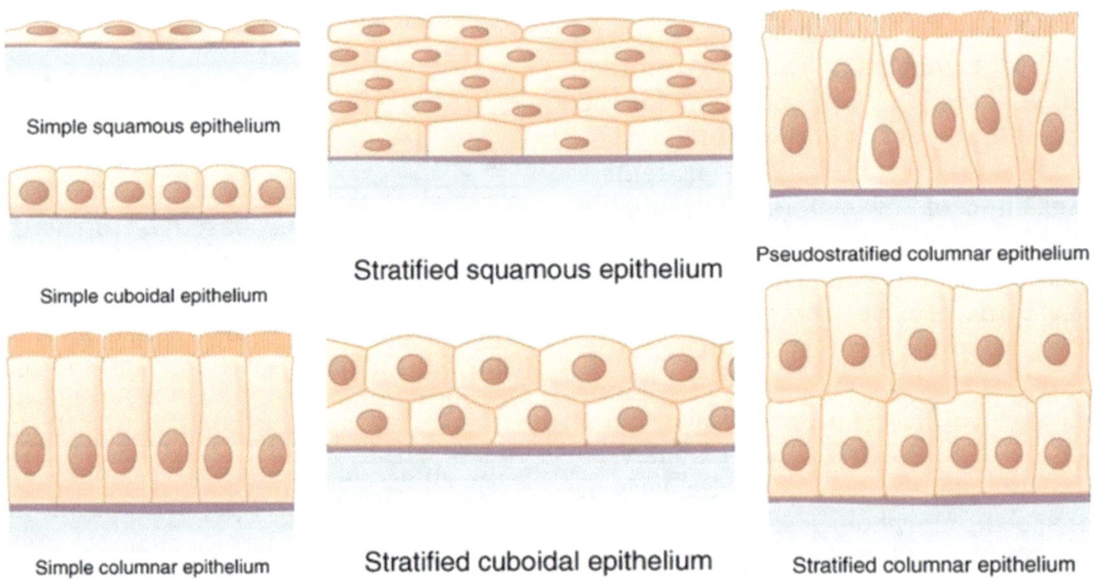

Figure 1.11. Types of epithelial tissue.

Source: https://microbenotes.com/wp-content/uploads/2020/05/Epithelial-Tissue-Types.jpg.

1.3.3. Role in Organ Systems

It is necessary to understand the roles of tissues within organ systems to accurately understand how they work together to support overall body function. Organs are made up of two or more tissue types that all serve individual roles to make up the efficiency of the organs as a whole. For example, in the respiratory system, the airway epithelial tissue serves protective and secretory roles, and connective tissues provide structure to the lungs and facilitate gas exchange. The discrimination of these tissues, on the basis of microscopic morphology, allows for specialized functions necessary for the operation of the organs in the system.

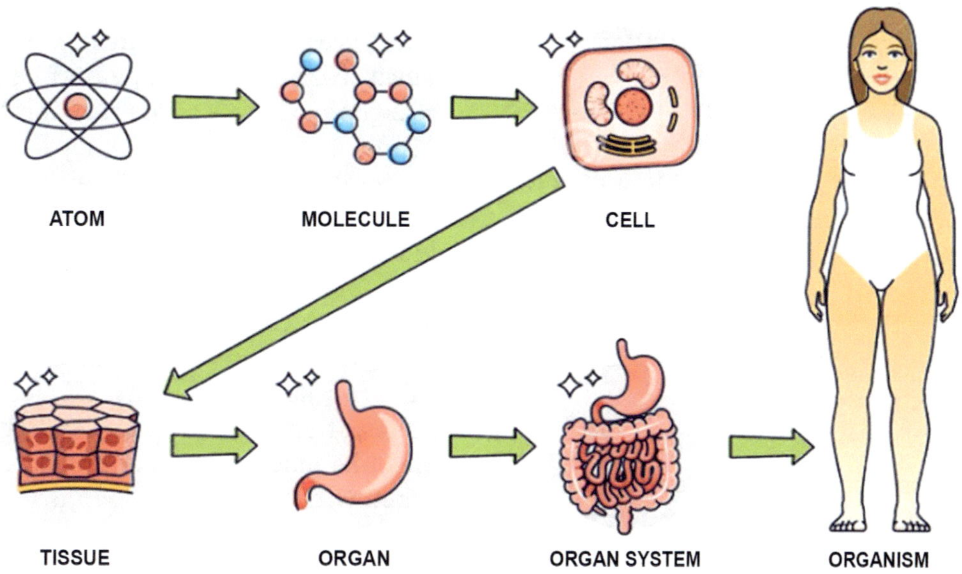

Figure 1.12. Role in organ systems.

Source: https://thumbs.dreamstime.com/z/organisation-organisms-hierarchical-level-structure-outline-diagram-organisation-organisms-hierarchical-level-252942090.jpg.

This sophisticated interaction is not of mere theoretical significance; it is necessary to provide homeostasis, and therefore, tissue morphology is a significant area of study within the field of biology. Moreover, the interaction of tissues among organ systems illustrates the complexity of their function in disease as well as in health. For instance, in muscle tissue, the arrangement of fibers and the nature of connective tissue are essential for transmitting force and its production. The mechanisms of altered histology in these tissues during disease or injury can give insights into variations in organ function. Besides, model research breakthroughs, for instance, into the virus-host tissue interaction as described in equine herpesvirus type 1 research, show how it is possible that *in vitro* models provide significant information approximating true tissue interaction conditions (Azab et al., 2019). These breakthroughs not only make it easier to understand the tissue role but also minimize animal testing requirements. The investigation of tissue functions is not limited to animal and human systems, but it also provides information regarding plant biology. In plant organ systems, *in vitro* tissue culture approaches have played a major role in understanding genetic diversity and metabolic processes. For instance, researchers have employed plant tissue morphogenesis for increasing crop vigor and productivity (Caretto et al., 2019). Differentiation of various tissues of plants, such as xylem and phloem, accounts for how they cooperate in transport and nutrient distribution. These findings not only enrich knowledge of plant physiology but also suggest deeply within plant agricultural biotechnology. The study of tissue morphology, both in animal and plant systems, therefore, brings to fore the universal function of tissues to sustain life and respond to the environment (Figure 1.12).

1.4. Connective Tissue Functions

Amidst the diverse scenery of tissue morphology, connective tissues are crucial in providing for the structural continuity and function of organs and systems within the human body. They serve as a scaffold that ties and supports the other tissues so that overall body architecture can be established and maintained. One of the most significant roles of connective tissue is its ability to transfer mechanical forces. For instance, compact connective tissues like ligaments and tendons are well suited to support tensile stress in attaching bones to muscles and maintaining joints stable. This biomechanical process is also demonstrated by proteins such as Tenomodulin (Tnmd), which enhances cell adhesion and plays a significant role in periodontal ligament development, highlighting the complexity of connective tissue processes in the musculoskeletal system (Chung et al., 2013). Connective tissues also have significant functions in providing metabolic support and transport of nutrients in the body. Composed of highly specialized cells in a rich extracellular matrix, these tissues facilitate the exchange of material between blood and other tissues. For cartilage, a particular form of connective tissue, avascular status necessitates reliance on diffusion to supply nutrients and remove waste. This characteristic demonstrates the flexibility and functional variability of connective tissues. Furthermore, the recent investigation has brought to light the presence of multipotent stem/progenitor cells, such as those of cranial neural crest, within connective tissues. Dental neural crest-derived progenitor cells (dNC-PCs) are a good example of the regenerative potential of connective tissues since they have established that they were able to differentiate into various lineages, such as neurogenic and osteogenic cells, elucidating their multifunctional role (Degistirici et al., 2008). Lastly, their immunological role cannot be underestimated as they have a vital function in the inflammatory response and process of repairing tissues. Connective tissues offer protection to a variety of immune cells, like macrophages and mast cells, that are tasked with responding to injury and infection, thus playing a vital role in homeostasis and protection. Their ability to produce and secrete immune signal molecules such as cytokines also illustrates the importance of their role in the modulation of both systemic and local immune responses. Moreover, the architecture of the extracellular matrix can modulate immune cell function, illustrating the intricate interrelationship between connective tissue structure and function. Thus, understanding of multifunctional functions of connective tissue is indispensable in explaining their impact on overall health and disease, and hence becomes a topic of relevance within tissue morphology.

1.4.1. Types of Connective Tissue

Connective tissue, which is one of the four main tissues in the human body, consists of a heterogeneous group of subtypes, all having specialized functions. Broadly classified into loose and dense connective tissues, they vary in form and function. Loose connective tissues, such as areolar and adipose tissue, provide strength and elasticity, acting as padding around organs. They are aggregates of elastin and collagen fibers with a few cells that assist in carrying out their function of transporting nutrients and supporting immune responses. Dense connective tissues like ligaments and tendons possess greater tensile strength due to closely packed collagen fibers that are capable of withstanding significant mechanical stress.

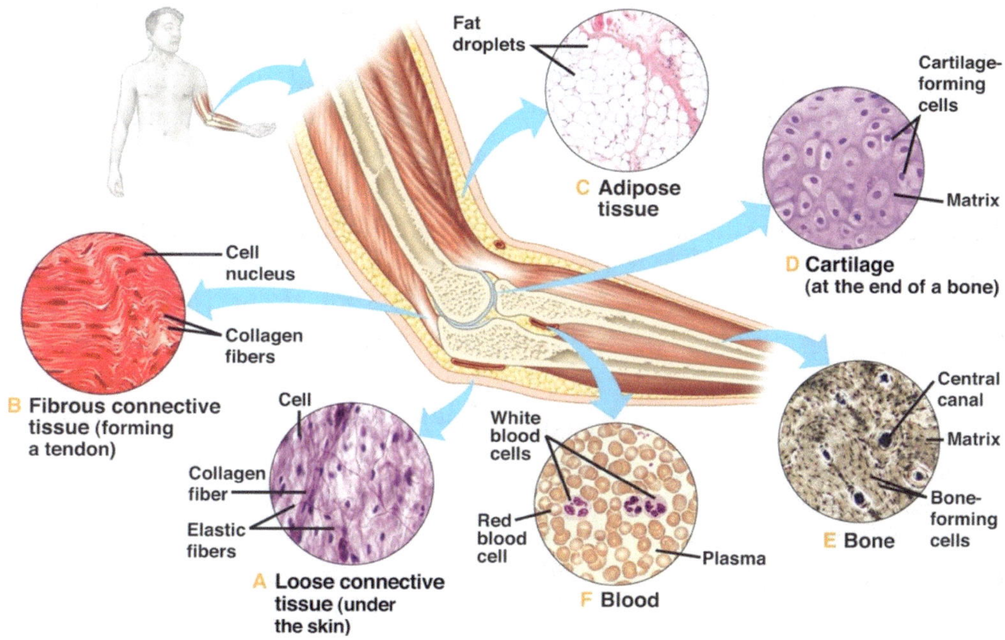

Figure 1.13. Connective Tissue

Source: https://www.slideserve.com/drew/tissues

The architectural differences of these subtypes not only reflect their functions but also indicate the vital role of connective tissue to maintain body integrity and facilitate mobility. Further subclassification of connective tissues reveals specialized types that have specific physiological roles. Cartilage, for example, a specialized type of connective tissue, appears in joints, the respiratory apparatus, and ear structures. Composed primarily of chondrocytes surrounded by a gelatinous extracellular matrix, cartilage is used to give flexibility and shock-absorbing properties with little friction among articulating surfaces. Bone, on the other hand, is a highly mineralized form of connective tissue with a rigid matrix composed of collagen fibers and hydroxyapatite crystals. Hardness brought about by these forms of tissue allows bones to support body weight and protect vital organs. Notably, certain connective tissues, such as adipose tissue, do not provide merely structural support but play a central role in energy storage and metabolic control, emphasizing the multifunctionality of categories of connective tissue to health in general. The role of connective tissues is more than structural support; they play a part in physiological functions and tissue repair. For instance, the periodontal ligament, a specialized connective tissue covering the tooth root, has multipotent stem cells of dental neural crest origin referred to as dental neural crest-derived progenitor cells (dNC-PCs). Such cells have been reported to possess the potential to differentiate into osteogenic and chondrogenic lineages and are key to the healing process following dental trauma. In addition, tenomodulin (Tnmd) has been found to increase cell adhesion in periodontal ligament cells and plays a crucial role in ensuring the structural integrity of the latter, especially during the process of tooth eruption when occlusal forces act upon it. These observations highlight the dynamic functions of connective tissue types, showing how they influence tissue resilience, repair mechanisms, and overall organismal functioning, making them pivotal in the discipline of tissue morphology (Figure 1.13).

1.4.2. Extracellular Matrix Composition

The extracellular matrix (ECM) is a crucial structural and biochemical matrix in tissues that has a profound influence on tissue morphology. It is composed of a non-uniform array of macromolecules like collagen, glycoproteins, and proteoglycans, which are not only responsible for providing mechanical support but also for regulating cellular behavior and intercellular communication. This complex matrix varies significantly from tissue to tissue, with various compositions reflecting the specific functional requirements of each tissue type.

For instance, the skeletal muscle ECM is tailored to facilitate contraction and regeneration of the muscle, while cartilage ECM is developed to withstand compressive forces and stabilize joints. The composition and architecture of the ECM have to be understood in order to realize in full how tissues are formed, maintain their architecture, and respond to various physiological and pathological stimuli, and this forms the central element of tissue morphology. The ECM is actively remodeled upon either physiological or pathological conditions, and remodeling of the ECM is a key function in the health and disease of tissues. Under pathological conditions, like osteoarthritis (OA), the ECM is radically altered, leading to cartilage degeneration. Chondrocytes, the intrinsic cells of cartilage, reorganize the ECM during inflammation, and this triggers a cascade reaction that erodes tissue integrity and function. Specifically, the disruption of key components in the ECM destabilizes the biomechanical properties of the tissue and makes the microenvironment not conducive for mesenchymal stem cells to participate in cartilage repair. This type of ECM remodeling not only inhibits the acceleration of OA evolution but also prevents regenerative processes, underlining the critical interplay between matrix composition and tissue morphology in health and disease, as noted in the literature (Maldonado, M, & Nam, J., 2013).

Studying the extracellular matrix also provides new pathways to therapeutic interventions in the treatment of various diseases, including peripheral artery disease (PAD), where ECM hydrogels have been shown to be promising. Using decellularized tissues to create biomaterials that are analogous to native ECM can facilitate better tissue recovery and regeneration. For example, recent research has assessed the efficacy of skeletal muscle-derived hydrogels, demonstrating their ability to stimulate arteriogenesis and improve blood flow in ischemic tissues. The findings revealed that tailored ECM composition may initiate the recovery of function through the recruitment of progenitor cells and enhance a favorable tissue repair microenvironment. The findings call for understanding ECM composition during the generation of targeted therapy that capitalizes on the body's inherent ability to heal, as well as managing the complexity of tissue morphology, as seen in studies aimed at PAD (Braden et al., 2016) (Figure 1.14).

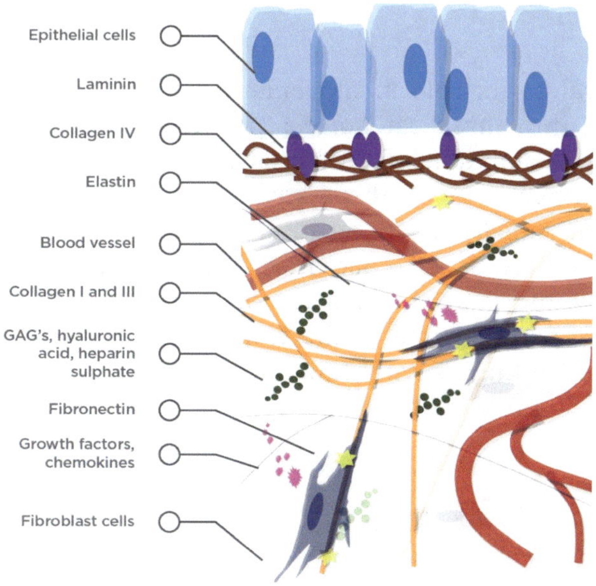

Figure 1.14. Extracellular matrix composition.

Source: https://jkhealthcare.in/wp-content/uploads/2022/07/tissue-network.jpg.

1.4.3. Role in Support and Protection

The complex tissue patterns in the human organism have vital roles to perform both for protection and support, as are exemplified in connective tissue structures such as bone, cartilage, and fat. Bone provides a rigid structure that supports the entire body, protecting important organs, e.g., the lungs and heart, from mechanical damage. Composed of collagenous matrix and mineralized deposits, bone is very hard but has room for movement by its attachment to muscles. Cartilage is not as hard but functions as a cushioning tissue among bones within joints, being a shock absorber and a flexibility increaser. Moreover, adipose tissue, besides being an energy store, is also an insulator and a protector of organs against external pressures, which underscores the multifaceted role of connective tissue in providing structural integrity and homeostasis. On the other hand, epithelial tissues function primarily for protection by forming barriers against physical and biochemical traumas. The skin, which is the largest organ, is one such typical example of this function through its structure that is multilayered and composed of keratinized epithelial cells, providing cover to inner tissues from infection, UV radiation, and drying. Collectively, epithelial layers not only provide physical protection but also contribute to immune defense, actively fighting microbial invasion. The gastrointestinal tract epithelium, for instance, regulates the uptake of essential nutrients while playing a barrier role against harmful substances. The active balancing between protection and the uptake of essential components highlights the complexity of epithelial morphology in health and disease, justifying the importance of tissue morphology studies towards understanding the nuances of protective mechanisms. In disease conditions, the integrity of protective and supportive tissues can be compromised, and severe health conditions arise. Diseases such as intestinal ischemia illustrate how breakdown of the epithelial barrier can render the epithelium more permeable so that too much enters the bloodstream and causes systemic problems. Investigation of this phenomenon indicates that protease activity and apoptosis may contribute to the increased transmural permeability that follows ischemic events, further complicating the protective role of the intestinal wall (Altshuler et al., 2014). Interventions to address these mechanisms, such as the giving of glucose and protease inhibitors, have proven to possess the potential to prevent tissue damage and restore functionality, demonstrating the utmost importance of acquiring knowledge on tissue morphology during disease (Alcazar-Fuoli et al., 2014). Through the analysis of these correlations, scientists can develop effective treatment protocols to enhance the support and protective roles of various tissues, which will ultimately enhance medical knowledge and treatment protocols.

1.5. Muscle Tissue Overview

The intricate architecture of muscle tissue is central to its role in movement and stabilization within the body. Muscle tissue is primarily divided into three categories: skeletal, cardiac, and smooth muscle, each possessing distinct structural and functional characteristics. Skeletal muscle, under voluntary control, consists of multinucleated fibers that exhibit a striated appearance due to the regular arrangement of actin and myosin filaments. This organization allows for powerful and regulated contractions necessary for movement and other daily activities. The cardiac muscle, the composition of the heart, functions involuntarily and is specialized for rhythmic contraction to ensure that blood circulation is effective. Smooth muscle found in the walls of hollow organs is also involuntary in function and is tasked with controlling internal functions, such as digestion and the widening of blood vessels.

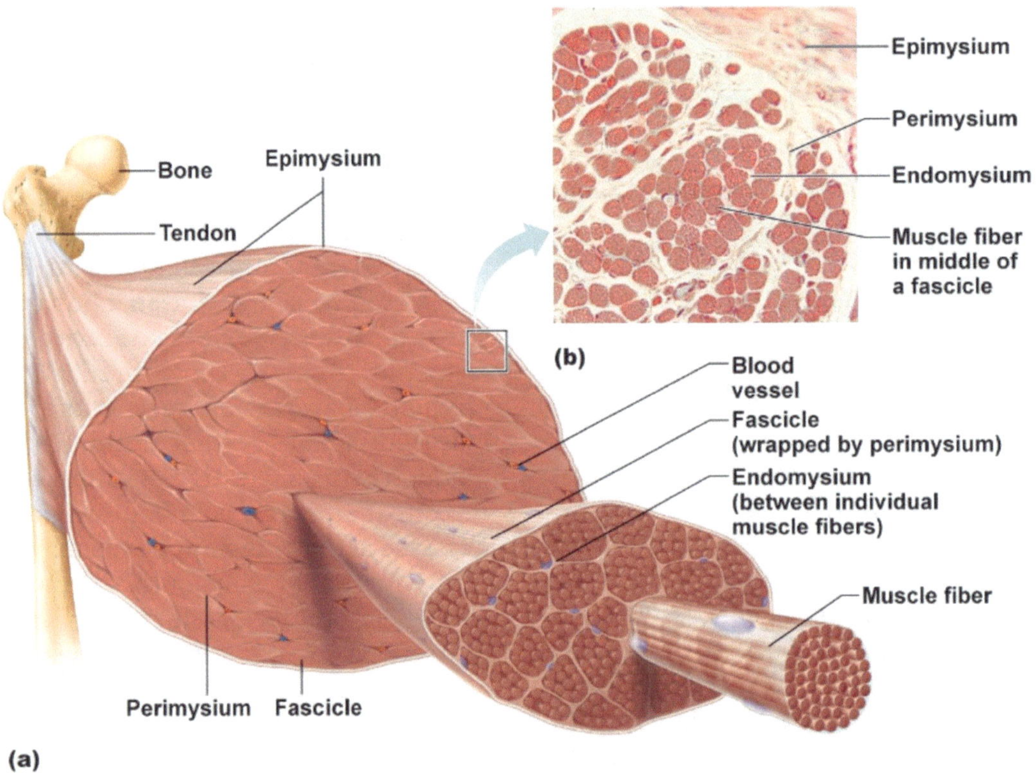

Figure 1.15. Muscle tissue overview.

Source: https://3.bp.blogspot.com/-rvggdQEFl50/XCTH2r0WlMI/AAAAAAAAHWs/B3jwXsFgYUgXxKZFtLcdJwYfkKLqZmm-wCLcBGAs/s1600/muscular-tissue-678x381.jpg.

These kinds of muscles, taken together, demonstrate the remarkable plasticity and specialisation of tissue morphologies needed for a range of physiological functions. The structural composition of muscle tissue not just facilitates movement but also serves as evidence of evolutionary adaptations to specific functional demands. For instance, new research on muscle-tendon interactions illustrates how exercise and disuse can dramatically change both muscle and tendon morphology. Research has established that alterations in training protocols are capable of eliciting changes in tendon structure and alignment that, in turn, influence recovery and muscle performance. Specifically, Aldini et al. (2016) point to how sudden withdrawal from training undermines tendon properties, capturing the delicate dance between activity and rest to maintain muscle-tendon integrity. This interaction embodies the importance of a smart understanding of muscle tissue's biomechanical properties, as they are directly associated with the entire musculoskeletal system's functionality and endurance. Furthermore, the diversified morphologies of muscle tissue also include specialized adaptations within specific species, embodying the evolutionary implications of muscle structure. An example is well known from the bat wing, as the unique composition of muscle and elastin bundles provides flexibility for flying. Studies indicate that the structural arrangement of such components is critical in controlling wing shape and enabling aerial movement and enhancing aerodynamic efficiency. Specifically, Fenton et al. (2017) outline the manner in which the intricate architecture of wing membrane muscles contributes to flight mechanics through a demonstration of an evolutionary response to environmental stress. In the process, studying these peculiar types of muscle tissue not only contributes to our understanding of muscle structure but also evokes additional questions about the relationship between structural adaptations and functional capabilities across species (Figure 1.15).

1.5.1. Types of Muscle Tissue

Muscle tissue, an integral component of the human body, is coarsely categorized into three major types: skeletal, cardiac, and smooth muscle. Each one is distinct in its function and has characteristic histological features depending on its role in the movement and functioning of skeletal muscles. Skeletal muscle, or striated muscle, is responsible for voluntary movements such as locomotion and posture. It is composed of long, rod-shaped fibers with a defined striation pattern due to filamentous packing of actin and myosin. Furthermore, the occurrence of more than one nucleus per cell distinguishes skeletal muscle and allows for a cellular response promptly during physical activity. Morphologically, as far as tissue structure is concerned, it is important to have knowledge of the architecture of skeletal muscle fibers because such structural specificity directly affects the performance of the muscle and its response to varying physiological demands. Cardiac muscle, found only in the heart, exhibits a unique hybridization of skeletal and smooth muscle characteristics. In contrast to skeletal muscle, cardiac muscle fibers are interlinked and branched and create a networked three-dimensional complex that enables coordinated contractions essential in efficient blood pumping. These striated muscle fibers share one nucleus and specialized intercalated discs that facilitate electrical conduction, allowing for synchronized heartbeats. Cardiac muscle is involuntary, as well, with its contractions governed independently by the heart's own conduction system, separate from consciousness. This organization illustrates how muscle tissue morphology directly determines its physiological function, highlighting the significance of structural alterations to meet organ-specific demands, e.g., rhythmic contractions in the heart. Smooth muscle, the most variable and least known of the three types, is comprised of non-striated fibers that function in involuntary movements in various organ systems. Smooth muscle can be found in hollow organs such as the intestines, blood vessels, and bladder, and is characterized by spindle-shaped cells and a single centrally located nucleus. Smooth muscle fibers differ from skeletal and cardiac muscles in that they lack the orderly striation pattern and therefore have a more uniform look under microscopic examination. These fibers relax slowly and have sustained contractions that can support gradual, rhythmic movements required in processes like peristalsis and blood vessel control. It has been shown that the structure of smooth muscle is not rigid; rather, it varies based on mechanical conditions or conditions of pathologies, as seen in research studying tendon structural adaptation during detraining and rehabilitation periods (Aldini et al., 2016) (Figure 1.16).

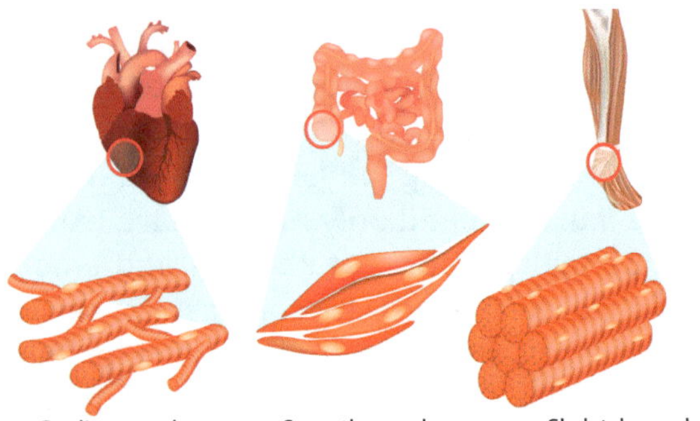

Figure 1.16. Types of muscle tissue.

Source: https://humanbio.org/wp-content/uploads/2020/04/muscle-tissues.jpg.

1.5.2. Mechanisms of Contraction

The contraction mechanisms within tissues, particularly muscle tissues, are complex and closely associated with their morphological characteristics. The crux of this phenomenon is the interaction between myosin and actin filaments, which form the basis of muscle contraction in a mechanism known as the sliding filament model. This mechanism demands that upon stimulation, myosin heads bind to actin to create cross-bridges that make the filaments slide over one another, resulting in shortening and muscle contraction. The dynamic interaction is supplemented by calcium ions, which bind with troponin, bringing about a conformation change that exposes binding sites on actin filaments. In addition, the arrangement of muscle fibers and their connective tissue environment significantly influences the muscle's contractile efficiency and functional capacity, underscoring the role of morphological structures in contraction and tissue function. In the study of actomyosin contractility, it is worth understanding its valuable contribution to cellular processes like migration and tissue morphogenesis. The contractile nature of the cell cortex, an actomyosin network beneath the cell membrane, reveals critical information regarding tissue morphology. Actomyosin networks present reversible aggregation with pulsatile contraction, a process that recurs in large-scale biological processes such as embryogenesis and tissue remodeling. Computational model research shows that such pulsatile behavior arises from a highly orchestrated balance among force generated by molecular motors, force relaxation via actin turnover, and force preservation through network connectivity. Through further investigation of the parameters that regulate such dynamics, scientists can enhance their understanding of the underlying mechanisms of contraction in cells, therefore illuminating their essential functions in tissue structure and integrity (Kim et al., 2017). Fighting the impact of aging on mechanisms of contraction provides critical correlations between morphological changes and muscle function. As humans age, a decline in muscle force generation is observed, influenced by alterations in both muscle fibers and the extracellular matrix (ECM). Notably, the mechanics governing force generation differ under varying contraction modes: concentric and eccentric. Studies demonstrate that while the stiffness of connective tissues increases with age, resulting in diminished force capacity during concentric contractions, the ability to generate force during eccentric phases remains relatively intact. This bipartiteness emphasizes the importance of establishing the intricate relationship between functional outcomes and microstructural modifications in muscle tissues. In addition, innovative modeling methods, such as pixel-based Reproducing Kernel Particle Method (RKPM), enhance understanding of these relationships by illustrating the extracellular and cellular components of muscle tissue and emphasizing how morphology influences contractile performance with age (Basava et al., 2020).

1.5.3. Importance in Movement and Stability

The intricate interaction among movement, stability mechanics, and tissue morphology is central to understanding how biological structures function optimally in their environments. In various living organisms, tissues are organized into specific forms that not only ensure structural integrity but also dynamic functionality with neighbouring elements. For instance, within a perfusion bioreactor used in tissue engineering, tissue construct reaction to mechanical loading is an important factor in its development and growth. The use of flow in the system is able to create huge effects on cell structure and function because mechanotransduction mechanisms regulate cell response according to environmental conditions and therefore are the foundation for the importance of movement and stability in tissue development (Byrne et al., 2008). One aspect of brokering in the debate over movement and stability is the morphology of cranial sutures, particularly in dynamic structures such as the growing skulls of primates. A case in point is the zygomaticotemporal suture, wherein not only does it allow the growth that the skull must have, but also stability despite movement between bones. New imaging technology indicates that the suture is not merely a simple linkage but rather interdigitating facets that confer structural stability against shearing forces. The architecture of the suture changes with age, so in younger individuals, there is freedom of movement, but with added complexity, it is restricted and hence achieves harmony between flexibility and stability (Curtis et al., 2014). Lastly, adaptation of tissue to achieve stability and movement is required for function in a range of biological contexts. Insight into the importance of morphological structure in tissues can yield further understanding of the effect of mechanical forces upon growth and stability in living systems. As research advances, particularly through computational modeling of tissue development, understanding the essential roles of mechanical environments will enable more sophisticated applications in biomedical fields, such as regenerative medicine and prosthetic design. The unification of adaptive responsiveness and structural stability in tissues thus forms a basis of both evolutionary biology and tissue morphology, stressing the significance of these factors within the broader scheme of anatomical and functional development.

1.6. Nervous Tissue and Its Role

Nervous tissue is a key component of the body's overall function, primarily via its two major cell types: neurons and glial cells. Neurons are the fundamental units that transmit information via electrical impulses, enabling communication between different parts of the body. This transmission is facilitated by the complex nature of neurons, which contain a cell body and dendrites where signals are received and an axon that carries signals to other neurons or muscles. The glial cells, on the other hand, have supporting roles like supplying nutrients, insulation, and protection to the neurons. They outnumber neurons many times over, which indicates the complex interrelationship in nervous tissue. The structural complexity of these cells mirrors their specialized roles, making them important for establishing homeostasis and facilitating responses to stimuli at various speeds across different environments, highlighting the significance of nervous tissue for tissue morphology. The morphology of nervous tissue is not an anatomical novelty but is closely related to its ability to function. Different neurons exhibit different shapes and sizes that are characteristic of their specific functions in the nervous system. The pyramidal neurons of the cerebral cortex, for example, are characterized by their triangular cell bodies and extended dendritic trees, which enable them to integrate and process complex information. Similarly, the morphology of glial cells contributes to their functions; astrocytes, for instance, possess star-shaped morphologies that allow them to engage with blood vessels and neurons to regulate blood flow and the delivery of nutrients to active populations of neurons.

This glial cell-neuron network architecture is the ultimate structure-function correlation, where the differing morphological characteristics enable the nervous system to properly process and respond to information, stressing the significance of nervous tissue within tissue morphology. Further understanding of the morphological features of nervous tissue has implications for various clinical conditions as well as for research purposes. Structural abnormalities of nervous tissue can have severe effects, including those involving neurodegenerative diseases and brain tumors. The interactions among cell morphology, growth habits, and the tumor microenvironment in gliomas can influence prognosis and treatment outcomes. Correlating cellular and tissue-level changes with clinical presentation is a crucial field of research, as highlighted in studies of glioma behavior and morphology. Through the application of advanced models that integrate molecular data and structural data, researchers can explain the complex relationships that regulate tumor invasiveness and growth. This could enhance the diagnosis and treatment of neurologic diseases, indicating a strong relationship between nervous tissue morphology and its life-critical functions in health and disease, emphasizing its importance when deciding tissue morphology (Adam et al., 2007; Fiegel et al., 2012).

1.6.1. Structure of Neurons and Glial Cells

Neuronal structure is complex and enables their unique role in the nervous system. Each neuron possesses differentiated parts: the soma (cell body), dendrites, and an axon. The soma holds the nucleus and is responsible for maintaining the cells' health. The dendrites branch off from the soma and serve to receive input from other neurons for communication within the network. The axon transmits electrical impulses from the soma to other neurons, muscles, or glands. Schwann cells and oligodendrocytes in the central nervous system wrap axons in a myelin sheath to make the signal conduction more efficient. Thus, the intricate structure of neurons allows them to develop extensive networks required to coordinate the body's functions, underscoring the importance of cellular form in nervous system organization and function. No less important than the function of the nervous system are glial cells, which are far more numerous than neurons. These glial cells have a range of essential functions like structural support, metabolic assistance, and homeostasis within the neural environment. Among various glial cells, astrocytes are highly multifunctional, and they play key roles in the development of the blood-brain barrier, the provision of nutrients to neurons, and contribute to the healing process following CNS trauma. Their highly complex branching structure enables them to directly communicate with numerous different elements of a neuron, successfully communicating and assisting. Oligodendrocytes also supply myelination to CNS neurons, whereas microglia are the immune responders of the central nervous system. The diversity of functions of glial cells makes them crucial in tissue morphology and the functioning of the neural tissue. Recent work highlights the dynamic organization of neurons and glial cells, revealed to be of utmost significance in neuroplasticity. Such evidence is demonstrated by the observation that synaptic remodeling, crucial to the formation of memory, is controlled through changes in astroglial organization. Ultrathin astroglial protrusions are generally discovered near synapses in experiments, suggesting a significant role in synaptic function and connectivity formation over time. Nonetheless, attributes such as the electrical activity of neurons are also able to cause morphological alterations in glial cells, e.g., their responsive ability in the neural environment (Heller, J. P. & Rusakov, D. A., 2015). In addition, the heterogeneity of radial glial cell types indicates that glial structures can exhibit heterogeneity suited to functional demands across species, as seen in studies of turtles and mammals. It is critical to understand these structural subtleties in order to appreciate how neural tissue responds to different physiological and pathological states (Clinton et al., 2014) (Figure 1.17).

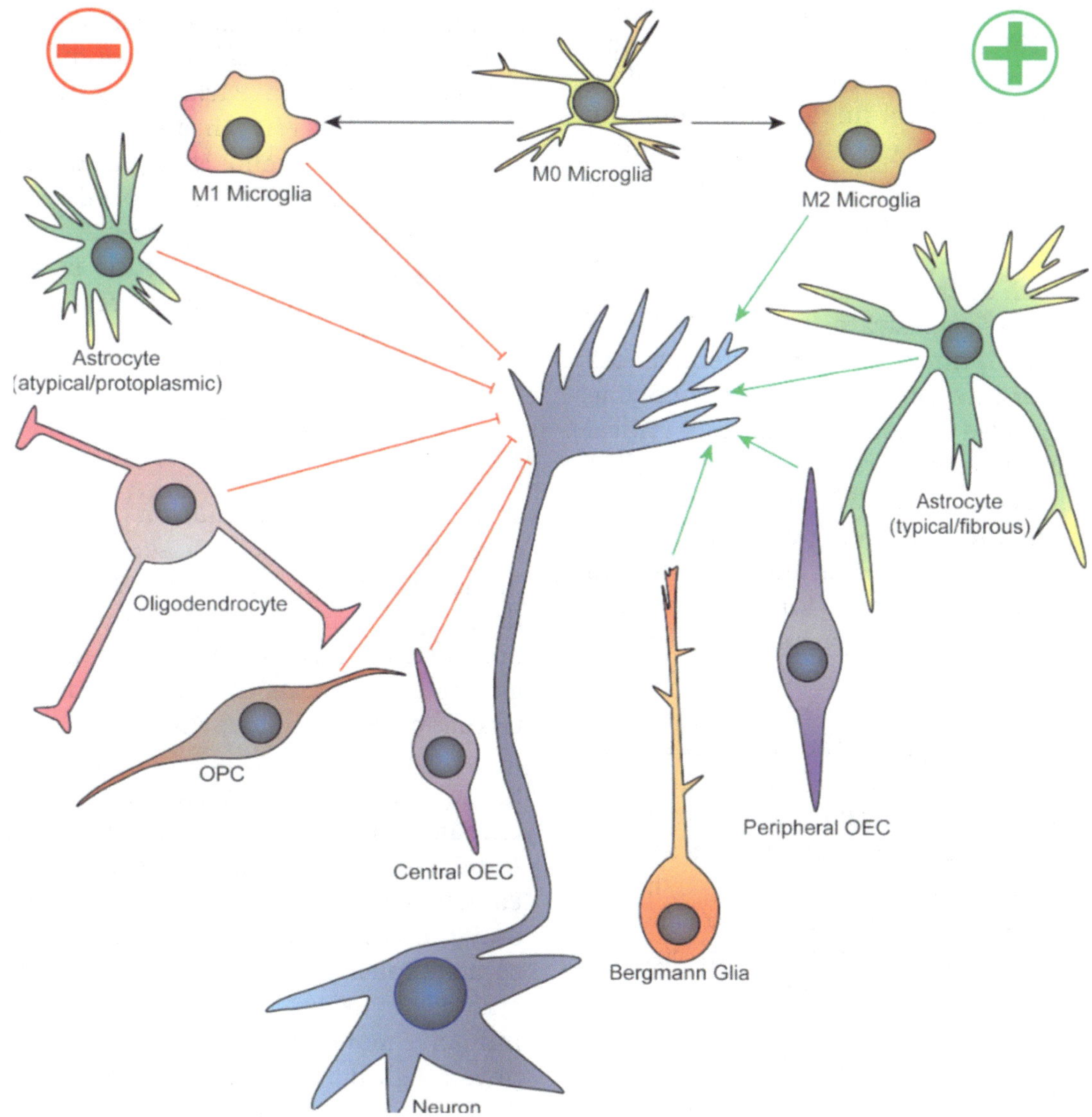

Figure 1.17. Structure of neurons and glial cells.

Source: https://www.frontiersin.org/files/Articles/528417/fnins-14-00203-HTML/image_m/fnins-14-00203-g001.jpg.

1.6.2. Function in Signal Transmission

The intricate tissue structures are also the first targets of signal transmission in the body, with intercellular communication the basis of maintaining homeostasis. At the cellular level, signal transmission is primarily carried out by glial cells and neurons, which together cooperate to pass information via the nervous system. Neurons utilize specialized synapses, where neurotransmitters are released and detected by post-synaptic receptors, enabling stimulation of electrical impulses. In addition, astroglial cells have been identified as central components of the process, as they enable synaptic function and modulate neural signaling cascades. The morphological features of the astroglia, such as their constricted protrusions around synapses, illustrate the complexity of their role in optimal signaling effectiveness and neuronal integrity preservation, implying a highly organized formative architecture critical for effective transmission of signals (Heller, J. P. & Rusakov, D. A., 2015). Furthermore, tissue's dynamic morphological features are crucial in responding to varied physiological requirements, particularly for learning and memory. Remodeling of synaptic connections plays a key role in memory acquisition and recall that arise from tissue structural plasticity due to functional requirements. Current studies have shown that morphological adjustments in astrocytes, including their ultrathin protrusions, are involved in regulating synaptic plasticity. This plasticity is significant in stabilizing synaptic contacts and, consequently, the efficacy of overall signal transmission within neuronal circuits. Understanding such morphological changes provides insight into the cellular mechanisms underlying memory and learning, with a primary focus on the tissue morphology's role in facilitating functional processes of signaling within the nervous system (Heller, J. P. & Rusakov, D. A., 2015). Moreover, the function of some signaling pathways towards tissue morphology is also central to the understanding of most neurodegenerative disorders. p38-mitogen-activated protein kinase (MAPK) signaling pathway is among the pathways that have been of interest for their role in synaptic plasticity as well as neuroinflammatory responses. By regulating substrates like MAPKAPK 2 and tau protein, p38 MAPK influences the actin remodeling that is involved in the maintenance of the structure and function of the synapse. Dysfunction of this signal-transducing pathway can lead to pathological states of disease, such as Alzheimer's and Parkinson's disease, and therefore to the relevance of the relationship between tissue morphology, signal transmission, and neurodegeneration. Improved insight into these signal-transduction processes is essential for designing future therapeutic strategies to preserve or restore normal communication within neural networks.

1.6.3. Role in Coordinating Body Functions

The intricate coordination of the body's functions is essentially based on the various tissues that constitute the body's structure. Each tissue type contributes uniquely to the body's homeostasis and coordination of communication among organ systems. For instance, epithelial tissue creates a covering and is involved in selective absorption and secretion. This tissue is of major importance to regulate the exchange of substances and signals that are required for body processes. Furthermore, connective tissues such as adipose tissue not only provide support but also act as regulators of metabolism. Adipose tissue also acts as an endocrine organ, secreting adipokines that influence metabolism and are involved in many physiological functions, thereby showing the diverse functions tissues possess to coordinate body activities (Gutierrez et al., 2017). Muscle and nervous tissues are particularly significant when it comes to coordinating body activities. Muscle tissue influences movement and can be divided further into skeletal, cardiac, and smooth muscle, which carry out specialized functions to aid in the process of physiological activity as a whole. Skeletal muscles allow for voluntary movement, while internal organs contain smooth muscle that regulates involuntary activities such as digestion and blood flow. By contrast, nervous tissue deals with communication within the body, transmitting messages that regulate and coordinate events. The interaction between nervous tissue and muscle shows how different tissue types work together to ensure that body functions are performed effectively and efficiently, highlighting the complex interplay required for responses and homeostasis to internal and external stimuli (Baban et al., 2019). The role of adipose tissue in obesity and metabolic disease also demonstrates how morphological characteristics of tissue influence the coordination of body functions. Adipocytes are engaged in storing and releasing energy through their endocrine functions that affect not just metabolic processes but also inflammatory responses in the body. Adipose tissue dysfunction, as seen in obesity, may lead to adverse effects such as insulin resistance that, in turn, makes metabolic regulation even more difficult. The endocrine function of adipose tissue underscores its significance in regulating responses to energy demands and hormonal signals. An understanding of these interactions within tissue morphology shows how changes in tissue structure and function can significantly affect overall health and the body's ability to maintain its numerous functions at optimal levels (Gutierrez et al., 2017).

SUMMARY

In brief, tissue morphology is an important cornerstone of comprehending the intricate structure and function of biological tissues. By employing a range of histological techniques, researchers are able to uncover the structural complexity that underlies tissue function. This research not only illuminates our current knowledge of normal physiological processes but also provides information regarding pathological conditions that are the consequence of tissue dysfunction. As imaging technologies and molecular biology drive the discipline forward, the uses of tissue morphology extend beyond biology into fields such as regenerative medicine and cancer research, highlighting its relevance and value within the wider scientific community. Additionally, implications of tissue morphology also extend into therapeutic areas, where morphological assessment can provide input for clinical intervention. Understanding cellular organization and disease interaction can facilitate the design of targeted therapies that normalize tissue architecture. Besides that, one must appreciate that tissue morphology is not static; it is being modulated by environmental factors, signaling pathways, and cell-to-cell interactions. This dynamic nature of tissue organization underscores the need for continued research to deepen understanding of the complex relationships between structure and function, enabling innovative prevention and treatment modalities for many diseases, as suggested by the data cited by Brown et al. (2014) and Gruhl, A. & Okamura, B. (2016). In essence, the field of tissue morphology is poised for revolutionary growth, stimulated by cross-disciplinary collaborations and technological advances. All future research endeavors must embrace a uniform integration that entwines genetic, biochemical, and biophysical information with tissue structure. This holistic strategy, aside from broadening our understanding of tissue biology, will further enhance our capacity to manipulate and engineer tissues for therapeutic purposes and make substantial contributions to organ transplantation and tissue engineering, among others. As science continues to strip away the secrets of tissue morphology, the potential for groundbreaking developments in medicine becomes increasingly obvious, ultimately favoring our understanding of life itself and human public health.

One of the fundamental elements of tissue morphology knowledge is the definition of cellular structure and its significance. Satellite cell analysis in adult skeletal muscle, for instance, demonstrates their essential role in tissue repair and regeneration following trauma. These stem cells resident in tissues undergo a lengthy process of migration, which is central to enabling rapid tissue recovery. Present evidence suggests satellite cells exhibit a two-step movement, first migrating beneath the basal lamina and subsequently accelerating along the myofiber surface. Interestingly, the locomotion of their cells is characterized by an atypical blebbing mechanism that contrasts with the typical lamellipodia-based model. These findings are relevant to therapeutic maneuvers as well, with recognition of satellite cell behavior influencing methods employed to induce skeletal muscle regeneration (Collins-Hooper et al., 2011). In the context of neurodevelopment, particularly of neonates, understanding cerebral anatomy makes a significant contribution to the overall tale of tissue morphology. With advances in imaging technologies, especially Magnetic Resonance Imaging (MRI), researchers have been able to investigate vascular development and cortical architecture in more detail. Specific algorithms for automatic vessel tree extraction and modeling have been formulated, in which more information regarding vascular growth during infancy can be obtained. At the same time, segmentation of the neonatal cortex also requires sophisticated techniques, as usual methods are inadequate due to differing characteristics in grey and white matter in brain development. Expectation-maximization techniques have been newly suggested to address these limitations and better reconstruct the cortex, with demands for specific methods in developing tissue analysis (Xue, 2008). The study of tissue morphology encompasses diverse cellular, vascular, and structural characteristics essential for growth and function. The precise understanding of satellite cell migration dynamics and cerebral neuroanatomy is symptomatic of how morphology intersects with regenerative medicine and developmental biology. Continued research will witness sophisticated steps to investigate these tissues, and in this process, lay open a treasure chest of comprehension that can potentially transform medical procedures. By analyzing the precise dynamics of cell behaviors and their spatial organizations, scientists can uncover the latent principle of tissue development and tissue repair. Thus, such information is crucial in achieving effective therapies for numerous diseases, emphasizing the importance of the morphology of tissues as a cornerstone in the life sciences (Xue, 2008; Collins-Hooper et al., 2011).

A LOOK TO THE FUTURE

PERIVASCULAR ADIPOSE TISSUE (PVAT):

Perivascular adipose tissue (PVAT) has emerged as a dynamic and influential component of the cardiovascular system, reshaping traditional views of fat solely as an energy storage depot. PVAT refers to the adipose tissue immediately surrounding most blood vessels, positioned in direct contact with the vascular adventitia, and distinct in structure and function from other fat depots such as subcutaneous or visceral adipose tissue. What was once considered a passive cushion for vessels is now recognised as an active paracrine and endocrine organ that directly participates in vascular physiology and disease processes. Under normal physiological conditions, PVAT exerts anticontractile and vasoprotective effects by releasing a variety of bioactive substances, including adipokines, gasotransmitters, and perivascular-derived relaxing factors. These molecules modulate vascular smooth muscle cell tone and endothelial function, helping regulate blood flow, vascular resistance, and overall tissue perfusion in accordance with metabolic demands. This local signalling network illustrates how PVAT contributes to fine-tuning vascular tone and maintaining vascular homeostasis.

PVAT is also characterized by a heterogeneous cellular composition that includes adipocytes, immune cells, endothelial cells, mesenchymal cells, and stromal cells, which collectively shape its secretory profile and functional impact on the adjacent vessel wall. These secreted factors influence not only vasodilation and vasoconstriction but also inflammatory responses and vascular remodeling processes.

However, when metabolic balance is disrupted—as in obesity, diabetes, and hypertension—PVAT can undergo phenotypic and functional changes that contribute to disease progression. In these pathological states, PVAT becomes a source of proinflammatory adipokines and chemokines, loses its anticontractile properties, and promotes endothelial dysfunction and vascular smooth muscle proliferation, processes that are implicated in atherosclerosis and vascular inflammation.

Research into PVAT is now focused on unravelling its molecular mechanisms, including how changes in lipid metabolism, immune cell infiltration, and adipokine signalling influence cardiovascular risk. This evolving understanding holds promise for novel diagnostic and therapeutic strategies that leverage PVAT biology to predict and mitigate vascular disease. As PVAT continues to be recognised as a critical regulator of vascular function, integrating its biology into broader cardiovascular research and clinical practice underscores the importance of adipose–vascular interactions in human health and disease.

REFERENCES

1. Mirzapoiazova, T., Li, H., Nathan, A., Srivstava, S., Nasser, M. W., Lennon, F., Armstrong, B., Mambetsariev, I., Chu, P. G., Achuthan, S., Batra, S. K., Kulkarni, P., & Salgia, R. (2019). Monitoring and determining mitochondrial network parameters in live lung cancer cells. *Journal of Clinical Medicine*, *8*(10), 1723. https://doi.org/10.3390/jcm8101723Adam, M., Ambrosi, D., Anderson, A., Anderson, A., Anderson, A., Anderson, A., et al. (2007). Computer simulation of glioma growth and morphology. *https://core.ac.uk/download/20446267.pdf* (accessed on 6th August 2025).
2. Adur, J. F., Bianchi, M., Carvalho, H. F., Casco, et al. (2014). Colon adenocarcinoma diagnosis in human samples by multicontrast nonlinear optical microscopy of hematoxylin and eosin-stained histological sections. *https://core.ac.uk/download/159290534.pdf* (accessed on 6th August 2025).
3. Agarwal, A., Alfano, R., Pradhan, A., Biswal, B., Boustany, N. N., Choi, W., Choi, H., et al. (2011). Differing self-similarity in light scattering spectra: A potential tool for pre-cancer detection. *http://arxiv.org/abs/1107.2519* (accessed on 6th August 2025).
4. Agustin Gutierrez, J., Freeman, D. J., Jayabalan, N., Lappas, et al. (2017). Cross-talk between adipose tissue and placenta in obese and gestational diabetes mellitus pregnancies via exosomes. *https://core.ac.uk/download/96883015.pdf* (accessed on 6th August 2025).
5. Alcazar-Fuoli, L., Armstrong-James, D., Bertuzzi, M., Bignell, et al. (2014). The pH-responsive PacC transcription factor of *Aspergillus fumigatus* governs epithelial entry and tissue invasion during pulmonary aspergillosis. *https://core.ac.uk/download/30435716.pdf* (accessed on 6th August 2025).
6. Aldini, N., Nicoli, D., Della Bella, E., Fini, M., Frizziero, et al. (2016). The role of detraining in tendon mechanobiology. *https://core.ac.uk/download/53528699.pdf* (accessed on 6th August 2025).
7. Alexander, R., Baker, A., Baraibar, M., Beale, B., Beale, G., Benjamin, M., Biggs, et al. (2014). Structure, ontogeny, and evolution of the patellar tendon in emus (*Dromaius novaehollandiae*) and other palaeognath birds. *https://core.ac.uk/download/36778015.pdf* (accessed on 6th August 2025).
8. Altshuler, A. E., Kurre, L., Lamadrid, I., Li, et al. (2014). Transmural intestinal wall permeability in severe ischemia after enteral protease inhibition. *https://core.ac.uk/download/323065462.pdf* (accessed on 6th August 2025).
9. Anderson, R. H., Ho, S. Y., Mazgalev, T. N. (2001). Anatomic-electrophysiological correlations concerning the pathways for atrioventricular conduction. *https://core.ac.uk/download/1676746.pdf* (accessed on 6th August 2025).
10. Andrén, P. E., Caprioli, R. M., Castellino, S., Charkoftaki, et al. (2018). Yale School of Public Health Symposium on tissue imaging mass spectrometry: Illuminating phenotypic heterogeneity and drug disposition at the molecular level. *https://core.ac.uk/download/152438977.pdf* (accessed on 6th August 2025).
11. Arafa, E. (2016). Determining cellular and biochemical function of a novel adhesion molecule in kidneys. *https://open.bu.edu/bitstream/2144/16062/1/Arafa_bu_0017N_11077.pdf* (accessed on 6th August 2025).

12. Asadian, M., De Geyter, N., De Moor, L., Declercq, et al. (2020). Hybrid bioprinting of chondrogenically induced human mesenchymal stem cell spheroids. *https://core.ac.uk/download/323232718.pdf* (accessed on 6th August 2025).

13. Azab, W., Kamel, M., Osterrieder, K., Pavulraj, et al. (2019). EHV-1 pathogenesis: Current in vitro models and future perspectives. *https://core.ac.uk/download/227044277.pdf* (accessed on 6th August 2025).

14. Baban, A., Calcagni, G., Dallapiccola, B., De Luca, et al. (2019). Atrioventricular canal defect and genetic syndromes: The unifying role of sonic hedgehog. *https://core.ac.uk/download/188826922.pdf* (accessed on 6th August 2025).

15. Bácsy, E., Bálint, K., Fazekas, I., Hegedűs, et al. (2005). Characterization of human pituitary adenomas in cell cultures by light and electron microscopic morphology and immunolabeling. *https://core.ac.uk/download/11856052.pdf* (accessed on 6th August 2025).

16. Basava, R. R., Chen, J.-S., He, Q., He, et al. (2020). Microstructural analysis of skeletal muscle force generation during aging. *https://core.ac.uk/download/286361329.pdf* (accessed on 6th August 2025).

17. Becker, M.-B., Begemann, G., Meyer, A., Sanetra, et al. (2005). Conservation and co-option in developmental programmes: The importance of homology relationships. *https://core.ac.uk/download/pdf/3800618.pdf* (accessed on 6th August 2025).

18. Berry, C. C., Davies, R. L., O'Boyle, N., Sutherland, et al. (2017). Temporal dynamics of ovine airway epithelial cell differentiation at an air-liquid interface. *https://core.ac.uk/download/84591468.pdf* (accessed on 6th August 2025).

19. Braden, R. L., Christman, K. L., Dzieciatkowska, M., Elhag, et al. (2016). Extracellular matrix hydrogel promotes tissue remodeling, arteriogenesis, and perfusion in a rat hindlimb ischemia model. *https://core.ac.uk/download/323065138.pdf* (accessed on 6th August 2025).

20. Brown, A. J. P., Brown, G. D., Chen, K., Drummond, et al. (2014). *Candida albicans* colonization and dissemination from the murine gastrointestinal tract: The influence of morphology and Th17 immunity. *https://core.ac.uk/download/29151197.pdf* (accessed on 6th August 2025).

21. Byrne, H. M., O'Dea, R. D., Waters, S. L. (2008). A two-fluid model for tissue growth within a dynamic flow environment. *https://core.ac.uk/download/pdf/6185199.pdf* (accessed on 6th August 2025).

22. Caretto, S., Frugis, G., Giannino, D., Iannelli, et al. (2019). Plant cellular and molecular biotechnology: Following Mariotti's steps. *https://core.ac.uk/download/188831409.pdf* (accessed on 6th August 2025).

23. Chung, U.-I., Docheva, D., Hiraki, Y., Hojo, et al. (2013). Tenomodulin expression in the periodontal ligament enhances cellular adhesion. *https://core.ac.uk/download/12175517.pdf* (accessed on 6th August 2025).

24. Clinton, B. K., Cunningham, C. L., Kriegstein, A. R., Martínez-Cerdeño, et al. (2014). Radial glia in the proliferative ventricular zone of the embryonic and adult turtle, *Trachemys scripta elegans*. *https://core.ac.uk/download/323069618.pdf* (accessed on 6th August 2025).

25. Collins-Hooper, H., Dash, P. R., Otto, A., Patel, et al. (2011). Adult skeletal muscle stem cell migration is mediated by a blebbing/amoeboid mechanism. *https://core.ac.uk/download/9077.pdf* (accessed on 6th August 2025).

26. Corrêa, S. A. L. & Eales, K. L. (2012). The role of p38 MAPK and its substrates in neuronal plasticity and neurodegenerative disease. *https://core.ac.uk/download/9257821.pdf* (accessed on 6th August 2025).

27. Curtis, N., Fagan, M. J., Witzel, U. (2014). Development and three-dimensional morphology of the zygomaticotemporal suture in primate skulls. *https://core.ac.uk/download/151157048.pdf* (accessed on 6th August 2025).

28. David, C. N. (1973). A quantitative method for maceration of *Hydra* tissue. *https://core.ac.uk/download/12164238.pdf* (accessed on 6th August 2025).

29. de Wiljes, O. O., Keijzer, F. A., van Elburg, R. A. J. (2017). Short and random: Modelling the effects of (proto-)neural elongations. *https://core.ac.uk/download/518732509.pdf* (accessed on 6th August 2025).

30. Degistirici, O., Götz, W., Jaquiery, C., Martin, et al. (2008). Defining properties of neural crest-derived progenitor cells from the apex of human developing tooth. *https://core.ac.uk/download/18240097.pdf* (accessed on 6th August 2025).

31. Di Cataldo, S., Ficarra, E., Acquaviva, A., & Macii, E. (2010). Achieving the way for automated segmentation of nuclei in cancer tissue images through morphology-based approach: A quantitative evaluation. *https://core.ac.uk/download/pdf/11412919.pdf* (accessed on 6th August 2025).

32. Fenton, M. B., Gray, P., Holbrook, K. A., Humphry, G. M., Maisonneuve, P., Meyer, W., Schumacher, S., et al. (2017). Diversity in the organization of elastin bundles and intramembranous muscles in bat wings. *https://core.ac.uk/download/76981004.pdf* (accessed on 6th August 2025).

33. Fiegel, H. C., Gfrörer, S., Metzger, R., Ramachandran, et al. (2012). Changes of smooth muscle contractile filaments in small bowel atresia. *https://core.ac.uk/download/14530388.pdf* (accessed on 6th August 2025).

34. Fischer, W. W. & Wilson, J. P. (2011). Geochemical support for a climbing habit within the Paleozoic seed fern genus *Medullosa*. *https://core.ac.uk/download/4889973.pdf* (accessed on 6th August 2025).

35. Forasiepi, A. M. & Sánchez Villagra, M. R. (2017). On the development of the chondrocranium and the histological anatomy of the head in perinatal stages of marsupial mammals. *https://core.ac.uk/download/161784436.pdf* (accessed on 6th August 2025).

36. Fujinaka, T. (2019). Comparison of osseointegration in piezoimplants versus cylindrical implants. *https://open.bu.edu/bitstream/2144/37058/7/Fujinaka_bu_0017N_14844.pdf* (accessed on 6th August 2025).

37. Gruhl, A. & Okamura, B. (2016). Development and myogenesis of the vermiform *Buddenbrockia* (*Myxozoa*) and implications for cnidarian body plan evolution. *https://core.ac.uk/download/42046060.pdf* (accessed on 6th August 2025).

38. Guzik, T. J. & Nosalski, R. (2017). Perivascular adipose tissue inflammation in vascular disease. *https://core.ac.uk/download/77600990.pdf* (accessed on 6th August 2025).

39. Hamid Reza Noori. (2009). Averaging transformations of synaptic potentials on networks. *https://core.ac.uk/download/pdf/288559.pdf* (accessed on 6th August 2025).

40. Heller, J. P. & Rusakov, D. A. (2015). Morphological plasticity of astroglia: Understanding

synaptic microenvironment. *https://core.ac.uk/download/29412340.pdf* (accessed on 6th August 2025).

41. Hill, G., Holcombe, M., Hose, D. R., MacNeil, et al. (2004). The Epitheliome: Agent-based modelling of the social behaviour of cells. *https://core.ac.uk/download/59287.pdf* (accessed on 6th August 2025).
42. Kim, T., Li, J., Yu, Q. (2017). Intrinsic regulators of actomyosin contractility engendering pulsatile behaviors. *https://core.ac.uk/download/85120290.pdf* (accessed on 6th August 2025).
43. Kirkland, M., Lin, T., Sutti, A., Tang, et al. (2011). Three-dimensional tissue scaffolds from interbonded poly(ε-caprolactone) fibrous matrices with controlled porosity. *http://hdl.handle.net/10536/DRO/DU:30032936* (accessed on 6th August 2025).
44. Klepzig, A., Kucherenko, M. M., Marrone, A. K., Rishko, et al. (2010). Paraffin-embedded and frozen sections of *Drosophila* adult muscles. *https://core.ac.uk/download/pdf/8608659.pdf* (accessed on 6th August 2025).
45. Maldonado, M, & Nam, J. (2013). The role of changes in the extracellular matrix of cartilage in the presence of inflammation on the pathology of osteoarthritis. *https://core.ac.uk/download/323067992.pdf* (accessed on 6th August 2025).
46. N/A. (2025). *Musculoskeletal discipline science plan. https://core.ac.uk/download/pdf/42808673.pdf* (accessed on 6th August 2025).
47. Preziosi, L. & Scianna, M. (2013). Modelling the influence of nucleus elasticity on cell invasion in fiber networks and microchannels. *https://core.ac.uk/download/pdf/11431730.pdf* (accessed on 6th August 2025).
48. Xue, H. (2008). Computerized analysis of magnetic resonance images to study cerebral anatomy in developing neonates. *https://core.ac.uk/download/295780.pdf* (accessed on 6th August 2025).

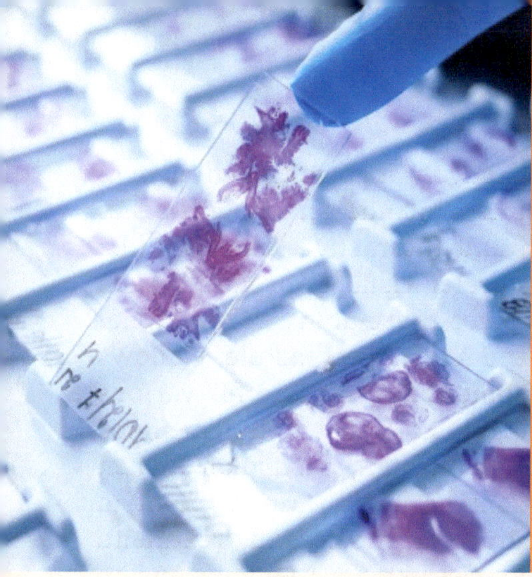

Chapter 2

PRINCIPLES OF HISTOLOGICAL TECHNIQUES

Contents

Introduction

Histology is a fundamental building block in the investigation of tissue structure and function, providing insight essential to the investigation of normal as well as disease states. Histology is the microscopic study of tissues based on principles incorporating cellular organization, composition, and physiological functions. The evolution of histological techniques, including staining, sectioning, and imaging, has markedly enhanced the visual portrayal of cellular traits, shedding light on the complex interactions among varied tissue types. Their use is at the heart of most areas of study, ranging from basic biology to advanced medical diagnosis. Understanding histology is crucial for medical professionals as it guides them in the process of diagnosing diseases and developing treatment protocols based on tissue properties, making it so vital in first-year classes of health-related educational programs. The introduction of new pedagogic techniques in histology programs can significantly enhance students' engagement and comprehension. The use of didactic guides, according to recent studies, may enable a model of learning through self-discovery in which students are actively involved in their own learning rather than acquiring knowledge passively. The guides often include an integration of theoretical texts, visual materials like drawings and illustrations, and interactive materials like quizzes and self-testing questions. Research indicates that students prefer visual approaches, such as diagrams and photographs, for learning histology and that they place these above conventional text-based presentations. The integration of such approaches into the teaching of histology allows teachers to create a more effective and interesting learning environment appropriate for various learning needs and attitudes, improving comprehension and recall of histological facts (Alaminos et al., 2013). Within the clinical environment, histology is even more relevant, particularly when dealing with pathological tissues. Sarcomas of soft tissue, for example, are a case in point in demonstrating the key role histological examination plays in accurate diagnosis and treatment. The tumors in question, comprised of tissue of mesenchymal origin, can exhibit a wide spectrum of histological features with important implications for the management of the patient. Histological examination of the specimen allows doctors to grade tumors, determine their malignancy, and apply effective therapeutic regimens. The relationship between histological findings and clinical data, as highlighted in case reports, is important for achieving optimal patient outcomes. Thus, an understanding of histological principles not only provides added richness to medical learning but also equips future medical professionals with the necessary skills to meet real-world problems in diagnostics and in the treatment of patients (Brincat, 1990) (Figure 2.1).

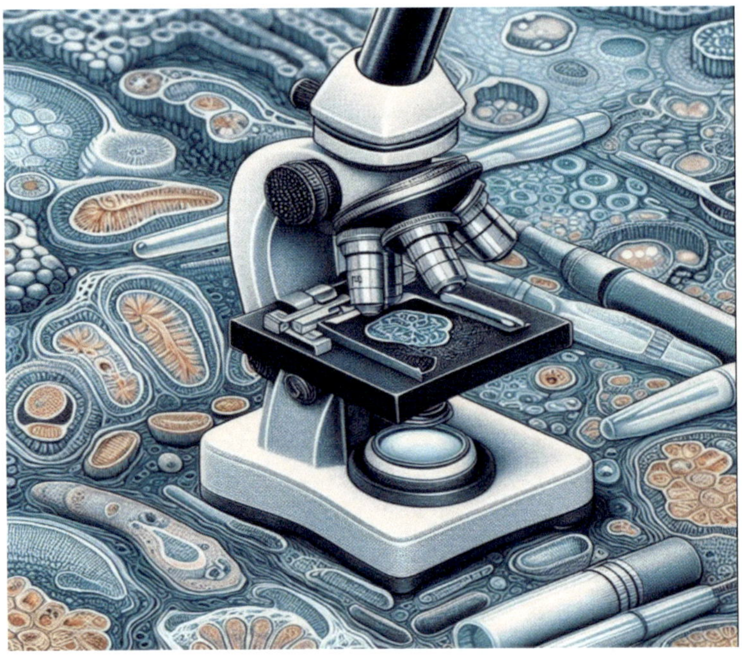

Figure 2.1. Principles of histological techniques.

Source: https://wiseias.com/wp-content/uploads/2024/09/Designer-41.webp.

Definition and Importance of Histology

Histology, the study of the microscopic structure of tissues, is a basic science to the biological and medical sciences. By studying cells and their arrangement in various tissues, histologists can learn a great deal about normal physiological functions, as well as identify pathological changes that indicate disease. This level of microscopic observation deepens our understanding of tissue structure and function, enabling us to construct specific medical treatments and diagnostic procedures. The data gathered by the histological study provides the basis for advances in clinical practice, offering a foundation on which to introduce histological principles into the training and education of doctors. Therefore, the definition of histology goes beyond tissue examination; it encompasses the vital tools by which we interpret biological systems and how they respond to environmental changes. The significance of histology is also illustrated with the aid of pathological diagnosis. Through the facility of being able to examine histopathological slides, practitioners are able to detect abnormalities that are typical of diseases such as cancers and inflammatory illnesses. For instance, malignant and benign tissue differentiation is based on histological analysis. In addition, advancement in histological techniques—like immunohistochemistry and molecular histology—has significantly enhanced the precision of diagnoses, which has provided opportunities for personalized medical therapies.

Such new methods enhance understanding of the tissue microenvironment at the functional level, allowing for in-depth examination of disease progression. Hence, the interfacing of histological techniques with clinical applications presents the primordial position this discipline has to assume in contemporary medicine, and how clinical management practices and laboratory findings are interrelated. Incorporating histological techniques into the curriculum for instruction is not only beneficial but inevitable in formulating an integrated perception among students and medical practitioners. Practical histology manuals, such as those commonly used, employ a range of educational methodologies to support self-discovery learning, an essential method for understanding complex tissue architecture and function. The application of a range of tools, from visual aids like drawings and pictures to hands-on exercises and self-assessment questions, supplements the learning process and encourages engagement. Moreover, the approach is consistent with contemporary education models that emphasize active learning and autonomy, as evidenced in studies on the effectiveness of various didactic resources (Alaminos et al., 2013). Through fostering creative thinking and advancing conceptualization, well-balanced histology education enhances the professional capacities of future medical professionals, eventually giving rise to improved patient outcomes and successful research processes (Huang et al., 2016) (Figure 2.2).

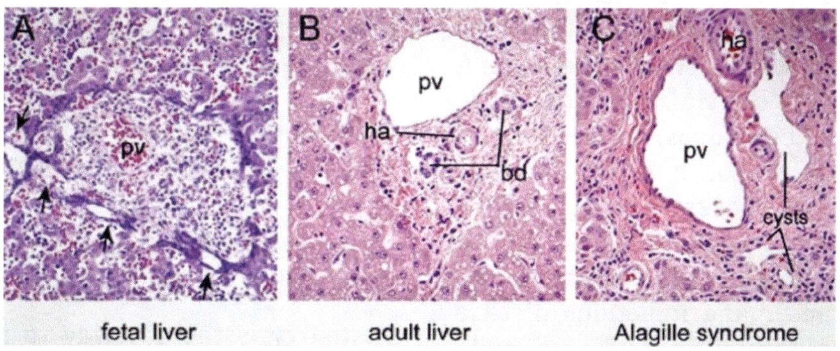

Figure 2.2. Definition and importance of histology.

Source: https://anatomynotes.org/wp-content/uploads/2020/01/Introduction-to-Histology-Applications-Importance-1024x418.jpg.

Historical Development of Histological Techniques

The development of histological methods transformed the disciplines of biology and medicine and gave new, unparalleled insights into cellular structure and tissue architecture. The historical emergence of these methods dates back to the end of the 19th century, when microscopy became advanced enough for researchers to view minute cellular details. These early investigators, such as Camillo Golgi and Santiago Ramón y Cajal, used silver nitrate staining techniques, which enabled them to distinguish among cell types in tissues. These studies laid the foundation for modern histology as it highlighted the importance of stain specificity and techniques of preparation in revealing cellular detail. These initial contributions highlighted that the comprehension of tissue pathology is inherently tied to histological methods and, as such, set a pivotal precedent for subsequent breakthroughs that would further our understanding of intricate biological systems. The early 20th century introduced additional innovations, including formaldehyde fixation and paraffin embedding, methods that would become cornerstones of histological laboratory procedures. Formaldehyde fixation preserved tissue morphology without diminishing artifacts, resulting in more accurate portrayals of cellular structures. Thin sections of embedded tissue were able to be cut because of this, and these were examined in the microscope for their histological characteristics. This improvement, combined with the development of more advanced staining techniques, enabled more precise investigations of a large number of tissues and the diseases that develop in them. For instance, the employment of special stains during this time greatly facilitated the investigation of cancer and infectious disease pathologies so that targeted treatments could be formulated on the basis of meticulous histological examination. Over the past few decades, advances in imaging techniques have ushered histology into a new era by integrating traditional morphologic examination with functional assessment. Methods such as multimodal two-photon microscopy and optical coherence tomography are among the significant developments in imaging tissue architecture at previously unattainable resolutions. These new techniques not only reveal to us the fine morphological details of cellular architecture but also assist us in gaining greater insight into physiological functions, as well as pathologically induced alterations such as those occurring in cholestatic liver disorders, primary biliary cirrhosis, and primary sclerosing cholangitis, which are characterized by unique histological features. The transition from basic staining procedures to modern imaging technologies captures the dynamic history of histological techniques and their important role of bridging basic research to clinical use, leading to improved patient care and outcome as knowledge is enhanced with new technology and more precise techniques (Leuschner, U. & Schlichting, J., 2013; Huang et al., 2016) (Figure 2.3).

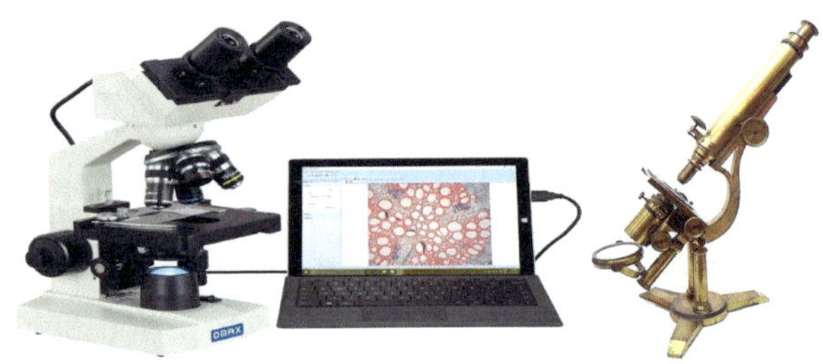

Figure 2.3. Historical development of histological techniques.

Source: https://i.ytimg.com/vi/CqJTpdxStUg/maxresdefault.jpg.

Applications of Histology in Modern Science

Histology is the gateway to modern scientific inquiry, particularly biomedical inquiry and clinical diagnosis. By the detailed dissection of tissue structure and cellular organization, histological techniques provide insightful information into disease mechanisms and tissue development. For instance, the advent of machine learning and data-driven methods has revolutionized histopathological analysis to allow researchers to leverage advanced computational techniques in order to categorize and assess voluminous amounts of histological data efficiently. This innovation fulfills the need for speed and precision in disease diagnosis as stipulated in research underscoring the crossroads of data mining and histology in modern biomedical research (elsey, T. W. & Wallace, W. H. B., 2010). As a result, histology not only further informs our understanding of disease but also speeds up diagnostic processes and thus improves outcomes for patients. Advances in imaging technologies have also supplemented applications of histology by facilitating comprehensive investigations of biological tissue at unprecedented resolutions. Techniques like three-dimensional reconstruction of histological sections have dramatically improved traditional histopathological assessments. By using high-precision layer-by-layer grinding of frozen biological tissue, new software is now available that reconstructs tissue images in full color and high resolution. This is especially beneficial because it enables scientists to observe complex tissue architecture at a resolution of 5–10 μm and enhances their ability to study complex biological systems (Brazina et al., 2017). Then, the integration of such technologies into histological methods not only enhances the level of detail to be reached for inspection but also assists in the building of accurate models that reflect the intricate behaviors in biological contexts. Additionally, histological techniques are applied in clinical settings, where tissue sample preparation and analysis are essential in disease diagnosis and guiding treatment protocols. Histological procedures rely heavily on pathologists to identify cellular abnormalities and provide crucial information on tumor type and stage, ultimately informing therapeutic management. The more complex the nature of diseases such as cancer, the greater the need for proper histological examination, which cannot be overstated. Histology aids in the identification of different tumor variants, their histological grades, and the evaluation of responses to therapeutic treatment. This submission emphasizes the crucial role of histological techniques in bridging the gap between clinical practice and research, thereby translating scientific progress into improved healthcare delivery and specialized patient management.

2.1. Basic Principles of Histological Techniques

An understanding of the basic principles of histological techniques is essential for anyone in the line of biological sciences, particularly medicine and pathology. Histology refers to the microscopic examination of tissues and lies at the heart of disease diagnosis, including cancer and infection. Histological techniques involve a series of significant steps, beginning with tissue fixation, which helps preserve cellular structure and composition. Fixatives, most often formaldehyde or glutaraldehyde, fixate proteins and nucleic acids, preventing decomposition and enabling the structure of the tissues to be held in place for microscopic examination. It is this first crucial step that opens the way for additional procedures like embedding, sectioning, and staining, which further enhance the distinctness of structural details and cellular components on the microscope. Following fixation, the embedding process transforms the fixed tissue to a hardened matrix that permits thin sectioning required for close examination. Paraffin wax is widely applied for this purpose because its properties make it easy to cut sections without damaging the samples. This embedded tissue is then sectioned at micrometer thickness, typically using a microtome, and mounted on glass slides for staining. Hematoxylin and eosin (H&E) staining techniques are significant for the imaging of numerous cellular components. These dyes change the color of particular structures, allowing pathologists to distinguish between cell types and identify abnormalities. With the advent of modern staining techniques, more sophisticated methodologies are utilized employing fluorescent markers, which significantly enhance the diagnostic value and allow the exploration of molecular pathways in tissues (Bishop et al., 2017). Improvements in histological techniques, including emerging imaging technologies, have transformed the science, making it possible to gain more acute information regarding tissue morphology and function. Such advanced techniques as microscopy with ultraviolet surface excitation (MUSE) have been developed, allowing for high-speed, high-resolution histological imaging with no slide requirement. The slide-free process significantly simplifies the diagnostic process, allowing clinicians to obtain timely critical information crucial to the care of patients (Bishop et al., 2017). Additionally, the integration of newer imaging technologies, e.g., optical coherence tomography, enables improved visualization of tissue structure and dysfunction across a variety of medical disciplines, such as ophthalmology, as demonstrated by investigations of the aqueous humor outflow tract in glaucoma. All these developments in histological techniques are indicative of the interdependent synergy between technology and research, which eventually translates into patient care and therapy (Figure 2.4).

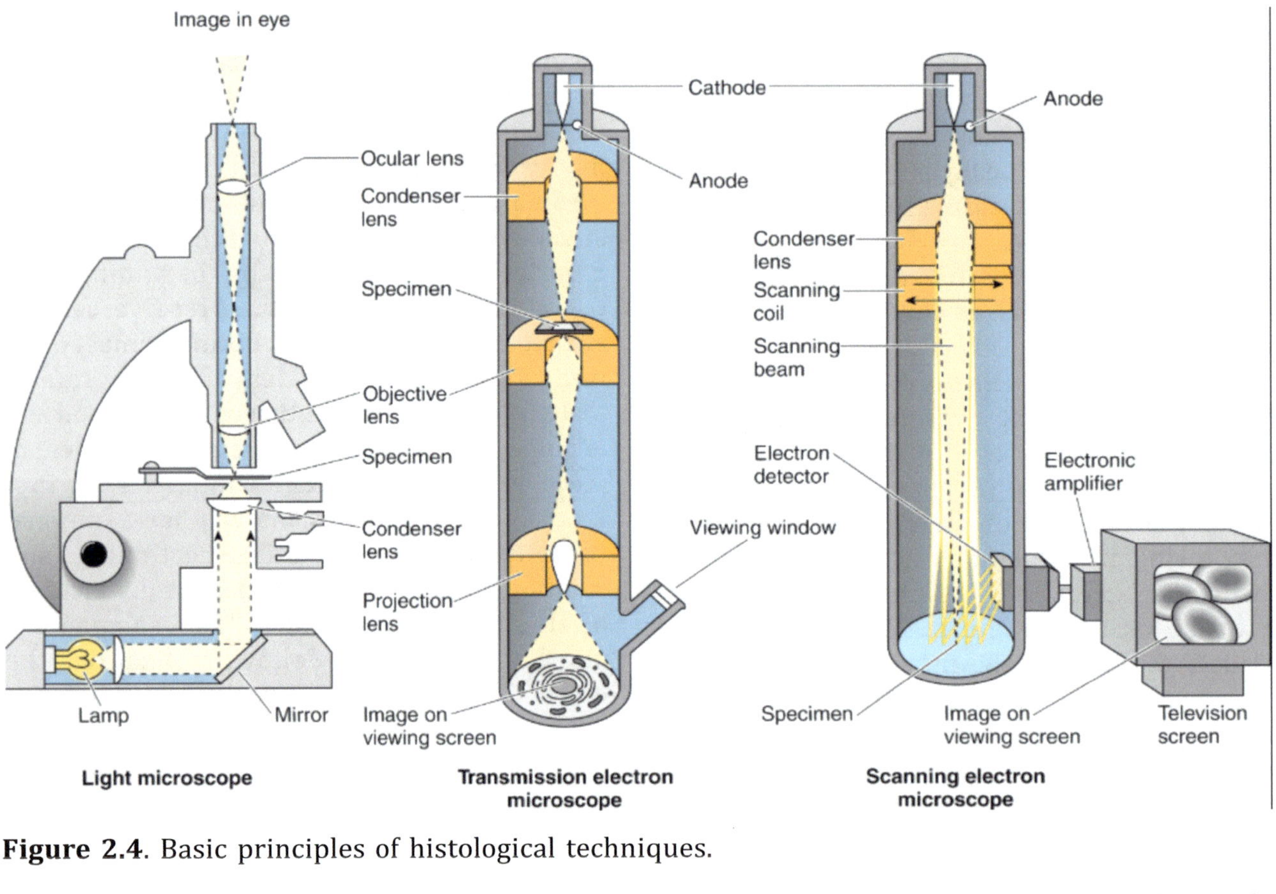

Figure 2.4. Basic principles of histological techniques.

Source: https://storage.googleapis.com/dl.dentistrykey.com/clinical/IntroductiontoHistologyandBasicHistologicalTechniques/0_3s20B9780323672726000011.jpg.

2.1.1. Tissue Preparation and Fixation

Preparation and fixation of tissues are a highly important process in histology, as they indirectly influence the quality and integrity of the microscopic examination of biological tissue samples. Fixation preserves the shape of cells and tissues by stabilizing proteins, halting autolysis, and preventing putrefaction. There are various fixatives available, the most common being formaldehyde and glutaraldehyde due to their ability to covalently cross-link proteins, making strong preservation of cell structure possible. The choice of fixative can then be made depending on the specific requirements of the study, such as tissue type and downstream processing. Lastly, effective fixation ensures that morphological characteristics are preserved, enabling accurate interpretation of histological details, which is crucial for disease diagnosis and research. Subsequent procedural steps to fixation in the processing of tissue include processing, embedding, and sectioning, all processes that are crucial to the attainment of quality histological slides.

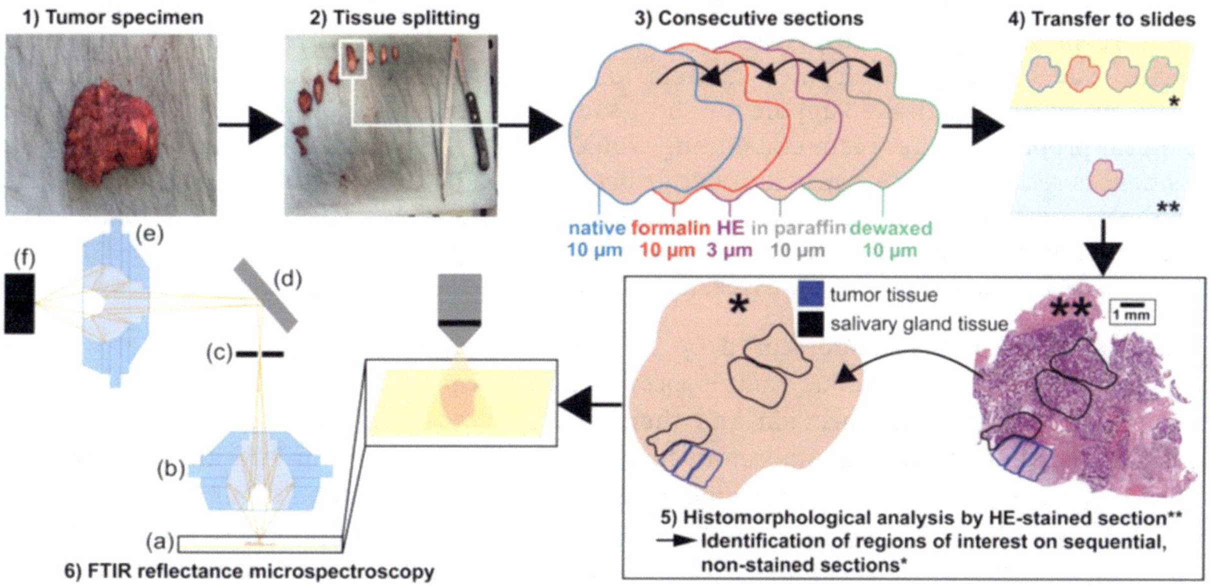

Figure 2.5. Tissue preparation and fixation.

Source: https://www.researchgate.net/publication/367025959/figure/fig1/AS:11431281212968439@1702925448043/Workflow-of-tissue-preparation-for-FTIR-microspectroscopic-measurements-Salivary-gland.tif.

Dehydration is usually done using graded alcoholic solutions to evaporate water, followed by clearing agents, which replace alcohol with a medium that is compatible with embedding material, e.g., paraffin. Good embedding is essential to support thin sectioning and facilitate the preparation of slices that are readily viewed under the microscope. Thin sections of 5-10 micrometers must be accurately cut and mounted on glass slides with care in order not to distort the tissue morphology. All these processes are crucial in preserving cellular structure integrity because any error might significantly hinder analysis and compromise the quality of histological examination. More sophisticated tissue preparation methods have enabled improved techniques that enhance the analytical capabilities of histological studies. Improved comparative genomic hybridization technology, for example, has enabled the detection and localization of chromosomal abnormalities in solid tumor samples from both frozen and formalin-fixed specimens to fulfill the need for reliable genetic analysis (Cremer et al., 1993). Furthermore, new stereotaxic equipment has been developed to improve anatomical accuracy in the preparation of neural tissue, enabling scientists to deliver precise positional information for neurophysiological applications (Andres et al., 1986). With such advanced techniques being integrated into routine histological practice, the accuracy of tissue characterization can be significantly improved, leading to enhanced diagnostic performance and greater understanding of complex biological processes (Figure 2.5).

2.1.2. Embedding Techniques

Among the fundamental principles of histological techniques, methods of embedding stand out due to their critical role in preparing the sample. Proper embedding is an important parameter to guarantee that tissues do not deteriorate in the following stages of slicing and staining. Paraffin wax and resin are typically employed as mediums of embedding, and each possesses distinct properties due to which it becomes suitable for specific types of tissue analysis. Paraffin, for instance, provides good tissue support for soft tissues and plays a very important role in standard histological preparation. Yet resin embedding would be more appropriate if precise ultrastructure assessment is required, since it provides better preservation of cell structure. With the use of these embedding methods, researchers anticipate improving cellular imaging resolution and accuracy, eventually translating to increased knowledge in tissue morphology and pathology, as highlighted in the need to improve histological assessment in bioengineered lung tissues (Silva et al., 2023).

Its significance is also underscored by the recent advances in mass spectrometry imaging (MSI) that necessitate meticulous sample preparation to optimize the analytical precision. Use of traditional fixation using formalin and then paraffin embedding has been proven to induce metabolite distributions to shift, therefore making the interpretation of MSI analysis data more complicated. Notably, recent research highlights the importance of maintaining the biochemical integrity of the tissue during embedding. For instance, the development of new embedding media such as hydroxypropyl-methylcellulose and polyvinylpyrrolidone hydrogels has provided alternatives that better preserve tissue biomolecules. These advances not only facilitate improving the accuracy of targeted analyses but also assist in integrating embedding strategies with orthogonal imaging modalities to obtain additional information regarding tissue function and composition (Dannhorn, 2020). Integration of embedding techniques and histological assessments underscores the importance of methodological consistency in the current tissue studies. As researchers strive to evaluate new bioengineered therapies, particularly regenerative medicine, the need for standardized embedding techniques has never been more acute. Standardization should be such that it takes into account compatibility with most biomaterials used in tissue engineering that will not tolerate the application of conventional fixatives. The conventional overreliance on traditional chemical moieties is thus a thing of the past, and the novelty introduced by synthetic and natural polymers must now be dealt with. As is explained in current studies, the quantification of cell-extracellular matrix interactions is an area that will greatly benefit from advances in embedding techniques, facilitating an enhanced comprehension of the intricate relationships within engineered tissues and enhancing their evaluation in preclinical models (Silva A., 2023) (Figure 2.6).

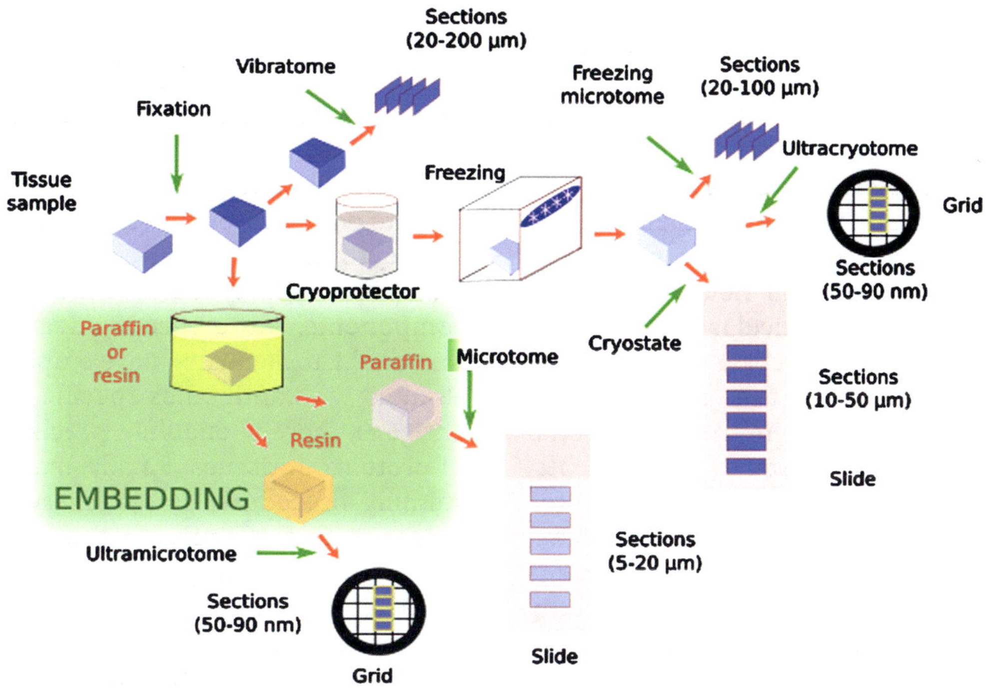

Figure 2.6. Embedding techniques.

Source: https://mmegias.webs.uvigo.es/02-english/6-tecnicas/imagenes/3-inclusion.png.

2.1.3. Sectioning Methods

Sectioning is a core histological technique, as it involves cutting tissue samples into thin sections that are best viewed under a microscope. The technique enables accurate visualization of cellular organization and tissue architecture, which is critical for diagnosis and research. There are several sectioning techniques with different levels of sophistication and application, including microtomy, cryosectioning, and laser capture microdissection. Microtomy is the most conventional technique that involves the use of a microtome to produce equal sections of embedded fixed tissues. The technique typically produces sections 3-10 micrometers thick, which are crucial for microscopic analysis. The precision of the procedure is extremely critical since any deviation can have a very significant influence on the interpretation of the tissue's histological characteristics. Cryosectioning is another method that is particularly useful for immediate intraoperative diagnosis. Fixation of the tissue sample is done by freezing and sectioning with a cryostat so that immediate examination can be conducted without chemical fixation. Even though cryosectioning provides faster results, it is disadvantageous in maintaining tissue morphology, which is altered in the process of freezing. The integration of these sectioning methods is crucial in clinical settings where there are emergent histopathological evaluations. The application of technology, such as microscopy with ultraviolet surface excitation (MUSE), offers more sophisticated functions in sectioning and imaging tissue specimens without the necessity for using traditional mounting on slides. MUSE demonstrates the potential for revolutionizing histological imaging by combining rapid tissue analysis with high-resolution diagnosticity, furthering patient care via maximally optimized histological assessment (Bishop et al., 2017). Moreover, advances in sectioning techniques have underscored the need for flexibility in histological protocols. For example, in experimental models, the utilization of sophisticated stereotaxic methodology in animal models has facilitated localizing tissue samples more specifically for sectioning. Such methods are imperative in neuroscience, as precise targeting of a particular brain area is required for reliable and reproducible results. Research suggests that this sophisticated stereotaxic system could improve positional accuracy, rendering it usable beyond bats, thereby providing new possibilities for histological investigation across various animal models (Andres et al., 1986). With advancements in histology, the addition of groundbreaking techniques of sectioning will not merely enhance the accuracy of tissue analysis but also expand the scope of research in both the preclinical and clinical settings (Figure 2.7).

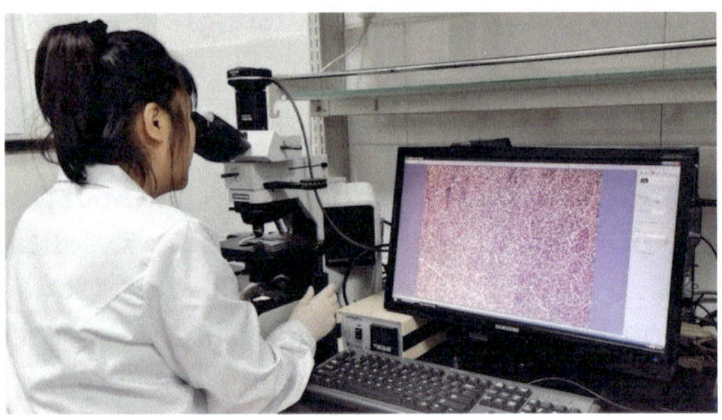

Figure 2.7. Sectioning methods.

Source: https://cloudfront.jove.com/CDNSource/teasers/61822.jpg.

2.2. Staining Techniques

The visualization of cellular architecture in histological preparations is greatly dependent on staining techniques, which are utilized to enhance the contrast between varying tissue constituents. These procedures play a fundamental role in providing cellular morphology clarity, enabling pathologists and scientists to differentiate between various tissue types, cellular parts, and pathological changes. Commonly used staining protocols are hematoxylin and eosin (H&E), staining nuclei and cytoplasmic detail, and special stains for specific cell types or extracellular matrix components. More recent advances, such as immunohistochemistry, have employed targeted staining with antibodies specific for individual antigens, thereby enabling precise localization of proteins in tissues. Finally, mastery of these staining procedures is necessary for accurate diagnosis and effective treatment regimens in contemporary histopathology. In histological practice, staining chemistry involves chemical reactions and adherence to standardized methods to ensure reproducibility and accuracy. The guidelines for HER2 laboratory testing, for instance, emphasize standardization of immunohistochemical examination of tissue specimens to support effective targeted therapy in the management of metastatic breast cancer. In recent recommendations, laboratories must employ a two-stage algorithm of testing, including preliminary immunocytochemistry analysis with subsequent follow-up fluorescence *in situ* hybridization for uncertain results. This systematic process enhances the validity of histological staining techniques to ensure diagnostic results reflect the true condition of tissues being examined. Strict quality controls and annual caseload determinations strengthen the integrity of staining procedures in clinical laboratories, affirming the important role that such principles play in histological practice (Bartlett et al., 2004). Furthermore, the development of novel staining techniques continues to advance in concert with advances in tissue engineering and regenerative medicine. Recent studies have demonstrated that hybrid bioprinting can be used to produce cartilage microtissues, integrating hybrid materials with properties that support cellular organization and viability. In this regard, the stain techniques employed are critical to assessing chondrogenic differentiation and overall tissue health using glycosaminoglycans and collagen markers as indicators of extracellular matrix integrity. With evolving bioprinting technology, the need for bespoke staining protocols that can keep pace with the complexity of three-dimensional tissue constructs becomes increasingly important. Observations, such as enhanced chondrogenic maturation facilitated by hydrogel properties, also illustrate the close marriage between stain techniques and successful tissue regeneration attempts. The continuous push-and-pull between innovation and technique supports an era in which staining techniques are integral to both diagnostic and therapeutic schemes in histology (Asadian et al., 2020) (Figure 2.8).

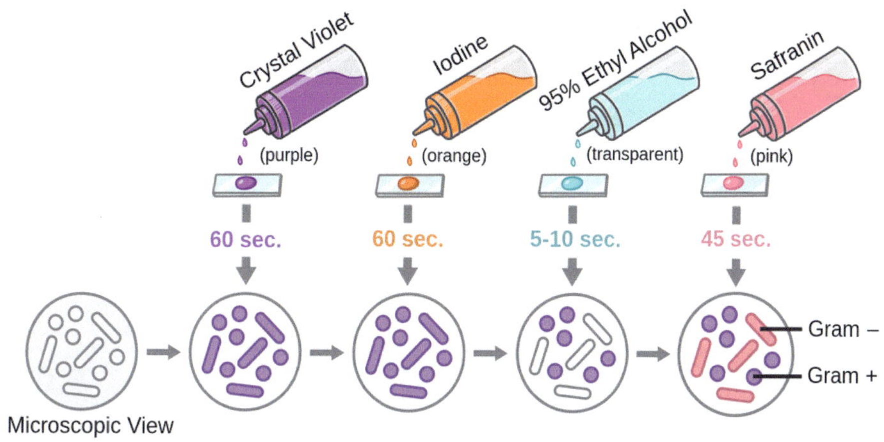

Figure 2.8. Staining techniques.

Source: https://labster-image-manager.s3.amazonaws.com/bd7be05a-dd65-4273-a739-ff9801800aad/GRM_The_Gram_stain_procedure_overview_THEORY.en.x1024.png.

2.2.1. Types of Stains: Basic vs. Acidic

In histology, staining techniques play a central role in visualizing cellular structures, and two prominent categories are basic and acidic stains. Basic stains such as methylene blue and toluidine blue O carry a positive charge and exhibit a select preference for negatively charged cellular constituents, especially nucleic acids and certain proteins. This affinity makes simple stains powerful in highlighting structures like the nucleus and ribosomes, thereby making them extremely useful for the appreciation of cellular morphology as well as function. Furthermore, the use of basic stains can highlight cellular changes associated with pathological states, facilitating diagnosis. For instance, in the examination of tissue that is diseased, characteristic staining patterns provided by basic stains can be a key guide toward the underlying cellular changes. On the other hand, acidic dyes, such as eosin, carry a negative charge and can bind to positively charged cellular components, primarily proteins and cytoplasmic structures. Acidic dyes play key roles in staining structures such as collagen fibers, cytoplasm, and granular structures in cells. Acidic stain techniques usually yield a color scheme different from that seen with basic stains, as they are capable of revealing detailed tissue architectural features not visible under a basic stain. This double staining not only facilitates enhanced histological examination but also paves the way to further insight into tissue pathology and physiology. Through the application of both types of stains concurrently, histologists are capable of producing a clearer picture of the tissue environment, thereby making for accurate diagnosis and research findings. Utilization of both basic and acidic stains also relies greatly on familiarity with how the stains react with the tissues' components chemically. Selection of the right staining procedure, therefore, relies on the specific cellular structures to be stained. For example, in ischemic stroke studies of thrombus composition, researchers have applied various staining approaches to distinguish among cellular constituents, as in recent histological and recanalization studies (Meher, 2020). Similarly, the multi-branching approach with the combination of traditional histology and modern techniques, including immunohistochemistry, can enhance diagnostic capabilities by enabling greater sophistication in the understanding of disease processes. Because histological techniques remain to be developed, incorporation of basic staining and acidic staining principles will be necessary continually, highlighting their rudimentary role in ongoing endeavors of cellular biology and pathology, as highlighted in the larger context of histological principles (Bochsler et al., 2007) (Figure 2.9).

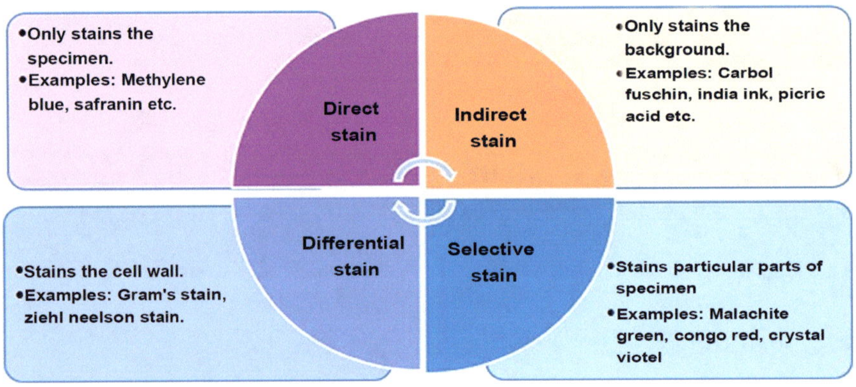

Figure 2.9. Types of stains: basic vs. acidic.

Source: https://biologyreader.com/wp-content/uploads/2018/11/staining-tech.jpg.

2.2.2. Common Staining Protocols

Histology is largely dependent on effective staining protocols, which are applied to optimize the visibility of cellular organization in tissue samples. Hematoxylin and eosin (H&E) staining, Massons trichrome, and immunohistochemistry (IHC) are the most frequently employed ones. H&E stain is particularly renowned, as it distinguishes cellular structures by staining nuclei blue and cytoplasm pink, with the capacity to perform quick yet thorough assessments of tissue morphology. This fundamental approach underpins more specialized applications, such as IHC, which employs antibodies to detect target proteins in tissue. Variations in staining protocols mirror their role not only to reveal anatomical structures but also to diagnose illness at the cellular level and thereby illustrate their fundamental position within the general principles of histological methods. For the sake of consistency and reliability of findings, strict adherence to standard staining procedures is essential. The development and advancement of staining methods have introduced quality control protocols to the forefront for enhancing reproducibility. Institutions usually adhere to guidelines by setting technical parameters, such as concentrations of reagents and incubation times. Recent advances in laboratory techniques underscore the importance of precise procedural adherence, as exemplified by algorithmic approaches, such as the two-stage test model used for HER2 testing that selects immunocytochemistry as the primary method, followed by fluorescence in situ hybridization for indeterminate results (Bartlett et al., 2004). This is not merely refining the testing procedure but also consonant with the overall mission of histological processes: to produce credible, interpretable data that directs clinical decisions. Moreover, the integration of advanced staining procedures has revolutionized histology practice such that elusive pathologies can be detected. Techniques such as multiplex immunofluorescence and *in situ* hybridization provide high spatial resolution by enabling visualization of multiple markers on a single tissue section. Such methods can potentially not only outline the presence or absence of specific antigens but also their relative locations with respect to the tissue architecture. As more researchers and clinicians make use of these state-of-the-art protocols, the need to continue educating and mastering laboratory procedures rises to a top priority (Bari et al., 2011). Following strict protocols and continuously adapting to new methods, laboratories can ensure not only that they are providing top-notch diagnostic services but also in making contributions to the future of histopathology (Figure 2.10).

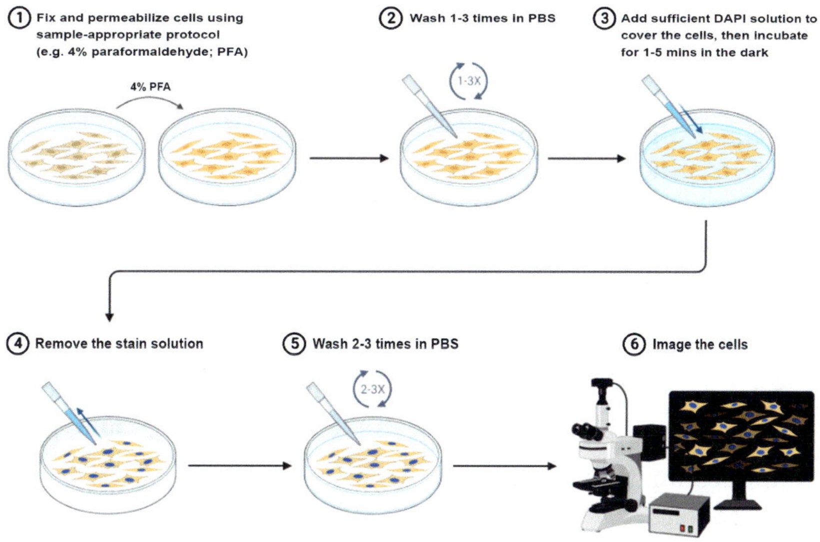

Figure 2.10. Common staining protocols.

Source: https://cdn.prod.website-files.com/621e95f9ac30687a56e4297e/64adcabdf5f044a8256e7f00_V2_1683511903512_a62bd581-5074-4cb0-bc2c-2ede5dfe3929_HIGH_RES.png.

2.2.3. Special Stains for Specific Tissues

Special staining in histology enhances the detectability of specific tissue components, which will be very difficult to identify using standard staining methods like hematoxylin and eosin (H&E). The specialized stains target specific cellular components or pathologic features and thereby facilitate additional discriminating assessment of tissue morphology. For instance, techniques like the Masson's trichrome stain are employed to isolate connective tissue components, especially collagen fibers, from muscle and epithelial tissues. Under pathological conditions, isolation is especially of interest, where the processes of disease are manifested in aberrant connective tissue. The development and application of such stains reflect an enhanced knowledge of tissue processes and disease pathology, and demonstrate the value of histological techniques to diagnosis, pathology, and inquiry. In addition to this, special stains are also pivotal in the assessment of microbial infections, particularly in the identification of specific pathogens in tissue samples. The Gram stain or Giemsa stain is an example of methods which allow the pathologist to differentiate bacteria and other microbes on the basis of their inherent cell characteristics. Such specificity is core in infection diagnosis and planning of therapeutic interventions accordingly. Furthermore, specialized staining can reveal abnormal cellular activity, e.g., the conversion of fibroblasts to myofibroblasts, which may indicate chronic inflammatory responses. As a specialty of general histological procedures, the utilization of special staining techniques serves to enhance the accuracy of diagnosis and therapeutic practice, attesting to the central position held by histology in modern medicine. Special stains are used in aquatic pathology for the histology of marine organisms, such as bivalve mollusks and crustaceans, which require specialized techniques.

It is evident from recent guidelines like the Histological Techniques for Marine Bivalve Mollusks book, which centers on techniques compatible with the special histological characteristics of marine invertebrates. Such adaptations ensure that histopathological preparations accommodate the distinctive anatomical features of such animals without compromising standards established in the study of vertebrate tissues. Such resources not only facilitate appropriate diagnosis but also encourage research into marine animal pathology, as observed by the necessity of specialized stains in facilitating histological applications to extend to broader areas, such as environmental health assessment and marine biology (Howard et al., 2004) (Figure 2.11).

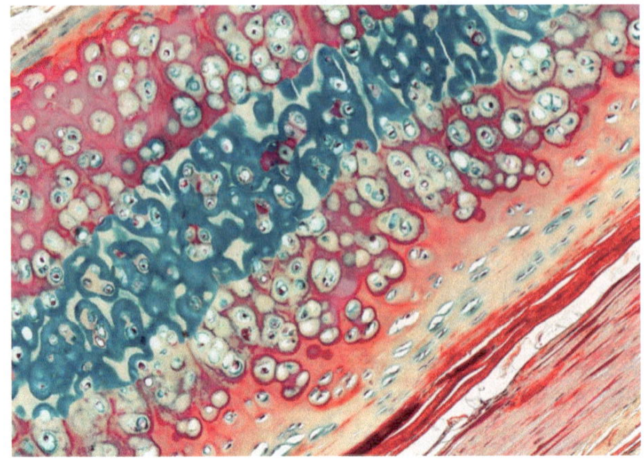

Figure 2.11. Special stains for specific tissues.

Source: https://www.leicabiosystems.com/sites/default/files/styles/720_tablet_portrait_fallback/public/media_image-file/2021-01/figure-10-special-stains.jpg?itok=4eWhp961.

2.3. Microscopy in Histology

The intimate relationship between histology and microscopy is the foundation of modern medical diagnostics and research. Microscopy is a key tool that allows pathologists and researchers to examine and research the microscopic tissue architecture. Traditional bright-field microscopy, which entails a lot of preparation of thin sections of tissue, has played a fundamental role in providing useful information regarding cellular morphology and pathology. But this kind of technique is time-consuming, and therefore, the timeliness of diagnostic information is compromised. It must be pointed out that the inclusion of advanced microscopy techniques can enhance the efficacy of histological investigations and thereby maximize the process of disease diagnosis, such as cancer and other pathological abnormalities, based on accurate analysis of tissues. Novel techniques such as microscopy with ultraviolet surface excitation (MUSE) are the epitome of the refinement of histological techniques designed to enhance efficiency and effectiveness. Unlike conventional processing-intensive microscopy, MUSE is capable of giving prompt, high-quality images from tissue samples without requiring rigorous processing. This new method employs ultraviolet light to excite the fluorescent stains only at the tissue surfaces, thus conserving preparation time and preserving future molecular assays. Such advances not only enhance the efficiency of the diagnostic process but also provide vital information earlier, thereby improving patient care across all aspects, particularly in low-resource settings (Alaminos et al., 2013). In addition to the technical developments, pedagogic approaches in histology have also involved effective didactic manuals to assist in an enhanced understanding of microscopic anatomy and pathology.

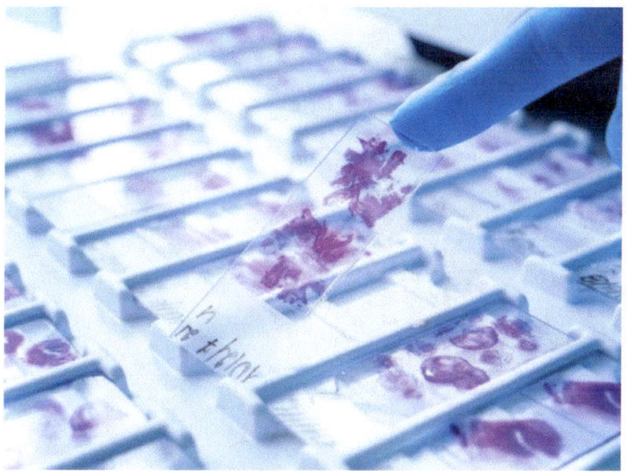

Figure 2.12. Microscopy in histology.

Source: https://d36nqgmw98q4v5.cloudfront.net/images/Article_Images/ImageForArticle_2183_16480257271579919.jpg.

These manuals provide an interactive learning environment where students engage with visual material, such as images and drawings, thus being able to better visualize complex histological structures. Studies indicate that visual strategies, including self-test questions and areas for students to take their own notes, significantly enhance student learning (Alaminos et al., 2013). Such learning programs emphasize autonomy and creativity, ultimately fostering a deeper understanding of histological principles. With a combination of innovative pedagogy techniques and modern microscopy methods, the field of histology is poised to progress in both academic success and clinical application (Figure 2.12).

2.3.1. Light Microscopy Fundamentals

Light microscopy is a starting technique in histology and can be applied to visualize cellular structures with high accuracy. Visible light passed through or reflected from the samples is utilized by this technique for enhancing knowledge regarding tissue structure and cell content. The light source, condenser, objective lenses, and eyepiece are the essential components of a light microscope that work in conjunction to magnify and resolve the small sample details. Its magnifying power is typically in the range of 40x to 1000x, allowing researchers to observe not only the gross morphology but also subcellular detail and organelles. In histological use, precise sample preparation, such as fixation and sectioning, is essential for tissue integrity and prevention of distortion upon viewing. Such a capability to truly represent biological tissues makes light microscopy pertinent to both research and clinical diagnostics. Advances in light microscopy techniques have also enhanced its utility in histological analysis. A good example is introducing a series of contrasting techniques to otherwise uncolored samples. Such common stains are hematoxylin and eosin (H&E), often utilized to separate various cellular components, thereby enhancing diagnostic accuracy in pathology. Moreover, methods like immunohistochemistry permit the imaging of single antigens within tissues, unveiling profound information about disease mechanisms and cell-to-cell communications. Coupled with digital imaging technology, these techniques enable quantitative analysis and the storage and distribution of microscopic images for educational and research purposes. While light microscopy continues to evolve, it remains a requirement to develop an understanding of the biology of biological tissues in basic research and in the clinic. Alongside conventional methodologies, newly developed technologies are defining the new era of light microscopy for histological methods. New technologies like optical coherence tomography (OCT) and photoacoustic tomography (PAT) are breaking imaging capabilities beyond conventional light microscopy restrictions. OCT, for example, uses distinct modes of few-mode fibers to generate high-resolution volume images of biological tissue, differentiating between different tissue types with greater contrast (Augustin et al., 2018). Alternatively, PAT provides multiscale imaging with increased depth of penetration but with high enough spatial resolution to greatly increase anatomical, functional, and molecular imaging capacities (Wang, L. V. & Yao, J., 2011). Such advances reflect the dynamic evolving capacity of light microscopy and its relevance in the ongoing discovery of biological systems, validating its role in research as well as in clinical diagnostics (Figure 2.13).

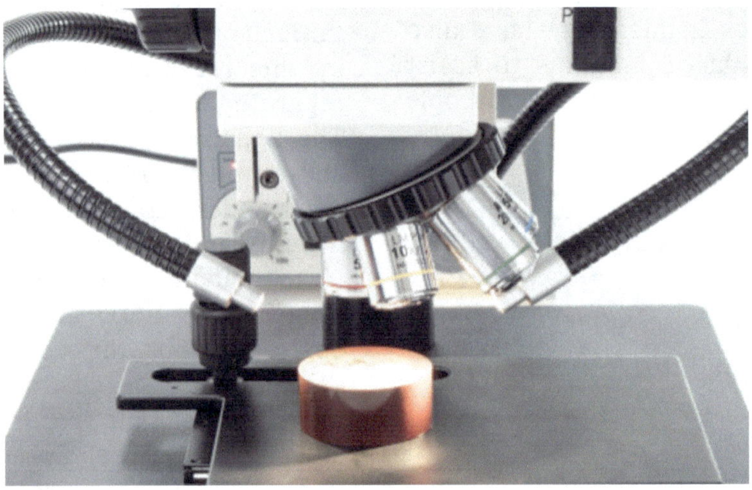

Figure 2.13. Light microscopy fundamentals.

Source: https://3.bp.blogspot.com/-_LtWamqoH60/W7cMMa3xfGI/AAAAAAAABkE/TCSGIN1Oao43hZ8nc995Ef6XUqoQ-IpHgCLcBGAs/s1600/201809_basics_light_microscopy_MET_2_11.jpg.

2.3.2. Electron Microscopy Applications

Electron microscopy in histological techniques significantly enhances the visualization of cellular fine structures at a resolution not previously possible. Electron microscopy cannot be replaced in most fields, from neurobiology to materials science, since it enables researchers to observe organelles and macromolecular assemblies at the nanometer scale. In histology, electron microscopy's high-resolution imaging capabilities are similarly invaluable for detecting pathological changes in tissues. For example, while examining neuronal tissues, electron microscopy can contribute valuable information about the structure and organization of dendrites and synapses. Such vital observations can enhance our knowledge in areas like neurodegenerative diseases, where alterations in axonal structures indicate functional deficits. The capacity of electron microscopy to provide precise morphological data thus constitutes an advancement in histological techniques, providing additional information on the microanatomy that is pivotal for research and clinical diagnosis. Moreover, electron microscopes' versatility of use is also evident in the examination of biological samples, particularly through the use of advanced imaging techniques such as micrographic video capture and editing (VCE). This new technique enables effective morphology recording with the capacity for virtual voucher specimen creation, which can be utilized in training and taxonomic collections. In nematological research, for instance, VCE systems enable specimens to be recorded without the constraints of traditional permanent slides. Not only does this facilitate accessibility, but it also ensures that morphological data is obtained in digital formats for future applications. The adoption of VCE represents a shift toward a unified digital approach in histology, reflecting the demand for methods capable of supporting both sophisticated morphological analysis and the ease of data sharing among study groups (Bert, W., & De Ley, P., 2002). Electron microscopy also contributes to sophisticated neuroimaging techniques, particularly with the calculation of the g-ratio—a significant element in the understanding of conduction velocity in neurons. By measuring the relative thickness of the myelin sheath covering axons, researchers can gain knowledge about neural tract functional integrity. Technical advancements in MRI enable in vivo g-ratio mapping, which integrates histological data with broader clinical correlations. These methods highlight the importance of precise calibration and methodological refinement to ensure consistency in linking MRI-derived markers and biological realities. These capabilities not only drive neurobiological research but also strengthen the relationship between histological techniques and imaging tools. Thus, the integration of electron microscopy with emerging technologies holds significant potential to elucidate the nature of the nervous system and its responses to various diseases (Callaghan, M. F. & Mohammadi, S., 2020).

2.3.3. Fluorescence Microscopy Techniques

Fluorescence microscopy techniques have transformed the history of histology by enabling the accurate visualization of cellular elements and processes at the molecular level. The technique employs selective fluorescent probes, which bind onto target molecules within biological specimens, and emit light with various wavelengths when excited by a light *Source.* Such selectivity is critical in histological analysis, where distinguishing normal tissue from pathological tissue becomes necessary. For example, fluorescence microscopy can account for the precision of cellular morphology and spatial distribution in diagnosing cancer, as shown by the use of combined multimodal nonlinear optical microscopies to distinguish between normal and cancerous tissues in patients with colon cancer. Besides enhancing diagnostic accuracy, this approach also provides a basis for the application of the same method to several disorders with abnormal cellular behavior (Adur et al., 2014). No less important among the fluorescent microscopy techniques is the ability to monitor dynamic biological processes in real time. Two-photon microscopy allows this by providing high-level imaging techniques that enable deeper penetration into the tissue without causing photodamage to the samples. Scientists are able to map and detect neuronal activity with high accuracy using the technique, as demonstrated in studies of the optic tectum of adult zebrafish. The dextran-conjugated calcium dyes used here illustrate the potential for single-cell activity to be followed without compromising the integrity of adjacent tissue. Such developments not only enhance our understanding of neuronal networks but also reflect the range of fluorescence microscopic techniques available to study complex biological systems (Engelmann et al., 2013). Furthermore, the ongoing development of fluorescence microscopy techniques is increasingly extending the boundaries of histological analysis. Methods such as super-resolution microscopy offer previously unattainable resolution beyond the diffraction limit, enabling scientists to observe nanoscale structures that may lie below the threshold of traditional approaches. These methods enable more quantitative studies of protein localization, interactions, and dynamics within cell environments. The increasing accessibility of genetically encoded fluorescent proteins also unveils the toolkit for scientists to examine living cells with previously inaccessible specificity in fixed samples. Thus, the application of such fluorescence techniques in histological processes not only enhances our ability to diagnose disease but also enables us to have better knowledge about biological processes at a fundamental level, revolutionizing existing histological technologies in research and clinical settings (Engelmann et al., 2013; Adur et al., 2014) (Figure 2.14).

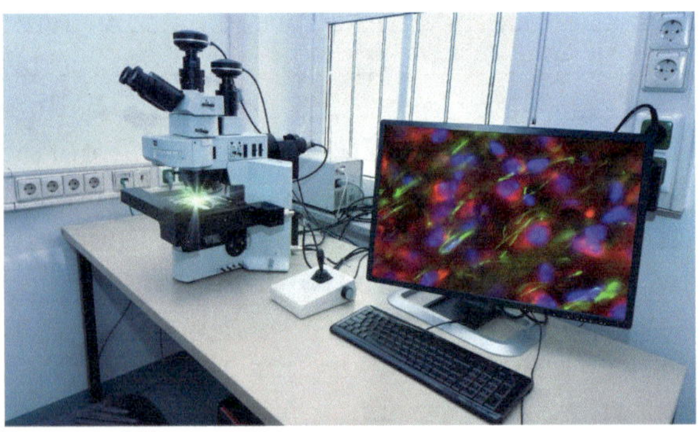

Figure 2.14. Fluorescence microscopy techniques.

Source: https://bitesizebio.com/wp-content/uploads/2017/04/Fluorescence-microscopy.jpg.

2.4. Histological Analysis

Histological analysis is a cornerstone in tissue architecture and cellular pathology examination, supplying information that is critical for disease diagnosis, especially cancers. Scientists can visualize the intricate structures in tissues to identify normal and disease conditions using various histological techniques. The method enables the assessment of morphological changes in tissues indicative of disease development. For example, sophisticated imaging techniques have demonstrated the efficacy of multimodal nonlinear optical microscopies for the investigation of microstructure in cancerous tissues, such as colon cancer. Such technologies reveal characteristic patterns that differentiate between normal and diseased tissues and enhance the diagnosticity of histological examination (Adur et al., 2014). Examples of such technologies include:. By the incorporation of these techniques in routine practice, pathologists can obtain greater insight into tissue-level changes in relation to malignancies and thereby ease the process of diagnosis and improve patient prognosis. In addition, the flexibility of histologic examination permits response assessment to extrinsic toxins and pathogens, aside from cancer diagnosis. A pertinent example can be seen in the study of the mycotoxin deoxynivalenol (DON) in pig intestinal tissues, an animal model for human health significance. Histologic examination of jejunal explants showed dose-dependent histological alterations indicative of exposure to the toxin, including villi architectural and cell integrity alterations. Histological techniques facilitated the identification of no-effect concentration levels of DON, ultimately contributing more insight into the impact of food contaminants on gastrointestinal histology (Bourges-Abella et al., 2009). This, besides making a contribution to the added knowledge of food safety, brings with it access to proper mitigation strategies of public health concern due to dietary toxins. Overall, histological analysis is an essential tool in the assessment of normal physiological function and the identification of pathological changes in tissues. Ongoing innovation in advanced histological techniques, such as multimodal imaging and *in vitro* culture systems, continues to advance the specificity and utility of this analytical technique. By reminding researchers and clinicians of the complex cell-microenvironment interactions, histological examination delivers to them critical information necessary for therapeutic and diagnostic efficiency. As well demonstrated in cancer diagnosis as well as the examination of food contaminants, the underlying principles that support histological methods are continually emerging, providing a testament to their continuing applicability in research and clinical contexts. This perpetual interplay between technological advancements and histological research holds promise for future breakthroughs in tissue-based diagnostics and therapies.

2.4.1. Qualitative vs. Quantitative Analysis

In histological procedures, the qualitative and quantitative analysis distinction will determine the nature and scale of research findings. Qualitative analysis deals with the characteristics and types of specimens, attempting to determine the pattern and context of cell designs and compositions. The procedure often involves complex observational studies, such as detailing the morphology of cells or tissue structure. For instance, examination of tissue samples using a microscope allows researchers to search for anomalies or special features that can indicate disease. Such qualitative results can be helpful to place within context the formulation of hypotheses and guide the ensuing quantitative research since they offer initial information that guides experimental design. On the other hand, quantitative analysis tries to provide numerical values that are quantitatively examinable, introducing a more objective platform to histological studies. In this case, measurements such as cell numbers, tissue area, and percentage of fat in liver tissues can be obtained using various imaging techniques, including magnetic resonance imaging (MRI). In accordance with (Kavanaugh, 2017), the quantification of liver fat percentages using MRI not only supports diagnosis but also assists in hepatic steatosis research, enabling greater understanding of the disease's prevalence and treatment. Quantitative analysis enables researchers to produce reproducible data that can validate or disprove hypotheses, eventually leading to evidence-based conclusions about cell and tissue conduct under varying conditions. Qualitative and quantitative analyses must be coordinated to achieve an integrated view of histological events. Qualitative analysis can influence the design of specific quantitative measures, and both analyses in a feedback cycle can enhance one another. In the context of advanced imaging techniques, as described in Matcher et al. (2009), qualitative assessments of articular cartilage structure can influence advances in treatment protocols for diseases like osteoarthritis. By integrating qualitative and quantitative methodologies, investigators can enrich their studies so that results are both descriptive and measurable. Through such a detailed method, better insight into biological phenomena is gained, subsequently increasing the application of histological techniques in clinical research and targeted therapies.

2.4.2. Image Analysis Software

In the recent past, the development of image analysis software has gone a long way in supplementing the capabilities of histological techniques to aid researchers in investigating tissue morphology and pathology with more sophistication. The sophisticated algorithms implemented in such software enable quantitative analysis of complex image data, thereby facilitating the inspection of cellular structure and the assessment of disease conditions. The new application of multimodal nonlinear optical (NLO) microscopies, as seen in recent studies, recognizes such a potential well. These techniques not only detect morphological changes in tissues but also permit exploration of disease-specific patterns for diseases like colon cancer and thus emphasize the role of efficient image analysis software in histopathology (Adur et al., 2014). Thus, the inclusion of image analysis software in routine practices can enhance diagnostic accuracy along with our understanding of disease evolution. In addition, image analysis software compatibility with various data sets remains prominent on the horizon of histopathological imaging methodology development. Normalizing such procedures is what is needed to make the integration of pathological image data with clinical and demographic information a reality. The Quantitative Histopathological Imaging Ontology (QHIO) here proposed addresses this challenge by providing a structured approach to the representation of imaging data as well as analysis procedures. Such integration promotes organized, multi-disciplinary partnerships among the pathology community to facilitate sharing of data and evidence enhancement reliability, particularly in advanced cases such as breast cancer hot-spot identification (Doyle et al., 2017).

Thus, the creation of image analysis software is an important milestone in histological practice, enabling pathologists to use reliable datasets to improve clinical outcomes. The impact of image analysis software extends beyond the lab, as it has the potential to affect clinical decision-making and patient care. By applying sophisticated imaging techniques coupled with analysis software, pathologists can detect subtle changes in tissues that might otherwise remain undetectable. This increased precision is particularly valuable in the diagnosis of cancer, where early detection and accurate staging can have a significant impact on treatment and patient outcome. The constant advancement of image analysis methods, as exemplified by the application of NLO methods to the identification of microstructural features in neoplastic tissue, illustrates the revolutionary nature of such advances in histological practice (Adur et al., 2014). Lastly, application of image analysis software not only enhances diagnostic histopathology quality but also has the potential to enhance personalized medicine strategies, tailoring interventions to patient profiles.

2.4.3. Interpretation of Histological Data

Interpretation of histological data is the focus of diagnosis in clinical pathology. Histology refers to the microscopic examination of biological tissue, allowing the identification of cellular structures and changes that may signal disease. Histopathologic assessment requires a step-by-step process, where the morphologic result is compared against patient history and clinical data. This convergence is not only basic to diagnosis but also to prognostication and therapeutic decisions. Furthermore, the convergence of histological observations with molecular and genetic data has become increasingly crucial, particularly in oncology, where precision medicine is largely based on understanding tumor biology. Interpretation of histological results is thus a pivotal element in generating clinically relevant findings, guiding therapeutic interventions, and improving patient outcomes. One of the particular uses of histological interpretation is seen in the treatment of male infertility, specifically in the case of testicular sperm extraction.

Studies show that factors like testicular histopathology play an important role in determining the prospects of sperm retrieval success. In one of the retrospective studies on patients subjected to this intervention, several histological categories from normal spermatogenesis to maturation arrest offered invaluable information that could be used to foretell the success of sperm retrieval. This correlation highlights the value of proper interpretation of histological features, as younger age, diminished FSH levels, and good testicular histology are associated with successful outcomes in sperm retrieval operations (Basciani et al., 2018). By proper utilization of histological data, clinicians can enhance the counseling provided to infertile men and ultimately contribute to male reproductive health care. Secondly, histological techniques have to be strictly standardized to ensure the validity and reproducibility of results.

For instance, HER2 status in breast cancer determines the greatest importance of adhering to standard testing protocols (Bartlett et al., 2004). A modified two-stage testing algorithm, emphasizing both immunocytochemistry and fluorescence *in situ* hybridization, mirrors the way a systematic method identifies the correctness of histologic interpretation. This standardization maximizes histopathological evaluation precision and also assists laboratories in maintaining expertise in terms of regular case load. In this way, enhancing histological interpretive expertise and adherence to methodological standards are central to providing accurate diagnoses and optimizing therapeutic plans across various clinical settings.

2.5. Common Histological Artifacts

Histological techniques are a staple of biological research, enabling examination of the structure and function of tissues. However, the risk of some artifacts forming during the processing and analysis of the sample should be known. Some artifacts, such as the formation of air bubbles, shrinkage of the tissue, and staining variability, can have severe impacts on the interpretation of histological findings. They can destroy visual coherence and spatial interrelations in tissue samples, lead to incorrect conclusions, and disrupt reproducibility in research outcomes. For instance, uneven staining can mask cellular detail and distort underlying histopathology. To give a proper result, histologists must detect and counteract these artifacts in the preparation stage and in the examination stage. Fixation is one of the primary reasons for histological artifacts. Weak fixation can result in artifacts such as vacuolization or distortion of cellular morphology. Fixatives that are too weak or too harsh can disrupt optimal preservation of tissue morphology and thereby yield false data. Furthermore, the embedding medium and sectioning process can also generate artifacts. Poor orientation of sections or incorrect cutting can generate uneven thickness and thereby regions with dissimilar stain uptake and visibility. According to these challenges, the application of standard histological procedures is absolutely necessary. Standardization of fixation and embedding techniques not only minimizes artifacts but also enhances the quality and validity of the histological study as a whole. Advances in histological techniques still provide ways of minimizing the occurrence of artifacts. As an example, modern imaging software has been a great tool for histological image processing, and researchers are able to eliminate some artifacts upon collection. Recent research has confirmed that utilization of high-precision layer-by-layer grinding techniques can improve section quality; this subsequently allows for reconstruction of high-resolution three-dimensional tissue structure (Brazina et al., 2017). Besides, sophisticated stereotaxic equipment has also been effective in achieving greater anatomical accuracy of positioning in anatomical studies, enabling more precise matching of data against brain atlas coordinates (Andres et al., 1986). Taking advantage of these technological improvements, along with adopting the best practices of histological technique, researchers are able to minimize the impact of artifacts and achieve more reliable histological interpretation (Figure 2.15).

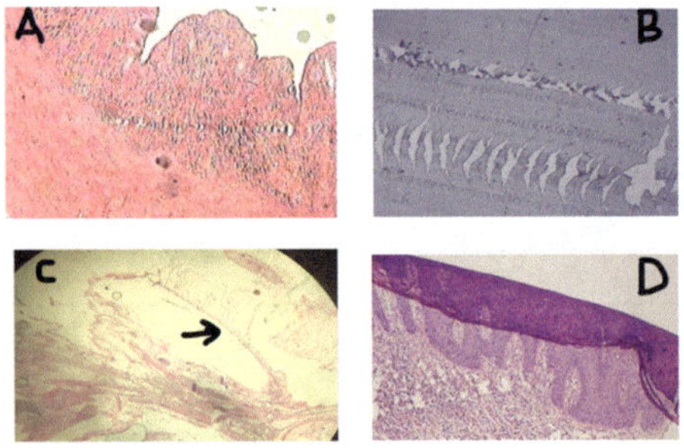

Figure 2.15. Common histological artifacts.

Source: https://html.scirp.org/file/2-7302052x5.png?20240318114847956.

2.5.1. Types of Artifacts and Their Causes

The examination of artifacts in histology provides vital information regarding the nature of changes that are brought about in biological tissues and why such modifications are effected. Artifacts may be produced by a number of factors, ranging from preparation procedures to the intrinsic nature of the biological materials under investigation. For example, specific staining techniques used in histology will cause certain artifacts, such as changing the color of tissues or warping the structures of cells. These adjustments emphasize the necessity to classify the potential impacts of each technique used throughout tissue processing. Since histological procedures enable researchers to monitor complex cellular associations, there is a need to raise awareness of how these procedures may introduce variability, ultimately affecting the interpretation of results and the conclusions of such research. Apparently, the procedures used in histological preparation can be responsible for huge artifacts. The embedding process, for example, often includes fixation and dehydration, which may result in shrinkage or swelling of tissues, leading to a discrepancy in the morphology observed. Moreover, some materials used for embedding may yield different results, influencing the analysis afterwards. When μCT is used as a tool for assessing bone integration against implants, comparison with traditional histomorphometry must be done in an effort to establish any difference occurring as a result of preparation artifacts. In a comparative study, researchers found μCT to be in good agreement with histology; however, quantification of bone area (BA) and bone-implant contact (BIC) at different time points was problematic, underscoring the need for strict methodological consistency (Coelho et al., 2013). Yet another facet of artifact analysis comes in the form of culinary residue studies, where taphonomic investigation reveals the processes employed to cook in ancient civilizations. Here, artifacts may be the result of the alteration of plant cell structures from processes such as boiling and cooking. Controlled laboratory tests on tubers indicated that cooking could lead to identifiable morphological and optical alterations at the microscopic level that researchers can subsequently analyze to make inferences about past human behavior and practices. On this basis, this study supports the use of integrating a broad range of techniques, including histological analysis, to infer the broader contexts of artifacts and their causes. By combining such approaches, researchers can discern underlying trends in artifact production in terms of cultural practice (Babot et al., 2014) (Figure 2.16).

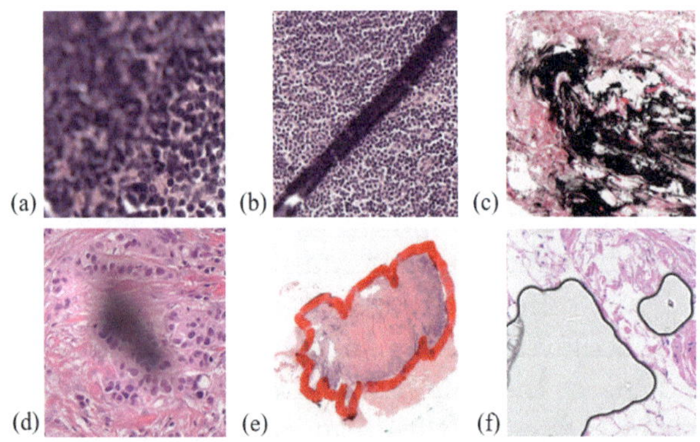

Figure 2.16. Types of artifacts and their causes.

Source: https://assets.diagnijmegen.nl/images/projects/pathology_artifact_detection_artifacts.png.

2.5.2. Impact of Artifacts on Analysis

The presence of artifacts in histological analysis provides significant information that interferes with the exact determination and reliability of diagnosis findings. Artifacts can occur at any stage of the preparation of tissues, including fixation, processing, and staining. These non-controllable changes can conceal the actual morphology of tissues, preventing pathologists from obtaining accurate results. For instance, in pulmonary edema, the artifacts from too much fluid infused can mimic or obscure actual pathological conditions, rendering diagnosis difficult. These errors illustrate the importance of careful technique in sample preparation to minimize artifact creation. Resolving these issues is essential, as artifacts not only deny clinicians an informed decision but may also lead to misdiagnosis, ultimately impacting patient management and treatment regimens. Of no lesser importance is the role that robust methodologies play in minimizing the risk of artifacts' effects on histological evaluation. Implementation of standardized protocols for tissue procurement, fixation, and embedding is crucial to ensuring uniformity among specimens. Pathologists should be trained to recognize common artifacts and distinguish them from true histopathologic changes. For instance, the discrimination of hydrostatic and high-permeability etiologies of pulmonary edema relies on accurate histological interpretation, which serves to underscore the importance of determining how artifacts can obscure important clues to underlying pathogenic mechanisms. Moreover, ongoing innovation in analytical and imaging techniques may enhance histological examination specificity and sensitivity, enabling clinicians to identify artifacts more accurately and confirm that histological findings align with clinical presentations (Assaad et al., 2018). The definition of artifacts extends beyond the level of preparation in histological workup and reaches into the field of clinical application. Other health professionals and dentists are often exposed to intraoral diseases where histological analysis is a component of diagnosis and treatment (Alonso et al., 2010). Familiarity with how artifacts affect histological analysis allows practitioners to look at biopsy and subsequent tissue review more skeptically. By being exposed to more balanced potentiating pitfalls, clinicians are able to make better use of more complete research practices, ultimately better serving the patient with accurate diagnoses. Furthermore, this information enables practitioners to address the medico-legal implications arising from such misinterpretations due to artifactual effects, thereby emphasizing the importance of precise histological techniques in clinical practice.

2.5.3. Strategies to Minimize Artifacts

Reducing artifacts is of paramount importance in histological methods, since artifacts can cause misinterpretation of tissue samples and inconclusive experimental results. Standardizing sample preparation protocols between experiments is an effective method of reducing artifacts. Having consistency in methods of fixation, embedding, and sectioning drastically cuts inter-sample variability that is likely to introduce artifacts. For instance, accuracy in the choice of a fixative is necessary because certain fixatives might act differently towards specific tissue types or biomaterials and cause structural distortions. Moreover, adherence to established protocols can enhance reproducibility such that investigations can be compared correctly. By enforcing rigorous procedural standards, researchers can create a more uniform histological context that minimizes the impact of extraneous variables on the outcome, ultimately increasing the quality of histological analyses and conclusions. Beyond standardization, improving the imaging techniques employed for histological analysis can play an important role in minimizing artifacts. Advanced imaging modalities, such as confocal microscopy and high-resolution electron microscopy, provide superior visualization, enabling scientists to resolve fine cellular architecture and interactions. For example, as discussed in the assessment of bioengineered lung tissue, histological examination must be adapted to accommodate variations in biomaterial chemical composition.

Ensuring imaging parameters are accurately calibrated to the exact requirements of each tissue type diminishes the risk of artifacts caused by overexposure, underexposure, or erroneous staining techniques. Calibration is essential, especially in establishing mixed cellular environments and extracellular matrices, as inaccuracy in imaging may obscure significant biological information, hence warping findings and inferences derived from the histological analysis. Additionally, further steps to eliminate artifacts consist of rigorous pre-analytical control and the incorporation of careful data processing methods. As indicated in the preclinical diffusion MRI (dMRI) example, protocols should recognize the multifaceted character of sample handling—spanning animal preparation and observation to data acquisition and processing (Acqua et al., 2023).

It should be observed that following these processes is important because errors at any of these stages might result in artifacts that destroy data integrity. Also, utilizing cutting-edge packages of imaging software can further enhance artifact detection and overall data fidelity. By developing new tests specific to biological and bioengineered tissues, scientists can enhance understanding of samples' structural and functional properties. Hence, adopting comprehensive strategies that include preparation, imaging, and analysis is crucial in order to minimize artifacts in histology, enhance robustness and reliability of outcomes in biomedical studies (Silva A., 2023).

2.6. Advances in Histological Techniques

The science of histology has undergone widespread evolution fueled by the integration of state-of-the-art technology that enhances diagnostic capacity. One of the most promising developments is the integration of Raman spectroscopy and Optical Coherence Tomography (OCT), which together provide complementary high-resolution chemical and morphological information about tissues. Traditionally, these techniques, used individually, were limited in achieving clinically useful sensitivity and specificity. However, newer research indicates that if one uses texture analysis to qualify OCT images and merges this data with Raman spectroscopy, scientists can enhance discrimination between normal and cancerous tissue, particularly in the case of Colonic Adenocarcinoma. This multimodal approach has resulted in improved diagnostic sensitivity, as indicated by 94% sensitivity when the two methods are combined, emphasizing the potential future of these new histological techniques in revolutionizing cancer diagnosis (Ashok et al., 2014). Furthermore, bioelectrical potential and metabolic profiling of tumor markers have provided a cutting-edge method for histopathological evaluation. Current studies highlight significant differences in biopotential measurements of cancerous and non-cancerous omental tissues, and the alterations are synonymous with tumor stage and progression-free survival. The ability to measure biopotential levels as well as metabolic markers provides a new paradigm for creating predictive algorithms to foretell surgical outcomes in patients with advanced epithelial ovarian cancer. This approach not only captures the biological processes occurring in tissues but also presents a platform where devices that can monitor the progression of disease in real-time can be developed. Ultimately, such advancements in histological procedures open doors to more tailored and efficacious treatment strategies (Boutelle et al., 2018). Apart from these advancements, ongoing enhancements in histological procedures identify the necessity of incorporating conventional practices with current technological developments. Fine-tuning methods of tissue processing and preparation, including automated slide preparation and enhanced staining protocols, has made it possible to achieve faster and more accurate diagnosis of diseases. Not only do these developments enhance the overall quality of histopathological reports, but they also reduce the time taken for diagnosis, which is essential in clinical practice where early intervention can make a huge difference to the patient's outcome. With advancing science, collaboration among pathologists, oncologists, and biomedical engineers will play a pivotal role in leveraging these advances to develop comprehensive and efficient diagnostic protocols that benefit patients and improve treatment outcomes (Figure 2.17).

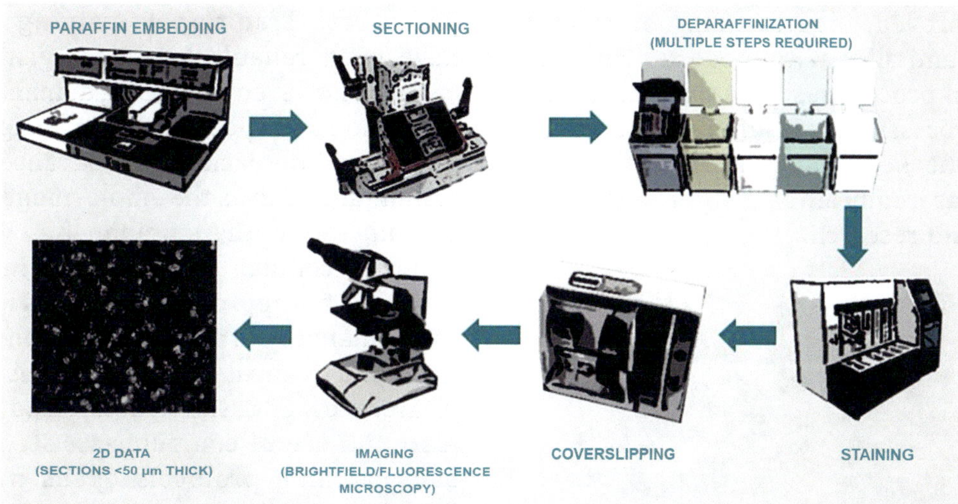

Figure 2.17. Advances in histological techniques.

Source: https://www.semanticscholar.org/paper/ Evaluation-Of-A- Field-Histology- Technique- And-Its- Branson/ ad46529a19204341 ea99c01862ad83cdfd534e23/figure/0.

2.6.1. Innovations in Tissue Processing

Technological innovations in tissue processing, accordingly, have significantly enhanced histology by improving the preservation, visualization, and analysis of biological specimens. Techniques like rapid freezing, vacuum infiltration, and microwave-assisted processing, for instance, have replaced traditional procedures, which were sometimes time- and resource-wasteful. Rapid freezing, for instance, preserves cellular architecture by inhibiting the formation of ice crystals, which can deform tissue morphology. In addition, microwave-assisted processing reduces the time for fixation and infiltration, making the workflow in histopathological labs easier. With such development into existence, it also inspires researchers to invent more sophisticated imaging techniques, making competitive comparison of cellular structures and functions possible, ensuring that researchers obtain the best results from their research. New imaging modalities' integration is vital in enhancing the outcomes of tissue processing. New methods such as multi-modal two-photon microscopy and optical coherence tomography allow researchers to investigate complex tissue architecture in greater depth than previously possible, bridging the gap between the structural and functional investigations. These methods not only yield information on healthy tissue architecture but can also be employed to investigate pathological changes. For example, in glaucoma, recent advancements have altered the focus from mere assessment of the trabecular meshwork only to a comprehensive exploration of the entire aqueous humor outflow (AHO) pathway. These developments are paramount for the development of treatment interventions, as they facilitate improved understanding of disease mechanisms and align with modern principles of histological procedures (Huang et al., 2016). New tissue processing methods are also bringing to the fore the need for standardization and automation as requirements for replicability and large-scale research.

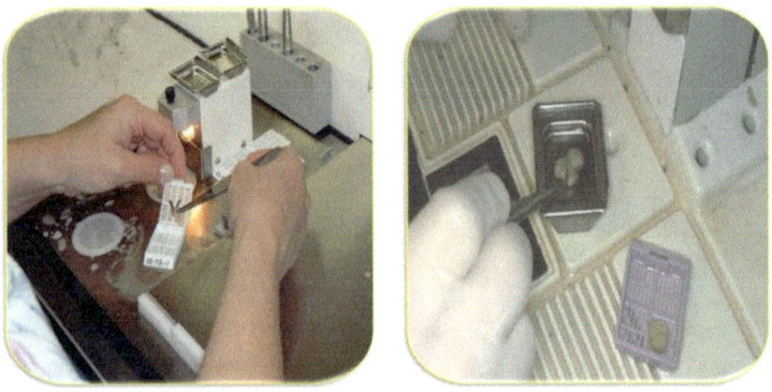

Figure 2.18. Innovations in tissue processing.

Source: https://tissuesampling.weebly.com/uploads/1/4/5/9/14590486/7586800_orig.jpg.

The quest for a centralized, open-access data repository can simplify the sharing of results and resources across disparate fields of research. It is particularly important in neurology, where structured mappings of neural circuits have to be made to unravel the complexities of brain function. Through the adoption of known experimental techniques that are extensible and transferable to current infrastructure, scientists are able to facilitate collaborations and innovations across the disciplines, basic as well as clinical (MacKenzie-Graham et al., 2009). Not only do these integrative approaches enhance the principles of histological methods, but they also help ensure that future research generates reproducible, actionable intelligence regarding health and disease (Figure 2.18).

2.6.2. Development of New Staining Methods

The discovery of new staining methods is leading histological technology progress, offering more capacity for visualizing cellular structure and processes. Traditional staining techniques have been reliable for histologists for half a century; however, increasing demands for higher resolution and specificity in imaging necessitate innovative approaches. New advances in staining techniques, such as the employment of multiplex staining, allow the simultaneous visualization of many cellular elements within one tissue section. This approach minimizes loss of tissue and enhances correlation between histological data and clinical outcomes, thus allowing a clearer view of tissue structure and pathologies. Also, the use of computer-assisted analysis in such staining protocols opens new avenues for precision in quantitative histopathological imaging, illustrating the direction towards more standardized techniques that can handle larger amounts of image data, as discussed during QHIO enhancement to foster data sharing and analysis (Doyle et al., 2017). In regenerative medicine, novel staining methods also become essential in the assessment of the effectiveness of novel therapeutic pathways. The advent of hybrid bioprinting technologies, where both biological and synthetic materials are employed, necessitates tailored staining methods to visualize intricate cellular patterns in bioengineered scaffolds. Protein- or glycosaminoglycan-targeted staining can be valuable to uncover information on engineered tissue function and developmental maturity. For instance, stem cell differentiation into cartilage is demarcated by the production of essential components of the extracellular matrix.

Hence, employing special dyes to track these modifications underscores the necessity to create new techniques synergistic with the goals of current regenerative therapies. These new methods not only aim to improve visualization but also to improve the comprehension of the cellular mechanisms that form the backbone of successful tissue regeneration (Asadian et al., 2020). Moreover, ongoing refinement of staining protocols integrates concepts from numerous distinct disciplines, both enhancing diagnosis and research potential. For instance, the use of fluorescent and luminescent tags within staining methods is an example of where molecular biology has intersected with histopathology, enabling dynamic imaging of cellular behavior in real-time. The developments enable the study of disease evolution at the molecular level, and the pathophysiological mechanisms are unmasked, which would otherwise have remained hidden. In addition, the creation of standardized staining protocols facilitates reproducibility across studies and helps in an enhanced understanding of disease and efficacy of therapeutic interventions. As the field progresses, novel staining methods will continue to evolve histological practices to keep pace with the increasing complexities and requirements of today's biomedical research and clinical practice, and ultimately bridge the gap between scientific rigor and practical health applications (Doyle et al., 2017; Asadian et al., 2020).

2.6.3. Integration of Molecular Techniques

The application of molecular techniques to histological processes is a remarkable advancement in biomedical research and diagnostic methods, pointing out the need for precise and fine-scale analysis of tissues. The meeting between molecular biology and histology has given rise to more effective protocols, which enable researchers to explore the pathological processes of disease at the detailed level. With techniques such as fluorescence *in situ* hybridization (FISH) or polymerase chain reaction (PCR), histologists are provided with useful tools to identify specific genetic markers and analyze gene expression in tissue samples. This synergy not only strengthens the diagnosis but also enables a deeper understanding of the pathological features of various diseases, including cancer, for which accurate identification is essential to achieve effective intervention. In turn, the recent adoption of multimodal imaging techniques has introduced a novel paradigm for tissue analysis, as evidenced by recent studies employing nonlinear optical (NLO) microscopies to differentiate normal from neoplastic tissues. These approaches allow for omnidirectional inspection of morphological changes that accompany disease progression and provide valuable information regarding stroma and epithelial conversions, particularly in conditions like colon cancer. These techniques can precisely quantify tissue microstructure, enabling pathologists to identify distinct patterns specific to malignancy. The simplicity with which it can be performed on fixed tissues enhances the validity of these techniques in clinical settings, pointing toward their application as diagnostic markers for a wide range of diseases characterized by deranged cell growth and collagen deposition (Adur et al., 2014). Finally, the integration of polarized-light methods into histological procedures again shows the multi-disciplinary approach that can be used to maximize tissue characterization. Second-harmonic generation microscopy and polarization-sensitive optical coherence tomography are examples of such methods that enable accurate interrogation of the extracellular matrix, which is necessary for understanding cartilage diseases, such as osteoarthritis, for example. Such advanced imaging modalities permit data on the structural integrity of tissues and tissue response to treatment protocols and thereby control treatment planning in tissue engineering. With advancing research, the application of such molecular approaches is likely to be therapeutic on a large scale, potentially leading to the development of tailored therapies targeting individualized molecular and structural abnormalities in tissues (Matcher, 2009). This is an indication of the necessity of embracing new techniques for better understanding and treating complex medical conditions (Figure 2.19).

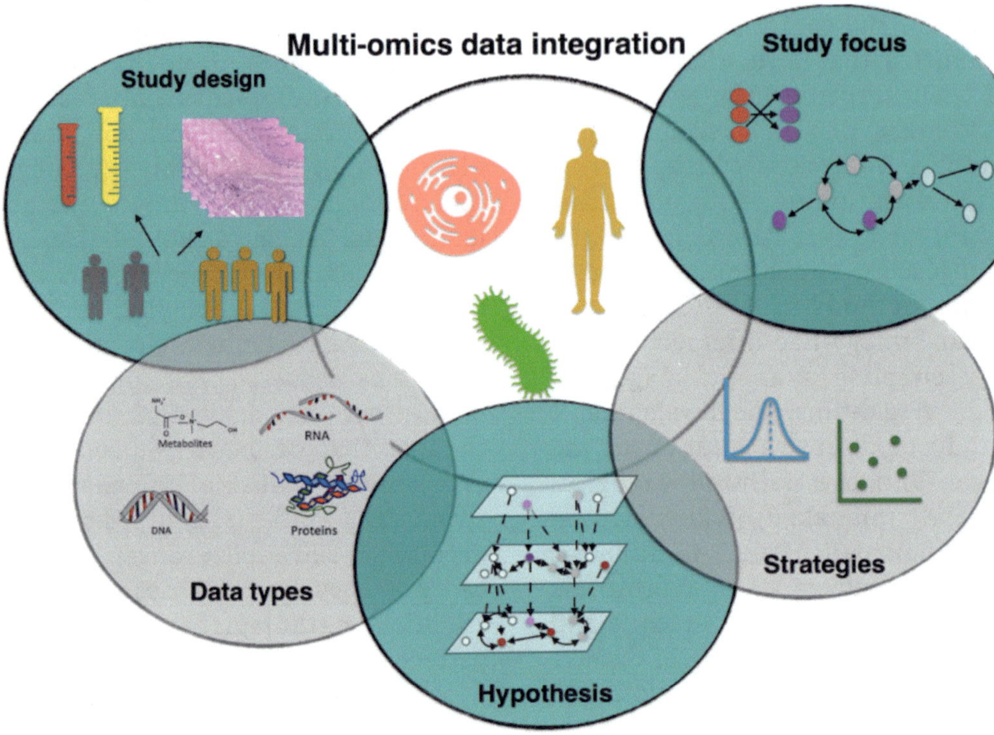

Figure 2.19. Integration of molecular techniques.

Source: https://media.springernature.com/lw685/springer-static/image/art%3A10.1007%2Fs10311-016-0581-3/MediaObjects/10311_2016_581_Fig1_HTML.gif.

SUMMARY

Overall, histological techniques are important to enhancing our understanding of tissue microstructures and their pathophysiological changes. Since histology is the foundation for disease diagnosis, applying systematic strategies in tissue preparation, staining, and examination enables pathologists to identify abnormalities at the cellular level. Methods such as immunohistochemistry and molecular imaging have transformed the discipline, enabling visualization of specific proteins and nucleic acids in tissues with exquisite detail. Not only does this added specificity contribute to diagnosing diseases like cancer, but it also enables investigation into mechanisms of disease, eventually leading to improved patient management techniques. For instance, the ability to observe morphological transformation, as shown in experiments employing nonlinear optical microscopies, accentuates the importance of careful histological observation in distinguishing normal and cancerous tissues, with a strong basis for clinical purposes and therapeutic decisions (Adur et al., 2014). In addition, histological techniques are continuously evolving, eased by the synergy of technology and innovation. Current studies highlight the application of newer models, such as the use and application of pig jejunal explants for the evaluation of the impact of dietary toxins like deoxynivalenol. The model not only gives information regarding morphological impact in intestinal tissue but also enhances our existing knowledge of food safety and its public health implications. By bridging the gap between experimental and applied histology, researchers are able to improve the formulation of safety standards and therapeutic interventions in response to empirically established facts. Histology's involvement in toxicological studies underscores the need for multidisciplinary approaches to address complex diseases while reaffirming the discipline's relevance in contemporary biomedical research (Bourges-Abella et al., 2009). Finally, the future of histological techniques is bound to rely on their ability to adapt and alter methods in response to technological and multidisciplinary scientific developments. When new diagnostic equipment and imaging modalities emerge, incorporating these developments into traditional histological techniques will likely continue to advance the precision of diagnoses and therapy planning. Apart from that, continuous education and training in these evolving techniques are necessary for health practitioners to be of the highest quality in tissue examination. The convergence of pathologists, biologists, and engineers will ensure that histology remains at the vanguard of not only disease diagnosis but also understanding biological mechanisms that control human health. Lastly, the dogma of histological techniques will continue to guide critical studies, clinical practice, and public health programs, enabling deeper insight into disease biology (Bourges-Abella et al., 2009; Adur et al., 2014).

In histological methods, there are a number of critical principles that direct tissue sample preparation and analysis toward gaining deeper insight into cell structures and functions. One of these underlying principles is fixation, where biological tissues are fixed to ensure that their structure is preserved and degradation is avoided. This process is important because it stabilizes proteins and nucleic acids in the tissue, enabling accurate interpretation during microscopic examination. Various fixatives, for example, formaldehyde or ethanol, are consistently applied, each with its own strengths and weaknesses in retaining cell morphology in an undamaged shape. Adhering to these routine fixation protocols is the way in which histologists are able to produce reproducible and reliable results that form a basis for further interpretation of histological morphology. Embedding of fixed tissues is an extremely significant principle, where the sample is impregnated using a hardening substance, usually paraffin or resin. This is a critical step for the production of thin sections for microscopic visualization. Sectioning tissue to microtome thickness (5–10 micrometers) enables high-resolution visualization of cellular morphology and tissue organization. Serving as the basis for subsequent staining techniques, embedding offers enhanced contrast and resolution in microscopic imaging. When coupled with appropriate embedding, sectioning procedures can minimize artifacts and improve the representativeness of the sampled tissue. This principle is supplemented with rigorous training and methodology to generate quality slides, which are crucial in crafting histological studies and understanding complex biological processes. Finally, the application of staining techniques is an imperative principle in histological practice because it signifies cellular elements and structures. Staining methods, such as Hematoxylin and Eosin (H&E) or immunohistochemical markers, are employed to differentiate tissue components, yielding critical information on cellular morphology and pathology. For instance, E-selectin targeted optical imaging has emerged as a promising technique in detecting inflammation in models of rheumatoid arthritis, showing the potential of high-tech staining procedures to elucidate disease mechanisms (Gompels, 2010). With the integration of these staining techniques into sophisticated imaging modalities, such as fluorescence microscopy, histologists can develop a better understanding of tissue dynamics and intercellular communication. These fundamental principles in histological techniques collectively provide a multidimensional approach towards understanding cellular structures and their functional relevance in disease and health.

A LOOK TO THE FUTURE:

UNDER PATHOLOGICAL CONDITIONS:

In biological and medical sciences, the phrase "under pathological conditions" is widely used to describe states in which normal physiological processes are disrupted by disease, injury, or other abnormal influences. Unlike physiological conditions—which refer to the normal functioning of an organism—pathological conditions encompass situations where cellular, tissue, organ, or systemic functions deviate from the healthy baseline due to intrinsic or extrinsic insults. These conditions include infections, chronic inflammatory processes, metabolic imbalances, genetic abnormalities, trauma, neoplasia, and a wide range of disease-associated dysfunctions. The term underscores that observed phenomena, molecular responses, or structural changes are occurring within a disease-altered biological context rather than representing normal biology.

At the cellular and molecular level, pathological conditions frequently trigger compensatory and maladaptive responses. For example, tissue hypoxia—insufficient oxygen delivery to cells—can activate stress-response pathways involving hypoxia-inducible factors, alter gene expression, and upregulate inflammatory mediators, contributing to disease progression rather than normal homeostasis. Similarly, chronic inflammation leads to the persistent presence of cytokines and immune cells that reshape local tissue environments, impairing repair mechanisms and promoting fibrosis or tumorigenesis. These processes illustrate how cellular signalling and gene expression can differ profoundly when organisms are challenged by pathological states compared with their behaviour under healthy physiological conditions. Understanding biological behaviour under pathological conditions is central to pathophysiology, the branch of science that investigates how normal physiological processes are altered in disease. Pathophysiological research seeks to elucidate mechanisms of disease onset, progression, and resolution, including identifying triggers, mapping cellular dysfunctions, and characterising how molecular networks and system-wide interactions are perturbed. This framework not only enhances scientific understanding of disease mechanisms but also informs therapeutic strategies aimed at restoring equilibrium or mitigating damage caused by pathological processes.

In experimental research, distinguishing results obtained under pathological conditions from those derived from healthy models is crucial for interpreting data correctly and translating findings into clinical relevance. For example, gene expression profiles, metabolite concentrations, or cellular stress markers may differ significantly when comparing tissues from diseased subjects to those from healthy controls. Without explicitly acknowledging the pathological context, conclusions about molecular pathways, treatment effects, or disease biomarkers may be misleading or incomplete. "under pathological conditions" refers to the deviation from normal biological function in response to disease-related perturbations, touching on alterations in structure, function, and regulatory networks across biological scales. Recognising this context—whether in bench research, clinical studies, or theoretical frameworks—is essential to accurately describe disease mechanisms, evaluate therapeutic interventions, and advance medical science's understanding of how organisms respond when health is compromised.

REFERENCES

1. Adur, J., Bianchi, M., Pelegati, V. B., Viale, S., Izaguirre, M. F., Carvalho, H. F., Cesar, C. L., & Casco, V. H. (2014). Colon adenocarcinoma diagnosis in human samples by multicontrast nonlinear optical microscopy of hematoxylin and eosin stained histological sections. *Journal of Cancer Therapy*, *05*(13), 1259–1269. https://doi.org/10.4236/jct.2014.513127Alaminos, M., Campos, A., Carriel Araya, V. S., Garzón, et al. (2013). Developing a practical guide for teaching histology: An evaluation of the didactic components. *https://core.ac.uk/download/55734395.pdf* (accessed on 6th August 2025).

2. Andres, B., Bock, B., Bures, F., De Valois, R., Schuller, G., Horsley, M., Betz, M., et al. (1986). A stereotaxic method for small animals using experimentally determined reference profiles. *https://core.ac.uk/download/12164086.pdf* (accessed on 6th August 2025).

3. Asadian, M., De Geyter, N., De Moor, L., Declercq, et al. (2020). Hybrid bioprinting of chondrogenically induced human mesenchymal stem cell spheroids. *https://core.ac.uk/download/323232718.pdf* (accessed on 6th August 2025).

4. Ashok, P. C., Bellini, N., Dholakia, K., Herrington, et al. (2014). Combined information from Raman spectroscopy and optical coherence tomography for enhanced diagnostic accuracy in tissue discrimination. *https://core.ac.uk/download/30317806.pdf* (accessed on 6th August 2025).

5. Assaad, S., Friedman, M. B., Kratzert, W. B., Perrino, et al. (2018). Assessment of pulmonary edema: Principles and practice. *https://core.ac.uk/download/145643671.pdf* (accessed on 6th August 2025).

6. Augustin, M., Baumann, B., Eugui, P., Harper, et al. (2018). Beyond backscattering: Optical neuroimaging by BRAD. *http://arxiv.org/abs/1712.00361* (accessed on 6th August 2025).

7. Babot, M. del P., Lund, J., Olmos, A. V. (2014). Taphonomy in the kitchen: Culinary practices and processing residues of native tuberous plants of the south-central Andes. *https://core.ac.uk/download/159287526.pdf* (accessed on 6th August 2025).

8. Bartlett, J. M. S., Dowsett, M., Ellis, I. O., Humphreys, et al. (2004). Updated recommendations for HER2 testing in the UK. *https://core.ac.uk/download/1568896.pdf* (accessed on 6th August 2025).

9. Basciani, S., Farcomeni, A., Franco, G., Gnessi, et al. (2018). Testicular histopathology, semen analysis and FSH, predictive value of sperm retrieval: Supportive counseling in case of reoperation after testicular sperm extraction (TESE). *https://core.ac.uk/download/188822501.pdf* (accessed on 6th August 2025).

10. Bert, W., & De Ley, P. (2002). Video capture and editing as a tool for the storage, distribution, and illustration of morphological characters of nematodes. *https://core.ac.uk/download/55790373.pdf* (accessed on 6th August 2025).

11. Bishop, J., Borowsky, A. D., Demos, S. G., Fereidouni, et al. (2017). Microscopy with ultraviolet surface excitation for rapid slide-free histology. *https://core.ac.uk/download/323068262.pdf* (accessed on 6th August 2025).

12. Bochsler, V. S., Galloway, S. B., Harley, R. A., Kramarsky-Winters, et al. (2007). Coral Disease and Health Workshop: Coral Histopathology II. *https://core.ac.uk/download/11017972.pdf* (accessed on 6th August 2025).

13. Bohland, J. W., Wu, C., Barbas, H., Bokil, H., Bota, M., Breiter, H. C., et al. (2009). A proposal for a coordinated effort for the determination of brainwide neuroanatomical connectivity in model organisms at a mesoscopic scale. *https://core.ac.uk/download/4881776.pdf* (accessed on 6th August 2025).

14. Bourges-Abella, N., Castellote, J., Joly, B., Kolf-Clauw, et al. (2009). Development of a pig jejunal explant culture for studying the gastrointestinal toxicity of the mycotoxin deoxynivalenol: Histopathological analysis. *https://core.ac.uk/download/12041537.pdf* (accessed on 6th August 2025).

15. Brincat, S. (1990). Multimodality management of soft tissue sarcomas. *https://core.ac.uk/download/46601735.pdf* (accessed on 6th August 2025).

16. Callaghan, M. F. & Mohammadi, S. (2020). Towards in vivo g-ratio mapping using MRI: Unifying myelin and diffusion imaging. *https://core.ac.uk/download/343121910.pdf* (accessed on 6th August 2025).

17. Coelho, P. G., Jimbo, R., Vandeweghe, S., Vanhove, et al. (2013). Utilizing micro-computed tomography to evaluate bone structure surrounding dental implants: A comparison with histomorphometry. *https://core.ac.uk/download/55848647.pdf* (accessed on 6th August 2025).

18. Cremer, T., Holtgreve-Grez, H., Lengauer, C., Manoir, et al. (1993). Molecular cytogenetic analysis of formalin-fixed, paraffin-embedded solid tumors by comparative genomic hybridization after universal DNA-amplification. *https://core.ac.uk/download/12170133.pdf* (accessed on 6th August 2025).

19. De Brazina, G., Uma Vetri Selvi, G., Papantoniou, I., Azinfar, L., Murino, L., Weber, L., Chiorean, L. D., et al. (2017). Software for full-color 3D reconstruction of the biological tissues internal structure. *http://arxiv.org/abs/1711.04118* (accessed on 6th August 2025).

20. Dannhorn, A. (2020). Improving spatially resolved MSI analysis of tissue sections for DMPK and toxicity studies. *https://core.ac.uk/download/542495172.pdf* (accessed on 6th August 2025).

21. De Bari, C., Kurth, T. B. (2011). Immunostaining of skeletal tissues. *https://core.ac.uk/download/4193241.pdf* (accessed on 6th August 2025).

22. Dell'Acqua, F., Aggarwal, M., Anderson, A., Bagdasarian, et al. (2023). Recommendations and guidelines from the ISMRM Diffusion Study Group for preclinical diffusion MRI: Part 1 – In vivo small-animal imaging. *http://arxiv.org/abs/2209.12994* (accessed on 6th August 2025).

23. Doyle, S., Gurcan, M., James, A., John, et al. (2017). Developing the Quantitative Histopathology Image Ontology: A case study using the hot spot detection problem. *https://core.ac.uk/download/131212651.pdf* (accessed on 6th August 2025).

24. Engelmann, J., Kassing, V., Kurtz, R. (2013). Monitoring of single-cell responses in the optic tectum of adult zebrafish with dextran-coupled calcium dyes delivered via local electroporation. *https://core.ac.uk/download/15979206.pdf* (accessed on 6th August 2025).

25. Gompels, L. (2010). In vivo fluorescence imaging of E-selectin: Quantitative detection of endothelial activation in arthritis. *https://core.ac.uk/download/1589084.pdf* (accessed on 6th August 2025).

26. Howard, D. W., Keller, B. J., Lewis, E. J., Smith, et al. (2004). *Histological techniques for marine bivalve mollusks and crustaceans* (2nd ed.). *https://core.ac.uk/download/19793342.pdf* (accessed on 6th August 2025).

27. Huang, A. S., Mohindroo, C., Weinreb, R. N. (2016). Aqueous humor outflow structure and function imaging at the bench and bedside: A review. *https://core.ac.uk/download/323065079.pdf* (accessed on 6th August 2025).

28. Kavanaugh, R. (2017). MRI overview for fat quantification in non-alcoholic fatty liver disease in the clinical and research settings. *https://open.bu.edu/bitstream/2144/24022/5/Kavanaugh_bu_0017N_12875.pdf* (accessed on 6th August 2025).

29. Kelsey, T. W. & Wallace, W. H. B. (2010). Machine science in biomedicine: Practicalities, pitfalls and potential. *http://arxiv.org/abs/1008.3795* (accessed on 6th August 2025).

30. Leuschner, U. & Schlichting, J. (2013). Drug therapy of primary biliary diseases: Classical and modern strategies. *https://core.ac.uk/download/14526202.pdf* (accessed on 6th August 2025).

31. Matcher, S. J. (2009). A review of some recent developments in polarization-sensitive optical imaging techniques for the study of articular cartilage. *https://core.ac.uk/download/50699.pdf* (accessed on 6th August 2025).

32. Meher, V. (2020). Analysis of thrombi from acute ischemic stroke patients using advanced imaging techniques. *https://core.ac.uk/download/304170202.pdf* (accessed on 6th August 2025).

33. Silva, I. A. (2023). Development of techniques to determine extracellular matrix alterations in acute and chronic lung diseases and bioengineered tissues. *https://core.ac.uk/download/576810689.pdf* (accessed on 6th August 2025).

34. Wang, L. V. & Yao, J. (2011). Photoacoustic tomography: Fundamentals, advances and prospects. *https://core.ac.uk/download/211389234.pdf* (accessed on 6th August 2025).

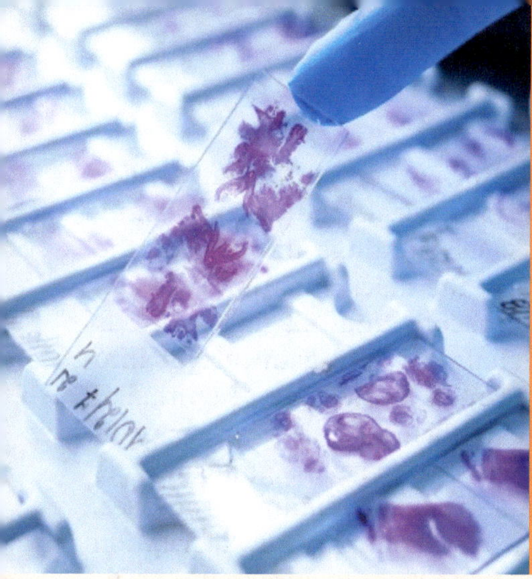

Chapter 3

EPITHELIAL TISSUE MORPHOLOGY

Contents

Introduction

Epithelial tissue is a fundamental multicellular animal structure, and it plays a crucial role in protection, absorption, secretion, and sensation. Epithelial tissue is a boundary against the external world and underlying structures and contributes to organ function and homeostasis. The morphology of epithelial tissue is diverse, consistent with the wide variety of specialized functions based on its location and what they perform in the organism. For instance, squamous epithelium is utilized for filtration and diffusion in locations like alveoli of the lungs, while stratified epithelium provides good protection to regions that are more likely to get abraded, e.g., skin. Morphology of the epithelium is important across many fields of research, including pathology and regenerative medicine, because alterations in epithelial structure can lead to diseases such as cancer and chronic inflammatory disorders. Morphological investigation of epithelial tissue is more than mere structural identification; it is a complicated interplay between cell structure and physiological impact. New developments detail how changes in the morphology of epithelial cells can be indicative of pathological changes. For instance, in pituitary adenomas, detailed cell culture characterization reveals the distinguishing characteristics of various tumor categories (Bácsy et al., 2005). These findings underscore the importance of morphological studies in clinical diagnosis, particularly the discrimination between benign and malignant pathology. Furthermore, the advances in microscopy and imaging methods allow researchers to observe the ultrastructural features of epithelial cells and gain insight into their functional dynamics and matrix interactions. In doing so, thorough knowledge of epithelial morphology paves the way for selective therapies aimed at re-establishing tissue integrity in disease conditions. Aside from its use in pathology, epithelial morphology plays a significant role in comprehending wider physiological processes, especially inflammation and immune processes. Chronic inflammatory gut diseases, which include those connected with HIV, exemplify how disruption of the epithelium can result in systemic impacts, including immune impairment (Arredondo et al., 2019). The interaction of microbial characteristics and epithelial integrity underscores the necessity of possessing a tight epithelial layer to support proper barrier function and immune response. The fascinating interaction between microbial metabolism and epithelial repair demonstrates the critical role of epithelial morphology in maintaining overall health. Therefore, studies elucidating the mechanisms of epithelial integrity are a promising area, providing insight into potential therapeutic interventions to restore tissue homeostasis and enhance resilience against a range of inflammatory diseases (Figure 3.1).

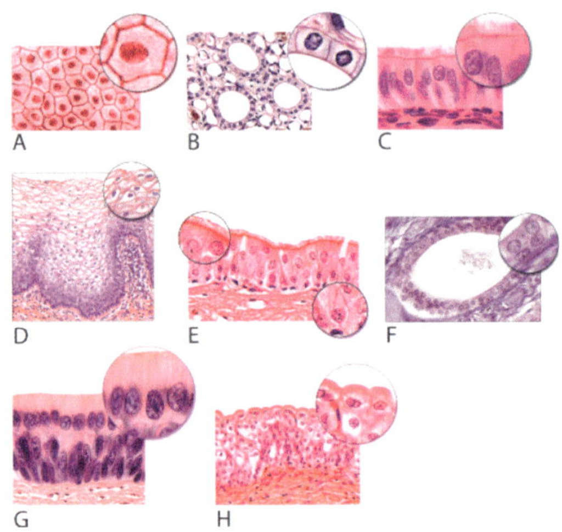

Figure 3.1. Epithelial tissue morphology.

Source: https://o.quizlet.com/d-ktuq1WXnpXop91AIUDlA.png.

Definition of Epithelial Tissue

Epithelial tissue is a primary tissue in the body, primarily a protective covering that invests body surfaces and lines organs and body cavities. It is made up of closely packed cells with minimal extracellular matrix, with which epithelial tissue carries out numerous essential activities like protection, absorption, secretion, and sensation. Epithelial tissue is typically divided by cell shape—columnar, cuboidal, or squamous—and layer number—simple or stratified. This variation in structure enables epithelial tissues to specialize for an array of functions in an extensive list of locations in the body, such as permitting nutrient absorption in the intestines or serving as a barrier to pathogens in the skin. The organization and morphology of such tissues are important for maintaining homeostasis and the continuity of function across various organ systems. Morphology of the epithelial tissue not just points to the varied functional roles but also to the tissue's adaptability to varying physiological conditions. For instance, the characteristic properties of transitional epithelium enable it to adjust to volume alterations of the organ, particularly in the urinary bladder, whereas cuboidal epithelium tends to be found in glandular structures where secretions occur.

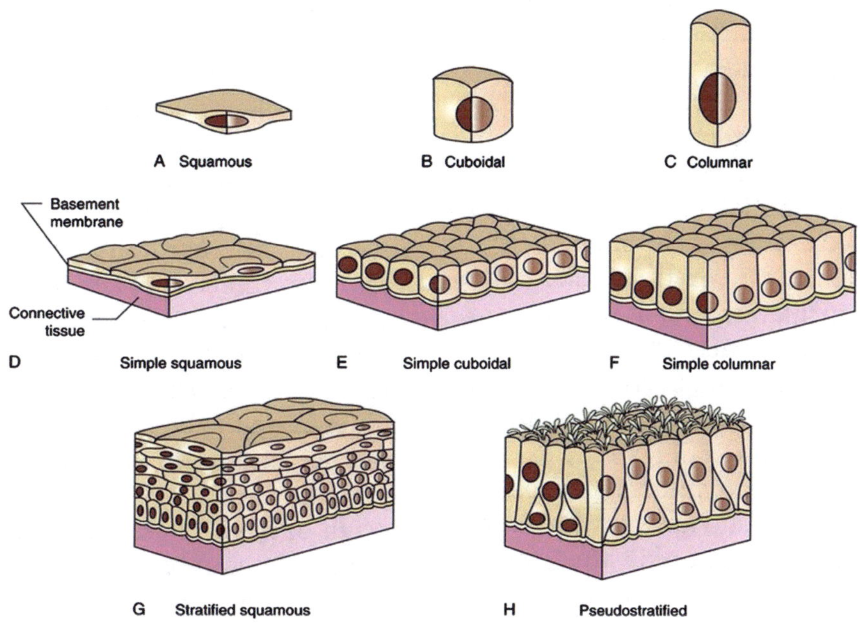

Figure 3.2. Definition of epithelial tissue.

Source: https://i.pinimg.com/originals/c0/34/cf/c034cf4e0b3f0aab4141338ff6ce283b.jpg.

Highly specialized properties of epithelial cells, including microvilli or cilia, enhance their functional efficiency; microvilli optimize surface area for secretion and absorption, whereas cilia are largely involved in the transport of substances across epithelial surfaces. Besides, epithelial cells possess a powerful regenerative ability from their high turnover rate, particularly in areas that experience abrasion or trauma. This potentiality towards regeneration is indicative of their function as an integral aspect of tissue maintenance and repair on a continuous basis. In terms of interaction with the other types of tissue, epithelial tissue is anchored by the underlying connective tissue with a basement membrane, which serves to anchor the epithelium and enable selective permeability. Such intricate association is vital for exchanging waste products and nutrients, highlighting the cooperative nature of the body's tissue systems. Studies have shown that alterations in epithelial tissue morphology can provide information about pathological states; for instance, progression from normal to hyperplastic or neoplastic states has largely been linked to changes in cellular structure and function (Chatdarong, 2003; Boucheron et al., 2009). Understanding epithelial tissue's multifaceted definitions and morphology is of the utmost significance in fields of study such as histopathology, where the recognition of cellular features can determine disease diagnosis and treatment (Figure 3.2).

Importance of Studying Epithelial Morphology

Epithelial morphology is the most significant part of structure-function studies in biological systems. Epithelial tissues, being extremely diverse in shape and arrangement, play important roles in protection, absorption, secretion, and sensation. From an examination of the shape of epithelial cells, researchers are able to discern how some shapes, e.g., cuboidal or columnar, mirror their functional capabilities. In particular, careful observation of epithelial layers is able to account for selective permeability mechanisms and barrier functions needed to ensure homeostasis. The analysis of these structures yields findings that extend beyond basic biology and inform pathology and treatment strategies. The knowledge of how morphological changes occur after states of disease, such as cancer or chronic injury, provides valuable information that can be employed to guide therapeutic interventions to reverse or recover normal function or to induce regeneration. Also, epithelial morphology changes represent a significant application in the study of many diseases, where these changes typically occur as precursors to corresponding pathological conditions. For instance, in situations such as acute kidney injury, the cell morphology of kidney epithelial cells can significantly influence overall organ function and the prognosis of the patient. As described in earlier studies, the regulation of cell morphology by particular receptors, such as TMIGD1, is essential for the survival and communication of cells. When the morphology of epithelia is changed, as it can be seen with experimental models, cell loss and functional compromise may be exacerbated, emphasizing the importance of maintaining the normal morphological features. This insight not only offers a greater appreciation of disease onset but also reveals windows for targeted interventions aimed at restoring or replacing morphological decline, underscoring the importance of examining epithelial tissue morphology in clinical practice. Also, the use of advanced models in studying epithelial morphology makes *in vitro* studies more valid, particularly in host-pathogen interaction. The best example is the three-dimensional lung epithelial cell model capable of mimicking *in vivo* characteristics and generating important information regarding bacterial activity, such as biofilm formation by *Pseudomonas aeruginosa*. By learning about how biofilms interact with epithelial cells and how well various antimicrobial agents work, researchers can develop more efficient ways of treating infections. The morphological environment provided by the epithelial cells has a significant influence on the behavior of pathogens and how they respond to therapy. Hence, understanding epithelial tissue morphology is integral to the design of novel therapeutic strategies that can effectively counter microbial virulence and improve patient outcomes in infectious diseases, underscoring its significance in both basic and translational biomedicine.

3.1. Types of Epithelial Tissue

Knowledge of the various kinds of epithelial tissue is vital to comprehend what they do in the human body. The tissues are primarily classified by numbers of cell layers and cell shapes. The first ones are simple epithelia, which consist of a single layer of cells, and stratified epithelia, consisting of layers upon layers of overlapping cells. Simple squamous epithelial flat cells, for instance, permit free diffusion and filtration that are significant in the alveoli of the lungs and the blood vessel lining. In contrast, stratified squamous epithelium, as seen in the skin, provides a tough barrier to physical and chemical damage, illustrating the adaptive nature of epithelial types to the functional requirements they have to meet. Besides layer categorization, epithelial tissues also occur in a variety of shapes encompassing squamous, cuboidal, and columnar forms that are specialized to serve specific functions like absorption, secretion, and protection. Simple cuboidal epithelium, for example, consisting of cells that are cube-shaped in form, normally occurs in kidney tubules, where the shape of its cells supports absorption and secretion activities. Conversely, the ciliated columnar epithelium, which is made of tall columnar cells, allows for the clearance of mucus and particles from the respiratory system. This difference not only illustrates the functional specialization of epithelial tissues but also their ability to adapt to special microenvironments in an effort to contribute to the integrity and effectiveness of organ systems under various physiological conditions. This remarkable plasticity of epithelial tissue is also brought into prominence by its response to pathological processes. For instance, in tumorigenesis, the morphological nature of epithelial tissue can be drastically altered, as in breast cancer, where different epithelial cell types respond differently to therapeutic measures. This reaction is not just an expression of cellular transformation but also proves the necessity of studying epithelial structure in the clinical setting. Various morphometric analyses have been developed to quantify these changes and examine how the shape of epithelia is connected with disease progression and treatment response. This is essential information as it not only broadens our understanding of tissue biology but also can guide therapeutic intervention to specific epithelial cancer types, thus emphasizing the most important connection between the structure of epithelia and outcome in disease and health (Bown et al., 2012; Cokus et al., 2019) (Figure 3.3).

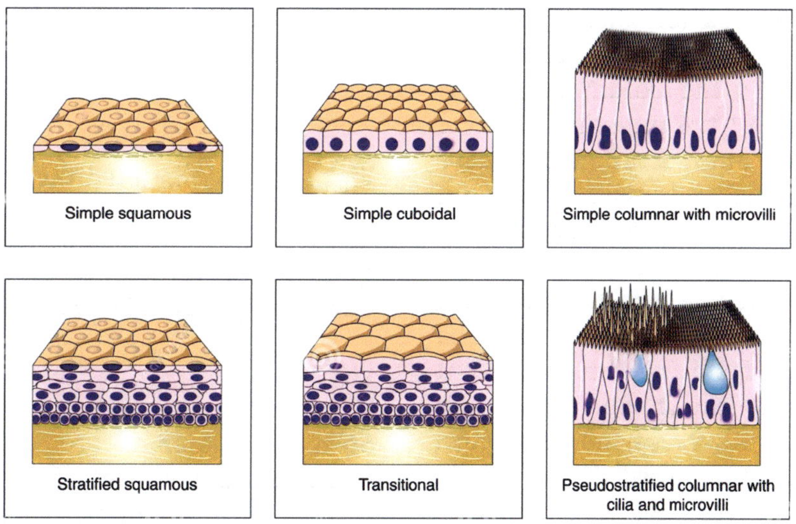

Figure 3.3. Types of epithelial tissue.

Source: https://thumbs.dreamstime.com/z/epithelial-types-12907649.jpg.

3.1.1. Simple Epithelium

Classification of epithelial tissue is vital in the comprehension of its structure and purpose in various organ systems, of which simple epithelium is significant. Simple epithelium is a single-cell layer that is in direct contact with the underlying connective tissues, as opposed to stratified epithelium, which consists of more than one layer. This one layer allows efficient functions such as absorption, secretion, and filtration in organs like the lungs, kidneys, and intestine. The simplicity of the simple epithelial cells allows a standardized environment to carry out these processes because they can be squamous, cuboidal, or columnar in shape and hence adapt to the individual needs of different physiological environments. For instance, the basic squamous epithelium, made up of flattened cells, aids in fast diffusion and filtration activities, which are essential in organs like the alveoli of the lungs and the kidney glomeruli. Morphologically, simple epithelium is quite versatile, as required by its diverse array of physiological activities. Simple cuboidal epithelium, made up of cubical cells, is primarily involved in secretion and absorption activities in glands and kidney tubules. This tissue's structure provides for a maximum surface area for such purposes, enabling the flow of substances across cell membranes. Similarly, the columnar shape, such as on the lining of the intestinal tract, is crucial to absorption and secretion of mucus and enzymes. Its taller cells usually possess microvilli, which enhance the absorptive surface area, rendering it more effective. Also, cellular specialization and the presence of cilia in certain simple columnar epithelia are adaptations that facilitate the movement of substances over epithelial surfaces, as in the respiratory tract. All these morphological features demonstrate the versatility of simple epithelium to meet diverse physiological needs. Current studies have highlighted the importance of understanding information about simple epithelium's morphology under both health and disease conditions, gaining insights into its functional adaptations. For example, a study using primary porcine oviduct epithelial cells (POEC) demonstrated that this simple epithelial model retains in vivo-like morphology for long-term culture, suggesting its physiological relevance (Chen et al., 2013). Through analysis of the POEC status of differentiation and functional properties, the scientists obtained valuable information pertinent to reproductive toxicology testing and basic research, emphasizing the significance of epithelial morphology in functional consequences. Besides, experiments on the cyclical changes of the reproductive organs show how simple epithelium responds to hormonal fluctuations, influencing fertility and overall health (Chatdarong, 2003). They demonstrate the dynamic nature of the simple epithelium, showing that its morphological properties are not only structural but also functional, supporting its wide variety of functions in the living organism (Figure 3.4).

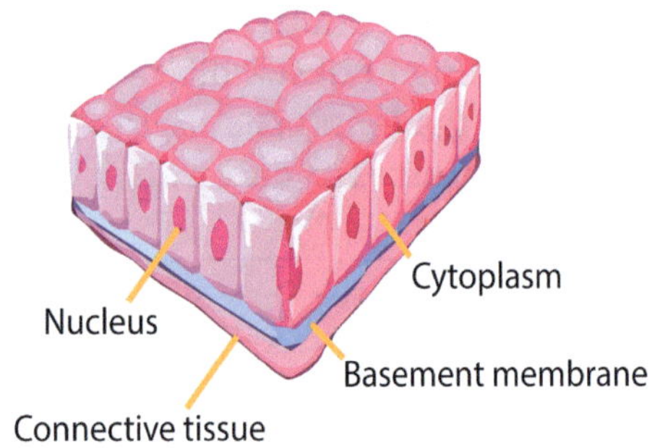

Figure 3.4. Simple epithelium.

Source: https://www.vedantu.com/question-sets/c7abe3ae-0d23-49b2-b1a2-e266d5669f7c6773703271504446528.png.

3.1.2. Stratified Epithelium

Stratified epithelium is a specialized organization of epithelial cells that offers vital protection in terms of layering in many tissues of the human body. This epithelium consists of several layers of cells and is strategically located to be able to resist mechanical stress while shielding underlying tissues from damage as well as infection by pathogens. The outer layer is typically made of squamous cells, which are flattened and scale-like to effectively cover vast surfaces, while inner layers may contain cuboidal or columnar cells. These structural modifications enable stratified epithelium to perform its basic functions, including abrasion protection in skin and contributing to barrier function in areas like the oral cavity and esophagus, where damage risk by mechanical and chemical forces is extensive. The function of stratified epithelium is more than structural defense; it is also crucial for maintaining the regulation of permeability and homeostasis in numerous organ systems. For instance, the stratified squamous epithelium of the skin is keratinized, which explains its impermeability and helps prevent transepidermal water loss, thereby enhancing hydration and overall skin integrity. Conversely, the non-keratinized types in the oral cavity and esophagus possess moisture retention that aids swallowing and digestion. Thus, the specific characteristics of different stratified epithelia are inextricably intertwined with their functional requirements according to their positions in the body, reflecting the delicate relationship between form and function in epithelial tissue structure. Science also indicates the plasticity of stratified epithelial cells exposed to various environmental conditions. For example, experiments indicate that growth factors in the epithelium play a significant role in regulating the differentiation and function of stratified epithelial cells. With the use of an air-liquid interface culture model, alterations in growth conditions elicited varying cellular responses with regard to ciliation and differentiation outcomes. These findings accentuate the dynamic nature of stratified epithelium, particularly in response to external stimuli with the potential to affect cell proliferation, barrier formation, and overall tissue integrity. As research examining the intricacies of epithelial interactions with pathogens, as in respiratory models, continues to emerge, further understanding of the versatility and relevance of stratified epithelia in health and disease can be gained (Berry et al., 2018; Baskin et al., 2019) (Figure 3.5).

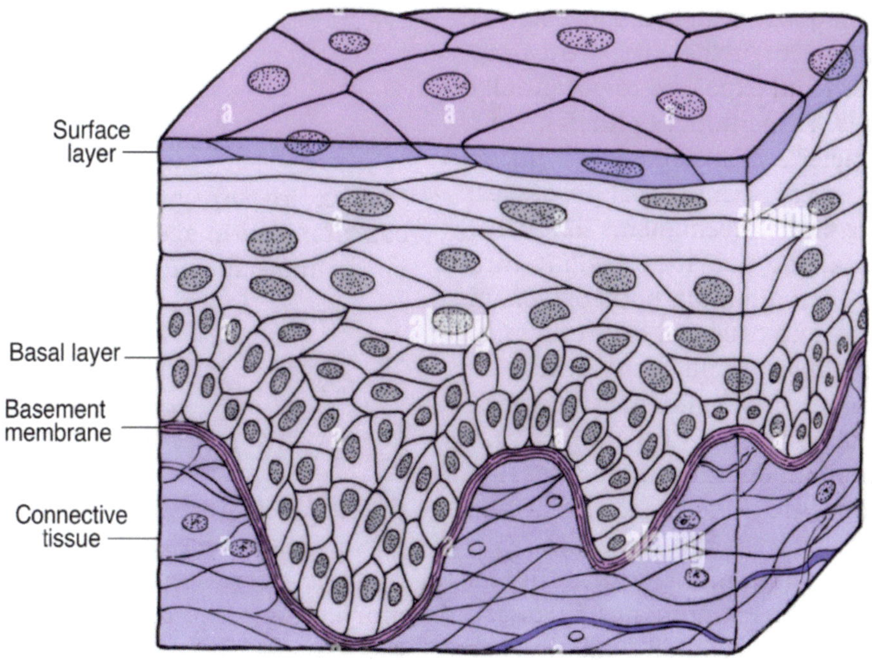

Figure 3.5. Stratified epithelium.

Source: https://c8.alamy.com/comp/HRJ4JF/illustration-of-stratified-squamous-epithelium-HRJ4JF.jpg.

3.1.3. Transitional Epithelium

Among epithelial tissue morphologies, transitional epithelium is a unique type with characteristic structural and functional properties, being predominantly lining the urinary bladder, ureters, and the urethra. Transitional epithelium is noted for its ability to stretch and be flexible to support variable amounts of urine to be stored and passed through. The feature of transitional epithelium is a multistratified organization that is able to transform from a relaxed state, in which cells are cuboidal and polyhedral, to an elongated state, in which the cells are flattened. Such dynamic morphological changes are required to maintain the integrity of the bladder wall during filling and voiding, provide a protective cover while allowing flexibility to internal pressure. Mechanistically, transitional epithelium relies considerably upon intercellular accommodations for its enhanced function. The apical surface of epithelial cells is protected by a unique layer of protein-rich plaques, which are crucial in preventing backflow of urine and protecting underlying tissues from exposure to potentially hostile substances. Transitional epithelial cells also reveal a characteristic nucleus-to-cytoplasm ratio, which varies with transitional processes. An understanding of the mechanisms that drive these cellular changes provides insight into how such a tissue can maintain homeostasis in fluctuating physical and chemical environments. The ability to exhibit this plasticity works to distinguish the character of epithelial structures, further corroborating the argument that transitional epithelium operates under a design optimized for specific functional intentions within the urinary system. Research into transitional epithelium pathology, including its response to carcinogenic stimuli, has produced significant findings on its cellular dynamics. For instance, it has been noted in research that when exposed to particular environmental stresses or genetic mutations, transitional cells will undergo alterations leading to bladder tumors. Chemical carcinogen-induced bladder cancer cells in model systems showed remarkable characteristics like loss of contact inhibition and elevated mitotic index, which are good markers for neoplastic transformation. Further, the chromosomal aberrations in these cells, ranging from triploid to tetraploid, point towards the susceptibility towards malignant transformation (Nishi., 1978). Therefore, ongoing research attempts to establish the molecular mechanisms behind controlling transitional epithelium, highlighting its importance not only in normal physiology but also in neoplastic disease (Gong et al., 2017) (Figure 3.6).

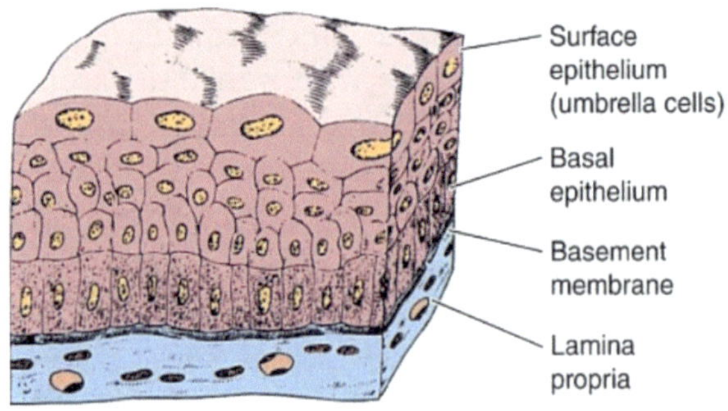

Figure 3.6. Transitional epithelium.

Source: https://jotscroll.com/images/forums-concatenated-images/1571698131-Transitional-epithelium-labeled-diagram-structure.jpg.

3.2. Characteristics of Epithelial Cells

Epithelial cells are characterized by their unique structural features, which are generally critical to their operation and contribution to tissue morphology. The cells stick tightly together in the creation of continuous sheets that form the covering of body surfaces and the lining of cavities. Such cohesive alignment is facilitated by specialized junctions such as tight junctions, desmosomes, and gap junctions. Tight junctions prevent the movement of substances from between cells, resulting in selective permeability of epithelial tissues. Additionally, the presence of microvilli on the apical surface of certain epithelial cells enhances their absorptive role, particularly in the intestines. The structural organization of epithelial cells is thus directly linked to their functional capacity, thus rendering them an important element in many physiological events. Besides structural characteristics, epithelial cells are functionally diverse.

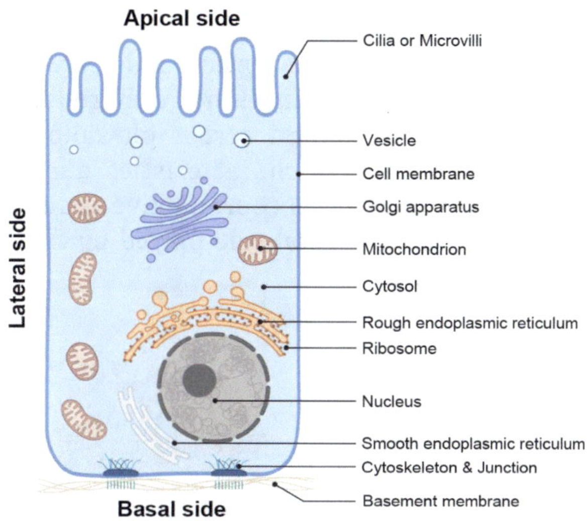

Figure 3.7. Characteristics of epithelial cells.

Source: https://rsscience.com/wp-content/uploads/2022/04/epithelial-cells-anatomy.jpg.

They are classified according to their shapes: squamous, cuboidal, or columnar, and the number of layers: simple or stratified. Such diversity in epithelial tissues permits them to have specialized functions that take place in organs. For example, the thinness of the simple squamous epithelium of the alveoli aids in gas exchange, while stratified squamous epithelium, which occurs in the skin, provides protection against mechanical forces and pathogens. Recent developments in computational modeling have also shed further light on the emergent behavior of epithelial cells, as evidenced by agent-based models that simulate cellular interactions and growth patterns under different conditions (Hill et al., 2004). These observations not only add to our understanding of epithelial tissue dynamics but also emphasize the importance of morphology to function. The characterization of epithelial cells also encompasses their response to environmental stimuli, which can have a significant influence over their growth and behavior. Rat diploid epithelial cell line experiments have been shown to maintain a normal diploid karyotype initially for extended periods in vitro; however, under certain conditions, morphology can change and heterogeneity increases (Masuji et al., 1974). Such flexibility is important in pathological conditions such as carcinogenesis, where the epithelial cells can undergo malignant transformation. Therefore, understanding the characteristics of epithelial cells is essential to addressing the complexity of tissue growth and development, particularly when disease is involved. Hence, further research on the control systems that govern epithelial shape will also enhance therapeutic interventions that aim to address disorders involving epithelial (Figure 3.7).

3.2.1. Cell Shape Variations

Morphology of epithelial tissue is characterized by the occurrence of specific cell shapes, which are crucial to their function and organization in the organism. The most frequent cell shapes among epithelial tissues include squamous, cuboidal, and columnar cells. Squamous epithelial cells, with their flattened and narrow morphology, facilitate rapid diffusion and filtration and are thus frequent in tissues such as blood vessel linings and alveoli. Conversely, cuboidal cells have a stronger profile that is suitable for secretion and absorption, usually found in glands and renal tubules. Columnar epithelial cells, being more in height than width, are likely to have microvilli or cilia and are involved in significant roles in absorption and secretion activities in the digestive and respiratory tracts. Cell morphological differences not only reflect functional adaptations but also signal refinements in homeostatic regulation across physiological contexts. Differences in cell shape are also underscored by distinctive characteristics during developmental processes and disease conditions, as indicated in studies on reproductive tissue. Studies in primary porcine oviduct epithelial cells (POEC) revealed the pivotal role played by the conditions of cell culture in the morphological characteristics of cells.

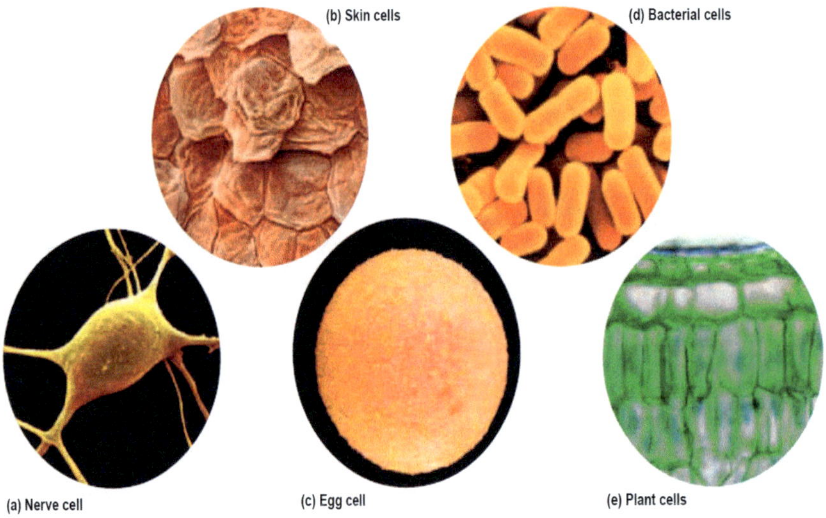

Figure 3.8. Cell shape variations.

Source: https://www.simply.science/images/content/biology/cell_biology/basic_unit_of_life/conceptmap/Cell_shapes1.gif.

This research found that considerable differentiation and retention of *in vivo*-like morphologies in POEC were achievable even when culture times were prolonged to six weeks (Chen et al., 2013). These results emphasize the adaptability of epithelial cells and the reality that they can re-evolve specialized morphologies under the influence of the environment. Understanding these dynamics in epithelial morphology is important to the understanding of reproductive biology and has the potential for application in reproductive toxicity testing and overall biomedical research. Additionally, the study of epithelial cell shape transitions beyond mere morphological description and into functional relevance in reproductive health. For instance, uterine luminal shape changes occurring in hysterography throughout the housecat's estrous cycle depict morphological and reproductive function correspondence. Some of these shapes, like coil-shaped lumens, demonstrated progestagenic effect and conditions such as endometrial hyperplasia (Chatdarong, 2003). Such morphological changes reveal how epithelial cells respond to hormonal stimuli and transform to facilitate reproduction effectively. The sophisticated relationship between cell shape variation and physiological functions underscores the value of such studies, providing a wider perspective for epithelial tissue morphology in terms of its dynamics and its reliance on intrinsic as well as extrinsic stimuli (Figure 3.8).

3.2.2. Cell Arrangement

The organization of cells in epithelial tissues is crucial to their function and taxonomy. Epithelial cells are organized according to their shape, i.e., squamous, cuboidal, and columnar, and also their layering, whether it is simple or stratified. Simple epithelia consist of one layer of cells and are usually engaged in processes such as absorption, filtration, and secretion due to their large surface area in relation to volume. Stratified epithelia, which are made up of layers, typically protect the exposed regions from abrasion, such as the skin and the lining of the mouth. This broad idea of cell pattern can be used to better understand how the shapes of epithelia are specialized to fulfill specific mechanical and physiological needs in organs. Aside from their shapes and stratification, the pattern of cell organization in epithelial tissues can indicate functional specialization. For instance, pseudostratified columnar epithelium appears stratified due to variations in cell height, but it is single-layered, utilizing cilia to propel mucus along its surface in the respiratory tract. This unique arrangement makes the respiratory system more effective through particulate trapping and elimination, as well as airway maintenance. In addition, the transitional epithelium is another notable arrangement, with several contractile, stretchable layers. Such adaptability is required in organs like the bladder, which must be capable of holding varying amounts of urine. The diverse arrangements within epithelial tissues demonstrate the correlation between cellular morphology and function. Exploring the significance of cell arrangement goes beyond the structural vocabulary; it intersects with pathologies and the effect of environmental stressors. As suggested by biological studies, changes in the organization of epithelial cells have compromised integrity that affects organ systems and well-being. For instance, research on coral diseases has shown that changes in cellular morphology have devastating effects on reef ecosystems, further demonstrating the greater value placed on cell arrangement. Specifically, the demand for accurate morphological diagnosis in coral pathologies is evidence of the complex interrelation between cell patterning and the toughness of the environment. By the integration of data from fields such as histology and cell biology, researchers can begin to develop more informed approaches to problem-solving resulting from cellular disorganization, both in corals and human health, and demonstrating the universal significance of epithelial tissue morphology in complicated systems (Bochsler et al., 2007; Gruhl, A. & Okamura, B., 2016).

3.2.3. Polarity of Epithelial Cells

Epithelial cell polarity is essential for normal function and organization. Epithelial cells possess distinct morphological domains, i.e., apical, lateral, and basal surfaces, and each of these has a specific role in tissue homeostasis and integrity. The apical membrane faces the lumen or the exterior environment, which allows absorption or secretion of molecules. The lateral surfaces provide for cell-cell adhesion through the presence of tight junctions, which support barrier functions and cellular signaling.

Concurrently, the basal surface is bound to the extracellular matrix, which provides support and stability. This compartmentalization is essential for the overall function of epithelial tissues because it allows for the specialized activities needed for functions such as nutrient transport and ion exchange. A recent review of the literature has highlighted the importance of quantifying transepithelial electrical resistance (TEER) as a cellular polarity and differentiation measure in epithelial cells.

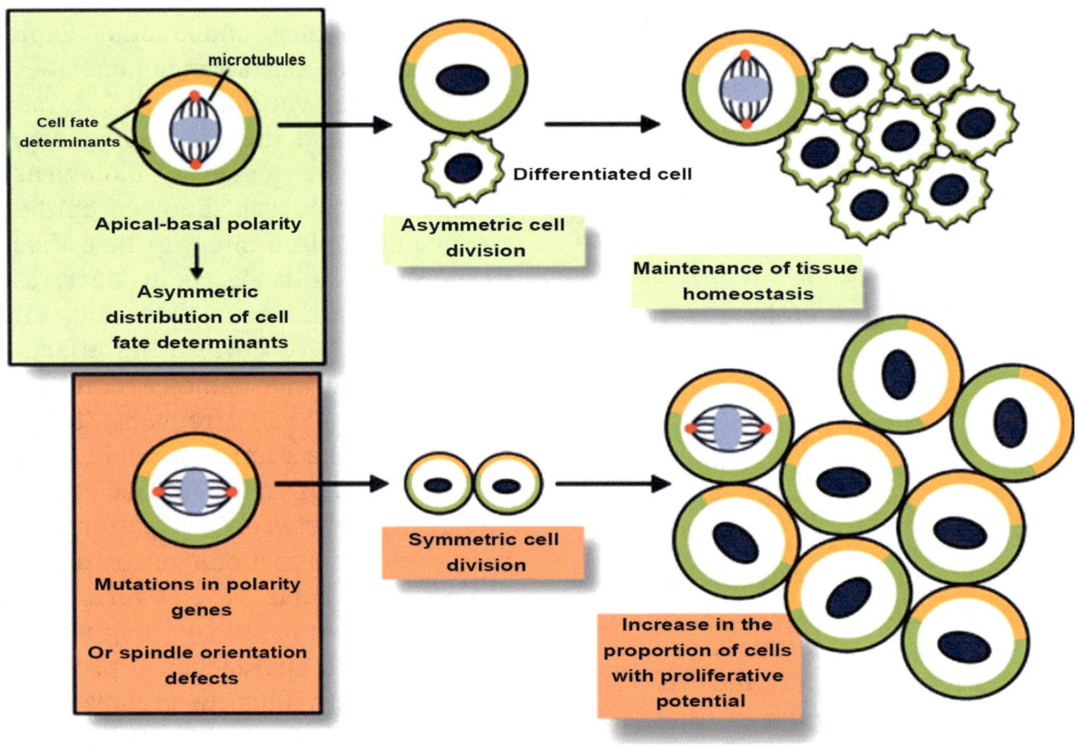

Figure 3.9. Polarity of epithelial cells.

Source: https://www.researchgate.net/profile/Christophe-Royer/publication/51170051/figure/fig4/AS:267690971496527@1440833909815/Loss-of-cell-polarity-in-epithelial-stem-cells-can-lead-to-asymmetric-division-defects.png.

Optimal levels of TEER have been found to be associated with defined cellular architecture and function, as is seen in porcine oviduct epithelial cells cultured under optimal conditions. Well-defined tight junctions at the lateral membrane, coupled with the maintenance of apical-basal polarity, are necessary to ensure effective barrier formation in epithelial tissues. (Chen et al., 2015) emphasizes this interaction by demonstrating that fully differentiated cultures exhibit medium TEER levels, which indicate high quality and proper polarity. Thus, TEER is not only a qualitative marker of epithelial cell integrity but also an indicator of the interaction between polarity and general cellular health. Epithelial cell polarity provides information about tissue morphogenesis and the dynamics of processes such as regeneration and tumorigenesis. This has been considered an active wetting transition in the case of forces by the cells themselves; however, morphological change in tissues, such as in the case of regeneration or malignancy, can be accounted for by the paradigm of active polar fluid dynamics, for example. This regard is based on the crucial fine balance between traction forces and cellular contractility. Ravasio et al. (2019) elaborate on this by demonstrating how these active cellular forces drive tissue architecture remodeling, placing emphasis on the importance of polarity in understanding the physiological and pathological remodeling of epithelial tissues (Figure 3.9).

3.3. Functions of Epithelial Tissue

Epithelial tissue plays a central role in maintaining homeostasis and overall health. Protection is one of its key functions; epithelial layers form defense barriers against physical damage, infection, and toxins that keep underlying tissues from being harmed. This function is evident in multilayered epithelia such as the skin and respiratory tract. Not only do these obstacles provide organization, but they also create a setting that avoids infection. For example, proteins such as MyD88 play a central role in protecting epithelial cells from invaders such as Pseudomonas aeruginosa and enable their survival during invasion (Evans et al., 2011).

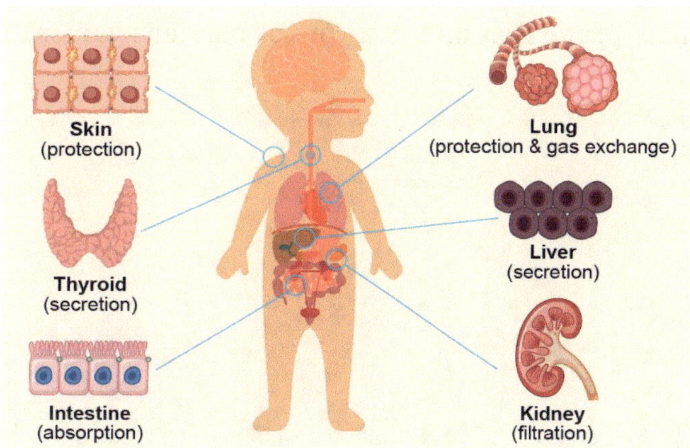

Figure 3.10. Functions of epithelial tissue.

Source: https://qsstudy.com/wp-content/uploads/2017/09/Epithelial-Tissue-1.jpg.

This protective function emphasizes the importance of epithelial morphology because tissue structure changes directly influence the effectiveness of such barriers in maintaining tissue integrity. Beyond protection, epithelial tissue is also of great importance for absorption and secretion. Epithelial cells can be specialized for selective nutrient absorption or waste product expulsion. The intestinal epithelium, for example, has adapted to maximize nutrient absorption by increasing surface area through microvilli that engage with the digested food. Moreover, glandular epithelium produces hormones, enzymes, and mucus in order to enable critical functions in various physiological processes. The cellular morphology and organization of the epithelial tissues directly support these processes, allowing for maximum transport mechanisms. The relation between structure and function demonstrates the capability of epithelial tissue to respond to the requirements of different environments as well as physiological needs, emphasizing its variability in the human body. Besides this, sensory perception is mediated by epithelial tissue, enabling organism-environment interactions. Certain epithelial cells, like those in the taste buds and olfactory epithelium, possess sensory receptors that perceive taste and smell. This sensory process is critical for survival, as it allows organisms to respond to their environment. Morphological characteristics of sensory epithelial cells, including their form and the arrangement of their microvilli or cilia, are extremely specialized to maximize detecting capabilities. Furthermore, these sensory processes can elucidate the pathology of certain diseases; morphological abnormalities of the epithelium can lead to impaired sensory perception. As shown by studies, the complexity of epithelial morphology, function, and contribution to host defense mechanisms is an indication of the complexity of these tissues as well as their multiple roles in general health (Alcazar-Fuoli et al., 2014) (Figure 3.10).

3.3.1. Protection

Epithelial tissue has a critical role in defense against environmental damage, pathogens, and physical trauma. Being the body's first line of defense, epithelial cells are tightly packed, forming a barrier with a controlled permeability that retains selective transport functions. Epithelial tissue's morphology, including its layering and cellular specialization, reflects its roles as protection. For instance, stratified squamous epithelium in friction-exposed tissues such as skin and the oral mucosa provides mechanical protection and is a robust barrier against damage.

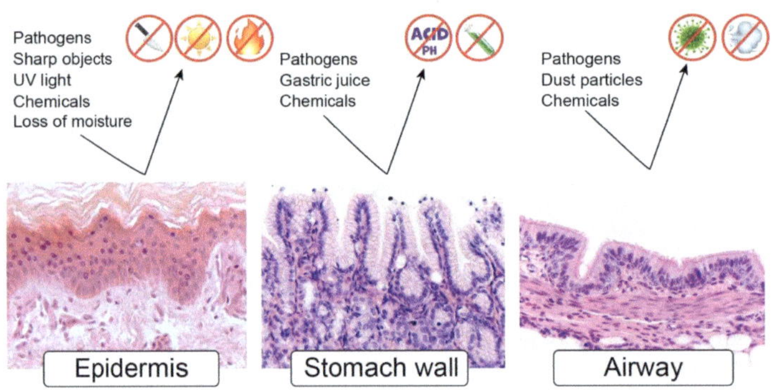

Figure 3.11. Protection.

Source: https://rsscience.com/wp-content/uploads/2022/04/epithelia-function-protection-1536x888.jpg.

Hence, morphological changes in epithelium structure are important to prevent the underlying tissue from harmful substances and thereby attain homeostasis and prevent infection. Moreover, the barrier of epithelial tissues is not merely physical; it involves biochemical processes that actively inactivate or react against pathogens. Epithelial cells produce various secretions, including mucus and antimicrobial peptides, which augment the overall protective function. These secretions create an environment against pathogens and also allow for debris removal. In the case of intestinal epithelial cells, for instance, as described in ongoing studies, ischemia-induced breakdown of the barrier may eventually lead to increased permeability with consequent tissue injury. This underscores the importance of epithelial morphology in enhancing protective roles, as the capacity of the system to respond to insult is irrevocably tied to its structural characteristics, thereby erecting both physical and immunologic defenses (Altshuler et al., 2014). Moreover, experimental approaches to interpreting epithelial protection have shown that it is multifactorial. It has been established that interventions, such as the supply of glucose in ischemia, can significantly cut down harm to the epithelial barrier by reorganizing metabolic requirements and enhancing barrier integrity. This knowledge aligns with research that suggests protective mechanisms are not structural in nature but rather encompass dynamic responses to injury and inflammation (Brown et al., 2014). The relationship between epithelial morphology and reactive function implies that a firm comprehension of these tissues requires attention to both structural components and the physiological mechanisms through which they function. Ultimately, the protective roles of epithelial tissues are essential not only in surface integrity maintenance but also in overall organismal homeostasis (Figure 3.11).

3.3.2. Absorption

Epithelial tissue plays an important role in the absorption of nutrients via the various organ systems, primarily the gastrointestinal tract. Morphological structures of the epithelial cells, such as increased surface area provided by microvilli, allow for increased absorption of necessary material. Microvilli are used to increase the epithelial surface area and thus the contact with the lumenal contents, which contain nutrients. Whenever nutrients like carbohydrates, amino acids, and fatty acids move through the epithelial barrier, their absorption directly influences the overall health and functionality of the organism. A number of diet-related adaptations are able to alter this process, initiating changes in gene expression and epithelial structure, as exemplified by the evidence supporting that nutrient supply plays a significant role in intestinal gene regulation post-weaning, leading to enhanced digestive function and metabolic processes required for optimum absorption (Bauer et al., 2011). Moreover, the interaction between epithelial morphology and absorption is not specific to the gastrointestinal tract. In the respiratory tract, for instance, the ability of epithelial cells to take up a variety of substances, including pathogens and environmental toxins, is indicative of their functional plasticity. As the epithelial cell layers differentiate, they acquire a more complex structure, which is crucial in a position to absorb efficiently and act as barriers. Differentiation leads to increased trans-epithelial electrical resistance (TEER), which indicates tight junction formation between cells, which is a necessary condition for selective permeability. Observations of ALI differentiated epithelial forms also explain this phenomenon, where the manner in which a highly differentiated epithelium enhances absorption capacity at the expense of protective functions is noted (Berry et al., 2017). Understanding these morphological adaptations is key to disease prevention strategies and restoring epithelial barrier function. Lastly, the absorption efficiency is not only dependent on morphological characteristics but also on the metabolic requirements of the epithelial cells themselves. Nutrient absorption is an energy-intensive process that consists of active transport mechanisms, including some involving certain proteins whose expression is regulated by diet. For instance, during disrupted feeding, such as weaning, the demand for specific transport proteins increases, thereby modulating the efficacy of absorption of various nutrients. The association between gene expression and nutrient absorption reflects an extremely responsive system in which alterations in diet profoundly affect epithelial function. Therefore, diet-specific treatments, founded on an understanding of epithelial morphology and absorption kinetics, would have the potential to optimize health outcomes and forestall absorption-related disease (Bauer et al.,

2011). This emphasizes the role of nutrition to optimize epithelial resistance and efficiency of absorption, underpinning overall physiological health.

3.3.3. Secretion

In morphological studies of epithelial tissue, secretion has an essential role to play in the maintenance of physiological processes. Epithelial cells, characterized by their polarity, contribute to various secretory functions that play a key role in maintaining homeostasis. The cells are tasked with synthesizing and secreting materials such as enzymes, hormones, and mucins that play significant roles in processes like digestion, maintenance of body fluids, and surface protection. For instance, mucin release is one of the factors involved in the build-up of protective mucus layers that cover a large number of organs, shielding epithelial tissue from mechanical trauma and pathogens. Morphological changes in cells, including alterations in microvilli and the plasma membrane, support their secretory function, with evidence of a close relationship between structure and function. The influence of external stimuli on secretion in epithelial tissues also requires consideration, particularly under pathophysiological conditions. For instance, the action of drugs such as Ketamine also puts into perspective the adverse reparative changes elicited in kidney epithelial cells. Recent research indicates that Ketamine induces severe cell shape alterations and disrupts renal proximal tubule epithelial cell function, in part through the regulation of important junctional proteins such as E-cadherin and β-catenin. This disruption leads to defective epithelial function and permeability, illustrating the profound influence of drug exposure on mechanisms of secretion. Understanding such mechanisms is paramount to the development of therapeutic approaches that avoid drug-induced injury and preserve epithelial function, emphasizing the importance of maintenance of integrity in secretory pathways. Furthermore, the development of standardized epithelial culture systems is of fundamental concern for the elucidation of secretion and its involvement in disease and health. Development of protocols for primary porcine oviduct epithelial cells (POEC) has provided a viable model for reproductive toxicology and tissue organization studies. In cooperation, the cultures exhibit a highly differentiated phenotype while maintaining key functions, including mucin secretion. The ability to reproduce *in vivo*-like morphology in the laboratory environment provides scientists with the opportunity to investigate the complexities of secretion free from the inconsistencies of live animal research. This knowledge is important in the study of the effect of environmental or drug agents on epithelial health, as part of the goal to establish the functions of secretion in epithelial morphology and functioning.

3.4. Epithelial Tissue in Different Organs

Epithelial tissue varies significantly in shape and function within different organ systems, illustrating the specific physiological function that it performs within a particular context. Within the gastrointestinal system, for instance, epithelial cells are organized into villi and microvilli, which maximize the surface area for nutrient absorption. Such a specialized structure not only facilitates effective digestion but also serves as a filter against pathogens and toxins. By contrast, the respiratory epithelium is of ciliated cells that are essential in mucociliary clearance, trapping, and expulsion of particles inhaled. Such differences reflect the fluidity of epithelial tissue as it bends to meet the demands of every organ to ensure homeostasis and well-being. The reproductive apparatus, too, has a unique expression of epithelial tissue and significant differences between the organs of the male and female reproductive apparatus. In the male, the testicular seminiferous tubules are occupied by stratified epithelium necessary for spermatogenesis, and the epididymis holds pseudostratified columnar epithelium that supports maturation of the sperm. The female reproductive system demonstrates simple columnar epithelium of the uterus, which is variable based on fluctuating hormonal influences during the menstrual cycle. Besides, the enhanced understanding of the morphology of epithelium in reproductive organ formation can be gained from mouse models, with anatomical and developmental differences highlighting the complex regulation of hormones and structural remodeling during puberty (Baskin et al., 2019). The overall picture presented increases the appreciation for the meticulous design of epithelial cells for their specific tasks. Recent advances in computational modeling have clarified the action of epithelial tissue, accounting for emergent properties that arise due to cellular interactions. Agent-based modeling of epithelial cell behavior has provided fundamental insights into growth patterns under varying environmental conditions, e.g., calcium concentrations (Hill et al., 2004). Through establishing a one-to-one mapping between biological cells and computational agents, scientists have been able to progress in the understanding of how such cells control their form and behavior based on external inputs. Such an approach not only confirms prior knowledge regarding the development of epithelial tissue but also makes new avenues of research into regenerative medicine and tissue engineering possible. Thus, the union of computational and biological understanding promotes the science and enables a firm examination of epithelial form throughout the body (Figure 3.12).

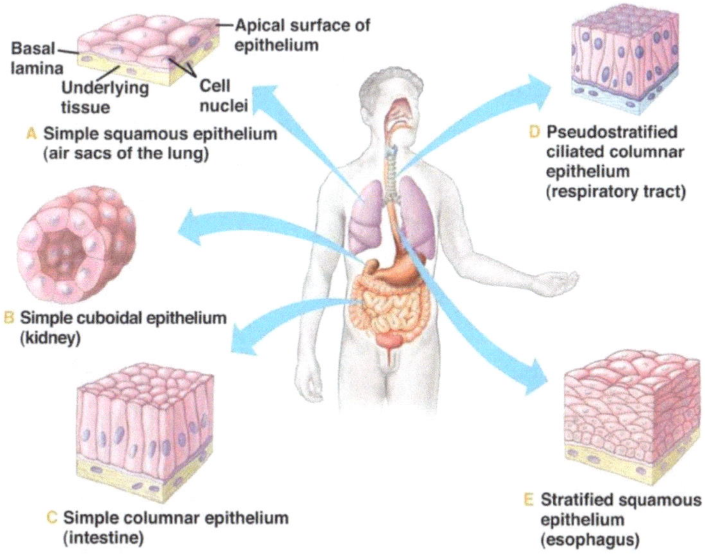

Figure 3.12. Epithelial tissue in different organs.

Source: https://medicinebtg.com/wp-content/uploads/2017/06/Epithelial-Tissues-In-Human-Body-tissue-is-classified-by-cell-shape-and-the-number-of-layers-it-therefore-found-1007x776.jpg.

3.4.1. Skin Epithelium

The skin's epithelium, or epidermis, is the strongest part of the integumentary system and acts as an essential barrier against external injury. The epidermal layer, primarily composed of keratinocytes, possesses the remarkable ability to regenerate in response to the varied conditions posed by UV exposure, infections, and physical abrasions. The epithelium is stratified and made up of layers of varying cell types and functions. The primary components are the stratum corneum, made up of dead keratinized cells that provide protection against water loss and host defense against the outside environment. Furthermore, the interstage between the inner layers, such as the stratum basale, is a reminder of the continuous process of cell turnover and differentiation characteristic of the integrity and tolerance of the skin. The physical and functional characteristics of the skin epithelium are thus pivotal to homeostasis and overall health. In developmental biology, the skin epithelium is involved in complex processes essential to its morphology and function. Gap junctional communication has been found to have an important contribution to chicken skin development, as illustrated by the preferential flow routes of dye transfer reported in experimental research. Specifically, it is stated that it exhibits limited gap junction coupling at its critical locations, such as feather buds, implying a complex regulatory process is involved in skin morphogenesis. The findings indicate that cell-to-cell communication in the epithelium is not necessarily passive but actively involved in the spatial and functional differentiation of skin structures, which presents the sensitivity of epithelial tissues to intrinsic as well as extrinsic stimuli. The impact of such research extends as far as understanding of skin diseases and the development of treatment procedures for epithelium-related illnesses (Chuong et al., 1993). Furthermore, skin epithelial research is also supplemented by interspecies comparative studies, for example, the investigation of porcine mammary epithelial cells showing similarities with human tissue. Through the use of advanced genetic technologies, researchers have created powerful models for manipulating porcine mammary tissue, unraveling mechanisms of epithelial transformation and tumorigenesis. Successful creation of a porcine model paves the way for human breast cancer study, underscoring the importance of epithelial tissue morphology in translational research. This comparative approach not only enhances our understanding of epithelial dynamics but also offers avenues for therapeutic investigation, particularly in cancer biology. Morphological features of skin epithelium, therefore, in addition to their functional significance, are key to basic and applied biosciences with broader implications for disease and health (Borowsky et al., 2015) (Figure 3.13).

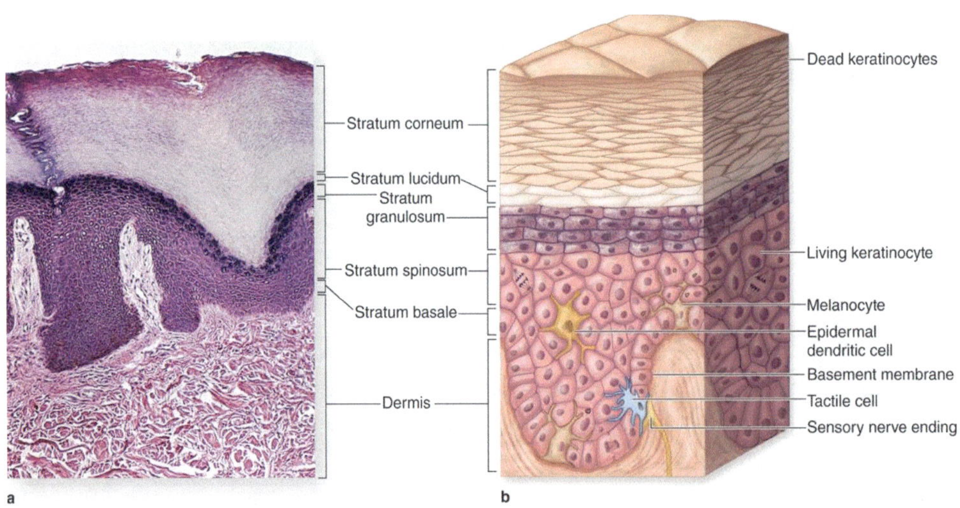

Figure 3.13. Skin epithelium.

Source: https://basicmedicalkey.com/wp-content/uploads/2017/04/00425-1.jpeg.

3.4.2. Lining of the Gastrointestinal Tract

The lining of the gastrointestinal tract is a mature, specialized epithelium that plays an important role in digestion and nutrient uptake. It consists of various types of cells and is liable for gut barrier maintenance and contacting luminal content as well as immune interactions. Particularly noteworthy is how the epithelial cells are organized along the gastrointestinal tract to enable each segment to be optimized for its specific digestive function. As an illustration, the small intestine contains a brush border of microvilli that maximizes the surface area for nutrient absorption and stomach columnar epithelial cells that secrete gastric juices essential in digesting food. Therefore, the morphology of these cells is intrinsically related to their function, which in turn justifies the significance of a well-formed epithelial layer in sustaining gastrointestinal health and effectiveness. The role of food components on the morphology of the gastrointestinal lining cannot be overestimated. New evidence indicates that the addition of some dietary fibers, such as chicory, has profound effects on gut morphometry and microbiota composition in most species, including chickens and pigs. For instance, research has proved that the addition of chicory does not just enhance good animal performance but also induces visible alterations to the gut lining architecture. Such alterations are of significant value as they contribute to improved nutrient utilization and gut integrity. Moreover, the intricate interactions between dietary fiber and epithelial lining may also modulate the expression of specific heat shock proteins, which also detoxify cells from stressors and enhance gut barrier function. Thus, it is important to understand these relationships to optimize dietary interventions for gastrointestinal health. Also, the vulnerability of the gastrointestinal lining to toxic substances, such as mycotoxins, highlights the need for ongoing studies on epithelial tissue morphology. A study on the impact of deoxynivalenol (DON) in porcine jejunal explants elucidates that exposure to this mycotoxin leads to detectable alterations in morphological characteristics.

The experiment confirmed dose-dependent changes, as evidenced by villus shortening and enterocyte lysis, highlighting the sensitivity of intestinal epithelial cells to environmental toxins. These findings highlight the importance of the epithelial lining both as a physical barrier to pathogens and as the primary defense against chemical attack. In this regard, a close understanding of determinants for the morphology of the gastrointestinal linings is critical for enhancing agricultural practices and raising food safety measures to the ultimate good of public health and well-being (Bourges-Abella et al., 2009; Liu, 2013) (Figure 3.14).

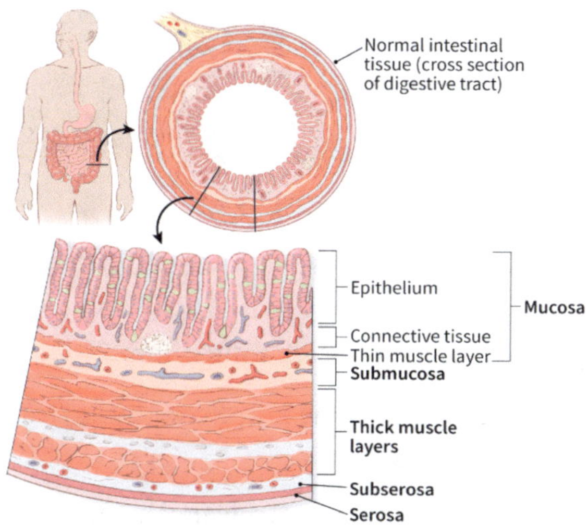

Figure 3.14. Lining of the gastrointestinal tract.

Source: https://www.cancer.org/cancer/types/gastrointestinal-carcinoid-tumor/detection-diagnosis-staging/staged/_jcr_content/root/main-container/center-container/column-1/center-right-container/content-container/textimage.coreimg.jpeg/1674504307404/normal-intestinal-tissue.jpeg.

3.4.3. Respiratory Epithelium

The respiratory epithelium is an unusual epithelial tissue covering the respiratory tract and is essential for the protection and operation of the respiratory system. It is primarily composed of pseudostratified ciliated columnar cells, and through this, the mucus and particles are able to be expelled from the airways, leaving it with a clear airway and sufficient gas exchange. The structural design of respiratory epithelium is extremely advanced, with ciliated cells supported by mucus-secreting goblet cells. The interaction is important in creating a barrier against particulates and pathogens, underscoring the tissue's role as a protector. Increased research has since determined that environmental determinants such as air pollutants play significant roles in influencing the morphology and functionality of this epithelium to result in numerous potential respiratory disorders and complications that highlight its significance in general pulmonary wellness. Modeling and characterization of the respiratory epithelium are crucial in understanding disease mechanisms and treatment interventions.

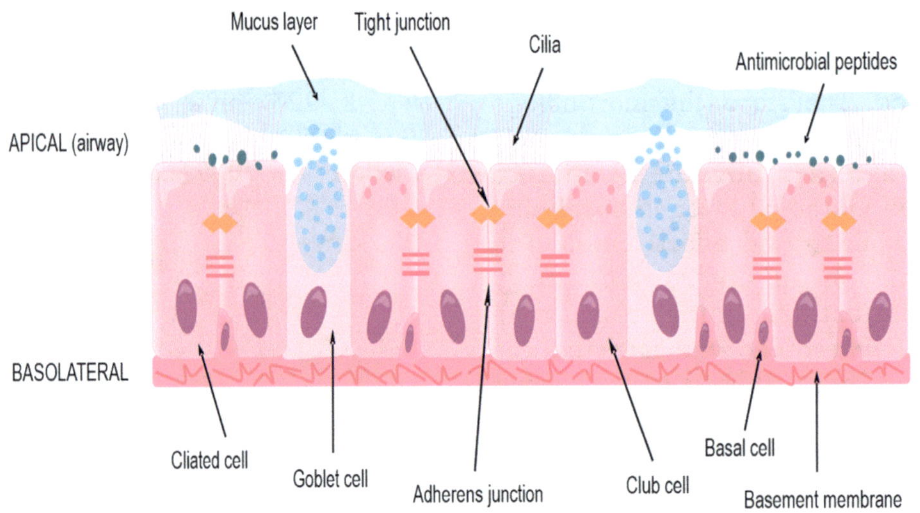

Figure 3.15. Respiratory epithelium.

Source: https://www.mdpi.com/ijms/ijms-21-08907/article_deploy/html/images/ijms-21-08907-g001.png.

The current technical advancements in cell culture techniques, particularly the use of air-liquid interface (ALI) culture, have enabled more accurate modeling of *in vivo* environments. One study using differentiated ovine tracheal epithelial cells confirmed the development of a pseudo-stratified epithelium with evidence of ciliary differentiation over an extended time course. This model presented a substantial increase in cell layer thickness and functionality as evidenced by rising trans-epithelial electrical resistance (TEER), an index of robust barrier formation. The ability to maintain the structural integrity and function of the respiratory epithelium *in vitro* enables extended experimentation with disease models, allowing scientists to examine pathological processes within this layer and to improve understanding of respiratory health and disease mechanisms (Berry et al., 2017). The respiratory epithelium is also the primary point of entry for many pathogens and is thus critical that its behavior with viral agents is known in minute detail. For instance, studies with porcine reproductive and respiratory syndrome virus (PRRSV) have documented discrete pathogenesis processes via polarized nasal mucosa explants. More significantly, disparity in virulence among strains defines discrete replication efficacies within the epithelial microenvironment; subtype 3 PRRSV strain demonstrated greater tropism compared to the less virulent subtype 1 strain. These findings reveal that the respiratory epithelium not only provides a barrier against toxic substances but also participates in viral entry and viral replication. This phenomenon testifies to the importance of understanding respiratory epithelial functional morphology in the course of infectious diseases, a thought-provoking exploration of potential therapeutic targets and prophylactic interventions (Cao et al., 2013) (Figure 3.15).

3.5. Microscopic Techniques for Studying Epithelial Morphology

Epithelial morphology has benefited greatly from advances in microscopy, which enable researchers to visualize intricate structures at the cellular level. Techniques such as light microscopy allow viewing of the cell arrangements and tissue architecture, providing valuable information about the structural function of the epithelia. Light microscopy is designed to enable one to ascertain morphological characteristics, i.e., cell shape and layering, which are basic in the distinction of different classes of epithelial tissues, i.e., simple and stratified tissues. In addition, immunocytochemistry, which uses antibodies to detect specific proteins, enhances the investigation of epithelial cells by illuminating their functional characteristics—such as the expression of surface markers associated with specific epithelial functions—and highlighting their physiological behavior under various conditions (Bácsy et al., 2005). Aside from the light microscope, electron microscopy, including scanning and transmission electron microscopy, is vital to the investigation of the ultrastructure of epithelial tissues. These techniques provide resolution that is unprecedented to enable one to see subcellular elements, such as organelles and cytoplasmic features, that are not visible with traditional light microscopy. Transmission electron microscopy, for instance, can identify the fine pattern of cell junctions and microvilli that characterize epithelial surfaces. Such high-resolution studies not only contribute to the appreciation of normal epithelial architecture but also to the identification of pathological changes in disease tissue. This is particularly beneficial in classification and studies of diseases like cancers, where the morphology may vary quite significantly from what is known to be normal patterns (Nishi., 1978). The application of culture techniques supplemented with microscopic examinations further enriches studies in epithelial morphology. Through the generation of primary cultures of cells from epithelial tissues, researchers can stock and conduct experiments on cells to observe changes in morphology over time. These cultures provide a dynamic system for the examination of epithelial cell responses to various stimuli, including hormonal signals and environmental insults. Monolayer cultures have been shown to maintain the physiological properties of epithelial cells, thereby serving as models for *in vitro* studies (Bácsy et al., 2005). Moreover, advances in imaging technologies, particularly live-cell imaging, have begun to expose the dynamic processes of epithelial cells in wound healing and tissue regeneration in recent years. Therefore, these microscopic methods overall enhance our understanding of epithelial tissue morphology, both fundamentally and for clinical use (Figure 3.16).

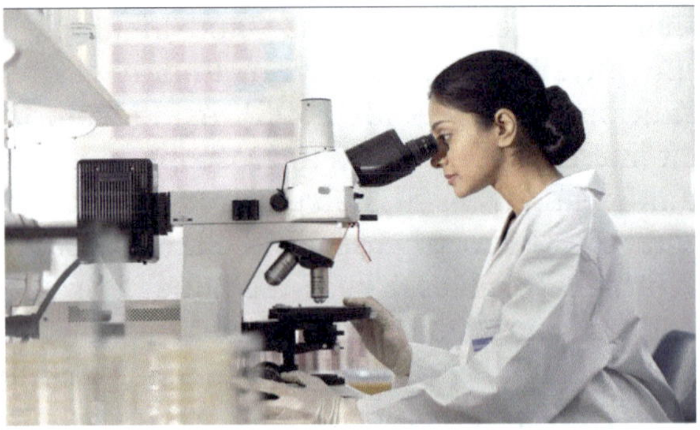

Figure 3.16. Microscopic techniques for studying epithelial morphology.

Source: https://cdn.shopify.com/s/files/1/0401/5452/9953/articles/ezgif.com-resize_1_6c94de05-8805-4bcb-bbdf-8cdfcbb151e7_1024x460.jpg?v=1592348469.

3.5.1. Light Microscopy

Light microscopy is a primary tool for studying the morphology of epithelial tissues, enabling accurate analysis of their characteristics. It allows researchers to observe the cellular pattern and structure of epithelial cells and learn about their functional relevance in organs. Through techniques such as immunocytochemistry and staining, one cellular component can be highlighted, unlocking valuable information on differentiation as well as pathology. As a case of cell cultures of pituitary adenoma, light microscopy has proved useful to study the morphology and endocrine activity of epithelial cells, thus gaining information that can be beneficial both to diagnostic and to therapeutic applications in oncological and neuroendocrinological research (Bácsy et al., 2005). The versatility of light microscopy is also utilized in examining tissue cultures from animal models, such as in bladder cancer. Tissue cultures derived from rat bladder tumors have a typical morphology that can be documented and examined using light microscopy. These experiments not only offer insight into the progression of cancerous alterations but also allow for comparison between normal and pathological conditions within epithelial tissues. For example, identification of microvillous density changes and alterations in cellular patterns can reveal significant information about tumor behavior and cellular interaction (Nishi., 1978). Light microscopy thus allows for the identification of subtle changes characteristic of malignancy, providing a visual framework for understanding epithelial tissue pathology. The morphology information obtained using light microscopy also contributes to the general understanding of epithelial tissue function. Epithelial sheets are interfaces and barriers in numerous biological systems, and their shape is directly associated with their purpose. For example, cellular orientation as well as the existence of specialized structures such as cilia or microvilli contribute to the efficiency of absorption, secretion, and protection as intrinsic to epithelial tissues. A detailed examination of these features by light microscopy provides a platform for correlating morphology and function, further underscoring that structure dictates cellular processes. Furthermore, with the integration of light microscopy with other imaging techniques, scientists are able to obtain a comprehensive image of epithelial tissues, bridging the gap between microscopic images and functional consequences during health and disease (Figure 3.17).

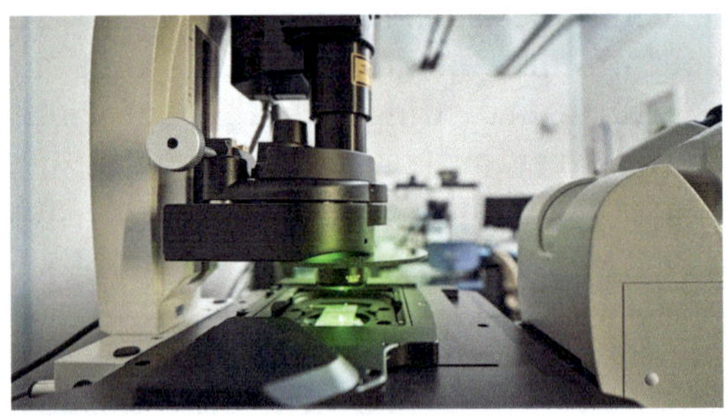

Figure 3.17. Light microscopy.

Source: https://media-cdn.oulu.fi/styles/main_image/s3/images/Biocenter_LightMicroscopy_MTO0750_HiRes.jpg?itok=6yiu3iKY.

3.5.2. Electron Microscopy

Morphology of epithelial tissue has been significantly enhanced by electron microscopy research, particularly in unveiling the ultrastructural aspects that are crucial in understanding the functional features of various epithelial cells. Electron microscopy provides far better resolution than regular light microscopy because it can display structures at the nanometer scale. This added definition permits examination of such cell features as microvilli, necessary to secure maximum surface area and absorption in intestinal epithelial cells, and junctional complexes that maintain tissue integrity and communication. Using techniques such as transmission electron microscopy (TEM) and scanning electron microscopy (SEM), researchers can describe the intricate architecture of epithelial tissues, thereby facilitating improved morphological and related pathological examination. Electron microscopy is a crucial diagnostic tool and technique for understanding various diseases of epithelial tissues in clinics. Therefore, with this approach, researchers have observed adenoma cells from pituitary tumors based on their morphological characteristics and ultrastructural details that distinguish the different tumor types. Detailed morphological analysis by electron microscopy helps pathologists relate in vitro findings to tissue biopsies, as in a study in which the viability and morphological characteristics of cultured adenoma cells were examined based on their histopathological appearances. These findings are a perfect example of how electron microscopy not only facilitates the diagnostic process but is also beneficial for generating directed therapeutic intervention based on the morphological data generated through patients' epithelial tissues (Bácsy et al., 2005). Moreover, the role of electron microscopy is not limited to diagnostic utility; it also facilitates understanding of the biological behavior of epithelial cells in various pathological conditions. For example, studies using a rat bladder cancer model illustrated the widespread alteration in the morphology of epithelial cells, e.g., keratinization, and the alteration in microvillus arrangements, as seen with scanning electron microscopy. These observations of nuclear-to-cytoplasmic ratios and cytoplasmic structure indicate the utility of electron microscopy in understanding the development and nature of epithelial carcinomas. By visualizing these changes at the ultrastructural level, researchers can gain critical information regarding tumor behavior and potential therapeutic targets, further solidifying the role of electron microscopy in the understanding of epithelial tissue morphology (Nishi., 1978).

3.5.3. Staining Techniques

Staining protocols are at the core of the understanding of epithelial tissue morphology because they provide valuable information about the structural and functional characteristics of cells. Different staining protocols can distinguish between different epithelial tissue components, uncovering concealed details of unstained tissues. This includes Hematoxylin and Eosin (H&E) staining, a commonly used method that highlights the contrast between cell nuclei and cytoplasm, thereby facilitating visualization of tissue architecture. Advanced techniques like Periodic Acid-Schiff (PAS) staining are particularly helpful for glycoprotein and mucin visualization in epithelial tissues, thus illuminating secreted cell functions in maintaining mucosal function and integrity. The choice of staining technique can directly influence the interpretation of morphological features, subsequently affecting conclusions drawn from histological evaluation of various epithelia. In addition to standard histological stains, immunohistochemistry has revolutionized the examination of epithelial tissue structure by allowing for the specific localisation of proteins in tissues. By attaching detectable tags to antibodies recognising target epitopes, researchers can quantify the expression of proteins at the centre of epithelial function, such as keratins and adhesion molecules. Such specificity enables one to comprehend tissue differentiation and cellular response to pathology more effectively. For instance, the study of ciliated epithelial cells in the respiratory tract widely employs immunostaining to identify markers associated with mucus secretion and ciliary function. These approaches are essential for determining how epithelial tissues become responsive to environmental stressors and develop pathologies, thereby informing normal function and disease, as established by studies using airway epithelial models (Berry et al., 2017). Additionally, the evolution of imaging methods has supplemented traditional staining techniques, enabling more advanced analysis of epithelial morphology. Techniques such as confocal microscopy enhance the resolution of stained tissue sections so that scientists are able to view subcellular structures in record resolution. Moreover, the pairing of fluorescent staining with high-resolution imaging techniques allows for studies of dynamic events such as cell migration and growth in epithelial layers. The ability to follow the reaction of epithelial cells to damage or stimulation is fundamental for learning about a variety of diseases, including cancers and chronic inflammatory conditions. As demonstrated through histological analyses of liver epithelial cells, delicate staining methods not only detect cellular architecture but also reflect functional alteration in response to pathologic change, demonstrating the importance of staining methods in epithelial tissue research (Masuji et al., 1974).

3.6. Pathological Changes in Epithelial Tissue

Pathologic alterations in epithelial tissue have a tendency to reflect underlying disease mechanisms that can influence health significantly. These changes are typically picked up by various diagnostic tests, one of which is optical coherence tomography (OCT). OCT is a non-invasive imaging technique that provides high-resolution cross-sectional images of tissue structure, which allows clinicians to differentiate between normal and pathological conditions with reasonable accuracy. With OCT, five important structures of the tissue were evaluated, which included the basement membrane and the keratin cell layer. By this method, the scientists had shown incredible accuracy at identifying the structural changes with a correct detection rate of 93.5% for the epithelial layer and 94% for the basement membrane, indicating the efficacy of OCT in the detection of oral disorders at early stages. Hence, the importance of identifying such pathological alterations becomes crucial since these are markers of early intervention and management strategies in clinical practice (Al-Delayme et al., 2012). Cell-cell interactions in epithelial tissues are complex and can be modeled to better understand their emergent properties under pathological conditions. Developments in computational modeling, such as agent-based models, facilitate this by modeling cellular interactions and biological processes. These models bridge the behavior of biological cells and software agents so that researchers can explore how changes in environmental conditions, for example, calcium levels, influence tissue morphology and patterns of cell growth. Indeed, this method has reported a qualitative correspondence between simulated growth patterns and *in vitro* cell models, indicating that computational paradigms can be a valuable asset for identifying cellular responses to pathological stimuli. By explaining cell behavior dynamics and their implications for epithelial tissue integrity, these models can be of use to offer a comprehensive overview of disease mechanisms (Hill et al., 2004). Explanation of pathological changes in epithelial tissues not only directs diagnostic maneuvers but also allows for the investigation of potential therapeutic approaches. Recognition of subtle changes, such as dysplasia or hyperplasia, aids in grading disease, particularly in oncology, where epithelial tissues are most often affected by malignancies. As an example, discrimination among various pathologies with the assistance of OCT has been discovered to provide a rich paradigm to understand disease development. The ability to classify and assess alterations in epithelial tissues is extremely useful in providing critical insights towards the development of targeted therapies. Moreover, the integration of advanced imaging techniques with computational modeling can enhance our insight into how epithelial cells respond to pathological stress, thereby enhancing clinical outcomes. Such an integrated approach underscores the need to maintain research on the morphological characteristics of epithelial tissues, as these play a pivotal role in health and disease management (Figure 3.18).

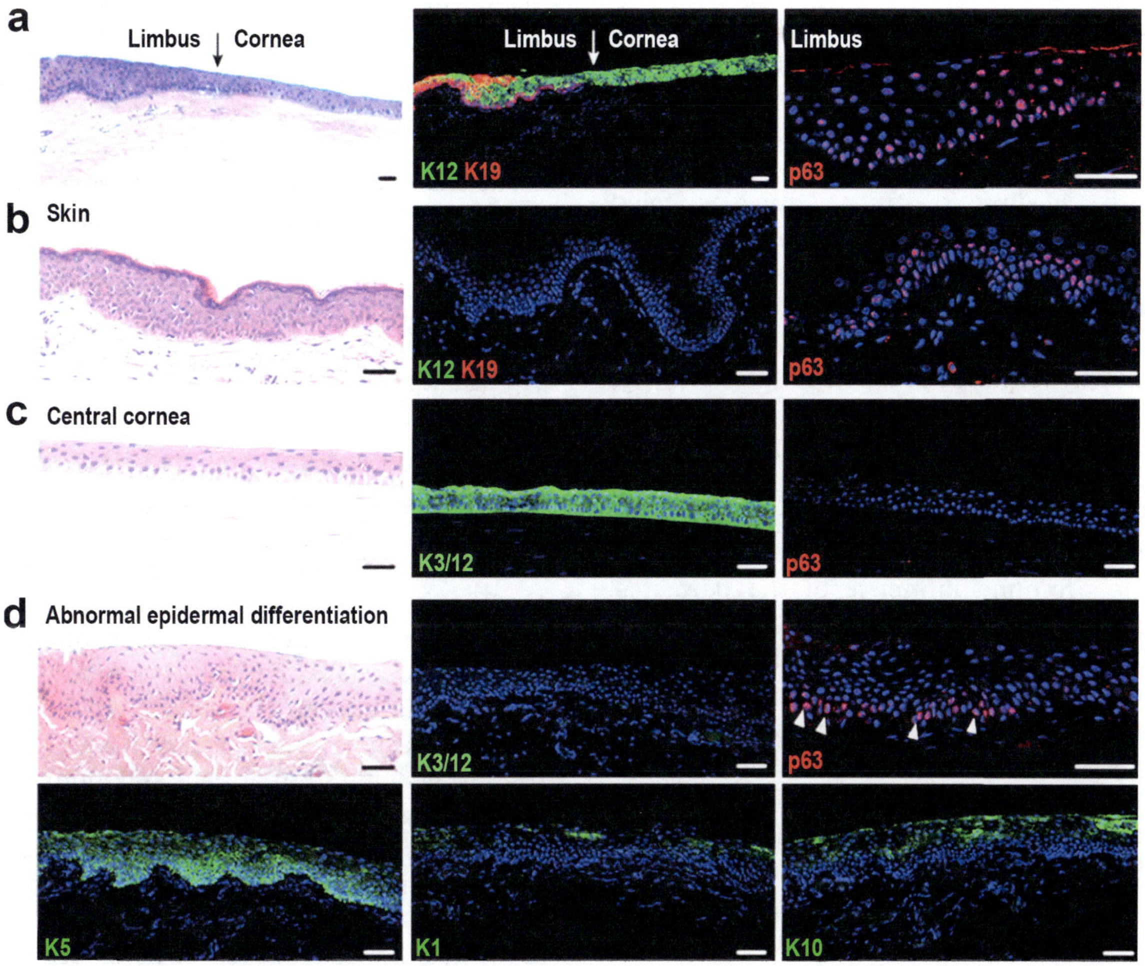

Figure 3.18. Pathological changes in epithelial tissue.

Source: https://www.researchgate.net/profile/Meixia-Zhang-4/publication/264056121/figure/fig4/AS:279022006226972@1443535438735/Normal-and-pathological-changes-of-corneal-epithelium-and-its-comparison-to-skin-a.png.

3.6.1. Hyperplasia

Hyperplasia, a cell-growing process that involves more cells in a tissue, is critical to maintaining and regulating epithelial integrity. Hyperplasia, referring to epithelial tissue morphology, typically refers to the body's response to stimuli that demand more cellular activity or repair procedures. The condition may take place as a physiological process, such as compensatory hyperplasia in the liver's regeneration following partial hepatectomy, or as a pathological characteristic in diseases such as chronic inflammation and neoplasia. The intricate balance between cell proliferation and apoptosis is instrumental in the normal function of tissues so that hyperplastic alterations do not result in malignancy. Study of these changes in epithelial tissues is critical to understand varying states of health and direct treatment strategies aimed at the restoration of normal tissue structure. In pathological hyperplasia, hormonal action and chronic inflammation are pertinent considerations. Gastric epithelium, for instance, can undergo extensive hyperplastic reaction to infection, e.g., that induced by the gastric nematode *Ostertagia ostertagi*. It has been shown by research that the developing cellular hyperplasia is attributable to enhanced transcriptional activity of signaling molecules governing epithelial cell homeostasis and the profound influence of the parasites' excretory/secretory products on gastric mucosa morphology. Inhibition of parietal cell function and consequent elevation in gastric pH also illustrates the sophistication of hyperplastic responses in that the body is attempting to acclimatize these foreign intruders as well as address its own homeostatic problems (Chiers et al., 2013). Hyperplasia is not simply a pathophysiological response; it is also a vital component of developmental biology. Implications from murine models with some relevance to human epithelial formation emphasize the significance of organogenesis in hyperplastic processes. For example, in the embryonic development of the male and female reproductive tracts, hyperplastic patterns are critical in dictating morphogenesis under the control of biological signals. While there are commonalities between murine and human developmental pathways, researchers must be cautious about disparities when making inferences across animal models and human biology (Baskin et al., 2019). This nuanced awareness of hyperplasia in epithelial tissues not only provides greater insight into normal physiology but also signifies the threshold to disease states.

3.6.2. Dysplasia

Dysplasia is a notable morphologic alteration in epithelial tissue, characterized by abnormal growth and maturation of cells. Dysplasia is a useful diagnostic sign, typically indicating an early neoplastic or precancerous state. Dysplastic tissue changes are expressed as abnormalities in cell form, size, and arrangement, which distort the normal architecture of epithelial layers. Studies using advanced imaging modalities, such as optical coherence tomography (OCT), have assisted in explaining these aberrations by illuminating the cellular structure involved. Specifically, OCT has been effective in distinguishing between dysplastic and regular tissues as well as pathological and regular tissues, highlighting the importance of identifying dysplastic alterations as a method for early detection of disease (Al-Delayme et al., 2012). This functionality is significant in clinical practice since early detection tends to lead to improved patient outcomes for dysplastic lesions. The effects of dysplasia go beyond its significance in diagnosis; they have significant roles to play in the treatment and monitoring of disease. Dysplasia, for instance, has a significant role in assessing the likelihood of developing into malignancy in the gastrointestinal tract, particularly for colorectal tissues. Rectal lesions identified on procedures such as endoscopic submucosal dissection (ESD) are usually subjected to histopathologic examination to determine the presence of dysplasia and the extent thereof. Existing evidence substantiates there to be a relationship between dysplastic changes and submucosal invasive cancer potential, necessitating careful follow-up in patients with such lesions (Aadam et al., 2019). This relationship not only influences clinical practice in management but also emphasizes the necessity of ongoing research in creating more accurate algorithms for the diagnosis of dysplastic tissues. Furthermore, the term dysplasia is used in numerous organ systems, such as oral, cervical, and cutaneous epithelia, each with a distinct specific clinical implication. For instance, dysplastic changes in oral tissues can be precursors of oral squamous cell carcinoma and therefore require thorough evaluation and, if indicated, treatment. The morphologic dysplastic changes of abnormal keratinocyte maturation and basement membrane integrity impairment can be adequately characterized with techniques like OCT, enhancing the specificity of dysplastic lesion identification (Al-Delayme et al., 2012). Increased understanding of dysplasia in epithelial tissue morphology is key to developing novel therapeutic options and improving early detection methods, ultimately informing patient prognoses across the various presentations of dysplasia.

3.6.3. Carcinoma

The study of carcinoma in relation to epithelial tissue morphology reveals the intricate changes at the cellular and architectural levels in cases where malignant conversions are made. Carcinomas, which originate from epithelial cells, typically exhibit cellular morphologic changes characterized by increased nuclear-to-cytoplasmic ratios, disorganized mitotic forms, and alterations in cellular pattern. Such morphological changes are significant in that they might indicate the degree of dysregulation and invasiveness of tumor cells. Cell atypia in carcinoma typically involves loss of contact inhibition, whereby transformed cells proliferate without restraint, leading to aberrant tissue architecture and a tendency to form tumor masses. This finding reaffirms the importance of understanding the basic morphological characteristics of epithelial neoplasia in diagnosis and treatment. The study of such characteristics tells us about the mechanisms by which carcinoma cells are able to become invasive, which is crucial for tumor development. One distinguishing characteristic is the role of molecular factors such as scatter factor, which can promote the invasiveness of carcinoma cells through its influence on cell motility and adhesion. In model systems, the scatter factor has been shown to promote epithelial cell invasiveness, increasing their ability to penetrate basement membranes and surrounding tissues. The invasive phenotype is typically accompanied by profound alterations in adhesion molecule expression, which further enhance the malignant properties of carcinoma cells. The interactive dynamics between these morphological changes and molecular cues shine light on the complexity of cancer formation, revealing routes that can be intercepted for therapeutic purposes in order to halt tumor invasiveness and metastasis. Additionally, the convergence of cellular and molecular data into carcinoma research calls attention to the necessity for ongoing studies in the morphology of epithelial tissues. With the findings of new facets of the way carcinoma cells display their malignant nature, it is essential that we enhance our understanding of the biological markers and the genetic determinants of the tumors. For instance, derivation of carcinoma *in vitro* cell lines can provide valuable models to explore neoplastic behavior and drug sensitivity. As illustrated in the research of cell lines from rat bladder tumors, the investigation of chromosomal abnormalities and aberrant cell behavior can provide more insight into carcinoma biology. By examining these features, we can develop more effective mechanisms of early detection, targeted therapy, and ultimately improve the patient prognosis in epithelial-derived cancers, influencing cancer treatment and research prognosis to a large degree.

SUMMARY

In conclusion, the intricate morphology of epithelial tissue reflects its diverse functions across organ systems. Epithelial cells are pivotal to protective barriers, absorption, secretion, and sensation, and form the foundation of physiological processes and structural integrity. The range of epithelial forms—simple squamous to stratified cuboidal—reflects an evolutionary adaptation to distinct functional demands imposed on various tissues. This diversity is not only anatomical but also involves complex biochemical mechanisms and regulatory processes, which in turn influence tissue structure and behavior. By comprehension of these morphological aspects, researchers can gain some understanding of the significance of epithelial function in physiology to health and disease. Furthermore, the refinement of histological techniques has enhanced our understanding of epithelial morphology, and significant observations across species, including humans and domestic animals, have been made. For instance, studies of the dairy cow mammary gland illustrate how deviations in involution can lead to histological changes that are not observed elsewhere in mammals. Such findings point to the necessity of incorporating modern-day agricultural practices into the evaluation of epithelial health because they inadvertently shape epithelial form and function. This highlights a critical juncture between veterinary medicine and human health, that the same will prove to be true for lactating human females regarding breast cancer risk, as has been noted by Anug et al. (2007). Lastly, recent research into steroidogenic potential in epithelial tissues, as indicated by the presence of such enzymes as P450c17 and P450aromatase, may yield important insights into local hormonal regulation. The dynamic pattern of these enzymes along various phases of the estrous cycle not only elucidates our understanding of reproductive biology but also has relevance for epithelial proliferation as well as differentiation. By examining how local steroid synthesis interacts with environmental and endogenous factors, researchers can disassemble the complexity of epithelial morphogenesis. The findings from such research not only enhance our knowledge of epithelial tissue but also suggest the potential for new therapeutic approaches to managing disorders related to epithelial dysfunction, as indicated by ongoing research (Neto et al., 2017).

The intricate morphology of epithelial tissues is pivotal to their activities in many organ systems. Epithelial cells are deeply specialized, with structures changing in accordance with position and physiological requirements. For instance, ovine tracheal epithelial differentiation in air-liquid interface culture illustrates extreme cellular responses to stimuli like epidermal growth factor (EGF) and retinoic acid (RA). EGF induces thickening of the epithelium and enhances ciliation, which is vital for the respiratory epithelium's mucociliary clearance function. Growth conditions, such as substrate pore density and oxygen concentration, can further optimize the epithelial phenotype, underscoring the necessity of specific culture environments for effective in vitro modeling of respiratory function (Berry et al., 2018). Besides growth factors, the plasticity of epithelial tissues has the highest importance in studying how they react to pathological states. Their capacity to acquire transitions, like EMT, highlights their versatility. Pharmacological modulation similar to what has been employed for human keratinocytes counteracted TGF-β-induced EMT in a form integral for fibrotic disease and cancer development. The identification of small molecule modulators, such as LXR agonists, illustrates the ability to manipulate the key pathways to alter epithelial behaviors. This not only identifies mechanisms underlying tissue plasticity but also suggests therapeutic applications for preventing malignancies and fibrosis (Bellomo et al., 2016). Epithelial tissue morphology extends beyond rudimentary biological processes; it encompasses key elements for disease prevention as well as for treatment interventions. The novel structure of epithelial cells gives them the ability to act as barriers, undergo absorption, and contribute to tissue signal pathways. Moreover, studies of conditions that promote maximal epithelial differentiation provide greater insight into their role in maintaining homeostasis. Environmental and cellular interactions in epithelial systems show the potential for therapeutic intervention in epithelial injury or disease responses. By elucidating significant developmental and pathological issues, we underscore the importance of epithelial tissue morphology as a top priority in both scholarly research and clinical practice.

A LOOK TO THE FUTURE:

CARCINOGEN-INDUCED BLADDER CANCER:

Carcinogen-induced bladder cancer represents a significant and well-characterized subset of malignancies in the urinary bladder that arise from long-term exposure to environmental, occupational, and lifestyle-associated carcinogens. Bladder cancer itself is the tenth most common cancer worldwide, with its etiology strongly linked to accrued genetic damage in urothelial cells that disrupts normal growth control and leads to uncontrolled proliferation and tumor formation. Much of this damage results not from random processes but from repeated exposure to specific carcinogenic agents that enter the body, are metabolically activated, and interact with bladder epithelium over time.

A key feature of carcinogen-induced bladder cancer is the role of chemical exposures that form DNA adducts, cause oxidative damage, and interfere with DNA repair mechanisms in urothelial cells. Aromatic amines, such as β-naphthylamine and 4-aminobiphenyl, historically identified in tobacco smoke and industrial dyes, are among the most studied bladder carcinogens. These compounds undergo metabolic activation in the liver and renal system, resulting in reactive intermediates that bind to DNA and inflict mutations, particularly in critical genes like TP53 and other tumor suppressor loci. Environmental contaminants such as polycyclic aromatic hydrocarbons (PAHs), nitrosamines, arsenic and chlorinated solvents further contribute to this process through similar genotoxic pathways, including oxidative stress and promotion of epigenetic dysregulation.

Lifestyle factors, especially tobacco smoking, remain the most significant modifiable risk factor for bladder cancer globally, accounting for a substantial proportion of cases. Combustion of tobacco generates a complex mixture of carcinogens that are absorbed, metabolized systemically, and eventually excreted in the urine, prolonging contact with the bladder mucosa and enhancing carcinogenic exposure. Occupational exposures, historically observed in workers in dye, rubber, and chemical industries, reflect the dramatic impact of carcinogen contact over decades, highlighting how repeated, chronic exposure elevates cancer risk far beyond that of the general population.

The molecular pathogenesis of carcinogen-induced bladder cancer is inherently multistep: DNA adduct formation, accumulation of somatic mutations, disruptions in cell cycle control, and alterations in gene expression all contribute to malignant transformation. As these changes accrue, the urothelial cells progress from normal epithelium through premalignant stages to full-blown carcinoma, characterised by genomic instability and dysregulated growth signalling.

Understanding the mechanisms of carcinogen-induced bladder cancer has profound implications for prevention, early detection, and intervention. Targeted risk reduction efforts—such as smoking cessation and occupational safety measures—combine with molecular profiling to identify at-risk individuals and potential biomarkers for early disease. Continued research also explores how host factors, including genetic susceptibility and metabolic enzyme polymorphisms, modulate individual risk and response to carcinogenic exposures.

REFERENCES

1. Yang, D., Aihara, H., Perbtani, Y. B., Wang, A. Y., Aadam, A. A., Tomizawa, Y., Hwang, J. H., Zou, B., Natov, N. S., Siegel, A., Khoshknab, M. P., Khashab, M. A., Ngamruengphong, S., Khara, H. S., Diehl, D. L., Maniere, T., Andrawes, S., Benias, P., Kumta, N. A., . . . Draganov, P. V. (2019). Safety and efficacy of endoscopic submucosal dissection for rectal neoplasia: a multicenter North American experience. *Endoscopy International Open*, *07*(12), E1714–E1722. https://doi.org/10.1055/a-1010-5663Al-Delayme, R., Hamdoon, Z., Hopper, C., Jay, et al. (2012). Structural validation of oral mucosal tissue using optical coherence tomography. https://core.ac.uk/download/16220461.pdf (accessed on 6th August 2025).
2. Alcazar-Fuoli, L., Armstrong-James, D., Bertuzzi, M., Bignell, et al. (2014). The pH-responsive PacC transcription factor of *Aspergillus fumigatus* governs epithelial entry and tissue invasion during pulmonary aspergillosis. https://core.ac.uk/download/30435716.pdf (accessed on 6th August 2025).
3. Altshuler, A. E., Kurre, L., Lamadrid, I., Li, et al. (2014). Transmural intestinal wall permeability in severe ischemia after enteral protease inhibition. https://core.ac.uk/download/323065462.pdf (accessed on 6th August 2025).
4. Anug, A.-M., Leitner, G., Silanikove, N., Merin, U. (2007). Pregnancy obstructs involution Stage II of the mammary gland in cows: General biological implications. https://core.ac.uk/download/pdf/287474.pdf (accessed on 6th August 2025).
5. Arafa, E. (2016). Determining cellular and biochemical function of a novel adhesion molecule in kidneys. https://open.bu.edu/bitstream/2144/16062/1/Arafa_bu_0017N_11077.pdf (accessed on 6th August 2025).
6. Arredondo, J., Cortopassi, G., Crakes, K. R., Dandekar, et al. (2019). PPARα-targeted mitochondrial bioenergetics mediate repair of intestinal barriers at the host-microbe intersection during SIV infection. https://core.ac.uk/download/323071923.pdf (accessed on 6th August 2025).
7. Assis Neto, A. C., Conley, A. J., de Oliveira, M. F., Dos Santos, et al. (2017). Immunolocalization of steroidogenic enzymes in the vaginal mucous of *Galea spixii* during the estrous cycle. https://core.ac.uk/download/323070725.pdf (accessed on 6th August 2025).
8. Bácsy, E., Bálint, K., Fazekas, I., Hegedűs, et al. (2005). Characterization of human pituitary adenomas in cell cultures by light and electron microscopic morphology and immunolabeling. https://core.ac.uk/download/11856052.pdf (accessed on 6th August 2025).
9. Baskin, L. S., Cao, M., Cunha, G. R., Ricke, et al. (2019). Reproductive tract biology: Of mice and men. https://core.ac.uk/download/323311356.pdf (accessed on 6th August 2025).
10. Bauer, E., Metzler-Zebeli, B. U., Mosenthin, R., Verstegen, et al. (2011). Intestinal gene expression in pigs: Effects of reduced feed intake during weaning and potential impact of dietary components. https://core.ac.uk/download/pdf/29230036.pdf (accessed on 6th August 2025).
11. Behrens, J., Birchmeier, W., Vandekerckhove, J., Weidner, et al. (1990). Scatter factor: Molecular characteristics and effect on the invasiveness of epithelial cells. https://core.ac.uk/download/237011392.pdf (accessed on 6th August 2025).
12. Bellomo, C., Bickle, M., Carthy, J. M., Gahman, et al. (2016). Chemical regulators of epithelial plasticity reveal a nuclear receptor pathway controlling myofibroblast differentiation. https://core.ac.uk/download/77017458.pdf (accessed on 6th August 2025).

13. Berry, C. C., Davies, R. L., O'Boyle, N., Sutherland, et al. (2017). Temporal dynamics of ovine airway epithelial cell differentiation at an air-liquid interface. https://core.ac.uk/download/84591468.pdf (accessed on 6th August 2025).
14. Bochsler, V. S., Galloway, S. B., Harley, R. A., Kramarsky-Winters, et al. (2007). *Coral Disease and Health Workshop: Coral Histopathology II.* https://core.ac.uk/download/11017972.pdf (accessed on 6th August 2025).
15. Borowsky, A. D., Cardiff, R. D., Hovey, R. C., Manjarin, et al. (2015). Neoplastic transformation of porcine mammary epithelial cells in vitro and tumor formation in vivo. https://core.ac.uk/download/323070390.pdf (accessed on 6th August 2025).
16. Boucheron, L. E., Can, A., Gurcan, M. N., Madabhushi, et al. (2009). Histopathological image analysis: A review. https://core.ac.uk/download/46378.pdf (accessed on 6th August 2025).
17. Bown, J. L., Eberst, A., Falconer, R. E., Harrison, et al. (2012). Characterising the tumour morphological response to therapeutic intervention: An ex vivo model. https://core.ac.uk/download/228177071.pdf (accessed on 6th August 2025).
18. Cao, J., Frydas, I., Nauwynck, H., Verbeeck, et al. (2013). Replication characteristics of porcine reproductive and respiratory syndrome virus (PRRSV) European subtype 1 (Lelystad) and subtype 3 (Lena) strains in nasal mucosa and cells of the monocytic lineage: Indications for the use of new receptors of PRRSV (Lena). https://core.ac.uk/download/55798902.pdf (accessed on 6th August 2025).
19. Chatdarong, K. (2003). Reproductive physiology of the female cat. https://core.ac.uk/download/11694645.pdf (accessed on 6th August 2025).
20. Chen, S., Einspanier, R., Schoen, J. (2013). Long-term culture of primary porcine oviduct epithelial cells: Validation of a comprehensive in vitro model for reproductive science. https://core.ac.uk/download/288114161.pdf (accessed on 6th August 2025).
21. Chiers, K., Claerebout, E., Geldhof, P., Goddeeris, et al. (2013). Analysis of cell hyperplasia and parietal cell dysfunction induced by *Ostertagia ostertagi* infection. https://core.ac.uk/download/55847013.pdf (accessed on 6th August 2025).
22. Chuong, C.-M., Fraser, S., Serras, F. (1993). Asymmetric patterns of gap junctional communication in developing chicken skin. https://core.ac.uk/download/4894070.pdf (accessed on 6th August 2025).
23. Coenye, T., Crabbé, A., Davis, R., De La Fuente-Nùñez, et al. (2017). Antimicrobial efficacy against *Pseudomonas aeruginosa* biofilm formation in a three-dimensional lung epithelial model and the influence of fetal bovine serum. https://core.ac.uk/download/84047108.pdf (accessed on 6th August 2025).
24. Cokus, S. J., De La Torre, M., Medina, E. F., Ramirez-Gutierrez, et al. (2019). Tissue-specific transcriptomes reveal gene expression trajectories in two maturing skin epithelial layers in zebrafish embryos. https://core.ac.uk/download/323076243.pdf (accessed on 6th August 2025).
25. Evans, D. J., Fleiszig, S. M. J., Herzmark, P., LeDue, et al. (2011). 3D quantitative imaging of unprocessed live tissue reveals epithelial defense against bacterial adhesion and subsequent traversal requires MyD88. https://core.ac.uk/download/323080710.pdf (accessed on 6th August 2025).

26. Gong, X., Li, S., Liu, K., Wang, et al. (2017). Roles of TGFβ and FGF signals during growth and differentiation of mouse lens epithelial cell in vitro. https://core.ac.uk/download/323080961.pdf (accessed on 6th August 2025).

27. Gruhl, A. & Okamura, B. (2016). Development and myogenesis of the vermiform *Buddenbrockia* (*Myxozoa*) and implications for cnidarian body plan evolution. https://core.ac.uk/download/42046060.pdf (accessed on 6th August 2025).

28. Hill, G., Holcombe, M., Hose, D. R., Mac Neil, et al. (2004). The Epitheliome: Agent-based modelling of the social behaviour of cells. https://core.ac.uk/download/59287.pdf (accessed on 6th August 2025).

29. Liu, H. (2013). Interactions between dietary chicory, gut microbiota and immune responses. https://core.ac.uk/download/11698989.pdf (accessed on 6th August 2025).

30. Masszi, A., Eddy, A. A., Farris, A. B., Ivanov, A. I., Moreno, A. P., Angres, B., Hills, C. E., et al. (2013). 'Special K' and a loss of cell-to-cell adhesion in proximal tubule-derived epithelial cells: Modulation of the adherens junction complex by ketamine. https://core.ac.uk/download/20442678.pdf (accessed on 6th August 2025).

31. Masuji, H., Nakabayashi, H., Sato, J. (1974). Long-term cultivation of two diploid epithelial cell lines derived from normal rat liver cells. https://core.ac.uk/download/12547369.pdf (accessed on 6th August 2025).

32. Nishi, M. (1978). A cell line derived from BBN (N-butyl-N-[4-hydroxybutyl]-nitrosamine)-induced rat bladder cancer: Establishment and scanning electron microscopic cell surface characteristics. https://core.ac.uk/download/12548657.pdf (accessed on 6th August 2025).

33. Ravasio, A., Mertz, A. F., Clark, A. G., Edwards, A. M. J., Harris, A. R., Smeets, B., et al. (2019). Active wetting of epithelial tissues. http://arxiv.org/abs/1902.08871 (accessed on 6th August 2025).

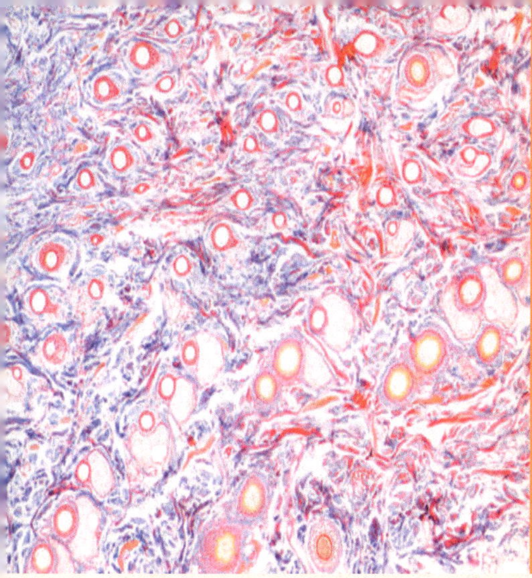

Chapter 4

CONNECTIVE TISSUE MORPHOLOGY

Contents

Introduction

Understanding the morphology of connective tissue is highly significant in the broader frame of biological science, particularly in the fields of histology and pathology. Connective tissue plays many significant roles, from structural support to energy storage and facilitating biological communication among cells. The variety of forms of connective tissue, ranging from loose to dense forms like tendons and ligaments, highlights the intricate relationships between form and function within the body. This morphology is not just the basis of normal physiological processes but can also be an indication of pathological conditions. While characterizing these features, researchers and medical professionals are able to gain some insight into tissue health, progression of a disease, and therapeutic approaches; this emphasizes the importance of connective tissue in preserving the overall integrity of the body. The specific proteins present in connective tissue confer its unique structure and function. For instance, Tnmd, a type II transmembrane protein, plays a critical role in dense connective tissues such as tendons and ligaments. It has also been found to be expressed in the PDL, but its timing and general functions of expression are not yet determined. Experiments have linked Tnmd's expression to developmental milestones, specifically tooth eruption, when mechanical stresses are placed in the surrounding tissues. Also, Tnmd modulation impacts cell adhesion in various cellular models, and this suggests that it plays a significant role in contributing to the maturation and maintenance of connective tissues. Such observations are fundamental for refining our knowledge of connective tissue morphology as well as its pathologic and physiological implications. In relation to systemic diseases, connective tissue morphology can be useful to offer insights into disease mechanisms and progression. For example, systemic sclerosis (SSc) is an autoimmune disorder characterized by significant changes in connective tissue, predominantly in the microvascular system. Nailfold microangiopathy, characterized by alterations in peripheral capillary morphology, is a significant disease marker that facilitates detection and assessment of disease progression at an early stage. Techniques such as nailfold videocapillaroscopy allow for up-close analysis of microvascular integrity to better elucidate capillary function in health and disease. The interplay between peripheral blood perfusion and connective tissue structure continues to be a rich area for study, particularly as newer imaging modalities advance our capacity to view and quantify these structural changes. These studies contribute to the literature on connective tissue morphology, how it correlates with global health outcomes and disease course (Figure 4.1).

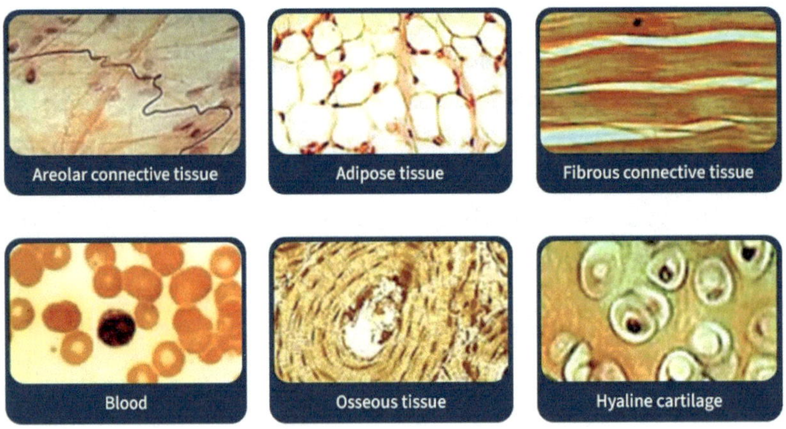

Figure 4.1. Connective tissue morphology.

Source: https://media.geeksforgeeks.org/wp-content/uploads/20240404111132/Diagram-of-Connective-Tissue.webp.

Definition of Connective Tissue

Connective tissue is a general feature of most biological systems and plays a critical role in providing structural support and facilitating intercellular communication. In its broad definition, connective tissue is a heterogeneous category of tissues comprising cells, fibers, and a ground substance that together bind, support, and defend other body tissues and organs. This tissue type is characterized by its varied shapes, ranging from loose connective tissue that fills the interosseous space between organs to dense connective tissues such as tendons and ligaments that withstand tensile stress. The composition and structure of connective tissue are critical determinants of its function, enabling it to accommodate the specific mechanical stresses exerted upon it in different anatomical settings. One of the most interesting aspects of connective tissue is that it is responsive to pathological changes. Such an example is systemic sclerosis, which results in profound morphological changes in connective tissue, arising from initial dysfunction of the microvascular system and subsequently affecting the tissue's overall function. Nailfold videocapillaroscopy is a technique of great importance in the evaluation of such vascular damage by allowing visualization of the morphology of capillaries, a very valuable disease progression predictor. Examining how connective tissue responds to environmental changes and disease provides insight into the mechanisms by which it maintains homeostasis and underpins repair.

Therefore, connective tissue morphology plays a central role in closing the gaps among function, structure, and pathology because it demonstrates how alterations at the cellular level have significant implications for overall tissue health. Furthermore, the interrelation between cellular behavior and mechanical properties in connective tissue is important to maintain physiological functions. Experiments have suggested that biophysical characteristics such as cell deformability and nuclear stiffness are important to regulate cell migration behavior in various microenvironments. This is more evident in tissue engineering, where scaffold-based constructs harness such physical characteristics to facilitate cell migration and incorporation. Observing cells navigate through constricted environments, such as those in diseased states or engineered matrices, underscores the extracellular matrix's role in regulating cellular processes. This knowledge gives not only our knowledge of connective tissue but also insight into pathways for therapeutic modalities aiming to control connective tissue dynamics to promote healing and regeneration in various clinical settings, as demonstrated through methods with cancer cell migration in remodeled extracellular settings (Preziosi et al., 2013; Cutolo et al., 2016).

Importance of Studying Connective Tissue Morphology

The structural architecture of connective tissue is important for understanding the architectural and functional complexities of most organs, particularly in developmental biology and clinical investigations. Connective tissues play vital roles in supporting and protecting organs and bring cellular function into the body. By examining the morphological characteristics of connective tissues, such as cellular organization and extracellular matrix structure, scientists can gain insight into fundamental biological processes in organogenesis and disease states. For instance, clarifying the distinct development of blood and lymphatic vessels in the pancreas underscores the importance of connective tissue architecture for organ function and overall physiology. These results are significant not only for basic science development but also for therapeutic intervention design in a very effective manner, particularly in the case of diseases such as diabetes, where the morphology of connective tissues governs metabolic health (Carlotti et al., 2014). Moreover, research in the morphology of connective tissues identifies major avenues for regenerative medicine, particularly concerning tissue repair and regeneration optimization. Advances in understanding how various elements of connective tissues, such as collagen and proteoglycans, construct tissue mechanics enable researchers to control them tactually. In diabetes, for example, the regeneration of beta cells that produce insulin relies heavily on a fine balance between the regeneration of the cells and the protective framework provided by connective tissues. Research on morphological changes in the pancreas during regeneration, such as those following pancreatic duct ligation, may inform techniques aimed at inducing tissue repair. The regenerative capacity underscores the significance of associative relationships within connective tissues and how they may have far-reaching consequences for the development of effective therapeutic regimens (Hao et al., 2013). Besides its use in regenerative medicine, understanding connective tissue morphology is also critical to understanding the pathogenesis of disease. Connective tissue architectural changes are typically observed with diseases such as fibrosis, arthritis, and vascular disease. By studying how connective tissues morphologically alter due to various stimuli—be it mechanical stress or pathological insults—it becomes feasible for scientists to obtain greater insight into disease mechanisms and validate putative therapeutic targets. For example, knowledge of the fact that particular collagen types are associated with tissue fibrotic responses can propel biomarker and therapeutic target discovery in chronic inflammatory disorders. Such information is crucial to the development of more specific and effective treatment strategies, maintaining the significant position of connective tissue morphology not only in health but in disease onset and recovery. Ultimately, the advancement of our knowledge in this field is of utmost importance for improving preventive and therapeutic interventions in healthcare.

Overview of Connective Tissue Types

Connective tissue is an integral component of the structure of the body and plays a significant role in the integrity and functioning of numerous systems. It is comprised primarily of extracellular matrix and other cell types and can be divided into several distinct types, including loose and dense connective tissue, supportive connective tissue, and specialized connective tissue. Loose areolar connective tissue, made up of adipose and reticular tissue, provides organs with cushioning and support, along with supporting the exchange of nutrients and waste between cells and blood vessels. Dense connective tissue, however, in ligaments and tendons, provides strength and resistance to stretching so structures can withstand mechanical stress. Understanding these categories allows for greater insight into the versatility of form and function of connective tissue in the organism. Supportive connective tissue consists of cartilage and bone, the fundamental structural elements of the skeleton. Cartilage, which is flexible and resilient, provides support to all joints and the respiratory system, and yet allows for smooth movement. Cartilage is a type of connective tissue that varies in form, including hyaline, fibrocartilage, and elastic cartilage, each designed to meet specific functional demands. Bone is a dense, mineralized, and rigid tissue that supports the body, encloses important organs, and acts as a storehouse of minerals. Bone is dynamic and undergoes continuous remodeling and reorganization to meet physiological needs, which is essential for maintaining skeletal health in its optimal state. The cartilage-bone interaction is a prime illustration of the fine structure of bone-supportive connective tissue, specifically highlighting its vital roles in homeostasis and biomechanics. Specialized connective tissues such as blood and lymph play a pivotal role in the transport of nutrients, gases, and wastes in various parts of the body. Blood, made up of its unique fluid matrix of plasma and cells, facilitates the exchange of oxygen and carbon dioxide and is a chief organ of immune functions. The morphology of red blood cells and leukocytes is altered to their functions in defense and circulation. Lymph, a specialized connective tissue, participates in the return of interstitial fluid to the bloodstream and aids fluid balance and immune monitoring. All these specialized connective tissues combined illustrate the diversity that occurs in connective tissue types and structure to function, directly impacting different physiological processes. The intricate architecture of connective tissues is responsible for their role in regulating health and disease within the overall plan of connective tissue morphology.

4.1. Types of Connective Tissue

Connective tissue is an essential component of the body's structural support and intercellular communication. It has been classified into different types, with most falling into the categories of loose and dense connective tissues. Loose connective tissue, such as areolar tissue, is characterized by loose fibers and extensive ground substance to facilitate flexibility and cushioning. This is found beneath epithelial layers and surrounding organs, allowing the passage of nutrients and serving as a reservoir for salts and water. The dense connective tissue, to which tendons and ligaments belong, consists of closely packed collagen fibers that give it strength and resistance to stretch. Variations in fiber organization and concentration contribute significantly to tissue function, underscoring the importance of connective tissue morphology in maintaining the integrity of various body structures. Specialized connective tissue is another large group, including adipose, cartilage, and blood tissue. Adipose tissue is not only an energy-storage reservoir but also an insulator and a cushion for organs, underscoring its multifunctional role in thermoregulation and protection against mechanical stress.

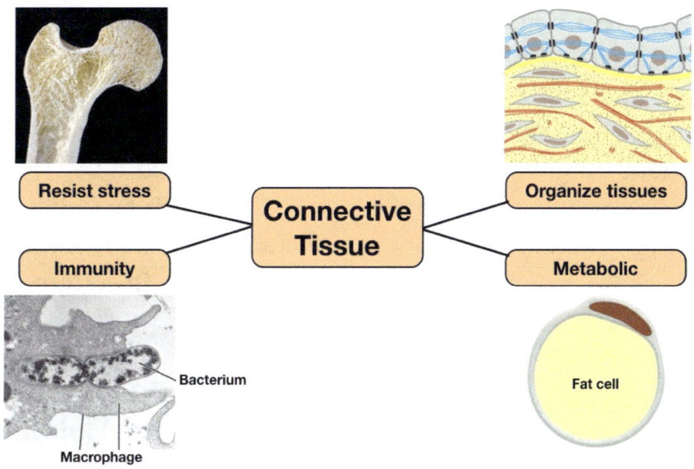

Figure 4.2. Types of connective tissue.

Source: https://yalehistology.s3.us-east-2.amazonaws.com/connective_tissue/connective_tissue_types.jpg.

Cartilage, another specialized tissue, is resilient yet flexible and supports structures such as joints and the respiratory system. Cartilage is avascular, receiving nutrients by diffusion only, which accounts for its slow healing. Blood, a fluid connective tissue, consists of cells in suspension within plasma and is essential for the transport of oxygen, nutrients, and waste products throughout the body. The diverse functions of such specialized connective tissues lead to the inference of the intricate correlation between their respective morphologies and functional significance. Additionally, the function of connective tissue morphology is further underscored by the analysis of hernias and their correlations with connective tissue integrity. Research has identified multiple forms of hernias to be linked to genetic variants in collagen and elastin, two essential components of connective tissue. Hernias are a protrusion of tissue or organ through its cavity, and the majority must be surgically corrected. In this article, we identify 65,492 cases for five forms of hernia within the UK Biobank and perform genome-wide association study scans on five forms and two combined groups. Our results demonstrate associated variants in all scans. Inguinal hernia contains the most associations, and we follow up with a study of 23,803 additional cases from four study groups, furnishing 84 independently associated variants.

This interaction illustrates the manner in which abnormalities in the morphology of connective tissue can lead to functional abnormalities and clinical disease, and emphasizes the need for continued research in this field, specifically the pathways involved in collagen and elastin synthesis and how they relate to overall tissue health and disease (Current results not only establish the existence of enzymes responsible for the synthesis of sex steroids in the vagina wall, but demonstrate that expression is dependent upon stage of the cycle, both as far as levels are concerned and the type of cells expressing.) (Figure 4.2).

4.1.1. Loose Connective Tissue

Loose connective tissue is an important structural component of connective tissue morphology. Characterized by loosely aligned fibers and high ground substance content, loose connective tissue also provides flexibility and cushioning to various organs in the body. Loose tissue stabilizes blood vessels, nerves, and organs, and can be seen from its role as a nourishment and support medium. The loose connective tissuethe movement of nutrients and waste products between cells and the proximal blood vessels.

The structural support role of loose connective tissue is therefore physiological because it includes active functions for transporting nutrients and defense mechanisms, hence maintaining tissue microenvironment homeostasis. The cellular composition of loose connective tissue is heterogeneous and contains fibroblasts, adipocytes, macrophages, and mast cells, each contributing a specific function to the tissue. Fibroblasts have a very important function as they secrete the various fibers and ground substances that constitute the extracellular matrix. Adipocytes or fat cells store energy and serve as insulators, repeating the versatility of functions of the tissues. The most important role of macrophages in the immune response is that these cells consume pathogens and dead cell debris, thereby indicating the presence of tissues in inflammatory reactions. Mast cells discharge histamines and other mediators that execute inflammatory reactions while facilitating healing. Such dynamic cellular interaction not only enhances the resistance of loose connective tissue but also enables it to respond effectively to environmental changes, thereby ensuring tissue integrity and function during healing and repair.

The findings indicate that loose connective tissue also has implications in medicine, particularly in wound healing and disease treatment. Experiments have begun to look at the possibility of changing the characteristics of this tissue to lead to improved clinical outcomes. Specifically, developments in biomaterials, such as electrospun poly(-caprolactone) scaffolds incorporating antibiotics, are illuminating for their compatibility with loose connective tissue during the healing of surgical wounds. These findings recognize the potential for modifying treatments utilizing loose connective tissue for effective management of adhesion formation and healing processes, as evidenced in the results of PCL membrane effectiveness in reducing postsurgical abdominal adhesions and promoting recovery (Bolgen et al., 2007). Thus, the discipline of loose connective tissue structure and function continues to be of prime significance to basic biological science as well as to clinical application (Figure 4.3).

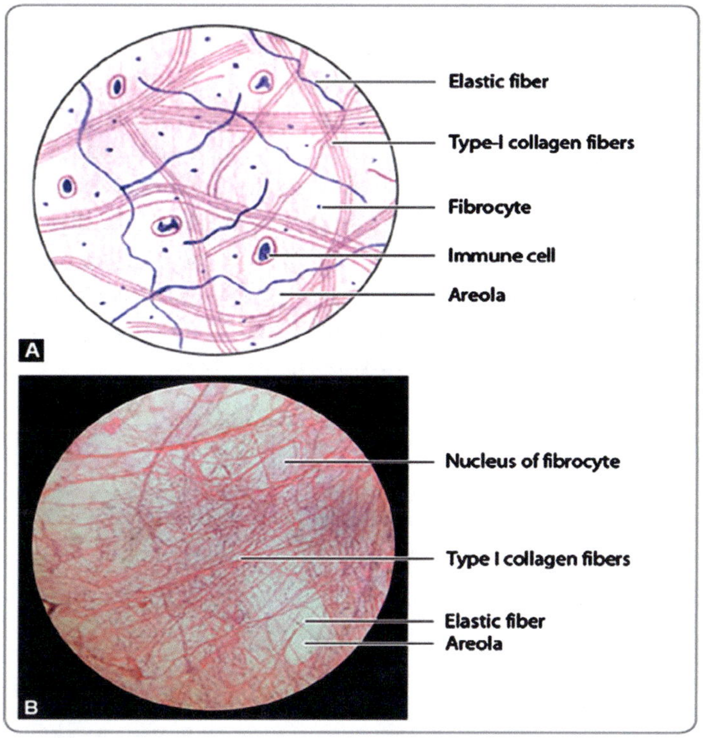

Figure 4.3. Loose connective tissue.

Source: https://d45jl3w9libvn.cloudfront.net/jaypee/static/books/9789352703548/Chapters/images/557-1.jpg.

4.1.2. Dense Connective Tissue

Dense connective tissue also provides structural support and stability to most organs and systems in the body. It is characterized by its high density of collagen fibers and is subdivided into two broad categories: dense regular connective tissue and dense irregular connective tissue. Dense regular connective tissue, including tendons and ligaments, features parallel orientation of collagen fibers, enabling it to withstand unidirectional tensile stress. Conversely, dense irregular connective tissue, found in tissues such as the skin dermis and organ capsules, contains a more irregular fiber structure, conferring multidirectional strength. Not only are structural components of dense connective tissue central to musculoskeletal element support, but they also contribute to the mechanics and resilience of many physiological systems in general. The physiological characteristics of dense connective tissue are, to a large degree, defined by the cell and biochemical makeup unique to its various subtypes. A case in point is tenomodulin (Tnmd), a type II membrane protein that is specifically expressed in dense connective tissues such as tendons and ligaments and appears to play a crucial role in cell adhesion and maintenance of structural integrity (Chung et al., 2013). Tnmd plays a supportive role in the assembly and stabilization of the extracellular matrix, thereby contributing to the mechanical stress-resisting capacity of the fibrous tissue. Such molecular specificity reveals dense connective tissue as more than a passive scaffold, as it actively participates in cellular activities and tissue homeostasis, demonstrating the complex interplay between morphological characteristics and functional outcomes in connective tissue systems. Chronic pathologies in connective tissue are often a result of structural and functional abnormalities within dense connective tissue. Conditions such as fibrosis, involving collagen deposition and hardening of the tissue, can extensively impair the working of connective tissue and cause chronic pain syndromes (Reis et al., 2011). This hardened condition can alter the mechanical properties of dense connective tissue, resulting in restricted movement and pain. An understanding of the mechanisms underlying such alterations is essential for the development of therapeutic strategies to restore normal function and relieve symptoms. Knowledge concerning the mechanisms of cellular response associated with fibroblast activity and collagen synthesis is necessary in relation to approaches towards controlling dense connective tissue-associated diseases, and hence indicating the need for ongoing study in connective tissue morphology and its impact on disease and health (Figure 4.4).

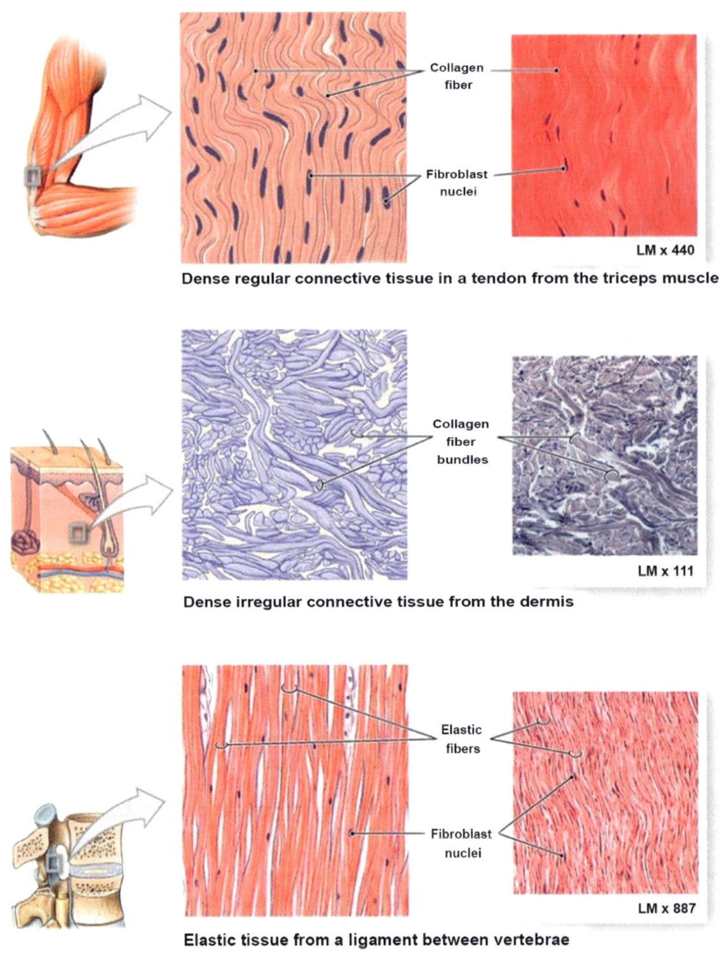

Figure 4.4. Dense connective tissue.

Source: https://i.pinimg.com/736x/38/13/c1/3813c121327c9ecef331f598c1211d68--tissue-types-anatomy-and-physiology.jpg.

4.1.3. Specialized Connective Tissue

In the context of the morphology of connective tissue, specialized connective tissues are of the utmost significance within the structural and functional diversity of the human body. These connective tissues, including tendons, ligaments, cartilage, and specialized adipose tissues, participate in various physiological functions required to achieve homeostasis. For instance, tendons attach bones to muscles to facilitate movement, whereas ligaments stabilize joints by connecting bones. It is the unique composition of these connective tissues—possessing specific types of collagen, elastin fibers, and an idiosyncratic extracellular matrix—that is accountable for their individualized mechanical properties. It has been shown that specialized connective tissues are not passive; they respond adaptively to mechanical stress and strain and exhibit the dynamic adjustability necessary for physical function and avoidance of injury.

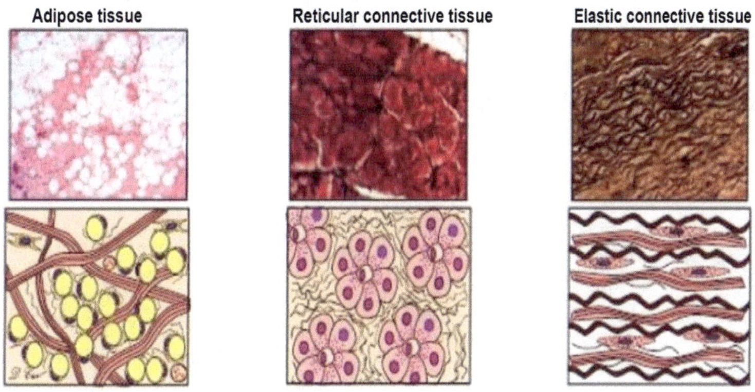

Figure 4.5. Specialized connective tissue.

Source: https://image.slidesharecdn.com/connectivetissue-170208053436/95/connective-tissue-23-638.jpg?cb=1506569643.

This adjustability raises important questions about the molecular mechanisms underlying tissue resilience and repair. One of the components of specialized connective tissue that is especially interesting is Tenomodulin (Tnmd), a type II transmembrane protein ubiquitously expressed in tendon and ligament tissues. It can be demonstrated that Tnmd is crucial to the maturation and maintenance of specialized connective tissues, specifically the periodontal ligament (PDL). Studies indicate that Tnmd expression is closely associated with developmental events, such as tooth eruption, in synchronization with the application of occlusal forces to the teeth and alveolar bone. Tnmd was also shown to enhance cell adhesion between NIH3T3 and human PDL cells, suggesting that its expression helps maintain the integrity of these tissues under mechanical forces. Understanding the role of Tnmd not only explains the cellular interactions in specialized connective tissues but also illuminates potential therapeutic targets for such tissue injuries (Chung et al., 2013). Studies on specialized connective tissues extend beyond their mechanical functions into their role in causing pathologies such as fibrosis, which can lead to chronic pain and reduced mobility. Excessive fibrotic reaction has been found to substantially increase the stiffness of tissues, resulting in conditions like drug-resistant chronic pain. This is particularly relevant in subcutaneous connective tissues, where collagen synthesis and tissue remodeling involve fibroblasts. The relationship between extracellular nucleotides and fibroblast activity is significant; for instance, the nucleotide UTP has been found to regulate the growth of the fibroblast and the synthesis of collagen type I. On the other hand, selective P2Y2 receptor activation does not affect proliferation but suppresses collagen synthesis, yet another demonstration of the complex pathways involved in the regulation of connective tissue homeostasis and adaptation. Exploration of these pathways has the potential not only to illuminate their function in fibrosis but also to lead to novel therapeutic approaches for chronic pain disorders (Reis et al., 2011) (Figure 4.5).

4.2. Components of Connective Tissue

The organization of connective tissue is complex, comprising a mix of cellular and extracellular elements that act together to confer function and morphological characteristics to the tissues. On a cellular basis, connective tissue comprises specialized cells, including fibroblasts, adipocytes, chondrocytes, and osteocytes. These cells are essential in terms of manufacturing and maintaining the extracellular matrix (ECM) that plays a significant role in providing structural support. The ECM is a complex assembly of fibers, ground substance, and diverse bioactive molecules that synergistically regulate tissue elasticity and flexibility.

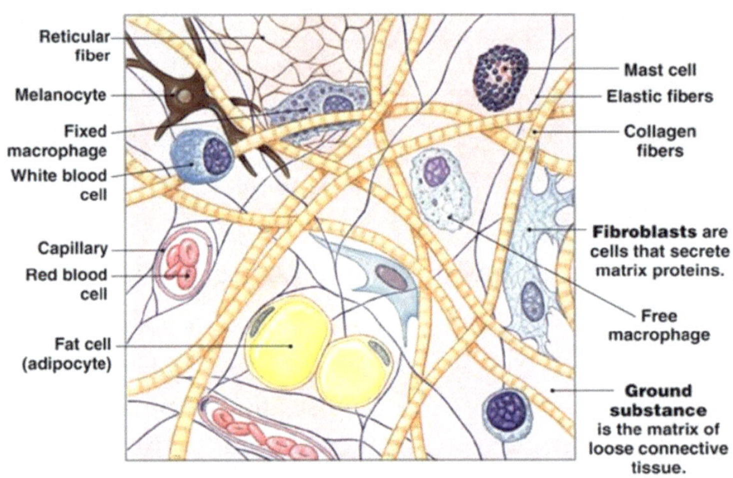

Figure 4.6. Components of connective tissue.

Source: https://medmuv.com/kafedra/internal/histolog/classes_stud/en/stomat/ptn/1/07%20Connective%20tissues.%20Loose%20connective%20tissue.%20Dense%20connective%20tissue.%20Connective%20tissues%20with%20special%20properties.files/image007.jpg.

Within the fiber categories, collagen and elastin are especially significant in terms of their tensile strength and elasticity, respectively. The particular organization and structure of these components have a direct influence on the physical properties of connective tissues and their suitability for various anatomical and physiological functions of the body. In addition to typical cell types, connective tissue possesses a dense extracellular matrix, a feature that distinguishes it from other tissues. The ECM is itself further divided into two broad categories: fibrous proteins and ground substance. Fibrous proteins such as collagen provide tensile strength to connective tissues so that they can resist stretch forces, while elastin is involved in their ability to recover their original shape after deformation. Ground substance, composed of proteoglycans, glycoproteins, and water, provides cell-to-cell communication and helps maintain the hydration of the tissues and nutrient transport. Functional flexibility and structural toughness of connective tissues are, for the most part, influenced by the fiber and ground substance content and arrangement. For instance, modifications in the components have led to the development of specialized connective tissues, such as cartilage, bone, and adipose tissue, each of which performs distinct physiological functions in the organism.

The relationships between the cellular components and the extracellular matrix are essential in maintaining the structural and functional integrity of connective tissue in the long term. Aging, for instance, triggers deep morphological and structural modifications in connective tissue. Evidence indicates that stiffening of connective tissues, such as the endomysium of striated muscle, is associated with aging-induced declines in force-generating capacity (Basava et al., 2020). These mechanical alterations affect not just the functioning of muscle but even the overall plasticity of connective tissues to dynamic mechanical environments.

Additionally, newer composite materials for biomedicine, which contain such substances as hydroxyapatite and gelatin, have shown promise in enhancing the function and regeneration of connective tissues (Bolshanina et al., 2016). These developments highlight the need to understand the complex morphology of connective tissue, which ultimately informs therapeutic interventions aimed at counteracting age-related degenerative changes (Figure 4.6).

4.2.1. Extracellular Matrix

The extracellular matrix (ECM) is essential to the structural and functional integrity of connective tissues. The ECM is a complex network of glycoproteins, proteins, and carbohydrates that not only provides physical support for cells but also biochemical signals for guiding cell behavior. The dynamic environment enables cells to interact with their surroundings and significantly influences cell proliferation, differentiation, and migration. In connective tissue morphology, the composition and structure of the ECM vary widely between tissues to suit their individual functional demands. The ECM of tendon, for instance, is replete with collagen fibers to provide tensile strength, whereas the ECM of cartilage is designed to withstand compressive load. Understanding these variations in ECM composition is key to understanding the complexity of connective tissue function and disease. Extracellular matrix studies have gained insight into the pathogenesis of connective tissue disease. Tendinopathy, a common condition in athletes, has been linked to alterations in the molecular pathology of the tendon matrix, with evidence indicating that changes in ECM composition may lead to significant functional impairment. The pathogenesis of tendinopathy can be challenging to study with the infrequent taking of biopsies before injury occurs. Nonetheless, advances in biochemical and molecular techniques have more clearly demonstrated how changes in the ECM lead to tendinopathy and healing. Through analysis of the ECM's role during locomotor functions, researchers have found prospective therapeutic compounds to reduce the incidence of tendinopathy and improve recuperation processes in patients, thus indicating the ECM's clinical importance in connective tissue morphology (Riley., 2004). Moreover, cell interactions with the extracellular matrix are crucial in maintaining tissue homeostasis and regulating remodeling. For instance, osteoclasts, bone-resorbing cells, engage with the bone matrix through a highly ordered lattice framework that coordinates the resorptive process. Computational modeling of these dynamics shows that parameters such as osteoclast interactions, vessel support, and cell fusion exert significant influence on the geometric features of resorption cavities in the bone matrix. Not only do such models further identify the function of bone remodeling, but they also emphasize the need to have a single approach when studying the ECM's role in various connective tissues. With more research in the field, it is increasingly evident that a comprehensive understanding of the ECM and how it functions is key to developing effective treatments for connective tissue diseases (Anderson et al., 2011) (Figure 4.7).

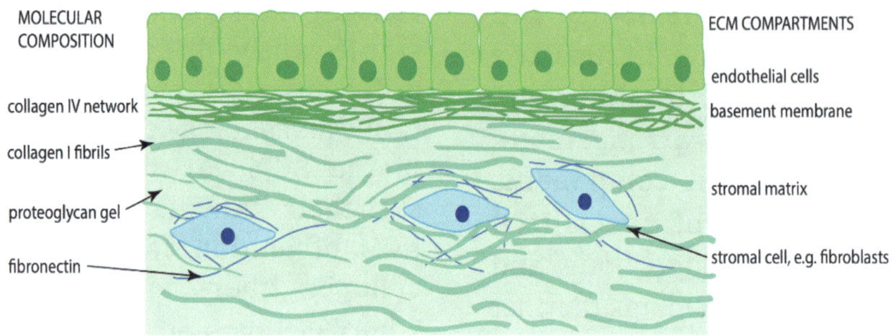

Figure 4.7. Extracellular matrix.

Source: https://www.ch.cam.ac.uk/group/duer/files/images/ecm.png.

4.2.2. Fibers (Collagen, Elastin, Reticular)

The structural components of the connective tissue fibers, specifically collagen, elastin, and reticular fibers, are responsible for the integrity and function of various tissues. The most common protein in the body, collagen, provides tensile strength to enable tissues to withstand stretching and mechanical stress. Each type of collagen has distinct structural characteristics that are required by specific tissues, such as skin, cartilage, and bone. Moreover, the function of collagen fibers is vital to healing; as seen in skin samples from various-sized Varanus salvator, thicker fibers predominated, indicating the mechanical strength and toughness of collagen in the dermis. The knowledge of the arrangement and distribution of collagen fibers is vital to the description of not only normal physiology but also the pathophysiology of connective tissue-related diseases (Agungpriyono et al., 2024). Elastin fibers provide connective tissue with elasticity such that structures return toward their resting form after deformation. Fibers play significant roles in the mechanical properties of tissues under constant tension, such as skin, lungs, and blood vessels. The abundance of elastin at the edge of the reticular dermis of the skin of lizards of various sizes demonstrates its role in allowing for dynamic change while maintaining structural integrity. Elastic fibers intermingle with collagen to form a compromise between strength and flexibility, thus facilitating the stability and mobility of various tissues. This gradual interaction between collagen and elastin fibers is critical for maintaining healthy function under physiological stress and ultimately affects outcomes in healing and tissue repair, underscoring the value of connective tissue morphology in disease and health management (Cherkas., 2023). Reticular fibers, which are a group of thin collagen fibers in a network, provide cells with a supportive framework in various organs, particularly in lymphoid and hematopoietic tissues. They establish a soft matrix that facilitates cellular interaction and the migration of immune cells, thus playing a major role in immune responses. The histological examination of various connective tissues shows that reticular fibers are usually conspicuous in organs like the liver, spleen, and lymph nodes, where they provide the organs' structural support with the ability to mobilize functional cells. The occurrence and distribution of the fibers correlate directly with the organ's capacity to execute its function effectively. Accordingly, an awareness of reticular fibers enhances our comprehension of the role of connective tissue and the implications for systemic disease that disrupts tissue architecture (Agungpriyono et al., 2024) (Figure 4.8).

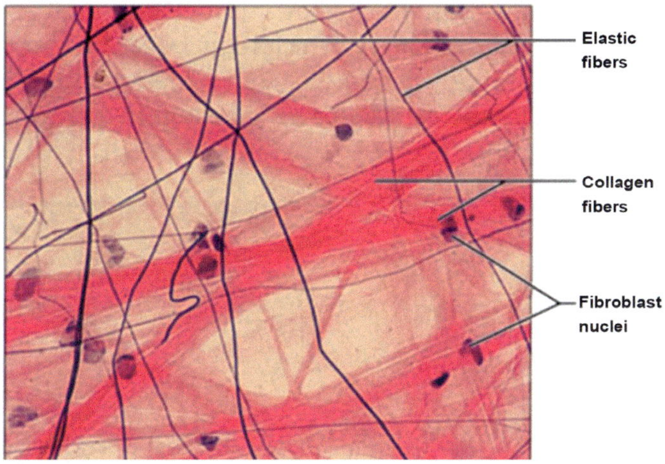

Figure 4.8. Fibers (collagen, elastin, reticular).

Source: https://o.quizlet.com/dx94aCMhC0xg90Jzt9zi9w.png.

4.2.3. Cells (Fibroblasts, Adipocytes, Immune Cells)

The organization of connective tissue is largely influenced by its cellular components, including fibroblasts, adipocytes, and immune cells. Fibroblasts, as the principal cells responsible for synthesizing the extracellular matrix, play a crucial role in maintaining the integrity of the structure of connective tissues. Fibroblasts produce collagen, elastin, and glycoproteins, which provide tensile strength and elasticity to various tissues. Fibroblasts also facilitate cell communication through the release of growth factors and cytokines that regulate various physiological processes. Notably, intercellular communication between adipocytes and fibroblasts is critical in tissue homeostasis, particularly in the mammary gland, where the two cells engage in communication to maintain mammary epithelium growth. These interactions are important for the maintenance of functional properties of connective tissues, highlighting the necessity to investigate the dynamics of fibroblasts in relation to the general morphology of connective tissues (Dzięgelewska, Ż. & Gajewska, M., 2018). Adipocytes, or fat cells, are not just energy reservoirs but active participants in the function of connective tissues. These cells play a crucial role in metabolic regulation by secreting adipokines that influence appetite, insulin sensitivity, and inflammation. Within connective tissue, adipocytes provide mechanical stability and facilitate the storage of nutrients, as well as contribute to the overall tissue environment. These cells play a significant role within the mammary gland, where they do not just interact with fibroblasts but also facilitate the control of the development and function of the adjacent epithelial structure. Moreover, studies have confirmed that adipocytes possess unique features that allow them to respond to hormones and influence cell behavior, thus emphasizing their intricate roles in the integrity and dynamics of connective tissues (Thomas, 2023). Immune cells also complicate the cellular profile of connective tissues by performing both protective and regulatory roles. Cells such as macrophages, mast cells, and lymphocytes play a role in the regulation of tissue homeostasis, especially in inflammation. They communicate with fibroblasts and adipocytes, therefore creating an interplay that is dynamic and can adjust tissue repair and regeneration processes. For instance, on injury, immune cells can secrete signaling molecules that stimulate fibroblasts to produce extracellular matrix components required for healing. In addition, immune cell infiltration into various tissues may underlie chronic inflammation, which impairs fibroblast function and adipocyte physiology. Describing the roles of such immune elements in connective tissue not only gives some clues to their pathologic significance but also holds out some prospect for therapeutic strategies to investigate tissue regeneration and repair mechanisms (Thomas, 2023) (Figure 4.9).

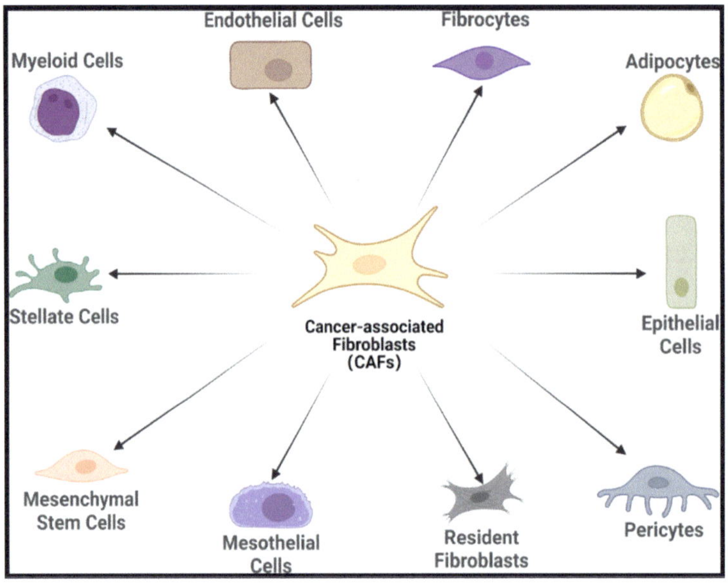

Figure 4.9. Cells (fibroblasts, adipocytes, immune cells).

Source: https://www.frontiersin.org/files/Articles/988295/fendo-13-988295-HTML-r1/image_m/fendo-13-988295-g001.jpg.

4.3. Functions of Connective Tissue

Connective tissue plays an essential role in maintaining the structural integrity of other biological systems within the body. Connective tissue performs various functions, including protection, support, and binding other tissues. One of connective tissue's primary functions is providing a scaffold that allows organs and systems to maintain form and position. This structural support is critical, particularly in dense connective tissue like tendons and ligaments, where muscles are attached to bones and joints are supported. The unique structure and organization of collagen fibers in these tissues contribute to the tissues' strength and resilience so that they can withstand a lot of mechanical stress and strain. In addition to providing structural support, connective tissue helps regulate numerous physiological processes in the body. For example, adipose tissue, a form of specialized connective tissue, plays a crucial role in energy storage and metabolism since it acts as a reservoir for mobilizable fats when energy is needed. Connective tissue has numerous cell types that play significant roles in immune responses, such as macrophages and mast cells. These cells aid in protecting the body against pathogens and facilitating healing processes. Further, the matrix formed by connective tissue is essential in cell signaling and communication, influencing cell behavior and enhancing tissue repair mechanisms.

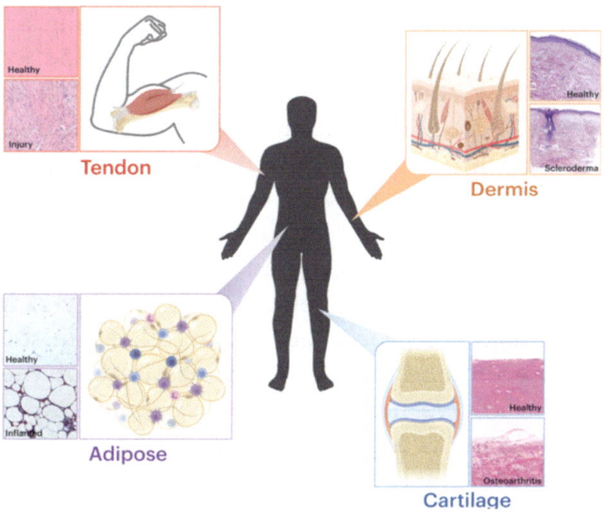

Figure 4.10. Functions of connective tissue.

Source: https://www.researchgate.net/publication/331990997/figure/fig1/AS:11431281173057220@1688743105117/Anatomy-and-disease-state-affect-connective-tissue-structure-function-properties-Adipose.png.

Cell proliferation of some cell types of the connective tissue highlights the dynamic nature of this tissue group, particularly in repair and regeneration. For instance, the expression of some proteins, such as Tenomodulin (Tnmd), highlights the regulatory functions of the connective tissue in cellular adhesion and growth. Tnmd plays a crucial role in dense connective tissues, contributing to the maturation of structures like the periodontal ligament (PDL) during tooth eruption (Chung et al., 2013). In addition, the presence of ectomesenchymal cells of cranial neural crest origin indicates the potential for connective tissue differentiation into various lineages, including osteogenic and chondrogenic cells (Degistirici et al., 2008). A function as versatile as this underscores the key roles connective tissue plays not just in homeostasis in physiology but also in regenerative medicine, where it holds promise to form an important part of tissue engineering and therapeutic strategy (Figure 4.10).

4.3.1. Support and Structure

The support and structural principle of connective tissue is primarily established by its composition and organization, which cooperate to give integrity and resistance to various tissues. The extracellular matrix (ECM) is the connective tissue matrix, containing proteins such as collagen that provide strength and elastin that provide elasticity. These fibers are embedded in a water-loving ground substance made up of glycosaminoglycans and proteoglycans that not only provide shock absorption but also permit diffusion of nutrients and waste products. In particular, the compact connective tissues such as tendons and ligaments possess a highly ordered structure, which enables them to support extremely high tensile loads corresponding to their significant role of transmitting mechanical loads. Moreover, the functional specificity of proteins such as Tenomodulin (Tnmd) underscores the dynamic interplay between structure and function within connective tissues, particularly in cell adhesion and periodontal ligament maintenance (Chung et al., 2013). With the development or degeneration of connective tissue, its structural properties shift, significantly affecting its mechanical support function. In skeletal muscle, for instance, ageing is associated with an increase in the content of connective tissue, such as the endomysium, which stiffens with age and reduces the force-producing ability. The rise in volume ratio of the connective tissue with ageing influences the reaction of the muscle under different kinds of contractions, particularly under eccentric and concentric conditions. The biomechanical changes engaged in the ECM are central to the process of how structural adaptation can affect the functionality of the muscle as a whole. Further, the cumulative changes in connective tissues capture the integration of cellular change and the microenvironment, highlighting the value of an extensive study of connective tissue morphology to understand the mechanisms underlying structural support and adaptive change (Basava et al., 2020). A study of the morphology of connective tissues yields significant insights into their roles in health and disease. Such heterogeneity as exists among the connective tissues, manifesting variability of matrix composition and shape, may influence tissue response to injury or mechanical stress. For instance, the novel biochemical properties of Tnmd are accountable for enhanced cell adhesion, which is a sign of its function to provide connective tissue homeostasis during a particular physiological stress, such as tooth eruption (Chung et al., 2013). Similarly, recognition of structural changes in tissues, including those in aging skeletal muscle, underscores the importance of an integrated approach to understanding how alterations in connective tissue structure contribute to function across the life course. Appreciation of the intricate association between structure and support in these tissues enables researchers to continue to explore therapeutic approaches to restoring or enhancing connective tissue integrity and function (Basava et al., 2020).

4.3.2. Storage of Energy

The concept of energy storage is directly related to the morphology of connective tissues, with adipose tissue serving as the primary reservoir for lipid energy. The adipose tissue cells, or adipocytes, store triglycerides that are released during states of energy deficit. This is not only crucial in maintaining metabolic homeostasis but also vital to the structural integrity of connective tissues as a whole. The lobular organization and vascular supply of adipose tissue dictate both its energy storage capacity and its functional responsiveness. Therefore, information on the microscopic composition of adipocytes and the extracellular matrix in which they are embedded is central to understanding how connective tissue morphologies vary with energy needs and metabolism in the body, demonstrating the salient interrelationship between structure and function in regulating energy. Furthermore, the capacity for energy storage by connective tissue is not limited to adipose tissue. Other connective tissues, such as cartilage and tendons, also indirectly contribute to energy metabolism. While not energy stores tissue, their structural components, such as proteoglycans and collagen, possess specific qualities that regulate how energy-rich substrates are processed and mobilized in the body. For instance, the viscoelasticity of the tissues allows mechanical energy absorption and release as a person moves, which is vital in facilitating locomotion and load-carrying functions. Biomechanical energy storage through such processes is vital in enabling the efficient functioning of the musculoskeletal system and is a testament to the fact that the morphology of connective tissue is vital not just in adding structural support but also in the facilitation of energy dynamics within physiological processes. Additionally, recent evidence has implicated specialized connective tissues in energy homeostasis through their regulation by body-wide metabolic pathways. For instance, certain connective tissues possess signaling molecules that regulate energy metabolism and inflammation and coordinate structural and metabolic functions of the body. The findings regarding nanocapsules in pharmaceutical use highlight how changes in formulation may affect the biological activity of drugs such as Selol, which influences cell metabolism and is associated with tissue morphology and responses to energy signals (Azevedo et al., 2014). The nature of these interactions underscores the importance of connective tissue morphology in the larger context of energy storage and utilization, reiterating the necessity of understanding how such tissues adapt at the cellular and molecular levels in order to perform their diverse functions within the body.

4.3.3. Transportation of Nutrients and Waste

Within connective tissue morphology, the transport of waste and nutrients plays a central role in maintaining homeostasis. Connective tissues, particularly ECM-rich ones, provide a channel through which essential substances are transported and metabolic wastes are removed. The ECM includes a number of proteins and glycosaminoglycans that not only provide support but also enable the free diffusion of nutrients such as glucose, amino acids, and lipids into adjacent cells. Additionally, the matrix facilitates the transport of cellular metabolic waste products, thereby preventing toxic accumulation and maintaining cell integrity. Hence, the effective function of connective tissues is essential for optimal nutrient supply and waste elimination, influencing tissue condition and functioning in general. In addition to physical movement, dynamic functions within connective tissues further contribute to the regulation of nutrient and waste management. Specialized cells of connective tissues, such as fibroblasts and adipocytes, play an active role in these activities. For instance, fibroblasts synthesize the various components of the ECM, which influences the form and, therefore, the permeability, regulating nutrient delivery. Adipocytes, besides serving as energy reservoirs, release biochemical messengers that have the capacity to influence the supply of nutrients as well as waste metabolism. Furthermore, the vasculature within connective tissue is tasked with supplying nutrients as well as eliminating wastes. Recent studies have shown that alterations in the organization of these vascular networks can affect nutrient supply (Deus, 2021). Hence, understanding the morphological intricacies of connective tissue allows for a deeper insight into the mechanism of nutrient and waste transport. Also, the consequences of defective nutrient transfer and waste removal within connective tissues could be of severe pathological consequences. Conditions such as obesity, diabetes, and inflammatory disease demonstrate that impaired connective tissue continuity and ECM function can generate systemic metabolic disturbances. For example, in the case of obesity, hypertrophy of the adipose tissue disrupts the circumscribing connective tissue structure and function, which impairs effective delivery of nutrients and removal of waste. Such a malfunction can exacerbate inflammation and cause comorbidities, thereby illustrating the interconnectedness of connective tissue anatomy with metabolic health. New treatments that aim to reconstruct or enhance connective tissue structure have the potential to mitigate the effects of reduced nutrient and waste transport (Abiuso et al., 2016). As such, there is an urgent need for a comprehensive understanding of connective tissue morphology to develop interventions that restore normal physiological function.

4.4. Connective Tissue in Different Organs

Connective tissue is an important component of various organs, providing their structure and function. Within the liver and other organs, not only does connective tissue maintain the architecture, but it also plays a role in the immune response. Recent research identified populations of dendritic cells within liver connective tissue, which are required for the liver's tolerogenic function. These cells possess a unique morphology that distinguishes them from others in organ systems because they have the capacity to activate T cells. These findings highlight the need to understand how connective tissue morphology influences immune dynamics, particularly in organ transplantation and tolerance mechanisms, and to further investigate the specific functions of these components across tissues and diseases (Li et al., 1994). The role of connective tissue morphologies is much different when contrasting different organ systems, particularly in their adaptations to functional demands. The case is the connective tissue associated with eccrine glands, particularly the footpads of animals like *Procavia capensis*, which has an impressive morphology well-suited to transport and secretion of fluids. Coiling tubular secretory parts, composed of discrete cell types such as clear and dark cells, is a form of connective tissue specialization for specific physiological purposes. Adaptation not only enhances glandular function but also enhances the organism's adaptation to its environment, e.g., traction on surfaces. This relationship between connective tissue form and function provides evidence of the evolution and adaptability of such tissues to specific ecological niches and activities (Stumpf et al., 2002). Finally, the diversity of connective tissue in various organs displays its multifunctionality in structure and function. Individuals studying connective tissue morphology must consider not just the form of the matrix and cells but also the dynamic interactions among the components and the overall physiological functions that they perform. Differences among connective tissues are not just historical or developmental but are directly related to the organ's particular needs, whether mechanical support, immune demarcation, or secretory efficiency. Comprehension of these relationships can allow for greater insight into pathology and tissue engineering and provide a unifying principle for the therapy of disease based on connective tissue dysfunction across a range of organs (Li et al., 1994; Stumpf et al., 2002) (Figure 4.11).

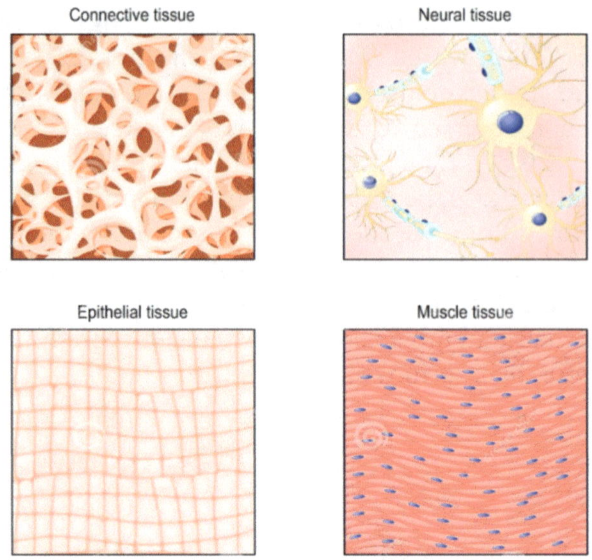

Figure 4.11. Connective tissue in different organs.

Source: https://thumbs.dreamstime.com/z/tissue-types-connective-muscle-nervous-epithelial-close-up-cells-different-tissue-anatomical-fiber-parts-epithelium-bone-205375511.jpg.

4.4.1. Role in the Integumentary System

The integumentary system is critical to homeostasis, as well as to the protection of internal structures, connective tissue forming the foundation in its organization and operation. The integumentary system, which consists of skin, hair, nails, and accessory glands, utilizes various types of connective tissue in providing support, elasticity, and delivery of nutrition. The dermis, a significant layer beneath the epidermis, consists primarily of dense connective tissue, supporting hair follicles, nerve endings, and blood vessels. The multilayered aspect not only accommodates barrier functions but also allows epidermal cells to be attached to deeper vascular systems to provide required nutrients and protective measures against outside perils. Hence, the role of connective tissue in the integumentary system is crucial in ensuring its protective and regulatory roles. Again, supporting the significance of connective tissue in the integumentary system is the evolutionary perspective observed in other animals. For instance, the integument of an enantiornithine bird shows a remarkably modern organization of connective tissue concerned with flight feathers, thereby indicating why the morphology of connective tissues has evolved to allow for functional needs over a period of time. The presence of specialized connective structures in the wing supported by very tiny muscles, tendons, and ligaments indicates a sophisticated relationship between structure and function in the mechanics of avian flight. This morphological complexity of connective tissue is more than a form adaptation; it is essential to the functional integrity of the wing in flight. The comparative morphology of connective tissues across species, therefore, sheds light on the evolutionary forces shaping the framework of the integumentary supporting system and broadens our understanding of its functional roles in different environments (Buscalioni et al., 2015). Also, the diversified connective tissue morphological adjustments in aquatic animals like catfish highlight their vital role in the integumentary system. The Neotropical family Trichomycteridae possesses diversified special adaptations that contribute to their survival within specialized ecological niches. For instance, their adaptations in the integument permit survival mechanisms like hematophagy and miniaturization, highlighting the multivariate contribution of connective tissues in facilitating diversified means of life. Morphological studies of these catfishes reveal that the integument, a composite made of layers of connective tissue, is an essential part of their unique behavior and environmental interactions. Morphological and functional adaptations of the integument enhance the role of connective tissues as structural elements and dynamic players in an organism's physiology. Thus, understanding the evolutionary significance of connective tissue morphology enhances the discourse on the role of the integumentary system in ecology (Adriaens et al., 2010).

4.4.2. Function in the Skeletal System

The skeletal system has myriad functions crucial to human mobility and overall health. It lends the most critical structural support, being the body to which muscles, tendons, and ligaments are attached. This structural feature allows for body shape and posture maintenance while allowing for movement through its articulation points. The bones also contain various types of connective tissues—among them cartilage and ligaments—that enhance toughness and flexibility. Additionally, the skeletal system protects vital internal organs; for instance, the rib cage protects the lungs and heart, and the vertebrae enclose the spinal cord. The integration of these connective tissues enables the skeletal system to resist stress and load, illustrating its dynamic nature through growth, repair, and remodeling activities inherent to connective tissue anatomy. Another of the body's vital functions of the skeletal system is the secretion and storage of vital substances such as phosphorus and calcium. These minerals are deposited in bone tissue, where they play a crucial role in several physiological functions beyond the skeletal system, including the conduction of nerve impulses and the contraction of muscles. When the body's stores of calcium decline, the skeleton mobilizes calcium into the bloodstream; when there is enough, mineralization within the bones occurs, a process that is mediated by osteoblasts and osteoclasts. Equilibrium is necessary to maintain homeostasis and optimize muscle function during exercise and other body activities. The intricate relationships within the connective tissue structure of bones reflect how these processes contribute to the overall morphology and function of the skeletal system, and they underscore the importance of connective tissue in maintaining stability and supporting dynamic metabolic activity.

Additionally, the responsiveness of the skeletal system is most apparent in its capacity to respond to biomechanical forces via modulation of connective tissue properties. As explained in current studies, for example, by taking into account age-related changes in the contractile ability of muscle, increased stiffness of connective tissue can influence force generation during different modes of muscle contractions (Basava et al., 2020). This relationship emphasized the need to not only understand the structural considerations but also understand the cellular responses within the skeleton. For instance, the role of cranial neural crest mesenchyme in bone and cartilage development indicates how different connective tissues participate in shaping the jaw, and how these structures have evolved adaptively over time (Abzhanov et al., 2019). This recognition of the dynamic roles of connective tissues within the skeleton serves to underscore the significance of their function in supporting structural requirements and reacting to functional requirements throughout life.

4.4.3. Contribution to the Circulatory System

The circulatory system, to a great extent, relies on the diverse functions that are performed by connective tissues, which provide structural support to blood vessels and circulatory organs. Connective tissue vessels that consist of a majority of connective tissue enable the body to transport nutrients, gases, and waste products efficiently. In particular, collagen fibers in vessel walls impart strength and elasticity to arteries, enabling them to withstand high pressures while maintaining sufficient elasticity to accommodate varying blood volumes. Such remarkable versatility is crucial in regulating blood perfusion to tissues and consequently orchestrating a subtle symphony of physiological reactions to internal and external stimuli. As studies progress, understanding the intricate morphology of connective tissues becomes increasingly important to the description of their specific role in the circulatory system's overall efficiency and functionality. Connective tissues provide more than mere structural support; they are also involved in metabolic processes central to circulatory health. For instance, interactions of endothelial cells with connective tissue elements like fibroblasts regulate inflammatory reactions and healing mechanisms following vascular injury. In addition, the vascular extracellular matrix contains reservoirs of growth factors and signaling molecules actively regulating vascular remodeling and repair processes. Recent discoveries illustrate the importance of these interactions in regulating vascular homeostasis and in resisting disease states such as atherosclerosis and hypertension. As illustrated by recent advances in modeling methods, understanding morphometric change in these tissues is necessary in order to predict the functional impact on vascular disease and health, representative of the profound interdependence of structure and function in the circulatory system. New techniques, including mathematical modeling and high-level imaging, have significantly enhanced our understanding of the morphological input of connective tissues in the circulatory system. Techniques such as 3D modeling from histological sections allow accurate visualization of tissue architecture, while molecular investigations can reveal cryptic species and functional subtypes that may otherwise remain undetected using traditional techniques (Jörger et al., 2011). Such unraveling not only aids in the diagnosis of various vascular pathologies but also guides therapeutic strategies towards restoring optimum vascular function. Additionally, these modeling procedures facilitate a deeper understanding of the influence of connective tissue morphology on hemodynamic parameters in both normal and pathological states (Audi et al., 2006). Thus, the integration of these various methodologies highlights the dynamic nature of vascular biology and underscores the extremely significant role played by connective tissues in the circulatory system's architecture and function.

4.5. Pathological Changes in Connective Tissue

The pathology of connective tissue is a significant area of study, particularly with respect to the processes underlying degenerative disorders, such as tendinopathy. Tendons, as key connectors between muscles and bones, are also very susceptible to pathological changes after repetitive micro-trauma that leads to acute or chronic degeneration. Current literature focuses on the difficulty of elucidating the precise etiology of tendinopathy, primarily due to the challenge of taking tendon biopsies before extensive tissue damage. While numerous articles address its treatment and diagnosis, few provide substantive scientific evidence. This emphasizes the need for further investigation of the biochemical and molecular changes that constitute the substrate for tendon disease, possibly towards more innovative therapeutic interventions to promote repair and enable functional recovery in such patients (Riley., 2004).

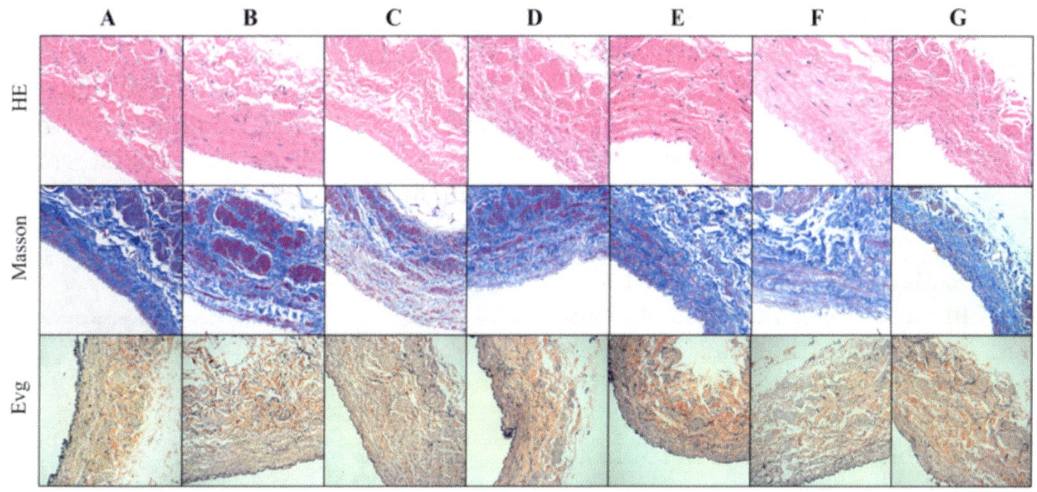

Figure 4.12. Pathological changes in connective tissue.

Source: https://www.laboratoryinvestigation.org/cms/10.1038/labinvest.2016.133/asset/22117ec2-4363-4b45-be6e-752744a7ee61/main.assets/gr1_lrg.jpg.

In elucidating the cellular and molecular mechanisms underlying connective tissue disease, the role of transforming growth factor-beta (TGF-β) in tendon healing is highlighted. TGF-ß has been indicated to be crucial in the process of tissue repair, and its various isoforms have been observed in normal and pathological tendons. Surprisingly, research indicates that chronic tendon lesions typically reflect a failure to properly repair or remodel the extracellular matrix following repeated micro-damage. Under pathological states, there has been an increase in reported levels of TGF-ß2, along with augmented cellular activity within the tendon matrix. This finding points to the complex interaction between cellular proliferation and the signal pathways controlling the healing process in degenerative tendons, and under conditions of elevated levels of TGF-ß2, the reparative responses that are desired might not be sufficient to correct the pathological state (Curry et al., 2001). Persistence of pathogenic changes in connective tissue raises grave questions about the effectiveness of current therapeutic measures in treating tendinopathy. Understanding the paradoxical action of TGF-β signaling, particularly the dissociation between TGF-β2 presence and TGF-βRI absence in chronic lesions, provides considerable insight into why treating these conditions is so challenging. Such insight leads us to suggest that exogenous TGF-ß administration may not be enough to induce recovery in degenerative tendons. Instead, a more differential approach from an integrative understanding of connective tissue morphology and pathology is required for the development of effective treatment paradigms. Therefore, further investigation is needed to elucidate the processes regulating TGF-β signaling and to explore additional therapeutic interventions that may more effectively promote tendon healing and restore normal connective tissue function (Figure 4.12).

4.5.1. Fibrosis and Scarring

Fibrosis is a pathological process resulting from the excessive deposition of extracellular matrix molecules, leading to changes in tissue structure and function. The condition is typically accompanied by scarring that can adversely affect the function of affected organs. The fundamental process of fibrosis is typically the activation of fibroblasts and myofibroblasts, which produce collagen and other matrix proteins. In chronic lesions, as in tendinopathy, dysregulation of growth factors, particularly transforming growth factor-beta (TGF-β), is of particular relevance. Overexpression of the isoforms of TGF-β has been found to be implicated in enhanced fibroblast activity and hence enhanced risk for the development of fibrosis. The chronicity of these conditions is reflective of the body's inability to heal tissue damage and points to the complexity of connective tissue morphogenesis within pathological processes (Curry et al., 2001). The fibrotic expression is often associated with changes in the morphology of connective tissue. In trachomatous trichiasis (TT), for instance, histologically there is an inflammatory infiltrate together with widespread collagen disruption, indicating pathologic healing processes. Higher levels of pro-inflammatory mediators, such as IL-1β, and growth factors, such as connective tissue growth factor (CTGF), were reported to promote fibrosis via mechanisms that cause epithelial-mesenchymal transition (EMT) of conjunctival tissues. The changes cause the scarring associated with TT, with dysregulated matrix metalloproteinase expression leading to increased breakdown of connective tissue architecture. By revealing the histological mechanism of fibrosis, researchers can design targeted interventions that can possibly arrest the progression of scarring and improve clinical outcomes (Burton et al., 2016). Notably, therapeutic approaches aimed at inhibiting fibrosis and scarring are increasingly recognized within the medical community. Interventions aimed at targeting the transforming growth factor-beta signal transduction pathway have been observed to alter the dynamics of fibrosis to a great extent.

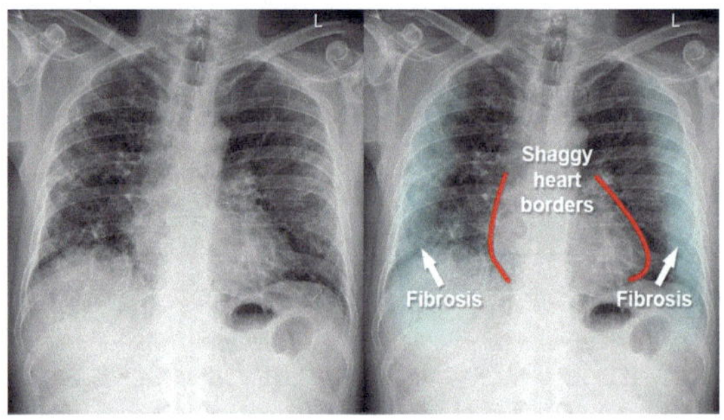

Figure 4.13. Fibrosis and scarring.

Source: https://www.radiologymasterclass.co.uk/images/chest-images/gallery-pulmonary/fibrosis.jpg?mtime=20210304211317&focal=none.

Therapies that manipulate inflammatory cytokine activity or inhibit pathological over-activation of fibroblasts can reverse, at least, balance the scarring process. As the morphology of connective tissue remains a core area of research interest, information on the dynamic interplay between inflammation and fibrosis is increasingly vital. By further characterizing the cell and molecular basis of it, therapy in the future can be made to prevent the detrimental effect of over-scarring, ultimately favoring more tissue repair and regeneration in such patients (Curry et al., 2001; Burton et al., 2016) (Figure 4.13).

4.5.2. Connective Tissue Disorders (e.g., Lupus, Scleroderma)

Connective tissue diseases such as lupus and scleroderma are a spectrum of autoimmune diseases that exhibit diverse morphological alterations in connective tissues. They most commonly appear in the skin, vessels, and other systems, as indicative of their systemic nature. Systemic lupus erythematosus (SLE), for instance, has been shown to entail microvascular structure, leading to its significant structural alterations demonstrable by advanced imaging techniques like nailfold capillaroscopy. This is a benign process that enables physicians to visualize capillary structure in detail and identify potential abnormalities that may not be detectable with standard diagnostic equipment. Detection of these capillaroscopic alterations is significant in that it has implications for the pathophysiology of lupus and informs clinical management interventions that are able to bring about optimal prevention of complications secondary to vascular involvement of the condition (Ariannia et al., 2016). Scleroderma, also known as systemic sclerosis, is another significant connective tissue disease defined by characteristic morphological features of connective tissues, more precisely in the skin and microvasculature. The capillaroscopic changes observed are usually classified into several patterns, one of which includes scleroderma-like changes that can overlap with other connective tissue diseases. Overlap necessitates a strict diagnostic workup because the appearance of similar changes in the capillaries in patients with lupus indicates that microvascular dysfunction is not specific to one disease. Instead, it points out the shared pathophysiologic mechanisms that can predispose to many of the rheumatic disorders. Thus, nailfold capillaroscopy has increasingly come to play a role in separating not only these two contrasting diseases but also in following disease course with time (Angelis., 2019). Knowledge of connective tissue disorder morphology extends beyond the vascular space, such as changes in cellular morphology and extracellular matrix components. In lupus and scleroderma, alterations in collagen deposition, fiber organization, and inflammatory cell infiltration may greatly change tissue integrity and function. Morphological changes are thus likely clinical manifestations, such as thickening of the skin in scleroderma or joint pain and stiffness in lupus. The measurement of connective tissue morphology, therefore, becomes an integral component of the diagnosis and management of such conditions, enabling the identification of particular treatments that might limit tissue damage and improve the prognosis of patients. The integration of sophisticated imaging with integrated morphological assessment improves understanding of the complex interplay among genetic, environmental, and immunological factors in connective tissue disorders (Ariannia et al., 2016).

4.5.3. Impact of Aging on Connective Tissue

With increasing age, there is a dramatic change in the structure and function of connective tissues and, as a result, the prevalence of many age-associated disorders. Connective tissue, like cartilage, tendons, ligaments, and the extracellular matrix (ECM), changes that could affect overall mobility and strength. Such structural changes are typically accompanied by increased production of collagen and other components of the extracellular matrix, leading to a stiff tissue matrix. This stiffening can jeopardize the cushioning capacity of joints and shock absorption by the tissues, and this is most evident in the elderly skeleton. The loss of connective tissue resilience is a very early indicator of degenerative conditions such as osteoarthritis and tendinosis, underscoring the importance of understanding these processes in reverse to mitigate their effects on health and function in the elderly. Aging also takes place in the cellular component of connective tissues, namely tenocytes in tendons and chondrocytes in cartilage. It was observed that with increased age, there is a shift in the phenotype of tenocytes such that they begin to exhibit characteristics that are similar to fibrochondrocytes, which otherwise produce cartilage. These alterations are associated with pathological conditions such as tendinosis, in which the tendon is degenerated due to diminished vascularity and altered biochemical milieus. Hypoxia, however, is shown to play a critical role in facilitating alterations that lead to abnormal tissue repair and maintenance. The interaction between senescence and impaired oxygen delivery in tendinous tissues thus sheds light on molecular mechanisms that are accountable for impairing connective tissue integrity and, by extension, global muscle function, lending evidence to the contention that intervention by tackling these mechanisms could be instrumental in managing age-related dysfunctions (Edwards et al., 2019). Furthermore, the mechanical properties of connective tissues in muscles also change with aging, which in turn impacts global muscle function. Studies have demonstrated that stiffening of connective tissue with age is particularly influential to muscle force production loss, most notably under concentric contraction, where the muscle contracts and becomes shorter. Stiffening of the connective tissues can reduce the ability of the skeletal muscle fibers to generate force under ideal conditions. Interestingly, this reduced ability to generate force is particularly pronounced under concentric contractions as opposed to eccentric contractions. Understanding muscle fiber-ECM interactions through advanced modeling techniques, as in recent studies, provides insight into the cellular and mechanical changes associated with aging. This relationship points out that the normalization of the morphological alterations in the connective tissues is a critical factor to address in an effort to create a probable method to enhance the function of the muscle in aged populations (Basava et al., 2020).

4.6. Techniques for Studying Connective Tissue Morphology

There is a growing appreciation of connective tissue morphology, which demands a multidisciplinary set of strategies to enable researchers to visualize and quantify structural attributes. Histological staining is one such strategy, in which tissues are prepared and processed in such a manner that specific components become apparent with a microscope. Masson's trichrome and hematoxylin-eosin are vital stains that facilitate differentiation of collagen fibers from the other cellular components, thus enabling the investigation of the extracellular matrix (ECM). This method allows the examination of the arrangement, density, and pathology of connective tissues. It is even feasible to use immunohistochemistry in order to localize proteins within the tissue and derive information regarding functional properties and cellular interactions. Therefore, the intersection of a range of various staining procedures is paramount to appreciating the intricate morphology of connective tissues and differentiating their distinctive functions during health and illness. Imaging techniques have also come a long way to enhance connective tissue morphology research. Techniques such as electron microscopy (EM) allow scientists to study tissues at the ultra-structure level, allowing them to closely examine cell organelles and ECM structures. Transmission electron microscopy, for instance, can reveal the organization of collagen fibers and their molecular arrangement, and this has implications for understanding mechanical properties and tissue integrity. On the other hand, scanning electron microscopy (SEM) can be used to produce 3D topographical images, which could delineate the surface architecture of connective tissues. The fine resolution is important for the evaluation of spatial relationships and cellular heterogeneity. With these new imaging tools, researchers can create a comprehensive view of connective tissue morphology that is beneficial for basic science and clinical needs. Integrated with histology and imaging techniques, molecular biology methods have emerged as important tools to explore connective tissue morphology. Techniques such as *in situ* hybridization and quantitative polymerase chain reaction (qPCR) allow exploration of the gene expression patterns of ECM components and signaling molecules.

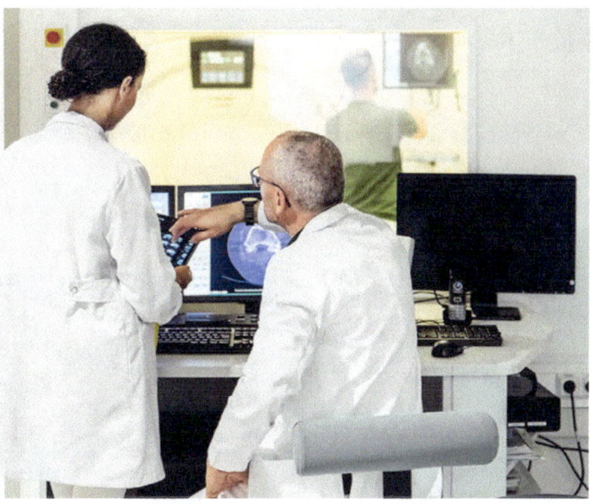

Figure 4.14. Techniques for studying connective tissue morphology.

Source: https://post.medicalnewstoday.com/wp-content/uploads/sites/3/2022/09/Doctors-CT-scan-732x549-thumbnail-732x549.jpg.

These molecular analyses enable the relationship between morphological information and functional changes in connective tissues. For example, the examination of collagenase gene expression in synovial fibroblasts is an illustration of overlap between cellular organization and biochemical signaling cascades, highlighting the work of genetic factors in tissue remodeling (Aggeler et al., 1984). Furthermore, methods such as proteomics have been utilized to clarify the protein composition of connective tissues and information about their functional states and responses to stimuli. By integrating molecular biology into connective tissue morphology, researchers can gain a deeper understanding of the dynamic principles governing the function and pathology of connective tissue (Figure 4.14).

4.6.1. Histological Staining Methods

Histological staining techniques are simple procedures used in connective tissue morphological research, enabling visualization of tissue architecture and intracellular structures. They may be employed to mark various structural elements, including collagen fibers, proteoglycans, and cell types that are components of connective tissue. The most widely used stain, hematoxylin and eosin (H&E), produces contrast among cell structures by staining nuclei a deep blue and cytoplasmic elements a pinkish hue. Differential coloration is significant in determining connective tissue architecture and the prevalence of specific cell types, such as fibroblasts and adipocytes. Also, the employment of specific stains can elucidate more nuanced details, i.e., elastic fibers with orcein or Masson's trichrome stain, that could further define extracellular matrix components, thereby contributing to tissue pathology as well as function. In addition to H&E, histochemical stains, such as Van Gieson and Alcian blue, are used to assess the localization of glycosaminoglycans and collagen in connective tissue. Van Gieson stain, for example, distinctly stains collagen red and enhances elastin and smooth muscle in yellow, so that it is simple to examine fibrous connective tissues. Alcian blue, on the other hand, stains acidic mucopolysaccharides and proteoglycans and reveals the presence of essential elements in cartilage as well as other connective tissue. The choice of staining method impacts the results of interpretation, especially in a comparison of materials for bone-forming potential, such as with certain calcium phosphate biomaterials in histological studies. Outcomes in this line emphasize the importance of appropriate staining methods for effective evaluation of tissue reactions to implants and biomaterials and for informing future research in regenerative medicine and tissue engineering (Barbeck et al., 2013). The effectiveness of histological stains also covers the assessment of cellular responses in connective tissues, particularly under pathological conditions. For instance, some staining techniques have been discovered to identify alterations in cell populations, such as differentiation and the occurrence of mast cells and globule leukocytes in various tissues. In terms of respiratory health, comparing the abundance and distribution of these types of cells via histochemical staining provides such critical data regarding their roles in immunity (Calonico et al., 1988). In addition, combining traditional staining methods with newer imaging technologies can provide a more complete picture of the dynamics of the connective tissue. By combining these methods, researchers are better able to elucidate the intricate relationships between cellular and extracellular components in connective tissues, thereby revolutionizing morphologic investigations in both health and disease (Figure 4.15).

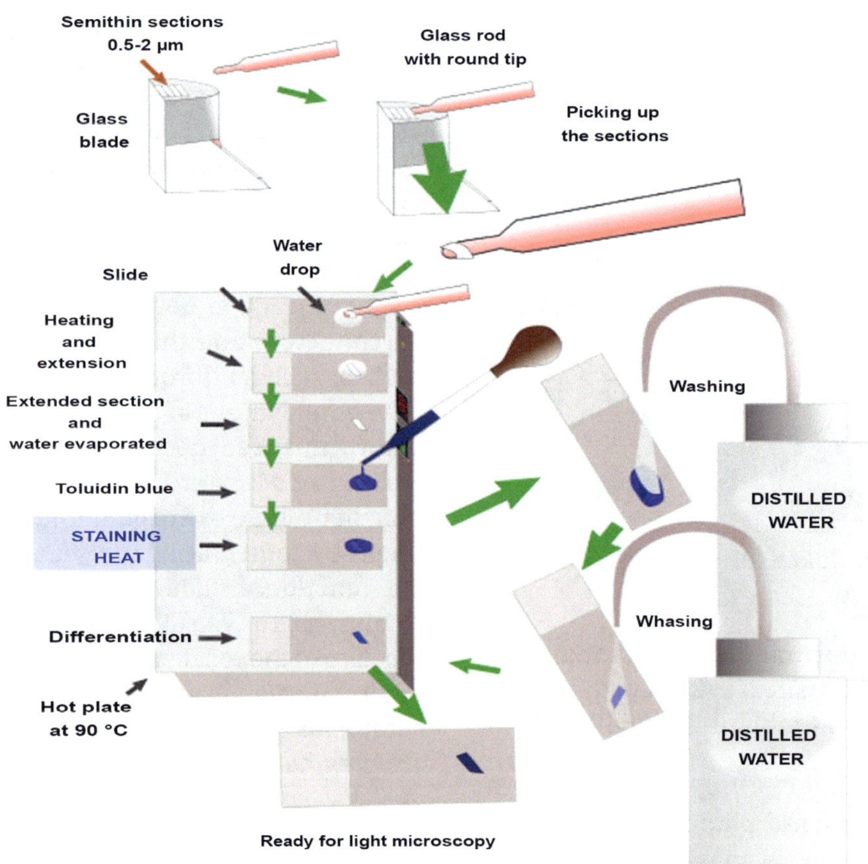

Figure 4.15. Histological staining methods.

Source: https://mmegias.webs.uvigo.es/02-english/6-tecnicas/imagenes/5-semifino.jpg.

4.6.2. Imaging Techniques (e.g., Microscopy)

The morphological examination of connective tissue is greatly facilitated by the use of high-tech imaging techniques, foremost among which are various forms of microscopy. Among these, second-harmonic generation (SHG) microscopy is noteworthy in that it can visualize collagen fibers directly, one of the key components of connective tissues. SHG utilizes the nonlinear optical response of collagen to give high-resolution three-dimensional images that reflect the fine structure and architecture of collagen fibrils. It is particularly useful in the study of pathologies characterized by collagen remodeling, providing information on how structural and functional changes are interconnected and relate to disease development. SHG microscopy thus expands our understanding of connective tissue architecture at the molecular level, providing significant information for basic science research as well as applied clinical applications such as tissue engineering. Polarized-light microscopy also further extends the role of imaging techniques in assessing connective tissue morphology. This method is used to study the preferred orientation and alignment of collagen fibers, which are of crucial significance to the mechanical properties of connective tissue. Data generated with the use of polarized-light microscopy can yield a clue to the influence of various biological parameters on the pattern of collagen organization, especially in pathological tissue. For example, the use of polarized-light methods in imaging articular cartilage highlights their potential for the evaluation of therapeutic outcomes in diseases like osteoarthritis. Not only do these imaging modalities add to our knowledge of the fundamental properties of connective tissues, but they also provide entry points into new therapeutic strategies that target specific structural abnormalities, as highlighted in recent developments in the field (Matcher, 2009). Moreover, sophisticated imaging technologies like SHG microscopy have broad implications for an understanding of the role of extracellular matrix components like proteoglycans in the structure of connective tissue. Studies have established that proteoglycans, particularly decorin, play a vital role in modulating collagen architecture and both fibril size and arrangement in tissues. Based on SHG microscopy parameters, researchers are able to characterize changes in collagen structure in various models, with distinctions in fibril organization correlated with proteoglycan presence or absence (Bushman et al., 2019). This sums up the broader applicability of imaging techniques to the investigation of connective tissue, emphasizing their potential to unveil the complexity of tissue morphology and its correlation with health and disease. These discoveries ultimately influence our overall understanding of tissue dynamics and direct future research into therapeutic intervention (Figure 4.16).

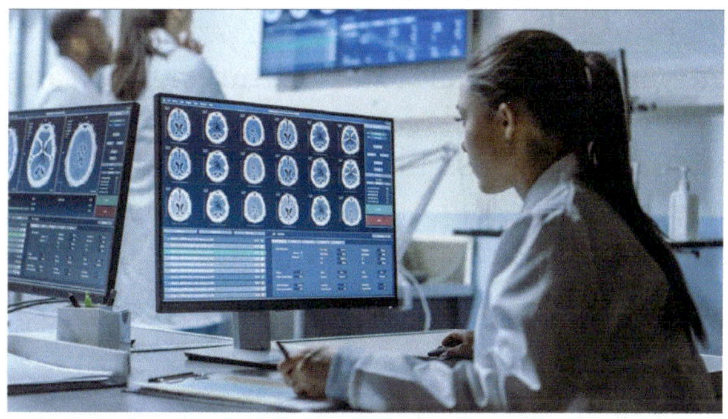

Figure 4.16. Imaging techniques (e.g., microscopy).

Source: https://www.healthcarebusinesstoday.com/wp-content/uploads/2020/07/image1.jpg.

4.6.3. Molecular Biology Approaches

Molecular biological techniques have played a significant role in understanding the morphology of connective tissue, as they provide information on the biochemical and genetic processes underlying tissue structure and function. The methodologies utilize techniques that, in most cases, involve gene expression analysis, protein profiling, and advanced imaging, and allow the scientist to decipher the intricate relationship between cellular components and their extracellular matrix (ECM). For instance, using the application of molecular markers, the cell differentiation of some of the cells in connective tissue, such as fibroblasts, osteoblasts, and chondrocytes, can be traced with the elucidation of their roles in tissue repair and development. Coupled with these methods, the information obtained has revealed the impact of mechanical signaling and biochemical signals from the ECM on behavior within cells, with significant implications for the morphologies of connective tissues in various biological processes. In addition to enhancing our understanding of molecular interactions, these techniques have also been crucial in investigating the pathological consequences of abnormal connective tissue formation. For example, genetic mutations involving the synthesis or regulation of ECM molecules, such as collagen and elastin, have been linked to several connective tissue disorders. By employing molecular biology techniques, researchers can model these genetic alterations in vitro, enabling close examination of how these alterations affect cellular signaling cascades and morphology. Furthermore, molecular data-based computational models, such as those investigated in the dynamics of bone resorption (Anderson et al., 2011), can simulate interactions between osteoclasts and bone matrix, hence modeling how disruptions of molecular processes might manifest as structural abnormalities in connective tissues. Furthermore, cross-species comparative molecular analysis over a broad range of species enhances the information richness pertaining to connective tissue evolution and adaptability. By studying molecular signatures specific to different connective tissues, researchers are able to trace evolutionary lines and study how morphological diversity emerges in response to environmental forces. The work on *Tritonoharpa* demonstrates how molecular data can help us navigate anatomical differences and functional adaptations in the context of neogastropods (Kosyan et al., 2009). Comparing the molecular features in a range of species, authors can explain the evolutionary significance of molecular innovation and provide a more general impression of connective tissue morphology across the biological range. This multi-faceted analysis then ultimately increases our understanding of both normal physiology and the pathophysiologic mechanisms underlying many connective tissue disorders (Figure 4.17).

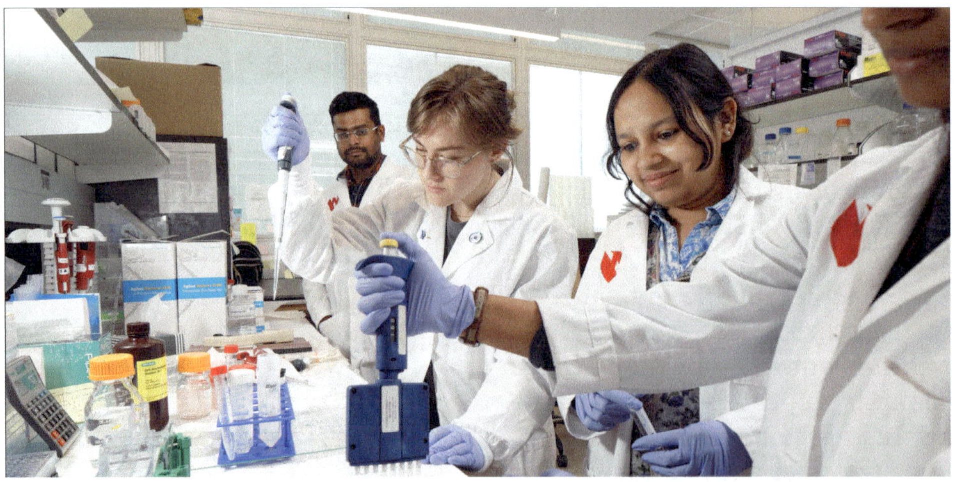

Figure 4.17. Molecular biology approaches.

Source: https://www.unmc.edu/biochemistry/_images/biochem-index-large2.jpg.

SUMMARY

In correlating findings on connective tissue morphology, it is evident that structural variations among connective tissues contribute significantly to their functions within the body. The diversity of connective tissues, illustrated through studies of such structures as tendons, ligaments, and vaginal mucosa, illustrates the manner in which some architectural organizations sustain mechanical strength and biochemical function. For example, the presence of steroidogenic enzymes in vaginal tissues varies across the estrous cycle, indicating that biochemical and structural adaptations are interconnected. These findings underscore the significance of learning about tissue morphology in the broader context of physiological function and developmental biology, towards an incentive for further research into the how and why of such associations in various types of tissues and conditions, as guided by study results (Neto et al., 2017). In addition, the role of proteins such as tenomodulin (Tnmd) in connective tissues such as the periodontal ligament highlights the extensive overlap between cellular functions and morphology. Tnmd is reported to be a principal cell adhesion mediator influencing the mechanical properties of the connective tissue in charge of tooth eruption. The expression of Tnmd during growth phases explains that connective tissues are not merely passive structures but dynamic structures that are involved in ongoing physiological processes. The compartmentalization of different domains in this protein, the BRICHOS domain among them, demonstrates how subtle molecular mechanisms are part of structural maintenance and functionality of connective tissues. Understanding of these processes enhances not only our knowledge of the function of connective tissue but also possibly provides therapeutic possibilities for disease states involving such tissues, validating the importance of connective tissue morphology to disease and health (Chung et al., 2013). In conclusion, connective tissue morphology yields invaluable information regarding both the structure and function of such tissues. The intricate interactions of cellular components, their spatial organization, and the consequent mechanical properties are evidence of the adaptive capability of connective tissues to physiological requisites and stressors. Additional research must keep demystifying the complexities of connective tissue morphology, particularly as related to hormonal regulation and cellular signaling processes. Understanding of these relationships will be essential to the development of directed therapy for connective tissue injury and disease, advancing the field of regenerative and reconstructive medicine. The knowledge thus gained from the investigation of the morphology of connective tissue is not only of fundamental biological importance but also of clinical importance in supporting tissue health and resilience across a variety of medical applications.

By investigating the intricacies of the morphology of connective tissue, it's clear that its structural components have a significant role to play in a variety of functional implications. One of them is the unique structure of connective tissue in the bat wing, consisting of thin skin over the forelimb bones, but facilitating flight. The organized bundles of elastin within this dermal layer not only contribute to the elasticity necessary for wing movement but also play a pivotal role in enhancing aerodynamic properties. The study of 130 bat species has revealed variations in these elastin bundles, ultimately informing our understanding of flight dynamics across different taxa. By including cross-polarized light imaging findings, scientists can illustrate how connective tissue architecture is directly related to species-specific locomotor adaptations and how morphology is important to the functional role of connective tissue in a more general biological sense (Fenton et al., 2017). Furthermore, the pathological aspect of connective tissue structure deserves critical scrutiny, particularly concerning disease development inclusive of such chronic pain syndromes.

Research has established that alterations in the stiffness of connective tissue resulting from fibrosis may have an important role in the processes underlying drug-resistant chronic pain. Fibroblast-to-extracellular nucleotides communication has been one of the main streams of research, linking collagen synthesis with the regulatory circuits of cell receptors. Specifically, nucleotide overgrowth due to UTP and ADP signifies pivotal biological processes in the subcutaneous connective tissue that bear witness to a sophisticated balance among various receptor interactions in modulating tissue repair and fibrosis. This kind of suggestion suggests an increased understanding of connective tissue morphology, not only clarifying its morphological characteristics but also uncovering useful information regarding the underlying causes of pathological states (Reis et al., 2011). Ultimately, the unfolding of knowledge regarding the subtleties of connective tissue morphology opens the doors to new therapeutic avenues to correct related diseases. Through an understanding of the molecular mechanisms driving connective tissue remodeling, researchers can now target particular receptors associated with fibroblast activity and collagen synthesis. For instance, regulation of P2Y receptor activity has great potential to control the fibrotic pathways involved in chronic pain. It is crucial to have an understanding of the diverse architectural elements of connective tissue and their functional roles in the development of specific interventions. The dependence of morphology on pathology demonstrates that connective tissue is an active participant in pathological and physiological processes, not merely a structural framework, thereby underscoring the relevance of its study in basic and applied biological sciences (Reis et al., 2011; Fenton et al., 2017).

A LOOK TO THE FUTURE:

BODY-WIDE METABOLIC PATHWAYS:

The body-wide metabolic pathways of a living organism represent a vast network of interlinked biochemical reactions that sustain life by converting nutrients into energy, building blocks, and signalling molecules essential for cellular function, growth, repair, and homeostasis. At every moment, trillions of enzymatic reactions take place within cells throughout the body, collectively forming metabolic pathways that break down substrates such as carbohydrates, lipids, and proteins, and then reassemble or transform these components to meet the biological demands of different tissues and organ systems. Fundamentally, metabolic pathways can be divided into catabolic processes, which degrade complex molecules to release energy, and anabolic processes, which synthesise new molecules and structures necessary for growth and maintenance. For example, glycolysis—a sequence of enzyme-driven reactions converting glucose into pyruvate—releases energy stored in chemical bonds and generates high-energy intermediates like ATP that power cellular activities. This pathway, like others in the metabolic network, does not operate in isolation but interfaces with processes such as the citric acid cycle and oxidative phosphorylation to support energy production throughout the body.

The interdependence of these pathways reflects a sophisticated system of regulation and coordination that ensures cells adapt to fluctuations in nutrient availability, hormonal signals, and physiological demands. Metabolic networks are highly complex, with many pathways branching, converging, and feeding into one another; intermediates produced in one pathway may serve as substrates or regulators in others. This interplay enables diverse tissues to collaborate—for instance, the liver mobilising glucose through glycogen breakdown during fasting and skeletal muscles utilising that glucose for contraction during activity.

Metabolic integrity is central to health: when the balance of pathways is maintained, cells efficiently harness energy and build essential molecules; when disrupted, common diseases such as diabetes, obesity, cardiovascular disorders, and metabolic syndromes can emerge from metabolic dysregulation. Understanding body-wide metabolic pathways not only deepens insight into fundamental physiology but also informs strategies for therapeutic intervention, biomarker discovery, and precision medicine. Research that maps and models these pathways at organismal scales—integrating genomics, proteomics, metabolomics, and computational systems biology—continues to reveal how systemic metabolic coordination underpins health and how its perturbation drives disease processes.

Body-wide metabolic pathways illustrate the remarkable orchestration of biochemical processes that sustain life, adapting to internal and external cues while integrating energy production, nutrient utilisation, and molecular synthesis across tissues and organs.

REFERENCES

1. Bednarczyk, M., Stadnicka, K., Kozłowska, I., Abiuso, C., Tavaniello, S., Dankowiakowska, A., Sławińska, A., & Maiorano, G. (2016). Influence of different prebiotics and mode of their administration on broiler chicken performance. *Animal, 10*(8), 1271–1279. https://doi.org/10.1017/s1751731116000173Abzhanov, A., Baggiolini, A., Baroffio, A., Beverdam, A., Chevallier, A., et al. (2019). Molecular and cellular mechanisms underlying the evolution of form and function in the amniote jaw. https://core.ac.uk/download/323079229.pdf (accessed on 6th August 2025).
2. Adriaens, D., Baskin, J. N., Coppens, H. (2010). Evolutionary morphology of trichomycterid catfishes: About hanging on and digging in. https://core.ac.uk/download/55867718.pdf (accessed on 6th August 2025).
3. Aggeler, J., Frisch, S. M., Werb, Z. (1984). Collagenase is a major gene product of induced rabbit synovial fibroblasts. https://core.ac.uk/download/323074870.pdf (accessed on 6th August 2025).
4. Agungpriyono, S., Kurniati, H., Nurhidayat, Phadmacanty, N. L. P. R., et al. (2024). Water monitor lizard (*Varanus salvator*) skin microstructure: Histochemical and morphometrical studies of fiber type characteristics. https://core.ac.uk/download/617724949.pdf (accessed on 6th August 2025).
5. Anderson, B., Beysens, D., Block, J., Boyce, B., Boyde, A., Britz, H., et al. (2011). Investigation of bone resorption within a cortical basic multicellular unit using a lattice-based computational model. http://arxiv.org/abs/1105.5093 (accessed on 6th August 2025).
6. Angelis, R. D. (2019). A practical overview of the role of capillaroscopy in rheumatic diseases. https://core.ac.uk/download/267929271.pdf (accessed on 6th August 2025).
7. Ariannia, S., Dehghan, P., Rajaei, A. (2016). Nail fold capillaroscopic findings in Iranian patients with systemic lupus erythematosus. https://core.ac.uk/download/483634926.pdf (accessed on 6th August 2025).
8. Assis Neto, A. C., Conley, A. J., de Oliveira, M. F., Dos Santos, et al. (2017). Immunolocalization of steroidogenic enzymes in the vaginal mucous of *Galea spixii* during the estrous cycle. https://core.ac.uk/download/323070725.pdf (accessed on 6th August 2025).
9. Audi, S. H., Clough, A. V., Krenz, G. S., Molthen, R. C., et al. (2006). Lung circulation modeling: Status and prospect. https://core.ac.uk/download/213071954.pdf (accessed on 6th August 2025).
10. Azevedo, R. B. de, Báo, S. N., Ganassin, R., González-Fernández, et al. (2014). PVM/MA-shelled selol nanocapsules promote cell cycle arrest in A549 lung adenocarcinoma cells. https://core.ac.uk/download/33550311.pdf (accessed on 6th August 2025).
11. Barbeck, M., Ghanaati, S., Kirkpatrick, C. J., Künzel, et al. (2013). Implantation of silicon dioxide-based nanocrystalline hydroxyapatite and pure phase beta-tricalciumphosphate bone substitute granules in caprine muscle tissue does not induce new bone formation. https://core.ac.uk/download/14525097.pdf (accessed on 6th August 2025).
12. Basava, R. R., Chen, J.-S., He, Q., He, et al. (2020). Microstructural analysis of skeletal muscle force generation during aging. https://core.ac.uk/download/286361329.pdf (accessed on 6th August 2025).

13. Bölgen, N., Korkusuz, P., Menceloğlu, Y. Z., et al. (2007). In vivo performance of antibiotic embedded electrospun PCL membranes for prevention of abdominal adhesions. https://core.ac.uk/download/pdf/11739273.pdf (accessed on 6th August 2025).

14. Burton, M. J., Derrick, T., Essex, D., Holland, M. J., et al. (2016). Increased epithelial expression of CTGF and S100A7 with elevated subepithelial expression of IL-1β in trachomatous trichiasis. https://core.ac.uk/download/42636526.pdf (accessed on 6th August 2025).

15. Buscalioni, Á. D., Chiappe, L. M., Marugán-Lobón, J., Navalón, et al. (2015). Soft-tissue and dermal arrangement in the wing of an Early Cretaceous bird: Implications for the evolution of avian flight. https://repositorio.uam.es/bitstream/handle/10486/672901/soft_navalon_SR_2015.pdf?sequence=1 (accessed on 6th August 2025).

16. Calonico, L. D., McDonald, D. M., Nadel, J. A., Tam, et al. (1988). Globule leukocytes and mast cells in the rat trachea: Their number, distribution, and response to compound 48/80 and dexamethasone. https://core.ac.uk/download/323079479.pdf (accessed on 6th August 2025).

17. Carlotti, F., Chuva de Sousa Lopes, S. M., de Koning, E. J. P., de Melo Bernardo, et al. (2014). Lymphangiogenesis and angiogenesis during human fetal pancreas development. https://core.ac.uk/download/55800083.pdf (accessed on 6th August 2025).

18. Cherkas, O. A., Kobeza, P. A., Marchenko, D. G. (2023). Basic principles of the structure and organization of connective tissue. https://core.ac.uk/download/588778720.pdf (accessed on 6th August 2025).

19. Chung, U.-I., Docheva, D., Hiraki, Y., Hojo, et al. (2013). Tenomodulin expression in the periodontal ligament enhances cellular adhesion. https://core.ac.uk/download/12175517.pdf (accessed on 6th August 2025).

20. Curry, V., Fenwick, S. A., Hackney, R., Harrall, et al. (2001). Expression of transforming growth factor-beta isoforms and their receptors in chronic tendinosis. https://core.ac.uk/download/2776656.pdf (accessed on 6th August 2025).

21. Curtis, K. C., Fischer, K., Fischer, P. U., Tkach, et al. (2017). Ultrastructure and localization of *Neorickettsia* in adult digenean trematodes provides novel insights into helminth–endobacteria interaction. https://core.ac.uk/download/83101037.pdf (accessed on 6th August 2025).

22. Cutolo, M., Llado, A., Paolino, S., Pizzorni, et al. (2016). Capillaroscopy in 2016: New perspectives in systemic sclerosis. https://core.ac.uk/download/74613576.pdf (accessed on 6th August 2025).

23. Degistirici, O., Götz, W., Jaquiery, C., Martin, et al. (2008). Defining properties of neural crest-derived progenitor cells from the apex of human developing tooth. https://core.ac.uk/download/18240097.pdf (accessed on 6th August 2025).

24. Deus, I. A. (2021). Preparação de um hidrogel a partir de membranas fetais humanas para cultura de células em 3D. https://core.ac.uk/download/325954045.pdf (accessed on 6th August 2025).

25. Dzięgelewska, Ż. & Gajewska, M. (2018). Stromal-epithelial interactions during mammary gland development. https://core.ac.uk/download/322438762.pdf (accessed on 6th August 2025).

26. Edwards, R. W., Maltenfort, M. G., McBeath, R., O'Hara, et al. (2019). Tendinosis develops from age- and oxygen tension-dependent modulation of Rac1 activity. https://core.ac.uk/download/213449831.pdf (accessed on 6th August 2025).

27. Fenton, M. B., Gray, P., Holbrook, K. A., Humphry, G. M., Maisonneuve, P., Meyer, W., Schumacher, S., et al. (2017). Diversity in the organization of elastin bundles and intramembranous muscles in bat wings. https://core.ac.uk/download/76981004.pdf (accessed on 6th August 2025).

28. Hao, E., Lee, S.-H., Levine, F. (2013). Efficient β-cell regeneration by a combination of neogenesis and replication following β-cell ablation and reversal of pancreatic duct ligation. https://core.ac.uk/download/287623694.pdf (accessed on 6th August 2025).

29. Jörger, K. M., Neusser, T. P., Schrödl, M. (2011). Cryptic species in tropic sands—Interactive 3D anatomy, molecular phylogeny and evolution of meiofaunal *Pseudunelidae* (*Gastropoda, Acochlidia*). https://core.ac.uk/download/12175392.pdf (accessed on 6th August 2025).

30. Kosyan, A., Modica, M. V., Oliverio, M. (2009). The relationships of the enigmatic gastropod *Tritonoharpa* (Neogastropoda): New data on early neogastropod evolution? https://core.ac.uk/download/54372429.pdf (accessed on 6th August 2025).

31. Leveson-Gower, D., Ly, D. (2025). *Bion-M2 PI 1-Pagers*. https://core.ac.uk/download/pdf/286393560.pdf (accessed on 6th August 2025).

32. Li, Y., Lu, L., Rao, A. S., Starzl, T. E., et al. (1994). Isolation, phenotype, and allostimulatory activity of mouse liver dendritic cells. https://core.ac.uk/download/12205069.pdf (accessed on 6th August 2025).

33. Matcher, S. J. (2009). A review of some recent developments in polarization-sensitive optical imaging techniques for the study of articular cartilage. https://core.ac.uk/download/50699.pdf (accessed on 6th August 2025).

34. Preziosi, L. & Scianna, M. (2013). Modelling the influence of nucleus elasticity on cell invasion in fiber networks and microchannels. https://core.ac.uk/download/pdf/11431730.pdf (accessed on 6th August 2025).

35. Reis, C. P. da S. e S. (2011). P2 purinoceptors signaling in fibroblasts of rat subcutaneous tissue. https://core.ac.uk/download/15568458.pdf (accessed on 6th August 2025).

36. Riley, G. P. (2004). The pathogenesis of tendinopathy: A molecular perspective. https://core.ac.uk/download/2776643.pdf (accessed on 6th August 2025).

37. Stumpf, P., Welsch, U. (2002). Cutaneous eccrine glands of the foot pads of the rock hyrax (*Procavia capensis, Hyracoidea, Mammalia*). https://core.ac.uk/download/16432898.pdf (accessed on 6th August 2025).

38. Thomas, S. (2023). An in vivo biocompatibility analysis of a novel tissue regeneration matrix using a pig model. https://core.ac.uk/download/568115992.pdf (accessed on 6th August 2025).

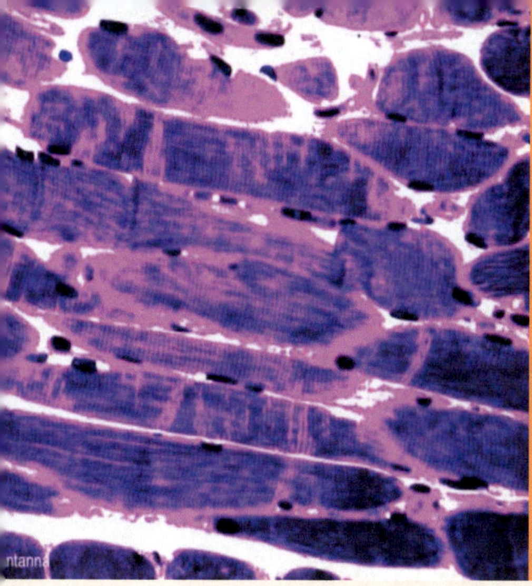

Chapter 5

MUSCLE TISSUE MORPHOLOGY

Contents

Introduction

Morphology study of muscle tissue plays an important role in the understanding of its elementary function in various biological processes across species. Muscle tissue, a specialized form of connective tissue, achieves its high performance due to its complex structural organization. Its structural pattern conditions the capacity of the muscles to contract and transmit forces, which is the basis for its importance in movement, as well as posture and stability. As studies have increased, an understanding of how a range of variables, such as training, aging, and hormonal changes, affect muscle morphology has become increasingly more important, especially in a clinical setting. Latest research indicates that structural qualities and mechanical properties of muscle tissues may alter significantly based on external stimuli, thereby making in-depth studies on such differences critical at this juncture. Muscle morphology is a fundamental concept that influences fields ranging from rehabilitation sciences to sports medicine and underpins effective treatment and training techniques (Aldini et al., 2016).

The one area that has been the focus of special attention in the morphology of muscle tissue is elastic structure studies across various organisms, particularly within the framework of their functional capabilities. One such example of such musculature would be the bat wing structural musculature that exhibits complex adaptations towards flight mechanics. Bats possess a specialized wing morphology, where the skin encloses the forelimb skeleton and extends between the digits, containing specially organized elastin and invested skeletal muscle. Experiments have proven that such elastic structures not only contribute to the aerodynamics of flight, but also to the fine control of wing shape during flight.

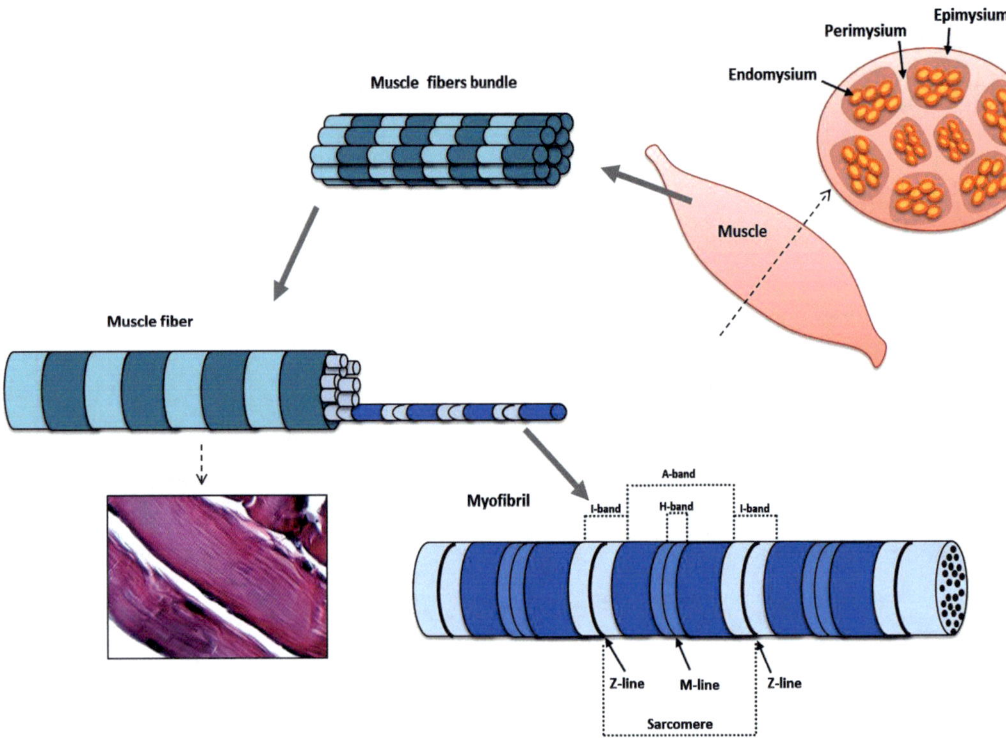

Figure 5.1. Muscle tissue morphology.

Source: https://www.mdpi.com/jfmk/jfmk-01-00289/article_deploy/html/images/jfmk-01-00289-g002.png.

This intricate architecture symbolizes the evolutionary significance of muscle tissue adaptation, highlighting how particular arrangements provide enhanced function. Accordingly, comparative morphological analyses of muscles across organisms are of immense value in gauging the evolutionary pressures shaping these adaptations and assessing their importance in ecological niches (Fenton et al., 2017). Additionally, the impact of training and detraining on muscle morphology is revealing of the dynamic nature of muscle tissues. Training regimens or de-training can bring about meaningful physiological change in the structure and function of muscles. Notably, understanding the biological response of muscle tissues to different conditions will inform rehabilitation interventions following injuries. These treatments are not only for the recovery of muscle strength but also for the corresponding tendon properties, which are crucial to maintaining musculoskeletal well-being. Recent findings show that acute detraining is, in fact, able to cause structural impairments in muscle tissues, so the attention to physical rehabilitation here is in order. By summarizing current evidence about muscle and tendon morphology, scientists can better elucidate mechanisms for recovery and performance in various athletic and clinical groups and finally provide more efficient training and rehabilitation programs (Aldini et al., 2016) (Figure 5.1).

Definition of Muscle Tissue

Muscle tissue is a specialized tissue that is mainly in charge of the movement and functioning of the body. Characterized by its unique ability to contract, muscle tissue enables both voluntary action, such as walking and lifting and involuntary movement, such as beating the heart and digestion. Muscle tissue is mainly categorized into three types: skeletal, cardiac, and smooth muscle. Voluntary control is present in skeletal muscle, which is typically attached to bones and enables locomotion. The cardiac muscle of the heart functions involuntarily and contains unique intercalated discs to provide synchronous contraction.

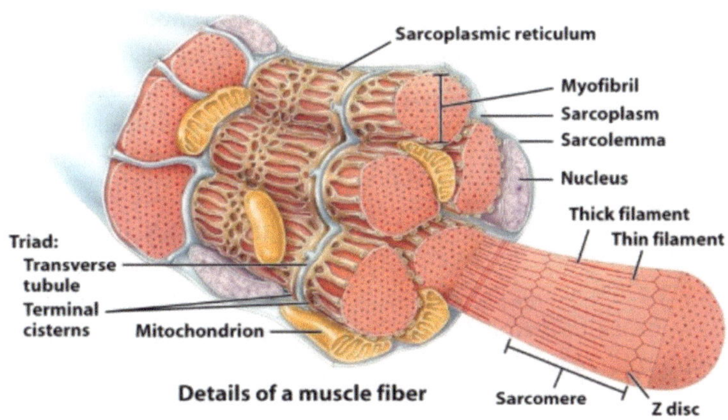

Figure 5.2. Definition of muscle tissue.

Source: https://duckduckgo.com/?q=Definition+of+muscle+tissue&t=h_&iar=images&iai=https%3A%2F%2Fwww.online-sciences.com%2Fwp-content%2Fuploads%2F2021%2F02%2Fmuscular-tissue-structure-34.jpg.

Smooth muscle in various organs is involuntary and plays a role in essential processes such as the regulation of blood flow and digestion. Gratitude for these differences highlights the richness and complexity of muscle tissue, enriching the study of its morphology. Additionally, the pattern, size, and shape of muscle fibers vary with the muscle type and its functional requirements. Studies have reported alterations in muscle morphology across various pathological conditions, including LBP, in which muscle fiber atrophy and degeneration can limit function and locomotion. These reports indicate the direct correlation among muscle structure and function under both health and disease conditions, as exemplified in conditions where derangements of the normal muscle tissue architecture occur (Danneels et al., 2016). Additional studies of muscle tissue morphology reveal that certain events, such as myofascial trigger points, also influence muscle integrity and function.

The theory of myofascial trigger points posits that localized regions of contracted sarcomeres can exist within normally relaxed muscle and may cause pain and reduced mobility. This was a specific observation in trapezius myalgia conditions, where biopsy sampling demonstrated foci of contracted sarcomeres in the muscle and created an interruption of the normal relaxation response. The fact that these contracted segments existed provides evidence of an understanding of deeper wisdom regarding muscular dysfunction and its implications on rehabilitation strategy (Cagnie et al., 2020). These observations underscore the importance of meticulous investigation of muscle tissue morphology in not only unraveling its varied structural characteristics but in tracing underlying processes of muscular pathologies, therefore informing effective treatment and management protocols (Figure 5.2).

Importance of Studying Muscle Morphology

Studying the structural features of muscle tissue helps us understand how muscles function at both the cellular and systemic levels." Closely examining muscle fibers, their composition, and their connective tissues, researchers can learn how different muscle types—skeletal, cardiac, and smooth—perform their unique physiological functions. This data is critical in developing targeted rehabilitation programs, improving sports performance, and informing surgical procedures. The identification of differences in muscle morphology also facilitates the diagnosis of muscular disorders and the design of effective treatments, underscoring the significant implications of studies in this field (Carlotti et al., 2014). More importantly, research on muscle morphology is relevant to understanding the body's adaptability to changes in physical demands or disease status. For instance, studying why muscle fibers hypertrophy in response to resistance training can inform strategies to maximize endurance and strength. In addition, understanding the changes in muscle morphology and composition with age can inform the better understanding of sarcopenia and other ageing conditions. It is increasingly necessary to study how factors such as exercise and diet influence muscle morphology. Such studies not only contribute to optimizing athletic performance but also continue to be vital in the advancement of longevity and quality of life with aging. Finally, ongoing investigation into muscle morphology permits additional understanding of the body's functional adaptations and resistance (Abourachid et al., 2014). Additionally, the significance of muscle morphology is a result of its applicability in biomedicine, particularly in relation to regenerative therapies. Examining the architectural and functional features of muscle tissue can shed light on regenerative potential after injury or disease. For instance, the knowledge gained from understanding how vasculature functions with muscle cells, as pointed out in recent studies of human organogenesis, can be used to develop tissue engineering and transplantation strategies. The knowledge generated by examining the interrelationship between muscle morphology and the vascular structures surrounding them, such as lymphatic vessels and blood vessels, is pivotal in the development of successful regenerative interventions. As investigators continue to unravel the complexity of muscle organization and its clinical relevance, they pave the way for new therapies to aid recovery and restore function, thereby emphasizing the necessity of comprehensive studies of muscle morphology (Carlotti et al., 2014).

Overview of Muscle Tissue Types

Muscle tissue can be broken into three broad categories: skeletal, cardiac, and smooth muscle. Each of these has distinct structural characteristics and physiological attributes that enable it to perform specific functions within the body. Striated skeletal muscle is voluntarily controlled and primarily serves movement and posture. Made of long, multinucleated fibers, the skeletal muscle shortens quickly and forcefully, which makes it crucial for tasks involving rapid energy bursts. It is fixed to bones using tendons, allowing for a tremendous variety of movements from basic gestures to intricate athletic movements. The aligned coordination of myofibrils within skeletal muscle fibers enhances the power and efficiency of contraction, a classic example of the intricate relationship between form and function in the architecture of muscle. Cardiac muscle, present only in the heart, possesses striations as well as intercalated discs, allowing for synchronized contractions to facilitate effective blood pumping. This involuntary muscle acts automatically via intrinsic pacemaker cells that create rhythmic contraction without the necessity for conscious control. The intercalated discs are critical junctions between the two adjacent cells, where electrical impulses are passed quickly to synchronise the contractions of the heart. The cardiac muscle fibers are shorter and extensively branched compared to skeletal muscle, which renders it with distinct functional properties. The effectiveness and endurance of cardiac muscle are of prime significance, as it must generate a life-long rhythm of contractions without fatigue. Understanding specialized cardiac muscle morphology is central to an understanding of how it functions in cardiovascular disease and the potential impacts of cardiac diseases, and consequently, the significance of greater study in the morphology of the muscle tissue. Smooth muscle, primarily in the walls of hollow organs and the circulatory system, plays a vital role in involuntary movements in the body. Unlike cardiac and skeletal muscle, smooth muscle lacks striations and comprises spindle-shaped cells that rhythmically and slowly contract. Smooth muscle is responsible for involuntary activities like respiratory processes, the control of blood flow, and digestion. The autonomic nervous system controls the contractions of smooth muscle, thereby enabling the delicate regulation of organ function. The morphology of smooth muscle enables it to contract in more than one dimension so that complicated movements are possible for organ function. The morphological study of smooth muscle makes us aware of the causes of diseases such as hypertension or gastrointestinal disease, and once again proves the need for diverse muscle tissue types for the maintenance of overall physiological homeostasis.

5.1. Types of Muscle Tissue

The body of human beings has three significant categories of muscle tissue, namely skeletal, cardiac, and smooth muscle, which possess a unique set of structural and functional properties. The skeletal muscle, attached to the bones through tendons, enables voluntary movements and is made up of long, cylindrical, multinucleated fibers. Striated muscle is controlled by the somatic nervous system, which allows for highly precise movement and coordination. In contrast, the heart muscle builds the heart walls and is involuntary and controlled by the autonomic nervous system. Its fibers are short, dichotomously branched, and interwoven, with the presence of specialized intercellular junctions referred to as intercalated discs for the purpose of facilitated contractions in harmony. Lastly, smooth muscle, which resides in the walls of hollow organs, such as the intestines and arteries, is also involuntary but has a non-striated appearance. Understanding these categories provides valuable information about their specialized functions in the human body and their contribution towards overall physiological functions. The morphology of skeletal muscle tissue is functionally linked to its functional requirements, with its striated nature attributed to the presence of actin and myosin filaments. Fibers in the skeletal muscles are organized into bundles, which are called fascicles, and are surrounded by connective tissues like epimysium, perimysium, and endomysium. This pyramidal structure not only facilitates muscle contraction but also enables efficient force transmission. The neuromuscular junction (NMJ) plays a crucial role in evoking muscle contractions, as motor neurons release neurotransmitters that stimulate skeletal muscle fibres. However, advances in tissue analysis techniques, such as MYOCLEAR, have enabled researchers to analyze NMJ morphology and density in whole-mount preparations, greatly aiding understanding of skeletal muscle function and how neuromuscular diseases affect contraction efficiency and overall muscle performance (Gretz et al., 2019). Cardiac and smooth muscle cells have significant roles to aid in developing homeostasis within the body, distinguished not only by their morphology but also in the way they are controlled. Cardiac muscle, with its highly organized anatomy, contains numerous mitochondria in order to supply sufficient energy for the continuous contractions of the heart. The intercalated discs of cardiac muscle cells enable electric impulses to be passed rapidly, as a result of which the coordination of heartbeats is highly efficient. On the other hand, smooth muscle tissue has a spindle and elongated shape with cells that are stimulus-sensitive from a wide range of sources, such as hormones and neural impulses. The muscle plays a significant role in involuntary movements like peristalsis in the gastrointestinal tract and vasodilation in arteries. The complex interplay among these muscle systems underscores their relevance to movement and circulation, as well as to pathology in cardiomyopathy and hypertension, areas that warrant ongoing research (Thiel et al., 2019) (Figure 5.3).

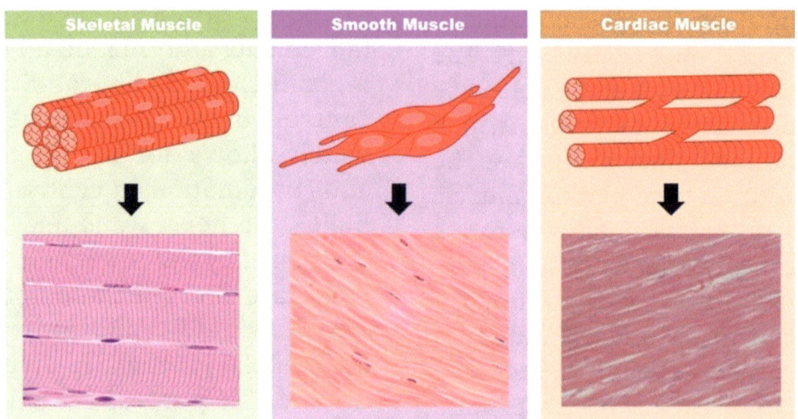

Figure 5.3. Types of muscle tissue.

Source: https://munnscience.weebly.com/uploads/3/8/0/6/38066171/852963235_orig.jpeg.

5.1.1. Skeletal Muscle

Skeletal muscle, characterized by its striated appearance and multinucleated fiber structure, plays a critical role in offering voluntary movement along the entire human body. This muscle is under the control of the somatic nervous system to offer precise motor functions ranging from simple postural alterations to complex motor activities. The morphologic organization of skeletal muscle is inextricably connected with its functional potential; every muscle fiber contains myofibrils arranged as sarcomeres, supporting the active units of contraction. The alignment of actin and myosin filaments within these sarcomeres provides the muscle with its striated look while optimizing force development throughout contractions. Understanding the unique morphology of the skeletal muscle offers insights into its flexibility, repair mechanism, and response to various physiological needs, which underlines its function in maintaining overall body function and mobility. Various cellular and molecular processes influence the formation and differentiation of skeletal muscle fibers, ensuring they acquire their specialized structures. Skeletal muscle is developed from myoblasts during embryonic growth, which are derived from somatic mesodermal cells. As these proliferating myoblasts combine, they form long multinucleated myofibers that exhibit exceptional morphological diversity based on their functional specialization. For instance, fast-twitch fibers, used in explosive movement, are significantly different in size and metabolic properties from slow-twitch fibers, more suited to endurance performance.

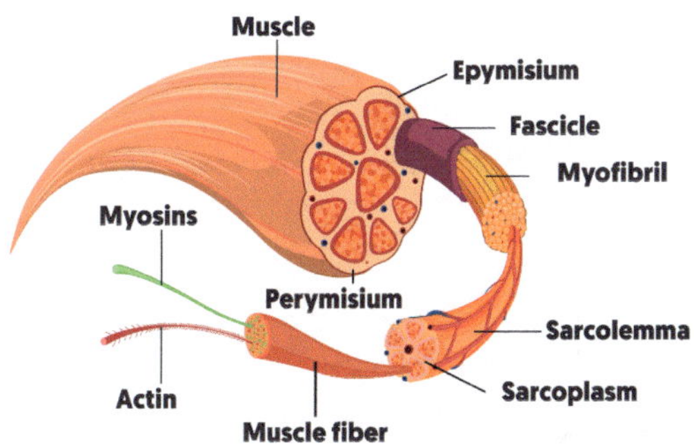

Figure 5.4. Skeletal muscle.

Source: https://www.worksheetsplanet.com/wp-content/uploads/2022/09/Skeletal-Muscle.jpg.

Myofibrillar protein synthesis and satellite cell proliferation are essential for the growth and recovery of skeletal muscle following injury. This dynamic relationship demonstrates how the morphology of skeletal muscle is not rigid but reflects continual adaptation to functional requirements and environmental stimuli. Second, the morphology of skeletal muscle can also be understood more effectively through evolutionary importance by comparing species. Research has highlighted that variability in the structure and function of the muscles is not merely an adaptation to diverse locomotor patterns but also indicates the evolutionary paths pursued by distinct lineages. For example, the plasticity of skeletal muscle fibers due to biomechanical stresses and motor patterns is highly relevant to species-specific evolutionary gain. Studies of the cranial neural crest mesenchyme illustrate the ability of the morphology of skeletal muscle to explain variance in vertebrate head and jaw morphology (Abzhanov et al., 2019). Additionally, studies on avian patellar tendons illustrate the evolutionary process by which skeletal muscle and associated structures have evolved specialized morphologies that enhance mechanical efficiency and advantage during locomotion (Alexander et al., 2014). The morphology of skeletal muscle is thus key to understanding functional adaptation as well as the broader evolutionary history (Figure 5.4).

5.1.2. Cardiac Muscle

Among various muscle tissues, cardiac muscle is unique due to its unique morphology and key physiological functions. Unlike skeletal muscle, which is multinucleated in appearance and under voluntary control, cardiac muscle fibers are linked together by intercalated discs and create a syncytial structure. Such a feature ensures speedy communication among myocytes, leading to coordinated contractions essential for the rhythmic beating of the heart. Additionally, striation of cardiac muscle is caused by ordered sarcomeres, and these render it efficient and strong. Understanding the structure of cardiac muscle is crucial for understanding how it maintains homeostasis and responds to metabolic needs; for these reasons, it is a focus of interest in cardiology studies of heart health and disease. Recent studies on cardiac muscle pathology have specifically targeted ensuring structural and functional integrity via new therapeutic regimes. For instance, investigations on the impact of angiotensin receptor blockade (ARB) in disease conditions like Duchenne muscular dystrophy (DMD) have contributed significant insight into the health of cardiac muscle. The study indicated that therapy with ARB guaranteed cardiac function for the long term without any marked influence on skeletal muscle morphology or function. These reports indicate that interventions do not always prevent muscular dystrophy progression but may have a significant role in preventing the myocardium from degeneration. This therapeutic approach is consistent with the development of new treatments for specific cardiac phenomena, underscoring the emphasis for future research on cardiac muscle preservation in dystrophic situations (Leask et al., 2011). Moreover, advances in genetic studies offer promising avenues for research and perhaps the treatment of cardiac muscle disease. Research into glycosylation mechanisms, and indeed into LARGE, has elucidated the interaction between glycosylation patterns in cardiac and skeletal muscles. Overexpression of LARGE has been found to restore functional glycosylation of alpha-dystroglycan, crucial in the stabilization of muscles. This approach not only highlights the importance of structural proteins in cardiac muscle but also suggests that understanding extracellular matrix interactions may pave the way for novel therapeutic regimens. Targeting the underlying molecular mechanism, researchers can increase the overall strength of cardiac muscle in dystrophies, paving the way for novel and safe therapies (Brockington et al., 2010) (Figure 5.5).

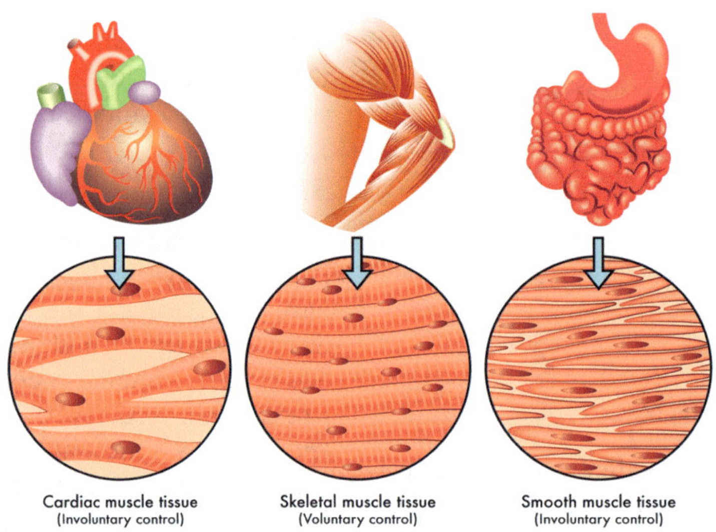

Figure 5.5. Cardiac muscle.

Source: https://weighttraining.guide/wp-content/uploads/2020/04/Muscle-structure.png.

5.1.3. Smooth Muscle

The mechanical properties of smooth muscle tissue are of fundamental significance in its operation throughout all organ systems. Contrary to skeletal and cardiac muscle, smooth muscle fibers consist of non-striated spindle-shaped cells that provide for involuntary regulation. This allows smooth muscle to sustain prolonged contractions without fatigue, facilitating body functions such as peristalsis in the digestive system and the regulation of blood vessel diameter. The differential morphology of smooth muscle cells is accountable for the alterations in shape and size of the cell following varied stimuli, so that it can adapt to the specific requirements of organs. The dense bodies of smooth muscle cells also serve as sites of attachment for the contractile proteins, facilitating force transmission during contraction, which is a critical requirement of the physiological functions they are modulating. The smooth muscle contractile apparatus is controlled through the interaction between actin and myosin filaments, regulated in a cascading fashion by calcium ion influx. Smooth muscle does not employ troponin in thin filaments for control, as in skeletal muscle, but instead, calcium binds to calmodulin, activating myosin light chain kinase, which phosphorylates myosin and enables cross-bridge cycling. This is particularly important at events such as vasodilation or vasoconstriction, where the ability of smooth muscle to contract and relax controls the overall blood pressure and flow. Additionally, smooth muscle tone being regulated by many biochemical pathways enhances its role in diverse physiological responses, mapping mechanical activity to the metabolic status of the tissue. Smooth muscle's plasticity, both morphological and mechanical, is required to guarantee homeostasis in various systems. Smooth muscle cells, apart from their physiological roles, are also very plastic and exposed to mechanical and biochemical stimuli emanating from their extracellular matrix (ECM). Such plasticity is required for the remodeling and regeneration of tissues after damage. As an example, smooth muscle cells can change their phenotype—transition from being contractile to the synthetic phase—enabling vascular tissue healing. Studying the interaction between smooth muscle cells and their ECM provides insight into such diseases as atherosclerosis, in which pathological remodeling occurs. Aging is associated with increased stiffness in connective tissue, which can negatively affect smooth muscle function. This increased stiffness also alters force generation during concentric and eccentric contractions." It is important to realize how smooth muscle architecture and ECM behavior are connected, as they play an essential role in the further advancement of therapeutic interventions aimed at cardiovascular disease or other diseases with smooth muscle dysregulation, shining the light on their significance in medical research and treatment development (Figure 5.6).

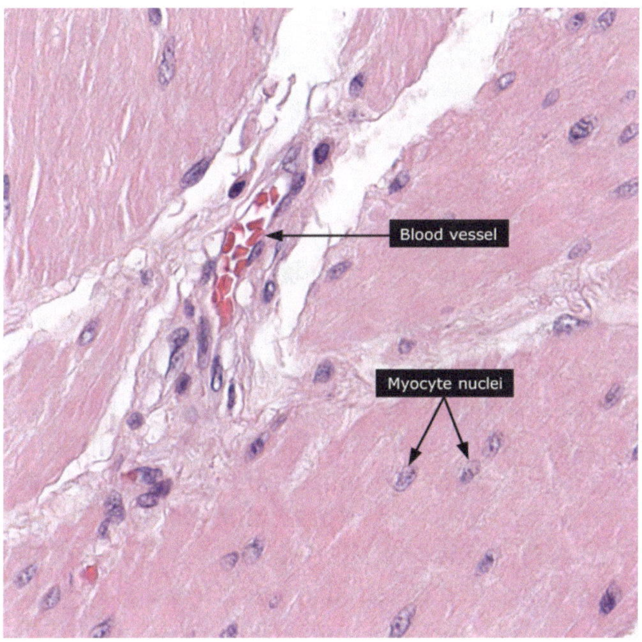

Figure 5.6. Smooth muscle.

Source: https://ibiologia.com/wp-content/uploads/2019/11/smooth_muscle__1__example_1__1_100_1.jpg.

5.2. Skeletal Muscle Morphology

The morphology of the skeletal muscle is characterized by its ordered structure, which is central to its function and adaptability. The ordered arrangement of the muscle fibers allows for force generation and efficient contraction. In skeletal muscles, the fibers are structured into fascicles that are encapsulated in sheaths of connective tissue. Each muscle fiber is a multinucleated cell whose length and diameter vary, contributing to the overall strength and function of the muscle. This hierarchical structure is duplicated in its fibrous composition, with collagen and elastin providing tensile strength and elasticity, respectively. Advancements in bioengineering and biomaterials have drawn inspiration from such a sophisticated architecture, highlighting its potential in the creation of biomimetic actuators with a similar performance and behavior as muscle, further reinforcing the need for studying skeletal muscle morphology in both biological and engineering contexts (Focarete et al., 2020).

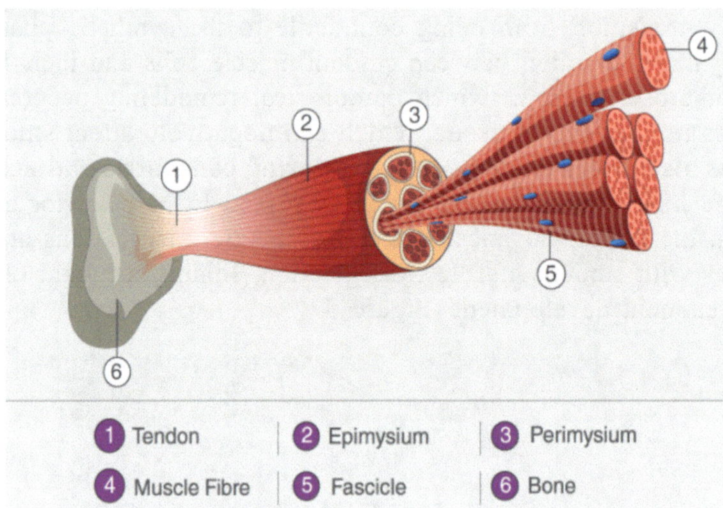

Figure 5.7. Skeletal muscle morphology.

Source: https://cdn1.byjus.com/wp-content/uploads/2022/02/structure-of-skeletal-muscle.png.

A significant component of skeletal muscle morphology is the biochemical and molecular processes that regulate the formation of muscle structure and the muscle's response to stimulation. Synthesis of glycosyltransferase enzymes is essential for the structural health of muscle cells, influencing the glycosylation of proteins such as alpha-dystroglycan, which is responsible for maintaining the attachment between muscle fibers and the extracellular matrix. Defects in the glycosylation process have the potential to lead to muscular dystrophies, suggesting the importance of molecular morphology in the health of muscles. Recent studies have identified that overexpression of enzymes like LARGE rescues glycosylation function, providing a therapeutic implication in the therapy of related muscular diseases. Studies indicate the complex interaction between the morphological nature of skeletal muscle and its biochemical environment, demonstrating that structural integrity directly influences muscle function and disease (Brockington et al., 2010). Also, the adaptation of skeletal muscle morphology through mechanical loading and disuse illustrates its dynamic nature.

Not only does repeated resistance training augment muscle fiber hypertrophy, but it also causes cellular adaptation, such as increased satellite cell activity and fiber-type shifting, which can improve overall muscle function and resistance. Conversely, muscle atrophy resulting from prolonged immobilization or disuse may result in major loss of muscle mass and strength. Understanding the morphological changes that result from various stimuli is of great importance for developing effective rehabilitation strategies and training protocols. This data allows for the optimization of interventions to preserve muscle function and prevent injury, thus validating the need for a comprehensive understanding of skeletal muscle morphology as part of the overall background of muscle tissue morphology (Figure 5.7).

5.2.1. Structure of Skeletal Muscle Fibers

The arrangement of skeletal muscle fibers is at the heart of their mechanism and is characterized by a complex array of proteins and organelles that enable contraction. Skeletal muscle fibers consist of multinucleated, elongated cells with numerous myofibrils aligned parallel to the length of the fibers. Myofibrils are made up of repeating units called sarcomeres, which are the basic contractile units of the muscle tissue. Within the sarcomere, thick filaments of myosin interdigitate between thin filaments composed primarily of actin and regulatory proteins such as tropomyosin and troponin. This highly ordered unit is required for the sliding filament mechanism of contraction, where the interaction of actin and myosin results in muscle shortening. Further, the overall architecture plays a vital role in defining the mechanical characteristics of the muscle, including its capacity to generate force and resist tension under different types of contraction. The pattern and composition of skeletal muscle fibers also differ based on their functional roles, leading to the identification of slow-twitch and fast-twitch fiber types. Slow-twitch fibers, with their high myoglobin and mitochondrial content, are specifically designed for endurance and sustained activity, depending on aerobic metabolism to produce energy. Fast-twitch fibers have lower levels of mitochondria but higher levels of glycogen and are suited for rapid, powerful contractions and quickly burn out. The structural heterogeneity has direct implications for muscle function and enables various muscles to be regulated according to the loading received in varying types of activity. Also, the distinct properties of each type of fiber are established by genetic, training, and environmental determinants, which are necessary to athletic performance and rehabilitation procedures. An awareness of these structural differences is necessary to appreciate the way skeletal muscle adapts to changing functional demands throughout life. Microstructural studies of the properties of skeletal muscle show that aging and other physiological changes can have sizeable effects upon muscle function and morphology. Notably, muscle force decline with advancing age involves both the muscle fibers and the extracellular matrix in which they are located. Studies indicate that the rigidity of connective tissue increases with age, thereby reducing the effectiveness of muscle contractions, particularly during eccentric movements (Basava et al., 2020). This stiffness may arise as an effect of changes in the microarchitecture of the muscle tissue, which underscores the significance of the extracellular matrix in muscle physiology. Additionally, changes in muscle fiber structure can impact functional implications in various patterns of movement, suggesting the complex interplay between muscle architecture, biochemical pathways, and mechanical capacities (Fenton et al., 2017). Knowledge of these factors is important in the development of successful interventions to counteract age-related muscle degeneration and maximize performance in various populations (Figure 5.8).

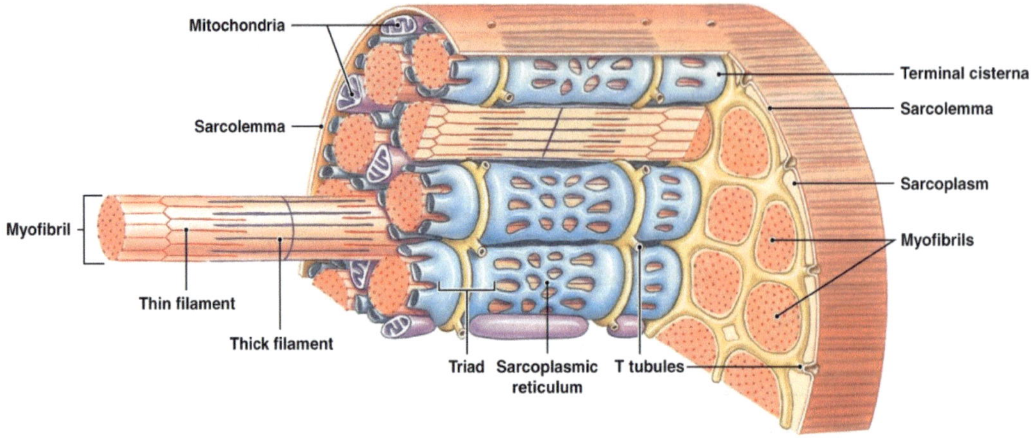

Figure 5.8. Structure of skeletal muscle fibers.

Source: https://i.pinimg.com/originals/48/ca/20/48ca20a70e4d1996385b21c2744d3a77.png.

5.2.2. Organization of Skeletal Muscle

The organization of skeletal muscle is highly ordered in order for it to accomplish its primary function of movement and force production. It consists of long, cylindrical muscle fibers, and it has a striated look because the myofilaments contained within each muscle fiber are arranged in an orderly manner. The myofilaments consist of actin and myosin, which contract muscle fibers via a complex mechanism known as the sliding filament theory. Each muscle fiber is encased by a sheath of connective tissue, the endomysium, which not only provides structure but also contains capillaries and nerve endings necessary for fiber maintenance and operation. Bundles of fibers possess outer layers of connective tissue, the perimysium, which are organized to create fascicles, or bundles. This ordered organization is responsible for the efficient transfer of force across muscle tissue of various lengths, making synchronized contraction and movement possible. More importantly, even the organization of skeletal muscle extends to its functional organization, which is specialized to the specific requirements it is exposed to. A good example of this is the organization of muscle fibers, which can vary greatly across muscle types, e.g., endurance versus strength muscles. In muscles that are primarily involved in long-term contractions, such as the soleus, fibers are typically oriented in parallel for higher efficiency for long-term activity. Conversely, for rapid and strong movements, such as the biceps brachii, pennate orientation of fibers offers greater cross-sectional area and hence maximum force. This dynamic relationship between structural organization and functional requirements demonstrates how evolutionary pressures have shaped muscle architecture to support diverse locomotor and postural functions across species, underscoring the importance of muscle organization within the broader context of muscle tissue morphology. An understanding of skeletal muscle organization also requires a discussion of cellular and molecular mechanisms that govern its development and adaptation. The embryonic development of the skeletal muscle from myogenic precursor cells illustrates the complex interaction between mechanical forces and genetic cues in the production of muscle. Ironically, cranial neural crest mesenchyme plays a critical role in patterning muscles and other related tissues, thereby influencing muscular diversity in animals. Similar to evolutionary development, varying molecular signaling is able to produce dramatic differences in muscle morphology, function, and injury. For instance, developmental aberrations may produce muscular dystrophies or other myopathies that interfere with skeletal muscle function, underscoring the need to identify these patterns of organization not only for biological insight but also for clinical purposes in the diagnosis and therapy of muscle-associated illnesses. Generally, the intricate organization of skeletal muscle elaborates upon a profound interface between structure and function, along with the molecular machinery responsible for muscle integrity (Figure 5.9).

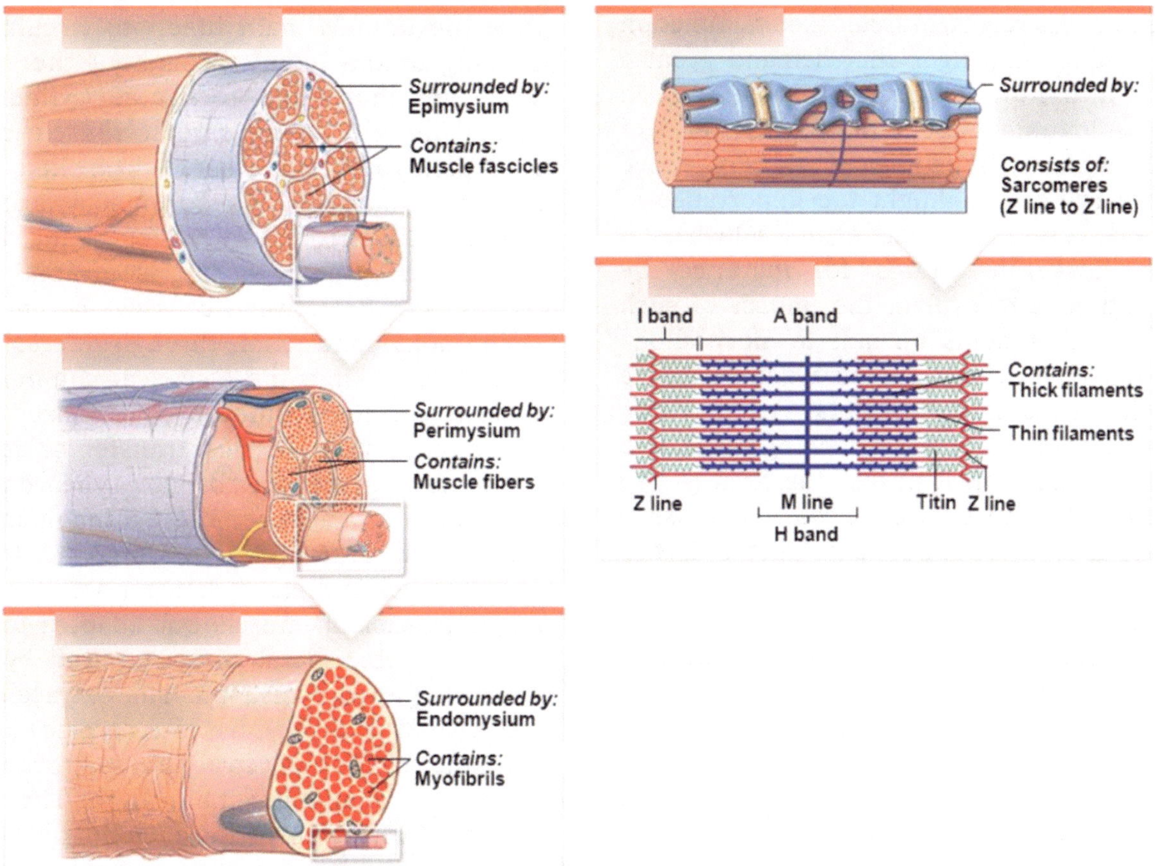

Figure 5.9. Organization of skeletal muscle.

Source: https://o.quizlet.com/phKcB88g1dqaGaYPevsE0w_b.png.

5.2.3. Role of Connective Tissue in Skeletal Muscle

Connective tissue is crucial to the skeletal muscle morphology and function as a significant supportive structure of the muscle fibers. It is comprised primarily of the endomysium, perimysium, and epimysium, and all these help contribute to the structure of the muscle as well as functioning in a unique manner. The endomysium envelops individual muscle fibers, providing structural support with the ability to communicate with the extracellular matrix. This interconnectivity is critical to the transmission of mechanical forces during muscle contractions, testifying to the interface between connective tissue and muscle function. Additionally, with age, the mechanical properties of connective tissues can alter significantly, e.g., stiffness, which can adversely affect the capacities of force generation, notably under concentric contractions. This has focused research on connective tissue dynamics in muscle morphology and function, particularly in aging populations (Basava et al., 2020). Furthermore, the sensitivity of skeletal muscle and its connective tissue to varying mechanical loads and kinds of stimuli has been seen. In the space environment, where weightlessness reigns, musculoskeletal function faces unique challenges that demand greater insight into how connective tissues adapt. Acute unloading affects the functional and structural integrity of muscle and connective tissue, serving to highlight the importance of these structures in maintaining musculoskeletal health. Research studies, for instance, by NASA, attempt to explain the impact of such adaptive adjustments on muscle morphology and connective tissue. Research admits to the plasticity of the musculoskeletal system, citing that adaptation to decreased loading can lead to functional impairment in the long term (N/A). This highlights the function of connective tissue not only as an inactive support structure but as an active participant in muscle adaptation and biomechanical health more generally. Finally, the intricate relationship between muscle fibers and connective tissues also provokes useful questions about performance and rehabilitation regimens. Understanding how connective tissues facilitate muscle function can guide the development of targeted treatments for injury, as well as age-related reduction of muscle function. Improved knowledge of the mechanical roles of connective tissues may guide rehabilitation exercise and strength training program development to oppose atrophic effects, particularly in the elderly or during disuse atrophy, as in individuals with prolonged immobility. By focusing on the dynamics of connective tissue, scientists will be in a position to provide a more encompassing explanation of muscle function, taking into consideration the intricate interactions between supportive structures and muscle fibers. This comprehensive understanding is vital to the development of musculoskeletal health interventions and their application across populations.

5.3. Cardiac Muscle Morphology

Cardiac muscle morphology is characterized by its clear-cut structural features that allow the organ's main function: circulatory pumping of the blood throughout the body. Unlike multinucleated, elongated, cylindrical skeletal muscle fibers, cardiac muscle cells, or cardiomyocytes are short, branched, and contain one nucleus. This morphology is useful for the simultaneous contraction of the heart tissue because the branching is advantageous for connectivity between cells, which enables synchronous contraction through intercalated discs. Discs enable the electrical coupling of adjacent cardiomyocytes by specialized gap junctions, so that the fast transfer of action potentials is made possible for synchronized heartbeats. In addition, the arrangement of myofibrils in cardiomyocytes contributes to the cardiac muscle's characteristic striated texture, similar to skeletal muscle but adapted to the chronic aerobic metabolism required by the heart's high-rate workload. The extracellular matrix (ECM) also plays a role in cardiac muscle morphology, providing structural support while facilitating cellular communication. The ECM consists of various proteins, including collagen and elastin, which, together, create a scaffold that supports the cardiac tissue's architecture. The network is also in charge of regulating cardiomyocyte function, including proliferation, differentiation, and mechanical properties. A study conducted with hydrogels indicates that it is possible to enhance the health and function of muscles in cardiac tissues by modulating the ECM, which will trigger regenerative processes upon injury. For instance, application of acellular extracellular matrix-based hydrogels has been promising not only for increasing tissue perfusion in cardiac treatments but also for further redeveloping muscle fiber morphology back to normal. Such interventions place great emphasis on ECM integrity to achieve maximal cardiac function and morphology, as shown in prior studies. Cardiac muscle morphology knowledge goes beyond mere structural review; it becomes vital in therapy design for cardiac-related conditions. Architectural failures in cardiac muscle, as in cardiomyopathies or heart failure, have a direct impact on the heart's capacity to pump, leading to critical health problems. Furthermore, the relationship between cardiac muscle cellular morphology and ECM composition warrants exploration for potential therapeutic interventions, particularly for post-injury normalization. The ongoing research on the promotion of cardiac muscle morphology via methods like gene therapy, including the upregulation of glycosyltransferases like LARGE for better glycosylation of alpha-dystroglycan, is reflective of the extent of innovation in treatments for the heart. By considering how cellular structure correlates with extracellular factors, researchers can develop holistic methods for reversing cardiac muscle dysfunction and improving prognosis in patients, as reflected in a series of pioneering studies (Figure 5.10).

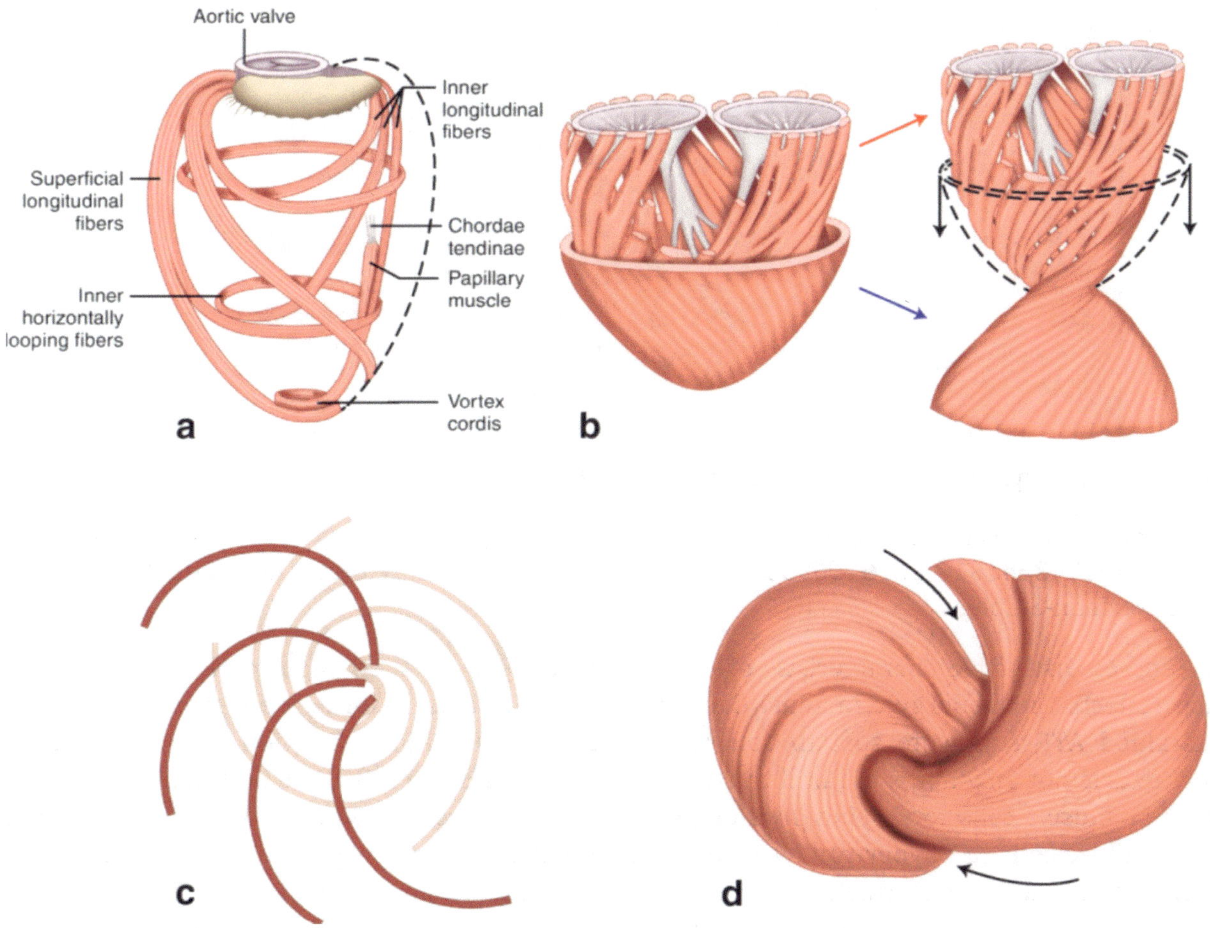

Figure 5.10. Cardiac muscle morphology.

Source: https://i0.wp.com/thoracickey.com/wp-content/uploads/2020/05/312524_2_En_13_Fig2_HTML.png?w=960.

5.3.1. Unique Features of Cardiac Muscle Cells

The unique features of cardiomyocytes are essential to the specialized role of the heart as a pump system that works in perpetuity. Compared to skeletal muscle, cardiac muscle possesses its striated appearance and inbuilt rhythmic contractions, primarily due to the specialized structure of its cells, or cardiomyocytes. The cells are intercommunicating and publicly branching, so that they can contract coordinately with each beat. This interconnectivity is facilitated by intercalated discs, specialized structures that connect adjacent cardiomyocytes. Intercalated discs contain gap junctions, which are direct cytoplasmic connections, and hence, electrical impulses are transmitted rapidly throughout the cardiac tissue. Hence, cardiac muscle cell morphology is exquisitely optimized for coordinated contraction, a crucial feature for effective blood circulation and general cardiovascular health (Cherkas., 2023).

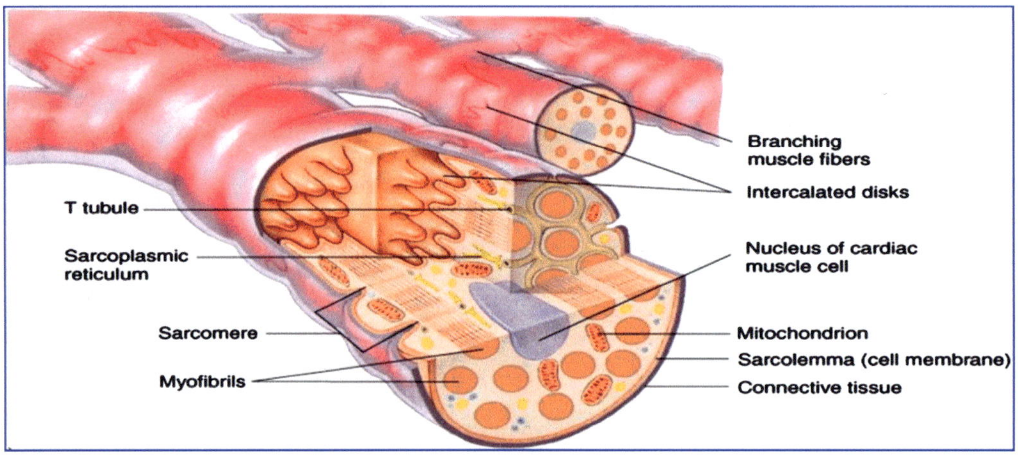

Figure 5.11. Unique features of cardiac muscle cells.

Source: https://www.researchgate.net/profile/Azza-Jabbar/publication/311274630/figure/fig42/AS:1003049124364301@1616156955462/Figure-610-Cardiac-muscle-cells-Reece-JB-Urry-LA-Cain-ML-Wasserman-SA.png.

Another distinctive characteristic of cardiac muscle cells is their high mitochondrial density, which reflects their energy demands. Cardiac muscle operates in an aerobic manner and needs a sustained ATP supply to sustain contraction as well as cellular function. The abundance of mitochondria not only helps to fulfill this energy need but also signifies the accommodative ability of cardiac muscle cells to varying physiological states. In increased workload, for instance, under exercise, these cells can hypertrophy, a condition in which cardiomyocytes increase in size in a bid to increase contractile performance. However, while good in the short term as an adaptive response, this can lead to pathological effects if sustained for an extended duration, usually predisposing a subject towards conditions such as heart failure (Brockington et al., 2010). It is therefore valuable to recognize the unique metabolic and structural features of cardiac muscle cells so that one may appreciate how they work in disease and health. The structural components of cardiac muscle also contribute to the functional superiority of cardiac muscle compared to other muscles. Such as the sarcomeres of cardiac cells, which are organized in an optimal fashion to support contractile function. These units possess a typical thick and thin filament organization that participates in muscle contraction. The desmosomal presence in the intercalated discs also provides mechanical strength through anchorage of neighboring cells, which is important in the high-pressure contractions of the heart. Besides, cardiac muscle cells contain an impressive ability to acclimatize to various stresses, which can be beneficial to fulfill possibly life-demanding needs, such as an increased requirement during severe physical exercise. By developing an understanding of these typical features, it can be better interpreted how they relate to cardiovascular disorders in terms of the intrinsic morphology of cardiac muscle (Cherkas., 2023) (Figure 5.11).

5.3.2. Intercalated Discs and Their Function

Intercalated discs are special cardiomyocyte junctions that form cardiac muscle tissue. They serve primarily to facilitate the transmission of electrical impulses for coordinated contractions of the heart that are necessary for adequate circulation. Intercalated discs have three main components: gap junctions, adhesive junctions, and desmosomes, all of which contribute significantly to myocardial function. Gap junctions permit direct electrical coupling between contiguous cells, enabling instantaneous communication required for synchronous contraction. By contrast, the mechanical strength provided by desmosomes helps anchor cardiomyocytes to one another, which is critical during the high-stress contractions of the heart. The highly engineered architecture of intercalated discs thus underscores their essential functions in maintaining both structural integrity and physiological function of cardiac tissue. The morphological organization of intercalated discs is directly related to the cardiac muscle's mechanical and electrical properties. Recent studies reveal that there is a strong correlation between the stability of intercalated discs and the heart's response to mechanical stress. The transient receptor potential vanilloid type 2 (TRPV2) cation channel, for instance, plays a pivotal role in maintaining cardiac architecture by supporting intercalated disc formation. Without TRPV2, cardiomyocytes exhibited gross disorganization of intercalated discs with consequent impaired myocardial conduction and reduction in cardiac function (Iwasaki et al., 2014). This suggests that intercalated discs are not only structural components but also play a pivotal role in mediating cardiac muscle adaptation to various physiological loads, making them an integral component of the heart's overall function. Moreover, the dynamic properties of intercalated discs are highlighted when cardiac hypertrophy is present, where they accommodate more mechanical load. As cardiomyocytes are undergoing hypertrophic adaptation—elongation and thickening—intercalated discs adapt to accommodate these changes. Research confirms that under mechanical stretch, cardiomyocytes exhibit a variety of responses relating to sarcomeric addition that occur at intercalated discs, such as Z disc formation and growth (Wei, 2021). The process not only underscores the significance of intercalated discs in muscle adaptation but also highlights the intricate interplay of signaling pathways activated by mechanical forces. In effect, intercalated disc function must be paramount in making the heart able to respond to increasing demand and maintain maximal physiological function.

5.3.3. Arrangement of Cardiac Muscle Fibers

The organization of cardiac muscle fibers is the key to appreciating the functional anatomy of the heart. In contrast to skeletal muscle fibers, cardiac muscle fibers are networked in a very organized pattern, creating a dense network that enhances synchronized contraction. This organization enables cardiac muscle cells, or cardiomyocytes, to work as one solid backbone during the rhythmic beating of the heart. They are arranged in a lattice or spiral configuration encircling the heart's chambers, enabling efficient contraction and relaxation. This specific arrangement optimizes not only the heart's mechanical function but also its electrical conduction, enabling rapid propagation of impulses through cardiac tissue and ensuring a synchronized heartbeat, which is essential for efficient blood circulation. This morphological cardiac fiber arrangement is also modulated by the presence of connective tissue elements, such as collagen, that contribute to the mechanical elasticity and strength of the heart. The structural support provided by this connective tissue complements muscle fiber organization into a shape that maximally takes advantage of their functional capabilities during systole and diastole. Research has indicated that thickening of the wall in the left ventricle plays an important part in efficacious systolic ejection, justifying the way in which myocardial architecture is structurally and functionally dependent. A coupling effect mechanism involving the muscle fibers and connective tissue has been proposed, whereby the collagen network surrounding the receptors helps stabilize the muscular fiber alignment (Bourdarias et al., 2008). This architectural design ensures that cardiac muscles can withstand the significant stresses generated during contraction while maintaining optimal performance. Moreover, the orientation of cardiac muscle fibers is not uniform throughout the heart; rather, it adapts to the specific functional demands of different regions. The fibrous nature of the cardiac fiber bundle allows variable arrangement, necessary for the differences in volumes and pressures found in different regions of the heart. The arrangement of the muscle fibers in a circular manner at the inlet and outlet of the ventricles, for example, provides for the proper constriction and dilation necessary in order to attain effective circulation of blood. Interestingly, it has been found through research that the organization of the fascicles can not only dictate the pumping ability but could also be responsible for the vulnerability of the heart to certain diseases. Knowledge of such intricate correlations, for example, that different fiber orientations are responsible for heart function, is paramount alongside examining the macrostructure of muscle tissues (Cheng et al., 2017) (Figure 5.12).

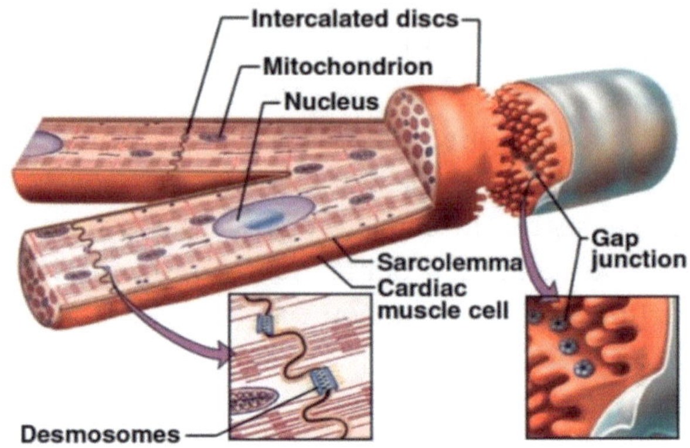

Figure 5.12. Arrangement of cardiac muscle fibers.

Source: https://external-content.duckduckgo.com/iu/?u=https%3A%2F%2Fwww.online-sciences.com%2Fwp-content%2Fuploads%2F2021%2F04%2Ffeatures-of-cardiac-muscle-fibers-2.jpg&f=1&nofb=1&ipt=fe344fce6e0337deab8693f14e7b5842041582d963fdcfdc8b006e853ab258cb.

5.4. Smooth Muscle Morphology

Smooth muscle morphology is characterized by typical architectural patterns that set it apart from cardiac and skeletal muscle tissues. Smooth muscle cells (SMCs) are spindle-shaped and elongated, and they are usually between 20 and 500 micrometers long. They possess only one centrally located nucleus, unlike the multinucleated fibers in skeletal muscle. Smooth muscle is deprived of striations due to the irregular arrangement of myosin and actin filaments, which contract in an indiscriminate, rather than linear, fashion. This type of structural organization makes smooth muscle capable of performing its primary task of involuntary contraction in various hollow organs, such as the gastrointestinal system and blood vessels, allowing vital physiological processes like digestion and maintenance of blood pressure. The morphology of smooth muscle cells significantly influences their functional capacity. For instance, SMCs are plastic with the capacity to be reshaped and refunctioned according to metabolic demand or development. Such plasticity is vital during tissue growth and repair, as evidenced by experiments involving the co-culture of fetal and adult smooth muscle cells. Results indicated that while each cell population maintained its phenotype, co-culture led to growth rate and protein profile alterations, highlighting that smooth muscle morphology is responsive and adaptable to the environment and consequently contributes to overall tissue homeostasis (Esen et al., 2024). These findings highlight the need for cellular interactions in the regulation of smooth muscle morphology and functionality. Understanding the morphology of smooth muscle is also vital from the pathology aspect. Pathological changes in the anatomy of smooth muscle may lead to a variety of diseases, such as hypertension or gastrointestinal disease, where the integrity of muscle tissue is lost. For example, cell architecture modifications under disease states can significantly impact contractility and responsiveness of smooth muscle, leading to organ dysfunction. Research has shown that the quality of histological preparation, such as fixation procedures used for analysis of smooth muscle tissue, plays a key role in the reliability of cellular assessments (Kandelouei et al., 2024). Better preservation processes are therefore required to bring about clarity about the complex smooth muscle morphology-function relationship, especially in a pathological context. Improved understanding of such interactions can provide windows of opportunity for treatment approaches aimed at restoring normal muscle function (Figure 5.13).

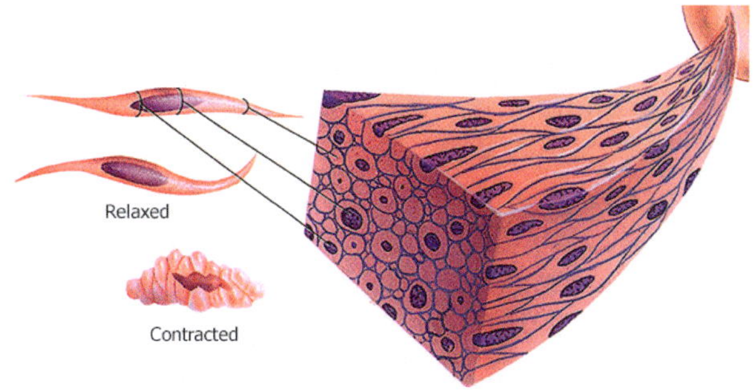

Figure 5.13. Smooth muscle morphology.

Source: https://www.lifelinecelltech.com/wp-content/uploads/2019/11/Vas-SMC-Contraction-right-blog.jpg.

5.4.1. Characteristics of Smooth Muscle Cells

Smooth muscle cells possess unique characteristics that set them apart from the other muscle cells, i.e., skeletal and cardiac muscle cells. Smooth muscle cells are non-striated, i.e., they do not possess the striations present in striated muscle due primarily to their filament organization of actin and myosin, which is more irregular in nature. This functional architecture produces a longer form, which allows smooth muscle cells to contract in multiple directions, something which is functionally necessary for mechanisms such as substance transport along hollow organs. Additionally, smooth muscle cells can be maintained for extended periods in a contracted state without fatigue, an effect partially attributed to their lower energy requirement compared to skeletal muscle (Aylott et al., 2014). This sustained contraction potential suits them well to be applied in functions like the maintenance of vascular tone in blood vessels and the control of gastrointestinal motility. The contractile machinery of smooth muscle cells is regulated strongly by their surroundings, particularly in three-dimensional environments that mimic physiological conditions. Research has indicated that in two-dimensional cultures, smooth muscle cells have altered contractile properties and morphologies compared to their in vivo equivalents (Aylott et al., 2014). Electrospinning technology, for instance, creates scaffolds that facilitate smooth muscle cell growth that is very similar to cell orientations in vivo and maintains cell alignment and a more functional phenotype. These tissue engineering advances not only account for smooth muscle cell behavior in response to different substrates but also underscore the necessity of realistic in vitro models to probe this behavior, with implications for disease modeling and therapeutic progress. Smooth muscle cell development and integration into function are essential to numerous physiological processes, including those that happen within the cardiovascular and gastrointestinal systems. In the pancreas, for example, smooth muscle cells play crucial roles in the vascular system that supports its complex endocrine and exocrine activities. In the development of the human pancreas, angiogenesis and lymphangiogenesis become absolutely necessary, and smooth muscle cell recruitment is a central part of such development. The presence of smooth muscle cells guarantees the functionality of new vessels so that there is an efficient supply of nutrients and hormones. These interactions highlight the importance of smooth muscle cells beyond their mechanical roles, their capacity to maintain organ homeostasis, and their potential therapeutic targets in regenerative medicine. Overall, knowledge about the nature of smooth muscle cells is essential in comprehending their multifaceted role in organ systems.

5.4.2. Types of Smooth Muscle

Its classification is essential to understanding its broad array of functions in the human body. Smooth muscle is primarily divided into two categories: single-unit and multi-unit smooth muscle. Single-unit smooth muscle in hollow organs such as intestines and blood vessels functions as a functional syncytium. This means contraction is simultaneous due to the presence of gap junctions, which allow for rapid communication between the muscle cells. Conversely, multi-unit smooth muscle, which occurs in organs such as the iris and large vessels, consists of separate fibers with independent functioning. These fibers are capable of being innervated by autonomic nerves, allowing for more precise control over contraction and relaxation. This variation is of great physiological importance since it implies the way in which various organs will respond to stimuli—synchronously or more coordinated, depending on the specific organ's needs. Smooth muscle's capacity to vary and respond to various stimuli is one of the main characteristics of smooth muscle and is revealed through its physiological functions. Single-unit smooth muscle is also characterized by spontaneous rhythmic contraction, which is seen in the gastrointestinal tract as peristalsis that facilitates digestion. This long-term involuntary contraction plays an important role in propelling contents effectively through the digestive system. Smooth muscle tone may also change due to hormonal control or the autonomic nervous system, demonstrating its flexibility. In comparison, multi-unit smooth muscle is also under considerable neural influence, but with the ability for more rapid modulation, such as in the pupil's contraction in response to light. This adaptability serves to emphasize the functional significance of smooth muscle types, relating their structural characteristics to broader physiological effects and to highlight their central roles in maintaining homeostasis in various body systems. Furthermore, smooth muscle tissue displays large morphological variations that correlate with its wide array of functions. The cells are spindle-shaped with a central nucleus and are not striated, unlike skeletal and cardiac muscle. The absence of striations is because the actin and myosin filaments' orientation is not into sarcomeres but distributed throughout the cell. In some pathological conditions, as in mucopolysaccharidosis (MPS-I), the morphology of the smooth muscle may be severely altered. In research work, alterations, such as intimal thickening and foamy macrophages and fibroblasts, may be found in the affected group.

These morphological changes have functional significance for the vasculature and highlight the role of smooth muscle within disease, further establishing its position in the study of muscle tissue morphology (Dickson et al., 2011; Carlotti et al., 2014).

5.4.3. Functional Implications of Smooth Muscle Structure

To examine the functional role of smooth muscle structure, it is essential to understand how its characteristic morphological features contribute to its functions across various physiological processes. Smooth muscle, by virtue of its non-striated morphology and involuntary regulation, is important in the regulation of the diameter of blood vessels as well as the motility of food through the gastrointestinal tract. The structure of smooth muscle fibers allows for continuous contractions with minimal energy utilized, necessary for the sustenance of organ activity over time. The physical properties, including the presence of gap junctions, facilitate synchronized contractions, which influence effective wave-like motions required for body functions.

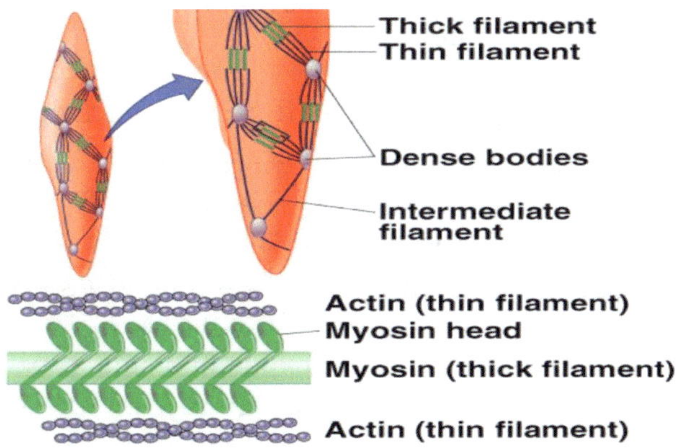

Figure 5.14. Functional implications of smooth muscle structure.

Source: https://image1.slideserve.com/2152265/structure-of-smooth-muscle-l.jpg.

The morphology of smooth muscle thus allows it to be effective in performing work requiring incessant, rhythmic contractions, ultimately influencing overall systemic homeostasis. The smooth muscle's flexibility distinguishes it from other muscles, enhancing its functional importance. Smooth muscle fibers, in contrast to other muscles, can vary significantly in length and size to be able to respond to varying physiological requirements. For instance, when the process of the gastrointestinal system is occurring, distension of the stomach triggers a reflex that augments the contraction of smooth muscle so that chyme is propelled along the digestive tract. Similar adaptability is observed in vascular smooth muscle, which adjusts tone in response to changes in blood pressure and flow. Once again, the viscoelastic properties of smooth muscle, dictated by the extracellular matrix, allow it to withstand mechanical stress while maintaining structural integrity. This dynamic regulation through the unique composition and organization of smooth muscle fibers is crucial for the normal physiology of various organs and body systems. Furthermore, smooth muscle structure plays a critical role in aging and disease. It has been observed that with advancing age, there occur changes in cellular composition and extracellular space of smooth muscle tissue, leading to altered contractile properties. Notably, increased stiffness of the passive tissues that surround smooth muscle can significantly influence its ability to produce force during different types of contractions. The disparate responses for concentric and eccentric contractions, wherein smooth muscle maintains partial function in spite of diminished force production, illustrate the complex relationship between structure and function. Understanding these morphological changes that occur with age provides evidence of potential therapeutic targets, enabling researchers to explore treatments that could potentially prevent smooth muscle dysfunction like that associated with hypertension and gastrointestinal disease. Generally, the structural significance of functional smooth muscle is intricate and critical for maintaining homeostasis and responding to physiological demands at all levels of life, as evidenced by studies documenting the microstructural modifications inherent in adaptation and muscle growth (Baskin et al., 2019; Basava et al., 2020) (Figure 5.14).

5.5. Muscle Tissue Development

Development of muscle tissue is a complex process beginning with the formation of myoblasts, the cells that will form muscles. Myoblasts are derived from mesodermal stem cells during embryonic development. As they develop and mature, they fuse together to form myotubes, significantly enlarging the muscle fiber. Such integration is required for the formation of the characteristic morphology of skeletal muscle, i.e., multinucleation and striated appearance. During this developmental process, regulatory factors and signal transduction cascades, such as the MyoD family of transcription factors, play crucial roles in guiding myoblast differentiation and fusion, ultimately resulting in the production of functional muscle tissues. Understanding of the mechanisms serves to explain how muscle tissue maintains itself, adapts to stress, and repairs following injury, and thus why the study of muscle development is a vital area of study. The function of the extracellular matrix (ECM) in muscle tissue formation cannot be overstressed. The ECM is a scaffold providing structure and biochemical signals necessary for myogenesis. It. supports cell adhesion and associates with muscle cells through various signal transduction pathways, which promote proliferation, differentiation, and maturation. Interestingly, recent findings have also shown that decellularized skeletal muscle-derived hydrogels have the ability to enhance tissue regeneration.

For instance, one study examined the efficacy of such hydrogels for the therapy of peripheral artery disease (PAD) by promoting tissue perfusion and muscle function through arteriogenesis, as compared to angiogenesis only, highlighting the distinct role that the ECM contributes to the process of muscle tissue expansion and repair mechanisms (Braden et al., 2016). By these interactions, researchers are able to develop new therapeutic strategies towards enabling muscle regeneration in the clinical setting. In addition, the morphology of muscle tissue is altered significantly throughout development and repair following injury. Skeletal muscle fibers have a typical pattern of myofibrils that enable them to carry out their function. Muscle morphology is changed by mechanical stress and hormonal regulation, which can change the type of fibers contained and muscle architecture. Specifically, skeletal muscle fibers can accommodate more work via hypertrophy, a process of enlarging existing fibers and not by increasing the number of fibers (hyperplasia). Therefore, muscle tissue structure is both a function of genetic predisposition and environmental influences, demonstrating the dynamic character of muscle growth over time. Studies of muscle tissue morphology across a range of contexts, including young people compared to older groups or across species, give insights into evolutionary modification in muscle structure and thus its significance in understanding muscle biology (Alexander et al., 2014) (Figure 5.15).

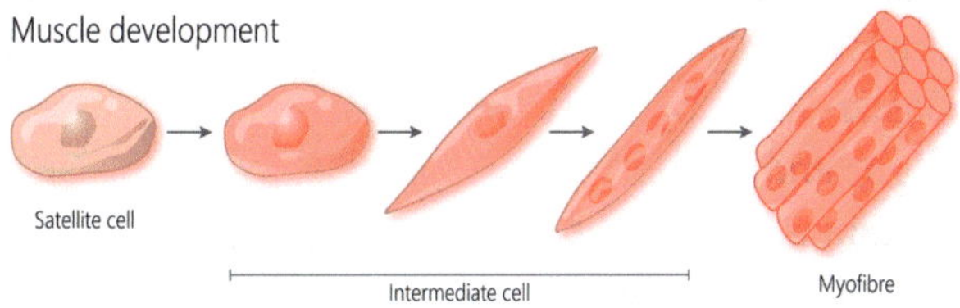

Figure 5.15. Muscle tissue development.

Source: https://as2.ftcdn.net/v2/jpg/02/39/86/01/1000_F_239860134_rXSl39mxfwynQgznFcL5O69DLOqVpELW.jpg.

5.5.1. Embryonic Development of Muscle Tissue

The developmental process of muscle tissue is a complex and strictly regulated phenomenon, regulated by environmental and genetic cues. Muscle development begins in the mesoderm, where the progenitor cells undergo a cascade of differentiation processes to give rise to various types of muscles, including skeletal, cardiac, and smooth muscle.

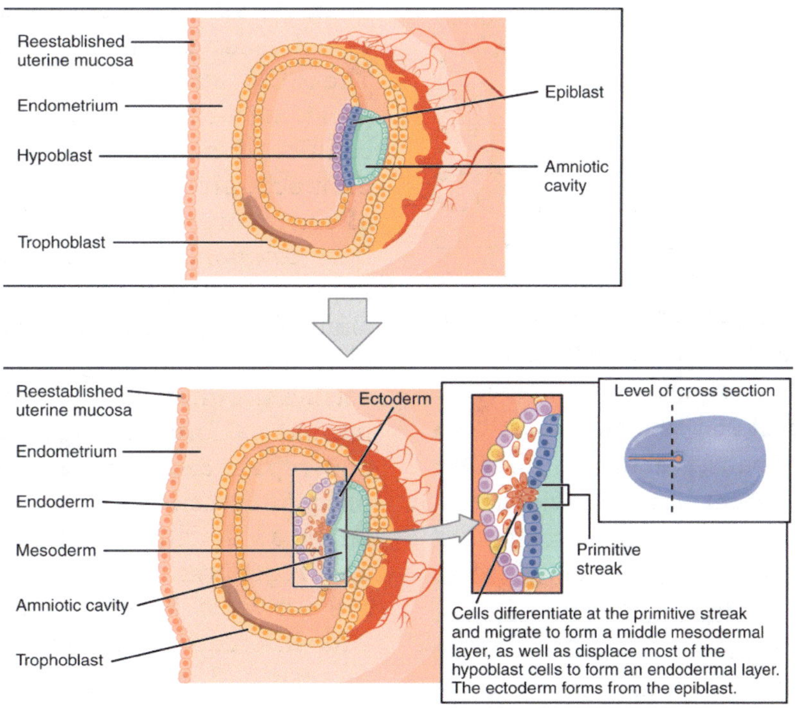

Figure 5.16. Embryonic development of muscle tissue.

Source: https://philschatz.com/anatomy-book/resources/2908_Germ_Layers-02.jpg.

Somites, which are derived from paraxial mesoderm, play an essential role in skeletal muscle development. As the progenitor cells proliferate and migrate, they form myoblasts, muscle fiber precursors. The early developmental stage is critical, as normal muscle tissue development is necessary for organ function and organism viability, highlighting the importance of accurate control during embryogenesis. Recent studies have elucidated the presence of myogenic cells capable of being cloned from the embryonic dorsal aorta, suggesting the potential that these cells may arise from non-somite sources. This is contrary to the traditional view of muscle tissue formation, which continued to be somite-focused and heavily focused on myogenic progenitors derived from somites. Researchers have suggested the potential transdifferentiation of vascular progenitor cells into myogenic lineages, creating an unanticipated cell fate determination plasticity in the embryo. In vitro experiments show that these aorta-derived cells are morphologically and marker-wise indistinguishable from adult satellite cells, and this suggests that they might follow a common developmental pathway. This new understanding of muscle progenitor sources suggests that muscle tissue regeneration after birth may involve the vascular system, further emphasizing the intricate interplay among tissue types during embryonic life. In addition, identification of double reporter mouse embryonic stem cell lines that express specific markers for endothelial and smooth muscle cells has also enhanced scientists' ability to visualize muscle tissue development in real-time. That is, these cell lines enable tracing of vascular and myogenic differentiation of cells, disclosing their spatial and temporal distribution. Coexpression of Tie-2 and α-smooth muscle actin markers during differentiation in this study lends support to the perception that embryonic muscle tissue arises from a shared progenitor pool. The new study not only explains the process of muscle formation but also opens up the avenues for producing targeted therapeutics for muscular degenerative disease. By this lucid understanding of the embryonic phenomena leading to muscle morphology, scientists are in a better position to counteract developmental anomaly-derived conditions (Figure 5.16).

5.5.2. Factors Influencing Muscle Growth and Repair

Implications for muscle repair and growth involve the discovery of certain important factors, including mechanical stimuli, nutrition, and ECM function. Mechanical loading from resistance training causes muscle hypertrophy through activation of a series of cellular signaling cascades. These signaling cascades allow for muscle protein synthesis, which leads to increased content of myofibrillar proteins in muscle fibers. In addition, proper nutrition, or more precisely, the availability of amino acids and adequate energy intake, is essential for optimizing recovery and growth. The ECM also facilitates muscle repair by providing a structural framework that regulates cellular dynamics, thereby modulating the biomechanical environment favorable for effective muscle repair. Therapies targeting ECM components, as demonstrated by recent studies, have been encouraging in inducing angiogenesis, a critical process for the delivery of nutrients and oxygen during repair, which verifies the interaction between biochemical and mechanical forces acting on muscle morphology and repair. Satellite cells are a population of progenitor cells that reside in muscle tissue and play a critical role in repairing muscles and regenerating muscle tissue. These cells are activated by muscle damage, proliferate, and differentiate to construct new myofibers or fuse with existing ones to induce muscle hypertrophy. The microenvironment of satellite cells, as determined by ECM composition and mechanical stress, plays a significant role in regulating their behavior. Recent advances in isolating single myofibers have provided valuable insights into how satellite cells interact with myofibers, making it possible for researchers to account for the various stages of muscle regeneration, including satellite cell activation and proliferation. This consciousness is essential because muscle regenerative potential is lost with age, and thus the maintenance of a permissive environment for such stem cells is crucial to facilitate effective repair and muscle growth with progressive age. In addition to that, inflammation and access to growth factors are critical determinants of muscle repair processes. With muscle damage, inflammatory signals govern the repair; they permit satellite cell activation and subsequent muscle regeneration. The balance of pro-inflammatory and anti-inflammatory cytokines is necessary for optimum healing; excess inflammation can inhibit the healing process. The growth factors, like insulin-like growth factor-1 (IGF-1) and fibroblast growth factor (FGF), are essential for muscle regeneration through the stimulation of satellite cell function and the facilitation of muscle protein synthesis. The therapeutic use of modulating such factors has the potential to unlock new pathways towards optimising muscle repair. Deploying interventions that exploit the positive attributes of inflammation and growth factor signaling has the potential to revolutionize muscle rehabilitation and sports medicine practice with the ultimate goal of improving muscle morphology and function during recovery.

5.5.3. Age-Related Changes in Muscle Morphology

Aging significantly affects the muscle morphology and consequent decrease in muscle mass and function, also referred to as sarcopenia. This is a result of a decrease in muscle fiber cross-sectional area and a decrease in muscle strength combined, leading to decreased physical performance. Most crucially, these changes are not merely surface-level; they represent reflections of more profound cellular alterations, such as muscle protein synthesis-degradation imbalance. Inflammatory markers increase with a catabolic impact, while drugs favoring anabolism in the muscle decrease. Thus, individuals become more vulnerable and more likely to experience falls and musculoskeletal trauma, highlighting the severe effect of aging on muscle composition and overall well-being in old age (Aniansson et al., 2009). With increasing age, physical activity declines on average, further contributing to muscle weakness. Due to a lack of activity, there is disuse of muscles, which augments the sarcopenic phenotype characteristic in the majority of older adults. However, research indicates that the degree to which adaptations in muscle morphology are altered is determined by the level of an individual's physical activity. For instance, there is a particular group of older adults with high physical activity levels whose muscle tissue quality, such as muscle fiber morphology and capillarity, is well maintained compared to their inactive counterparts.

This finding highlights the importance of physical activity in reducing the effects of ageing on muscle structure, thus suggesting that regular exercise might promote healthy ageing of muscle and preserve muscle mass and strength (Evans, 2015). The muscle biopsies of active older adults are taken for histochemical studies, which reveal that significant morphological alterations typical of ageing can be reduced or delayed by continuous physical activity. Unlike sedentary individuals whose muscle fibers are lost quickly with growing age, highly active individuals exhibit very minor changes within a decade. These findings suggest that physical training is beneficial in preserving muscle tissue structure and enhancing capillarization. The findings of this research have broader applications than physiological ones to muscle morphology; maintaining robust muscle tissue will maximize independent living in older age, reducing dependency and overall improving quality of life. The appreciation and prevention of changes in muscle morphology with increasing age are thus critical when formulating successful interventions to ensure healthy aging (Aniansson et al., 2009).

5.6. Pathological Changes in Muscle Tissue

Pathological changes in muscle tissue are interrelated complexly with multiple factors, like age, exercise status, and systemic disease. Notably, disease conditions like muscular dystrophy demonstrate the effects of genetic mutations through profound alterations in muscle morphology. Muscle fiber size, structure, and composition changes lead to functional deficits. For instance, in diseases such as Duchenne muscular dystrophy, fiber degeneration of muscles is followed by an increase of fibrous and adipose tissue progressively, significantly reducing muscle strength and endurance.

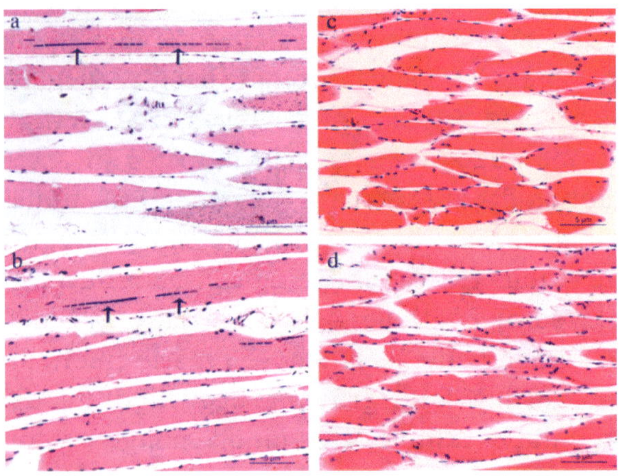

Figure 5.17. Pathological changes in muscle tissue.

Source: https://www.researchgate.net/publication/312103953/figure/fig1/AS:960122931130376@1605922553419/Pathological-changes-of-skeletal-muscle-cells-SkMCs-in-the-electric-death-The-nuclei.gif.

This particular fact places into perspective the importance of understanding the biological and anatomical variations in muscle tissue in relation to disease progression and therapeutic response. Furthermore, assessment of such pathological changes provides useful information on the rehabilitation processes that can mitigate the impact of such degenerative disorders on overall muscle function and structure. Apart from being genetically controlled, lack of activity can also produce formidable, unfavorable changes in muscle tissue. Experiments on tendon health, for instance, indicate that an acute detraining can lead to compromised structural organization in muscle tissue and impaired mechanobiological function of the damaged tissue. While skeletal muscle itself accommodates varying functional loads, sudden withdrawal of training can initiate a cascade of unwanted morphological events that include atrophy and compromised integrity of connective tissue. This connection applies in particular when one considers rehabilitation programs, as poor control of muscle disuse can completely reverse gains. As emphasized by recent research that discusses the effects of detraining, it is necessary for clinicians and coaches to apply evidence-based programs enabling less acute adaptation whenever exercise resumes, with emphasis on progressive reconditioning of the musculature. Furthermore, therapeutic advances open up promising lines to correct pathological muscle tissue alterations. Therapeutic strategies such as viral delivery of LARGE, which is a glycosyltransferase that is therapeutic in muscular dystrophies, have been shown to correct the glycosylation of alpha-dystroglycan on dystrophic muscle cells. Such glycosylation defects are correctable, and they can enhance the structural integrity and functional performance of muscle tissues with glycosylation defects. Transgenic animal models in experiments have demonstrated that such interventions can halt the progression of further pathological changes within muscle tissue, and thereby preserve muscle morphology through time. The significance of such results is profound, and they suggest that gene therapy and drug interventions may offer effective and safe means to reverse the pathological mechanisms of various myopathies and thereby improve muscle function and well-being (Brockington et al., 2010; Aldini et al., 2016) (Figure 5.17).

5.6.1. Common Muscle Disorders and Their Effects

Muscle disorders are a collection of conditions that significantly impair muscle function and morphology and induce a variable degree of disability. Conditions like muscular dystrophy and myasthenia gravis involve largely skeletal muscle and entail progressive weakness, muscle degeneration, and impaired functional ability. Muscular dystrophies, a family of genetic disorders, exhibit wide variation in their presentation and course, often resulting from mutations in genes encoding muscle proteins involved in protein synthesis. These mutations weaken the integrity of muscle fibers, causing not just muscle wasting but also profound alterations in muscle tissue morphology, including fibrosis and fatty infiltration.

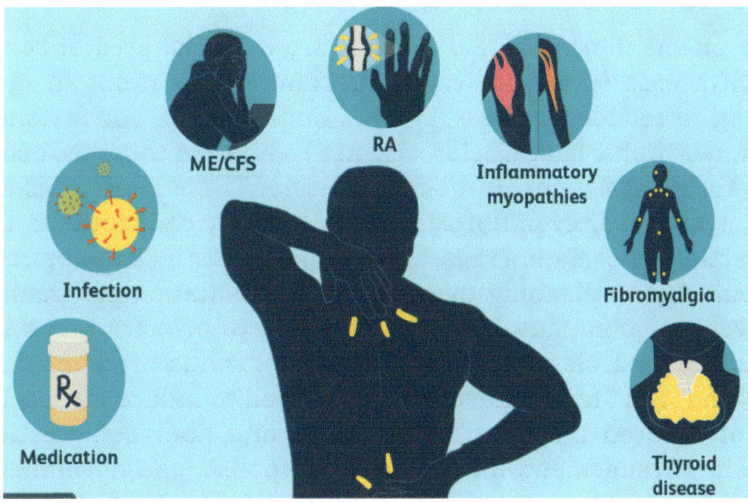

Figure 5.18. Common muscle disorders and their effects.

Source: https://www.verywellhealth.com/thmb/5oGmY7d-C7F2hOTimWANZVWs5tk=/1500x0/filters:no_upscale():max_bytes(150000):strip_icc()/musclepainfinal-01-5c86a54e46e0fb00010f1126.png.

Treatment of such disorders is generally most effective using a multidisciplinary treatment strategy that includes medical, physical, and therapeutic management to preserve muscle function and enhance the quality of life in affected people. Besides genetics, muscle disorders acquired through illness, like rhabdomyolysis and inflammatory myopathies, are good examples of how muscle morphology can be negatively affected. Rhabdomyolysis, often resulting from excessive physical exertion, trauma, or drug use, degrades muscle and overwhelms the blood with toxic protein. It is characterised by serious risks, notably renal failure due to secondary myoglobinuria, stressing the urgency of prompt medical intervention. In contrast, inflammatory myopathies consist of autoimmune muscle fiber destruction, with associated pain, weakness, and atrophy. These disorders disrupt the normal architecture of muscle tissue and may lead to scarring, further adding to muscular dysfunction. Understanding these disorders requires not just observation of clinical presentation, but careful attention to the molecular and cellular machinery responsible for muscle structure and function. Research has begun to uncover potential therapeutic interventions for the restoration of muscle integrity and function in patients with prevalent muscle disorders. Gene therapy technologies related to diseases caused by specific genetic mutations have also been promising in animal models, with their restoration of proper muscle protein expression having decreased disease effects. For instance, experimental over-expression of LARGE has been investigated to enhance alpha-dystroglycan glycosylation, with which it has been demonstrated to have protective roles in muscle function in the case of dystroglycanopathies, as indicated by research that tested long-term over-expression of LARGE in animal models. Moreover, pharmacologic strategies to promote muscular resistance and regeneration are constantly being sought. It is required to integrate new research with the traditional treatment procedures to offer comprehensive care to patients with muscle disorders in order to promote a positive outlook toward muscle health and well-being (Figure 5.18).

5.6.2. Impact of Diseases on Muscle Morphology

The effects of disease on the morphology of muscle are a crucial area of research in the field of muscle tissue. Several disease states can cause substantial alterations in muscle fiber anatomy and physiology, leading to reduced muscle function and mobility. For instance, diseases such as muscular dystrophy, amyotrophic lateral sclerosis (ALS), and even those associated with aging have been known to bring about alterations in the musculature. These alterations may be secondary to hypertrophy, atrophy, necrosis, or even fibrosis and collectively contribute to the overall decline of muscle quality and function. Information regarding the particular morphological alterations induced by these diseases is valuable in planning therapy and rehabilitation programs to improve muscle health as well as prevent ongoing muscle loss. In addition to primary muscle disorders, systemic disease severely influences muscle morphology through various mechanisms. Diabetes mellitus, chronic renal disease, and heart failure have been described to induce muscle atrophy and wasting with characteristics of reduced muscle fiber diameter and fiber compositional alteration. The association of metabolic derangement, inflammatory response, and hormonal imbalance in these conditions underlies the observed morphological alterations. Specifically, chronic inflammation can lead to increased fibrosis in muscles, which, in turn, hardens the muscles and further complicates muscle function. Understanding the role systemic disease plays in altering the morphology of muscles emphasizes the necessity of interdisciplinarity in science as well as clinical practice, where muscle health is considered under an integrated picture of body health. Recent studies have also begun to look at the effects of training and detraining on muscle morphology, with a specific focus on disease. When patients with muscle atrophy due to some disease undergo resistance training, they are capable of showing regenerative morphological responses such as increased myofiber cross-sectional area and enhanced mitochondrial density. However, abrupt cessation of training or inactivity, such as normally occurs with chronic disease or hospitalization, can result in profound structural backsliding. Evidence from preclinical studies indicates that abrupt elimination of mechanical loading leads to muscle structural and functional degradation, highlighting the precarious equilibrium between training stimuli and muscle adaptation (Aldini et al., 2016). Hence, the need for an interactive study of the correlation among disease, training, and detraining for building effective rehabilitation programs for muscle morphology improvement in the said population.

5.6.3. Regenerative Capabilities of Muscle Tissue

Muscle tissue also possesses excellent regenerative capacity, largely because of the unique characteristics of satellite cells, a pool of muscle stem cells between the basal lamina and muscle fiber sarcolemma. Satellite cells become activated to proliferate and differentiate into myoblasts for repairing and regenerating muscle upon muscle injury. This healing process is tightly regulated, with a huge range of molecular signals and growth factors guiding cell-to-cell communication and migration through phases of healing. The highly orchestrated coordination between various cell types, cytokines, and extracellular matrix molecules generates a hierarchical response to muscle injury. Such regenerative capability is of immense significance, especially within the realm of sports medicine, where muscle strain and tears are frequent incidents and their underlying mechanisms may result in improved therapeutic interventions with improved recovery periods and complete restoration of functional integrity of the muscular tissue (Litvinova et al., 2025). Furthermore, advancements in regenerative medicine have unveiled the potential use of mesenchymal stem/stromal cells (MSCs) as a new method of inducing muscle tissue regeneration. Adipose-derived MSCs, however, are of specific interest since they are relatively easy to obtain and possess great myogenic differentiation potential. Research indicates that the cells can differentiate into muscle cells effectively, with notable myogenic markers associated with muscle repair (Ngeun et al., 2024). The immunomodulatory characteristics of MSCs also present an added benefit since they can modulate inflammation during healing, potentially ensuring no complications arise that could disrupt recovery. With the exploitation of the potential of MSCs, researchers hope to develop targeted therapies that not only heal muscle better but also can serve as prophylactic medications for muscular degeneration against a variety of pathological conditions. Muscle tissue regeneration is also subject to the success of external factors, including age, nutrition, and comorbidities. With aging, the muscle tissue's inherent regenerative potential decreases primarily due to a decrease in satellite cell number and functional capacity, as well as changed inflammatory processes. This decrease in potential for muscle repair with age causes sarcopenia, or progressive loss of muscle force and mass. Nutrition also plays a governing role, and the supply of amino acids and some micronutrients is in favor of recovery within the muscle. In addition, environmental influences such as exercise and physical rehabilitation play a significant role in the process of regeneration by promoting a conducive environment for satellite cell activation and thus myogenesis. Comprehension of these diverse influences can potentially design comprehensive approaches for the purpose of fortifying muscle tissue rebuilding in different populations and for overall muscular health (Litvinova et al., 2025).

SUMMARY

In reviewing the study of muscle tissue morphology, it is crucial to admire the intricate structure and function of various muscle types, including skeletal, cardiac, and smooth muscle. The morphology of each is distinct and is directly linked to its corresponding functional adaptations. For instance, skeletal muscle fibers are organized into fascicles that permit precise control during movement, whereas cardiac muscle contains intercalated disks that facilitate synchronized contractions necessary for efficient cardiac function. In addition, knowledge of muscle tissue morphology not only enhances our understanding of physiological function but also forms a foundation for clinical practice, such as the diagnosis and treatment of muscular disease, thus relating form and function practically. Last but not least, recent scientific research, for instance, research on myofascial trigger points in human skeletal muscle, has enlightened us to the refinements of muscle morphology. The observation of segmentally contracted sarcomeres in both myalgic and nonmyalgic subjects supports the hypothesis of the formation of trigger points and the pathological alterations that occur at the level of the muscle fiber. In addition, this research educates rehabilitation practice by illustrating the mechanisms of muscular pain and dysfunction. These findings underscore the importance of extensive knowledge of muscle morphology as therapists develop intervention protocols to promote recovery and optimise muscle function, further emphasising the clinical value of morphological studies in muscle tissue. In addition to the functional and structural factors of muscle tissue, the significance of how external factors affect muscle morphology, such as training, aging, and detraining, is also considered. The literature illustrates that cessation of training can put tendon structure and properties to considerable test, such that rehabilitation and recovery are compromised. Understanding these consequences facilitates planning of judicious physical activity programs following injury, such that muscle and tendon integrity is not compromised during rehabilitation. As illustrated in recent studies, the interplay between muscle morphology and mechanical properties highlights the significance of holistic approaches to muscle training and recovery. A combined appreciation of muscle tissue morphology, therefore, is an important consideration within therapeutic settings as well as the maximization of competitive performance, and indicates the importance of continued research into this fast-developing discipline.

The architecture of muscle tissue is closely connected with its potential for function, and this is well demonstrated in skeletal muscle. One of the important aspects of skeletal muscle architecture is the inclusion of satellite cells, which are a resident stem cell population with a function in tissue repair in the event of injury. Experiments have shown that these cells migrate in two stages: initially beneath the basal lamina, and then they increase their migration when they reach the surface of the myofiber. The mechanism of migration is characterized by a new dynamic blebbing-based process rather than the traditional lamellipodia-mediated propulsion. The role of signaling pathways, including nitric oxide and non-canonical Wnt signaling, in regulating the migration of satellite cells indicates the complexity of muscle tissue morphology and underscores the possibility of therapeutic strategies for inducing muscle regeneration (Collins-Hooper et al., 2011). In addition to skeletal muscle, the muscle tissue morphology in other vertebrates, such as bats, exhibits spectacular adaptations that optimize functional performance. The wings of bats are made up of a specific membrane with ordered bundles of elastin and embedded skeletal muscles, which offer the accuracy required for aerodynamic maneuvering during flight. Researchers have found that, via cross-polarized light imaging, bat wing membranes show typical patterns of birefringence, which is related to their material structure. These elastin bundles are arranged in various directions, and the muscle architectures of the wings are diverse between families of bats, and this is evidence of evolutionary adaptations to various flight styles. Morphological diversity not only aids the mechanics of flight but also emphasizes the importance of anatomical features in muscle tissue functionality among species (Fenton et al., 2017). The morphology of the muscle tissue in different organisms provides the critical details about the evolutionary aspect of muscle repair and function. In as varied a group as rodents and bats, the presence of unique muscular features such as elastin bundles, which accommodate the flexible and dynamic demands of flight, or the regenerative capacity provided by satellite cells in skeletal muscle, illustrates the extent to which morphology is contingent upon the physiological functions that the muscles perform. These findings contribute to an integrated understanding of muscle tissue adaptation and underscore the relevance of morphological studies in de-mystifying muscular performance. By synergizing conceptualizations across these studies, researchers can better elucidate mechanisms of muscle growth and repair, which will provide novel therapeutic intervention avenues in treating muscular diseases and enhancing human and animal performance.

A LOOK TO THE FUTURE:

DUCHENNE MUSCULAR DYSTROPHY (DMD)

Duchenne muscular dystrophy (DMD) is a severe, progressive genetic neuromuscular disorder that stands among the most impactful and well-studied inherited diseases affecting children. As an X-linked recessive condition, DMD predominantly affects boys, arising from mutations in the DMD gene on the X chromosome that encodes dystrophin, a critical protein for maintaining the structural integrity of muscle fibres. The absence or near absence of dystrophin destabilises muscle cell membranes, leading to muscle weakness, degeneration, and replacement of functional muscle tissue with fat and fibrotic tissue, with profound implications for mobility and organ function over time. DMD typically manifests in early childhood, with symptoms often first becoming evident between ages 2 and 4 as motor delays, frequent falls, difficulty climbing stairs, and an abnormal gait emerge. Progressive lower-limb muscle weakness produces characteristic clinical signs such as enlarged calf muscles (pseudohypertrophy) and the Gowers' manoeuvre, in which affected children use their hands to push up from the floor due to weakness of proximal muscles. Without intervention, most boys with DMD lose independent ambulation by adolescence and develop involvement of respiratory and cardiac muscles, contributing to life-limiting complications.

At the molecular level, the DMD gene is one of the largest in the human genome, encoding multiple dystrophin isoforms. Frameshift mutations or large deletions that disrupt the reading frame abolish dystrophin synthesis, resulting in the classic DMD phenotype, whereas in-frame mutations producing truncated but partially functional protein lead to a milder form of the disease known as Becker muscular dystrophy.

Diagnosis is established through clinical evaluation, genetic testing, and biomarkers such as elevated creatine kinase, which reflects muscle breakdown. Early and accurate diagnosis is essential for management and family counselling, particularly given the X-linked inheritance and implications for carrier status in female relatives. While there is currently no cure for DMD, advances in supportive care, corticosteroid therapy, cardiac and respiratory management, and emerging genetic and molecular therapies have improved quality of life and extended survival into adulthood for many affected individuals. Novel treatments—including exon-skipping drugs and gene therapy approaches—aim to increase dystrophin production or slow muscle degeneration, reflecting an evolving therapeutic landscape. As research continues to translate genetic and pathophysiological insights into clinical applications, DMD serves as a powerful example of how precision medicine can reshape outcomes for rare genetic disorders.

REFERENCES

1. Chadwick, K. P., Regnault, S., Allen, V., & Hutchinson, J. R. (2014). Three-dimensional anatomy of the ostrich (Struthio camelus) knee joint. PeerJ, 2, e706. https://doi.org/10.7717/peerj.706Abzhanov, A., Baggiolini, A., Baroffio, A., Beverdam, A., Chevallier, A., et al. (2019). Molecular and cellular mechanisms underlying the evolution of form and function in the amniote jaw. https://core.ac.uk/download/323079229.pdf (accessed on 6th August 2025).
2. Adamo, S., Benedetti, A., Bouché, M., Moresi, V., et al. (2018). Culture conditions influence satellite cell activation and survival of single myofibers. https://core.ac.uk/download/158822304.pdf (accessed on 6th August 2025).
3. Aerts, P., Ayuso, M., Prims, S., Van Cruchten, S., et al. (2019). Does intrauterine crowding affect the force generating capacity and muscle composition of the piglet front limb? https://core.ac.uk/download/287940318.pdf (accessed on 6th August 2025).
4. Aguiari, P., Barbon, S., Bertalot, T., Conconi, M. T., et al. (2016). Nanopatterned acellular valve conduits drive the commitment of blood-derived multipotent cells. https://core.ac.uk/download/80154438.pdf (accessed on 6th August 2025).
5. Aldini, N., Della Bella, E., Fini, M., Frizziero, L., et al. (2016). The role of detraining in tendon mechanobiology. https://core.ac.uk/download/53528699.pdf (accessed on 6th August 2025).
6. Alexander, R., Baker, R., Baraibar, M., Beale, B., Benjamin, M., Biggs, J., et al. (2014). Structure, ontogeny and evolution of the patellar tendon in emus (Dromaius novaehollandiae) and other palaeognath birds. https://core.ac.uk/download/36778015.pdf (accessed on 6th August 2025).
7. Aniansson, A., Bertoldo, A., Bigot, A., Herbst, A., Hiona, A., Musarò, A., et al. (2009). Sarcopenia: Etiology, clinical consequences, intervention, and assessment. https://core.ac.uk/download/pdf/8385376.pdf (accessed on 6th August 2025).
8. Aylott, J. W., Bridge, J. C., Brightling, C. E., Eltboli, O., et al. (2014). Human airway smooth muscle maintain in situ cell orientation and phenotype when cultured on aligned electrospun scaffolds. https://core.ac.uk/download/42494297.pdf (accessed on 6th August 2025).
9. Basava, R. R., Chen, J.-S., He, Q., He, X., et al. (2020). Microstructural analysis of skeletal muscle force generation during aging. https://core.ac.uk/download/286361329.pdf (accessed on 6th August 2025).
10. Baskin, L. S., Cao, M., Cunha, G. R., Ricke, W. A., et al. (2019). Reproductive tract biology: Of mice and men. https://core.ac.uk/download/323311356.pdf (accessed on 6th August 2025).
11. Berghella, L., Coletta, M., Cossu, G., Cusella-De Angelis, M. G., et al. (1999). Skeletal myogenic progenitors originating from embryonic dorsal aorta coexpress endothelial and myogenic markers and contribute to postnatal muscle growth and regeneration. https://core.ac.uk/download/4875001.pdf (accessed on 6th August 2025).
12. Bourdarias, C., Gerbi, S., Ohayon, J. (2008). A pseudo-active kinematic constraint for a biological living soft tissue: An effect of the collagen network. https://core.ac.uk/download/47305500.pdf (accessed on 6th August 2025).
13. Braden, R. L., Christman, K. L., Dzieciatkowska, M., Elhag, D., et al. (2016). Extracellular matrix hydrogel promotes tissue remodeling, arteriogenesis, and perfusion in a rat hindlimb ischemia model. https://core.ac.uk/download/323065138.pdf (accessed on 6th August 2025).

14. Brockington, M., Brown, S. C., Cirak, S., Liu, L., et al. (2010). Transgenic overexpression of LARGE induces alpha-dystroglycan hyperglycosylation in skeletal and cardiac muscle. https://core.ac.uk/download/1730280.pdf (accessed on 6th August 2025).

15. Cagnie, B., Calders, P., De Meulemeester, K., Gerwin, R. D., et al. (2020). Foci of segmentally contracted sarcomeres in trapezius muscle biopsy specimens in myalgic and nonmyalgic human subjects: Preliminary results. https://core.ac.uk/download/322828773.pdf (accessed on 6th August 2025).

16. Carlotti, F., Chuva de Sousa Lopes, S. M., de Koning, E. J. P., de Melo Bernardo, A., et al. (2014). Lymphangiogenesis and angiogenesis during human fetal pancreas development. https://core.ac.uk/download/55800083.pdf (accessed on 6th August 2025).

17. Cheng, L. K., Kumar, D., Mittal, R. K., Zifan, A., et al. (2017). Three-dimensional myoarchitecture of the lower esophageal sphincter and esophageal hiatus using optical sectioning microscopy. https://core.ac.uk/download/323064197.pdf (accessed on 6th August 2025).

18. Cherkas, O. A. (2023). Methodological features of the presentation of cardiac muscle morphology in a histology course. https://core.ac.uk/download/604347224.pdf (accessed on 6th August 2025).

19. Collins-Hooper, H., Dash, P. R., Otto, A., Patel, K., et al. (2011). Adult skeletal muscle stem cell migration is mediated by a blebbing/amoeboid mechanism. https://core.ac.uk/download/9077.pdf (accessed on 6th August 2025).

20. Dae, M., Fang, Q., Feng, J., Gao, X., et al. (2010). Targeted in vivo extracellular matrix formation promotes neovascularization in a rodent model of myocardial infarction. https://core.ac.uk/download/323073026.pdf (accessed on 6th August 2025).

21. Danneels, L., Goubert, D., Meeus, M., Van Oosterwijck, J., et al. (2016). Structural changes of lumbar muscles in non-specific low back pain. https://core.ac.uk/download/84042457.pdf (accessed on 6th August 2025).

22. Dickson, P. I., Ellinwood, N. M., Kakkis, E. D., Lyons, J. A., et al. (2011). Arterial pathology in canine mucopolysaccharidosis-I and response to therapy. https://core.ac.uk/download/323076774.pdf (accessed on 6th August 2025).

23. Esen, H. K., Biltekin, B., Korkmaz, M., Güvenç, B. H. (2024). Population kinetics and protein profiles of co-cultured adult and fetus rabbit bladder smooth muscle cells. Urology Research and Practice, 50, 240–246. https://www.semanticscholar.org/paper/4feae9b136e359a0d5a8600182ebc125dd37aa24 (accessed on 6th August 2025).

24. Evans, M. E. (2015). Muscle disuse; the culprit of sarcopenia? A study in master athletes. https://core.ac.uk/download/161890624.pdf (accessed on 6th August 2025).

25. Fenton, M. B., Gray, P., Holbrook, K. A., Humphry, G. M., Maisonneuve, P., Meyer, W., Schumacher, S., et al. (2017). Diversity in the organization of elastin bundles and intramembranous muscles in bat wings. https://core.ac.uk/download/76981004.pdf (accessed on 6th August 2025).

26. Focarete, M. L., Fornaia, G., Gotti, C., Gualandi, C., Sensini, A., Zucchelli, A. (2020). Biomimetic hierarchically arranged nanofibrous structures resembling the architecture and the passive mechanical properties of skeletal muscles: A step forward toward artificial muscle. https://core.ac.uk/download/351906809.pdf (accessed on 6th August 2025).

27. Gretz, N., Hafner, M., Hörner, S. J., Reischl, M., et al. (2019). A novel optical tissue clearing protocol for mouse skeletal muscle to visualize endplates in their tissue context. https://core.ac.uk/download/197481021.pdf (accessed on 6th August 2025).

28. Iwasaki, K., Kanagawa, M., Katanosaka, K., et al. (2014). TRPV2 is critical for the maintenance of cardiac structure and function in mice. https://core.ac.uk/download/32591845.pdf (accessed on 6th August 2025).

29. Kandelouei, T., Zhang, W., Houghton, M. E., Knudsen, B., Edgar, B. A. (2024). Improved preservation of mouse intestinal tissue using a formalin/acetic acid fixative and quantitative histological analysis using QuPath. Current Protocols, 4. https://www.semanticscholar.org/paper/c2993e357d32d1a98030291c4355cd45cf9eb833 (accessed on 6th August 2025).

30. Leask, A., Bostick, B., Kuehn, B. M., Colussi, C., Van Erp, C., Gaetano, C., Spurney, C. F., et al. (2011). Chronic losartan administration reduces mortality and preserves cardiac but not skeletal muscle function in dystrophic mice. https://core.ac.uk/download/pdf/8583596.pdf (accessed on 6th August 2025).

31. Leveson-Gower, D., Ly, D. (2025). Bion-M2 PI 1-Pagers. https://core.ac.uk/download/pdf/286393560.pdf (accessed on 6th August 2025).

32. Litvinova, O., Kumetchko, M., Pavlov, S., Babenko, N., Kolisnyk, I. (2025). Problems of healing soft tissue injuries. Eastern Ukrainian Medical Journal. https://www.semanticscholar.org/paper/374fa30057b57b8364f998a15d4dec09e52f7be5 (accessed on 6th August 2025).

33. N/A. (2025). Musculoskeletal discipline science plan. https://core.ac.uk/download/pdf/42808673.pdf (accessed on 6th August 2025).

34. Ngeun, S. K., Shimizu, M., Kaneda, M. (2024). Myogenic differentiation and immunomodulatory properties of rat adipose-derived mesenchymal stem/stromal cells. Biology, 13. https://www.semanticscholar.org/paper/47df74b8208a744a146ec78191b34d95e904dcde (accessed on 6th August 2025).

35. Thiel, M., Williams, M. P. I., Reischl, M., Hafner, M., Rigon, M., Gretz, N., et al. (2019). A novel optical tissue clearing protocol for mouse skeletal muscle to visualize endplates in their tissue context. https://core.ac.uk/download/201249343.pdf (accessed on 6th August 2025).

36. Wei, A. (2021). Time-lapse observation of sarcomeric addition in hypertrophic models based on a tissue-like cardiomyocyte culture. https://core.ac.uk/download/524894872.pdf (accessed on 6th August 2025).

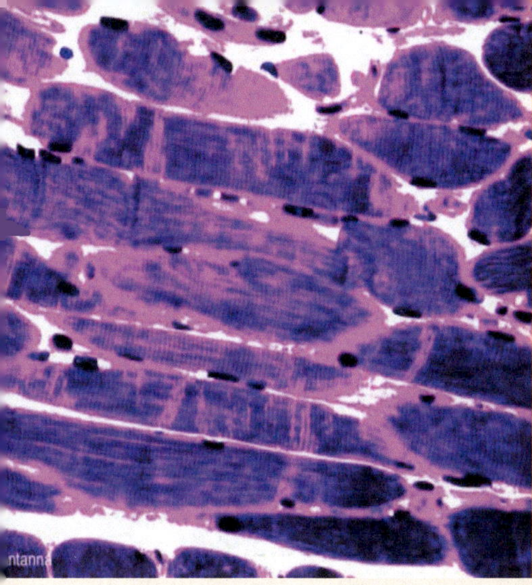

Chapter 6

NERVOUS TISSUE MORPHOLOGY

Contents

Introduction

The study of nervous tissue morphology is essential for understanding the structure and function of the nervous system, a key component of the human body. Nervous tissue is composed of various cellular components, primarily neurons and glial cells, which perform specialized yet complementary functions. Neurons, the system's main communicators, have unique structural features that facilitate synaptic transmission and information processing. In contrast, glial cells provide vital support for neuronal health and homeostasis. Understanding the significance of these cellular components is significant to comprehending the processes of neurological function and disease. Understanding the sophistication of nervous tissue morphology, in addition to providing insight into healthy neural networks, also underscores the changes that occur in states of disease, and thus, it is necessary to consider these changes in detail. Recent advances in neuroscience have initiated studies on the morphological changes that take place in populations of neurons upon exposure to a variety of stimuli or pathologies. The advent of primary neuronal cultures has been a landmark development within the field, offering the opportunity to study single neurons isolated from their native environments. This method makes it possible to study in detail how morphological alterations occur under physiological states, and as a response to neurodegenerative disease, to demonstrate its application in simulating diseases such as HIV-associated dementia. With the measurement of the changes, researchers can determine correlations between structural alterations and loss of function. The study of these alterations becomes especially relevant because we are attempting to find out how much neurodegeneration contributes to cognitive function. Procedures targeting cell viability and synaptic formation in such cultures will be prominent in future studies. As neuroscience has advanced, the inclusion of contemporary methods for the analysis of nervous tissue morphology is essential. The intricate correlation between neuron structure and function underlies our comprehension of neurobiological mechanisms in health and disease. Methodologies that can measure and describe the alterations of neurons play a fundamental role in enabling us to comprehend conditions such as neurodegeneration. The requirement for standard procedures in studying these alterations cannot be overstressed, as demonstrated by recent studies of HIV's impact on neuronal morphology (Saunders., 2009). In addition, research funding strengthens the ongoing interest in this field to address the complexities of nervous tissue (Canillas et al., 2017). As further research continues to unravel, centering on the significance of neuronal morphology, diagnostics, and therapeutics will be enhanced, as well as the foundation knowledge required to further the science of neuroscience as a whole (Figure 6.1).

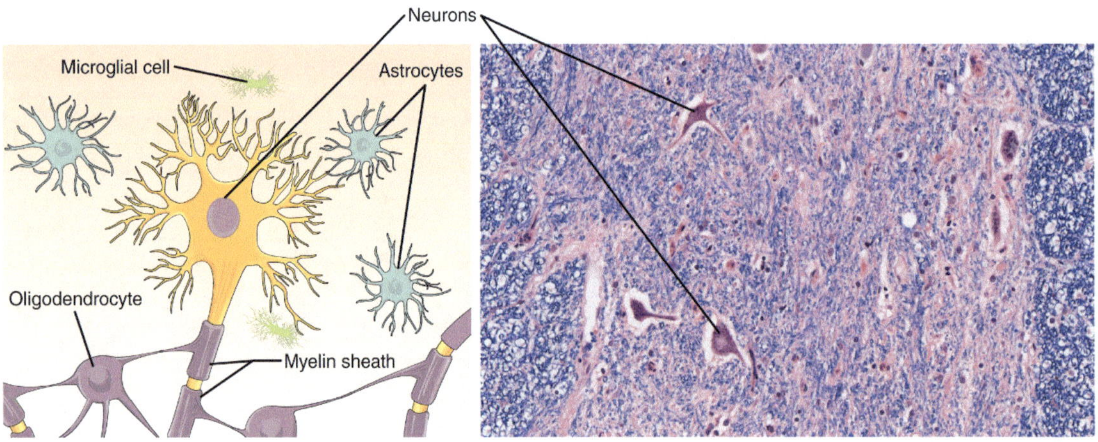

Figure 6.1. Nervous tissue morphology.

Source: https://philschatz.com/anatomy-book/resources/416_Nervous_Tissue-new.jpg.

Definition of Nervous Tissue

Nervous tissue is composed of specialized cells that transmit electrical impulses throughout the body." Composed of neurons and support glial cells, nervous tissue plays a vital role in the reception of stimuli, processing information, and integrating the response. Neurons, which are the building blocks of the nervous system, are physically organized for communication by having axons and dendrites that facilitate the transmission of impulses. In parallel, glial cells, which outnumber neurons, provide structural support, supply, and insulation to facilitate optimal neuronal function.

Organization of these cells is a reflection of the complexity of their function, calling to mind the manner in which they contribute to roles other than signal transmission, that is, to the general homeostasis of the nervous system. Such integration of cellular components underlies the analysis of the morphology and function of nervous tissue in both health and illness. It traces the history following the development of nervous tissue and offers interesting insight into its adaptive potential and evolutionary significance. Regardless of the body plan variety found within various organisms, the basic genetic makeup of nervous tissue is relatively constant. This implies nervous system evolution might be made possible by combinatorial processes such as gene regulation, the recruitment of existing genes to new functional roles, and overall changes in gene makeup. Understanding these mechanisms is paramount as it determines how nervous tissue is capable of varying over time to accommodate the physiological demands of different environments. By contrasting the homology relationships of various species, particularly with an interest in evolutionary developmental biology, researchers are able to establish the shared features comprising nervous tissue and its function across the animal kingdom, as suggested in Becker et al. (2005). Furthermore, recent advances in immunological techniques have enabled us to better understand certain cell types within nervous tissue, namely, Schwann cells of the peripheral nervous system. Their isolation and purification have been essential in elucidating their role in myelin formation and regeneration following injury. One such example is the peripheral myelin glycoprotein P_0, which is an integral part and illustrates the association between the Schwann cells and their respective axons to promote the development of effective electrical insulation. Schwann cell interaction with myelinated axons has been shown to induce meaningful growth factors for cellular proliferation and repair mechanisms, reflecting the dynamic elements of nervous tissue. Such morphological understanding of individual components improves our overall knowledge regarding the functioning of nervous tissue, particularly within the context of regeneration, as highlighted in Brockes et al. (1981).

Importance of Studying Nervous Tissue Morphology

Morphology of nervous tissue is an elementary aspect of neuroscience that explains the intricate architecture and organization of the brain and spinal cord. Understanding the structural aspects of neurons, glial cells, and their interaction is necessary to know how the nervous system functions and communicates. This knowledge not only informs us about healthy physiological processes but also throws light upon pathological processes like neurodegenerative diseases and mental illnesses. Employing advanced imaging devices and histological examinations, scientists can image and explore cellular orientations, synaptic mechanisms, and tissue integrity. This kind of study enables the early diagnosis of abnormalities, thereby facilitating interventions in a timely manner. The structural data from the studies of nervous tissue morphology are important to the spreading of neuroplasticity and the consolidation of efficient therapeutic treatments in reversing the destructive effects of neurological disorders (Buchner et al., 2009). In addition, the study of nervous tissue morphology is vital to the identification of the substrates of cognitive and behavioral events. Certain morphological changes in neural networks can have severe effects on information processing in the brain. For instance, variations in dendritic morphology and synaptic maturation have been associated with learning, memory, and mood regulation. Implications derived from knowledge of such morphological features can relate specific structural changes to subsequent behaviors, ultimately informing psychological and neuroscientific theory. The impact of psychological disorders, such as anorexia nervosa, demonstrates the need for greater understanding of structural neuroimaging and neural networks (Ehrlich et al., 2018). By studying morphological change within the context of various behaviors, researchers are better able to design interventions aimed at enhancing cognitive ability and emotional stability. Perhaps of greater importance, the results of nervous tissue morphology research overlap the specific confines of individual disease and enter into the general investigation of neurodevelopment and aging. As the nervous system develops, morphological changes occur that are required for successful function and for a measure of adaptability. By studying the morphology of nervous tissue at different ages of life, researchers can identify windows in neurodevelopment that are susceptible to environmental influences or genetic influences. Conversely, morphological changes in nervous tissue indicate the progression of neurodegeneration and a decline in cognitive capacity among aging populations.

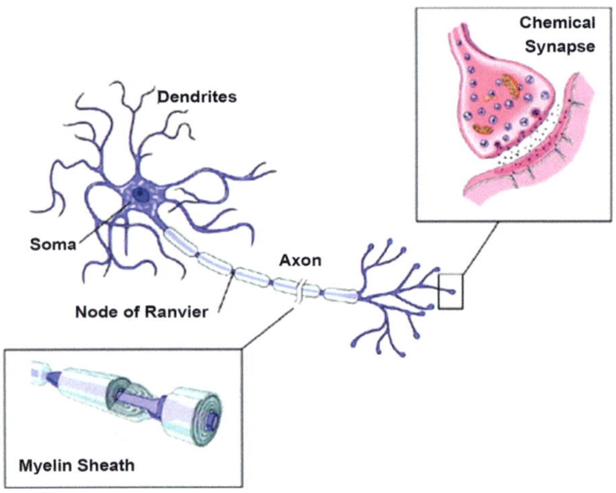

Figure 6.2. Importance of studying nervous tissue morphology.

Source: https://image.slideserve.com/1267945/nervous-tissue-l.jpg.

Perceiving these morphological transformations not only enhances our understanding of the life cycle of neural tissue but also directs brain aging promotion in healthy directions. Overall, the significance of the study of nervous tissue morphology is that it can unravel the complexities of neural function, development, and pathology, and its relevance offers a framework for the development of neuroscience and clinical practice (Buchner et al., 2009) (Figure 6.2).

6.1. Types of Nervous Tissue

The nervous tissue group is broadly separated into two major types: neurons and glial cells, each with distinct yet supportive functions in the central and peripheral nervous system. Neurons are the focal functional components of the nervous system and are responsible for the transmission of electrical impulses. Their structure, which consists of a cell body, dendrites, and an axon, is designed for signal conduction speed. Dendrites pick up incoming messages, and the axon transmits the messages to other neurons, muscles, or glands. Glial cells, on the other hand, are more often the background actors of the nervous system. They outnumber neurons several times over and are charged with maintaining homeostasis, structural support, and neuron-to-neuron communication. Phenotypic diversity of glial cells, astrocytes, oligodendrocytes, and microglia mirrors their specialized functions, from nutrient transport to myelination, evincing the complexity of nervous tissue morphology. Neurons are also classified on the basis of structure and function. Structural diversity is represented by unipolar, bipolar, and multipolar neurons, each of which is suited to specialized signaling functions. For instance, unipolar neurons, with a single axon arising from their cell body, are typically found in sensory pathways, whereas bipolar neurons, with one axon and one dendrite, play a critical role in sensory systems such as olfaction and vision. In contrast, multipolar neurons, with many dendrites and a single axon, are the most common in the central nervous system, enabling complex integrative functions. The morphology of glial cells is also diverse; astrocytes are star-shaped to allow them to surround neurons and regulate synaptic activity, while oligodendrocytes coil around axons and form myelin sheaths to enhance signal transmission. The morphological specialization of neurons and glial cells shows the fine structure that supports neural function. Research breakthroughs illuminate the plasticity of nervous tissue, particularly the potential of neural stem cells (NSCs) in development and also tissue repair. NSCs can self-renew and differentiate into glial and neuronal cells and are crucial for homeostasis as well as response to injury. Experiments indicate that the cells are isolatable from various tissues, such as adult brain and bone marrow, and that they are versatile in regenerative medicine. For example, human marrow-derived NSC-like cells (hmNSCs) can differentiate into astroglia, oligodendroglia, and neurons under specific conditions, thereby further supporting their therapeutic potential in neurodegenerative disease (Boehm et al., 2004). The capacity to replace missing tissue and restore function speaks volumes about the dynamic morphology of nervous tissue and raises important questions about the molecular mechanisms that control neural differentiation and repair (Canillas et al., 2017). Therefore, knowledge of the various forms of nervous tissue is important for promoting neurobiology and creating novel therapies (Figure 6.3).

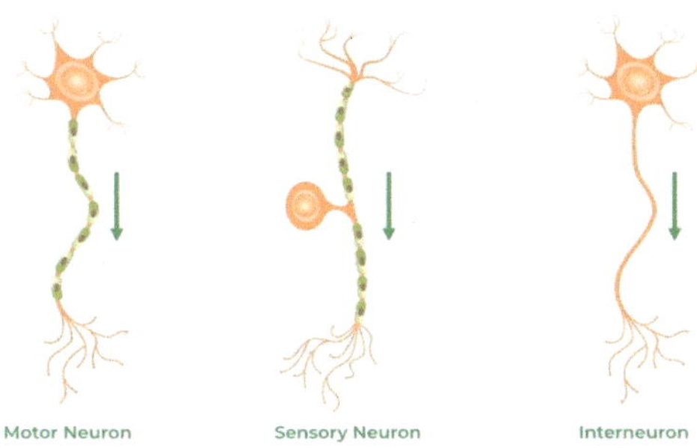

Figure 6.3. Types of nervous tissue.

Source: https://media.geeksforgeeks.org/wp-content/uploads/20230516133555/Types-of-Neurons.webp.

6.1.1. Central Nervous System (CNS)

The central nervous system (CNS) maintains the body's physiological balance, serving as the center for the receipt and interpretation of sensory information, reaction in terms of motor activity, and regulation of vital processes. Comprising the brain and spinal cord, the CNS is a complex system of neurons and their corresponding glial cells, featuring various morphological features conducive to its diverse functions. The complex organization of the CNS reflects the connection between structure and function; e.g., the brain cortical layers have unique cellular architectures suited to various cognitive processes. Morphological complexity enables a highly specialized communication system, which is necessary for integrating information from peripheral sensory pathways essential for homeostasis and for responding to environmental changes. The past several years have unraveled the relationship between adipose tissue and the CNS, particularly concerning energy homeostasis. The adipose tissue has not only come to be seen as an energy reservoir but as an interacting reservoir of energy with the CNS via sensory and sympathetic neurons. Notably, investigations using the latest imaging technology have unveiled a network of calcitonin gene-related protein (CGRP)+ sensory neurons in white adipose tissue (WAT). These sensory neurons, under selective regulation by the adipose mammalian target of rapamycin complex 2 (mTORC2), are responsible for playing critical roles in the mediation of signals reporting energy status and metabolic demand to the CNS. This complex interaction, revealed by emerging evidence, demonstrates the importance of sensory innervation in WAT and its impact on CNS signaling pathways involved in energy regulation, forming a highly complex feedback mechanism within the nervous system. Furthermore, the intricacy of sensory neuron morphology in WAT directly relates to systemic metabolic functions, i.e., insulin signaling. mTORC2's reliance on CGRP-positive sensory neurons for robust arborization implies that any impairment in such signaling would lead to reduced sensory innervation to the CNS, which has the potential to play a role in insulin resistance and other metabolic abnormalities. Most critically, this implies that the integrity of WAT—and its nerve connections—is utterly critical for whole-body metabolic homeostasis. Disruption of such sensory innervation has been associated with severe physiological consequences, highlighting a demand to explore CNS interactions with peripheral tissues further. By the knowledge of such interactions, researchers are able to explain therapeutic treatments for nervous tissue morphology to offset insulin resistance and related metabolic syndromes (Colombi et al., 2022).

6.1.2. Peripheral Nervous System (PNS)

Comprising sensory and motor neurons, the peripheral nervous system connects the central nervous system (CNS) with the body's organs and limbs, facilitating both voluntary and involuntary movements Its structure is separated into the somatic nervous system, which controls voluntary actions, and the autonomic nervous system, which controls involuntary functions such as heart rhythm and digestion. The PNS is specifically equipped to regenerate so that damaged nerves can heal and restore function. This regenerative capacity is in stark contrast to the CNS, where healing is impossible. Understanding the morphology and function of the PNS is essential to the progress of neuromedicine, especially in the treatment of nerve function-relevant conditions and the understanding of the impact of various environmental factors on nerve integrity. Current research points towards the significance of nicotinic acetylcholine receptors (nAChRs) in the PNS, particularly in early development and in response to external stimuli. These receptors, especially the α7 nAChR subtype, are overwhelmingly expressed in peripheral tissues, including dorsal root ganglia and sympathetic and parasympathetic ganglia, with expression as early as embryonic day 13 (Broide et al., 2019). Their early expression indicates that they are essential for neuronal plasticity and communication during critical developmental stages. Furthermore, alterations in nAChR expression are crucial in the growth and function of peripheral nerves, highlighting their role in developmental neurobiology. Elucidation of the temporal and spatial patterns of nAChR expression will enable an understanding of how environmental factors, such as gestational nicotine exposure, influence PNS growth and function and potentially impact long-term neurodevelopmental outcomes.

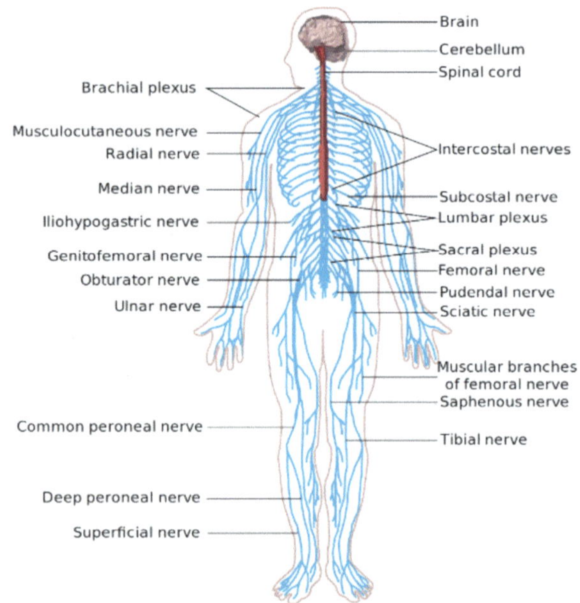

Figure 6.4. Peripheral nervous system (PNS).

Source: https://www.karunayoga.in/wp-content/uploads/2017/09/Peripheral-Nervous-System.png.

The PNS anatomy is also a potential point of concern regarding susceptibility to neurotoxic compounds that disrupt normal functioning and lead to neurodegenerative disease. Neurotoxicity is the array of adverse effects generated by chemicals that impede the structure and function of the nervous system. Some chemicals may kill neural cells outright, while others may inhibit critical metabolic processes for neuronal survival (Brust et al., 2014). The peripheral nerves of the PNSs are also variously sensitive to these compounds, influencing not only the occurrence of immediate effects but even the possibility of chronic deficits. Moreover, damage induced by neurotoxic chemicals may show as short-term symptoms or lead to permanent disabilities, which underscores the need for careful monitoring of exposure to the environment. Recognizing this danger underscores the need to develop therapeutic interventions that enhance PNS resilience and promote regeneration after neurotoxic insults (Figure 6.4).

6.1.3. Autonomic Nervous System (ANS)

The autonomic nervous system (ANS) is a vital system that regulates involuntary physiological functions, such as heart rate, digestion, and breathing, to maintain homeostasis. It is composed of two divisions: the sympathetic nervous system (SNS) and the parasympathetic nervous system. The intricate system is essential in regulating various body responses, including heart rate, digestion, and breathing habits. Studies have elucidated the function of respiration in modulating heart rhythm and autonomic modulation, revealing that the ANS is closely entwined with breathing rhythms. Physiological modulation of cardiac and vascular responses across respiratory phases can provide insight into numerous medical conditions, particularly respiratory conditions. In line with this, advancements in the knowledge of the ANS and its functionality can pave the way for new treatment avenues for diseases caused by autonomic dysregulation (Barnes et al., 2014). The morphological complexity of the ANS is emphasized by the characteristics of the morphological attributes of its axonal projections and neural connections. Sophisticated immunohistochemical techniques have been used recently to delineate the organization and distribution of sympathetic and parasympathetic fibers in the heart. Observations indicate the presence of a dense network of axons that not only innervate the cardiac tissues but also possess an intricate interplay between SNS and PSNS terminal structures. Interdigitation of the axons, alternating varicosities, may offer a means for antagonistic communication between these two branches to enable even more subtle regulation of cardiac activity. This intricate architecture underscores the importance of identifying the morphological characteristics of the ANS because it is the foundation upon which physiological function, as well as possible pathological alterations, can be further explored (Harden, 2009). In addition, intrinsic cardiac ganglia (ICG) are significant sites of integration of autonomic signals. These ganglia have an important role in modulating interactions between extrinsic sympathetic fibres and intrinsic cardiac neurons, and coordinating the heart's response to stimulation. Importantly, the presence of small intensely fluorescent (SIF) cells inside and outside the ICG suggests a distinctive group of interneurones possibly engaged in chemosensory function and regional communication within the cardiac microenvironment. Further, the morphological pattern of distribution of SNS and PSNS axons, as witnessed in different cardiac regions, works towards validating the proposition that the functional operations of the ANS have a deeply connected association with its structure. This precise description of the structural and functional relationships of the ANS provides an entrance through which understanding alterations related to age, illness, and other physiological conditions (Harden., 2009) (Figure 6.5).

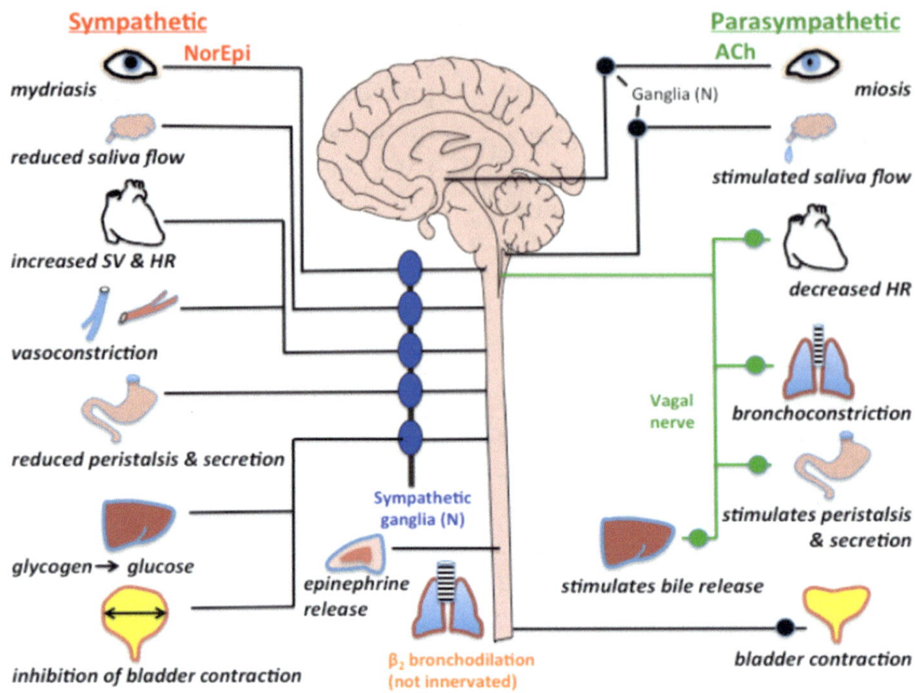

Figure 6.5. Autonomic nervous system (ANS).

Source: https://tmedweb.tulane.edu/pharmwiki/lib/exe/fetch.php/ans.png.

6.2. Neurons: The Functional Units

Neurons are the fundamental units of the nervous system, responsible for sensory experience, motor control, and intellectual functions. Their intricate anatomy includes specialized regions: the soma, dendrites, and axons. The soma, or cell body, houses essential organelles and is central to cellular metabolism. Dendrites branch off from the soma, creating a complex network that receives and consolidates synaptic input from other neurons. In comparison, the axon transmits action potentials from the cell body away, enabling faster transmission over longer distances. The morphological heterogeneity facilitates the neurons to modify their shape according to their functional requirements and mirrors the elegant diversity built into the neural network. The combination of various types of neurons and their unique morphology is an extremely crucial aspect of neural function. For instance, sensory neurons possess specialized morphology that renders them especially responsive to environmental stimuli, whereas interneurons tend to possess shorter axons for local communication within circuits. Research on non-mammalian preparations, such as olfactory centers of Coenobita hermit crabs, alludes to the complexity of neuron structure-function relationships. Experiments show that olfactory sensory neurons project to olfactory lobes, with local interneurons like those expressing orcokinin helping process odors by passing signals and regulating sensory input through lateral inhibition (Dircksen et al., 2020). This further supports the view that distinct neuronal morphologies enable distinct functions in sophisticated networks, ultimately contributing to the nervous system's evolutionary development. Neuronal functional unit study transcends traditional organisms into the realm of whole-brain emulation, particularly in simpler nervous systems. Insect brain emulation (IBE) is an accessible intermediate goal, mimicking the biological realism necessary to investigate cognitive processes. The proponents argue that the imitation of full insect nervous systems may lead to breakthroughs in artificial intelligence and robotics and hence demonstrate the efficacy of neuron structure in engineered systems (Collins, 2018). By prioritizing IBE, researchers have the potential to unlock doors to more widespread applications in neuroscience and even simulations of human brains. The pursuit of these goals lays bare not only the functional importance of neurons but also their role in explaining cognitive and behavioral phenomena across many species, ultimately advancing our understanding of nervous tissue morphology.

6.2.1. Structure of Neurons

The structure of the neuron is essential in understanding its role in the nervous system. Neurons are specialized cells and are responsible for information transport throughout the body via electrical signals and chemical messengers. Neurons have several different components: the soma (cell body), dendrites, and axon. The soma contains the nucleus and takes care of maintaining the cells' overall health. Dendrites, branching projections of the soma, receive signals from other neurons and thus render synaptic communication feasible. The axon, however, projects away from the soma, typically sheathed in myelin wraps that are adapted to speed signal conduction. These components form the elaborate information processing mechanisms used in neurophysiology, highlighting the importance of neuronal structure in both health and disease in their lengths and widths that are relevant to their respective functions. Sensory neurons, for instance, would typically have long dendrites in order to be able to accommodate the greatest surface area of input, whereby they are able to collect information from the external world effectively. Motor neurons, in turn, possess long axons that reach considerable distances, enabling them to carry signals between the spinal cord and muscles. These morphological characteristics are pivotal to the effectiveness of signal transduction within various neural networks. In addition, the knowledge of neuronal structure has also been greatly advanced by new techniques such as primary neuronal cultures, allowing for the fine study of single neurons without destroying their functional properties (Saunders., 2009). Thus, the intricate architecture of neurons becomes pivotal both in physiological and disease conditions. Not only is the operation of neurons established by their individual structure, but also by their synaptic associations within large-scale networks.

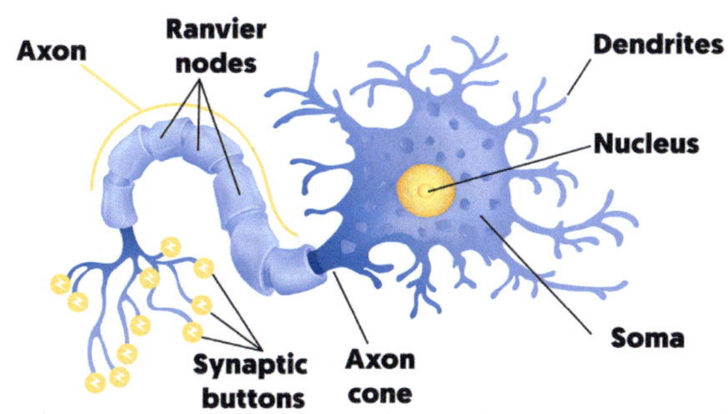

Figure 6.6. Structure of neurons.

Source: https://www.worksheetsplanet.com/wp-content/uploads/2022/08/Neuron-Structure-Diagram.jpg.

The synapse is the site of neuron-to-neuron contact where signals are conveyed by neurotransmitter release and reception. The complex dynamic at the synapse is controlled by the structural arrangement of presynaptic and postsynaptic neurons. Researchers have used histological techniques, like immunohistochemistry, to make synaptic proteins visible and understand the organizational patterns of such associations. Not only do these studies put into focus how the shape of synapses influences neurocommunication, but also how distortions in these organizational patterns lead to disease conditions (Dircksen et al., 2020). As neuroscience evolves, the comprehension of the intricate anatomy of neurons and their synapses continues to be crucial to developing therapeutic strategies for neurodegenerative diseases and to better understanding nervous system function (Figure 6.6).

6.2.2. Types of Neurons (Sensory, Motor, Interneurons)

Neurons are classified into three broad categories: sensory neurons, motor neurons, and interneurons. Sensory neurons are specialized for the reception of environmental stimuli and the encoding of physical or chemical stimuli as neural impulses that are transmitted to the central nervous system. These cells are endowed with receptors that can detect a range of stimuli, including light, sound, and temperature. Interestingly, their morphology is typically composed of long dendritic processes that enhance their capacity to store sensory information, bearing witness to functional specialization in nervous tissue morphology. Motor neurons, however, are responsible for transmitting messages from the central nervous system to effectors such as muscles and glands, facilitating movement and physiological response. These neurons possess a clear morphological plan, which is typically composed of long axons extending to peripheral targets, maximizing communication. In addition, the soma of motor neurons is found primarily within the spinal cord's anterior horn, reflective of their most basic function in somatic and autonomic pathways. The association and coordination of motor neurons reflect the highly structured nature necessary for coordinated control of the motor, which is fundamental to an organism's adaptability and survival in a dynamic environment. Interneurons are critical integrators of the nervous system, and they have a prominent role in the central nervous system. Interneurons connect sensory and motor pathways, processing information and transmitting communication between them. Interneurons have various morphological characteristics ranging from small local circuits to more complex forms extending over different brain and spinal cord regions. Research illustrates the role of interneurons in regulating sensory perception and motor output, with their involvement in reflex arcs as well as other integrative processes. To illustrate, research indicates that spinal circuit interneurons participate in many reflexes, underscoring their role in neural routing efficacy and response regulation during health and degeneration (Buchner et al., 2009; Amandusson et al., 2012).

6.2.3. Neuronal Communication and Signaling

Neuronal communication is central to the complex nature of the nervous system, and it is largely made possible through specialized structures to enable effective signaling. Neurons communicate via synapses, where neurotransmitters are released from presynaptic terminals and attach to receptors on postsynaptic membranes. **This** communication is critical for transmitting information. The morphology of neuron structures, including dendritic spines and axon branches, controls the efficacy and plasticity of transmission at synapses. Specifically, enhanced synaptic strength can lead to long-term potentiation, a process employed in learning and memory formation, and hence, the association between neuronal morphology and functional ability in signaling is highlighted. In addition, the enteric nervous system (ENS) demonstrates the association between neuronal morphology and functioning signaling. There was recent evidence implicating Toll-like receptor 4 (TLR4) in the regulation of vesicular signaling pathways that are crucial for gut motility and neuronal viability. For instance, TLR4 deletion has been reported to induce gliosis and decrease the overall number of neurons in the ileal myenteric plexus, demonstrating the essential relationships among receptor signaling, neuronal integrity, and gastrointestinal function. Besides, the altered cholinergic excitatory response observed in TLR4-deficient models highlights the manner in which neurochemical interactions can lead to significant alterations in the ENSs' structural and functional status. Hence, knowing the molecular mechanisms underlying neuronal communication is an obligatory step toward comprehending the systemic implications for both health and disease states within the nervous tissue system (Giulivi et al., 2017). In addition to this, dynamics in astroglial cell architecture are also essential in facilitating communication and signaling between neurons. Although astrocytes are very much known to play the support roles, it is also known that they participate actively in neural signaling by making contact with neurons in synaptic sites. It was only recently discovered that remodeling of astroglial protrusions, which are directly linked to synaptic architecture, is essential for orchestrating neuronal activity and modulating neurotransmission. This cellular function contributes to the neural plasticity necessary for memory encoding and cognition. Astrocyte involvement in neurotransmitter uptake and regulation of ion homeostasis further depicts their integrative function in neuronal communication. With continuous research progress, interactions will define the complexity of cellular structure behind neural communication, emphasizing the need for exploring astroglial morphology as an essential parameter within the larger context of nervous tissue morphology (Heller, J. P. & Rusakov, D. A., 2015).

6.3. Glial Cells: Support and Protection

Glial cells, also referred to as the forgotten heroes of the nervous system, play a significant role in neuronal maintenance and protection. Unlike neurons, whose primary function is to transmit signals, glial cells provide structural and metabolic support to ensure the neurological environment is optimal for neuronal functioning. They contribute to the maintenance of the blood-brain barrier, through which homeostasis and protection of the brain from dangerous substances are sustained. Glial cells are also involved in metabolic processes that enable neurons to function optimally in their signaling capacities. This variety of support attests to the central position of glial cells in nervous tissue integrity and indicates their importance not just in normal physiology but in disease as well. The interaction of glial cells with neurons is essential to the overall operation of the nervous system. Glial cells such as astrocytes and microglia, in addition to providing structural support, are themselves actively engaged in neurotransmitter recycling, modulation of the signal, and modulation of synaptic transmission. Astrocytes, for example, control the extracellular space by upholding ionic levels and eliminating excess neurotransmitters following the engagement of synaptic activity. Meanwhile, microglia are the resident immune cells of the central nervous system that are constantly on patrol for signs of damage or infection. The glial cells' ability to react rapidly to neuronal activity and stress stimuli is part of ensuring long-term neuron health and functional maintenance of neural circuits, thus highlighting their protective roles in a number of physiological conditions. Furthermore, novel evidence has led to a better understanding of the neuroprotective and repair roles of glial cells, particularly in relation to injury and neurodegenerative disorders. There has been evidence that destruction of specific glial signaling pathways can adversely affect neuronal survival and functional outcomes. For instance, modulation of TLR4 signaling is essential for maintaining the structural and functional integrity of the enteric nervous system, as evidenced by gliosis and reduced neuronal populations in knockout mice (Giulivi et al., 2017). This was an illustration of protective mechanisms glial cells employ under stress. Similarly, promotion of oligodendrocyte maturation and remyelination promotion have been linked to glial interactions, as demonstrated using pharmacological interventions enabling such (Díaz-Lucena et al., 2018). Such findings collectively point to the importance of glial cells in being keepers of neuronal integrity within the larger context of nervous tissue morphology (Figure 6.7).

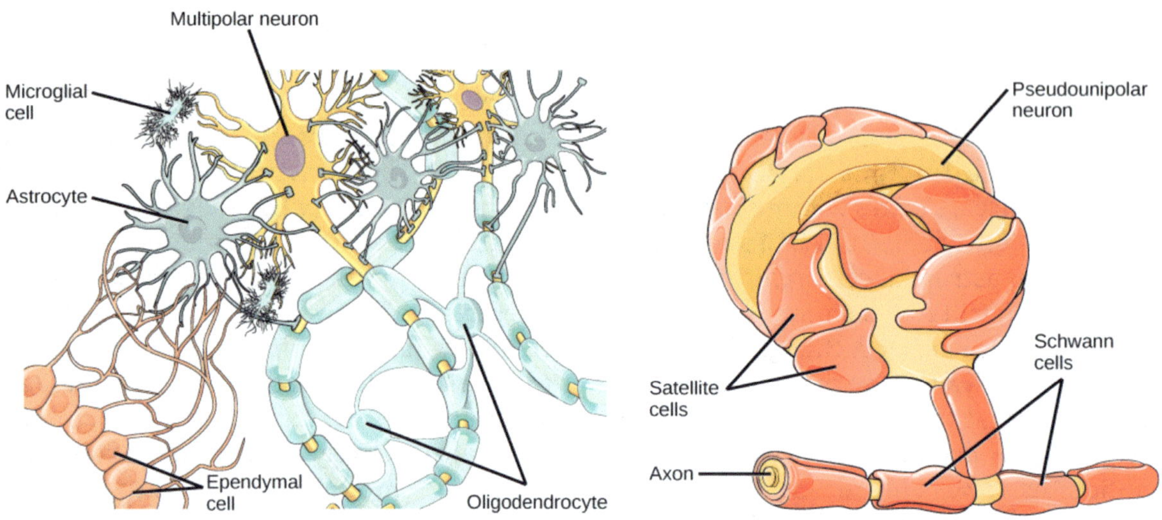

Figure 6.7. Glial cells: support and protection.

Source: https://opentextbc.ca/biology/wp-content/uploads/sites/96/2015/03/Figure_35_01_06.jpg.

6.3.1. Types of Glial Cells (Astrocytes, Oligodendrocytes, Microglia)

The intricate morphology of nervous tissue is mostly controlled by several types of glial cells whose functions in maintaining homeostasis and sustaining neuronal activity are vital to nervous system integrity. Among them, astrocytes are most likely the most versatile, comprising the greatest number of glial cells within the central nervous system. Their star-shaped shape enables them to physically embrace neurons and blood vessels, thus allowing for the delivery of nutrients and disposal of waste. This contact is essential for neuronal health and survival. In addition, astrocytes are involved in synaptic modulation by controlling neurotransmitter levels and maintaining the blood-brain barrier. Astrocytes have been demonstrated by more recent studies to exhibit dynamic changes in cellular shape, particularly in neuron-glia communication and myelination, which points to their essential function in the neurovascular unit (Anderson et al., 2014). Collectively, these actions show that astrocytes are an important part of nervous tissue structure and function. Oligodendrocytes are another important type of glial cell that contribute to nervous tissue morphology and efficiency through the formation of myelin sheaths around axons. This myelination is crucial for the rapid transmission of electrical impulses in neurons, allowing for efficient communication within the nervous system. Oligodendrocytes can myelinate multiple axons simultaneously, unlike the solitary Schwann cells that myelinate solitary axons in the peripheral nervous system. Their role extends beyond the simple insulation; they actively provide metabolic support and axonal integrity. The current research indicates that oligodendrocytes have complex interactions with astrocytes and axons and therefore respond dynamically to dynamic changes within their microenvironment

(Anderson et al., 2014). Understanding oligodendrocyte morphology and function is at the core of understanding the pathophysiology of demyelinating diseases, which shows how alterations in glial cell functions can significantly affect nervous tissue morphology and function. Microglia, resident immune cells in the central nervous system, are another crucial type of glial cells that are involved in the maintenance of nervous tissue morphology and homeostasis. These cells possess unique characteristics allowing them to track and respond to changes within the brain's microenvironment. Microglia are immune defense cells that respond to damage and infection by modulating inflammatory responses. They contribute to synaptic pruning in development and life, sculpting neuronal networks and enabling optimal connectivity. The specific morphological changes microglia undergo upon stimulation further highlight their active functions in disease and health. As further research explains intricate interactions between microglia and other glial cells, particularly in neurodegenerative disorders, the need for scrupulous morphological study becomes apparent, as highlighted by the systematic classification criteria for glial cell types. The glial cell connectivity eventually affects the overall functionality and shape of the nervous system.

6.3.2. Functions of Glial Cells in the Nervous System

The functions of glial cells in the nervous system are diverse and essential in maintaining neural homeostasis. Glial cells like astrocytes, *microglia*, *oligodendrocytes*, and Schwann cells have important supporting functions beyond structural support. Astrocytes, for instance, play an essential role in modulating the extracellular environment, maintaining ion balance, and providing metabolic support to the neuron. They also participate in the blood-brain barrier, which serves to supply the selective permeability that protects the brain from substances that could be harmful. Additionally, astrocytes participate in synaptic modulation, which is a crucial part of information processing and recycling of neurotransmitters. This intricate web of interactions is evidence of the importance of glial cells to ensure neurons perform optimally, assuring that their roles extend far beyond support to active participation in neural communication and health. Microglia, the microglial immune cells residing within the central nervous system, add still another layer of complexity to glial cell roles. These cells play a crucial role in scanning the neural environment and reacting to injury and infection.

Microglia are extremely plastic and adapt their function according to the local environment. For instance, during neuroinflammation, microglia get activated to clear debris and secrete pro-inflammatory cytokines, which help to defend the nervous system against invading pathogens and assist healing processes. Existing studies also suggest that microglia possess inherent heterogeneity, which allows them to perform various tasks based on distinctive features rather than environmental stimuli alone. Such inherent difference means that subtypes of microglia may play distinct roles in various neurological disorders, highlighting their central role in both homeostatic and pathophysiological function in neural tissue (Joseph et al., 2019). Oligodendrocytes and Schwann cells, the myelinating glial cells, also account for the diversity of glial cell functions. Oligodendrocytes myelinate axons of the central nervous system, which is very fast in conveying electrical signals. This is crucial to enable efficient communication between neural networks. Schwann cells, similarly, perform the same function in the peripheral nervous system and are important in nerve repair following injury. In addition to their myelinating role, oligodendrocytes and Schwann cells both release neurotrophic factors that promote neuronal survival and growth. Glial cells thus not only facilitate rapid signal transmission via myelination but also facilitate the health and repair of neurons, highlighting their pivotal role in the broader context of nervous tissue form and function (Giulivi et al., 2017).

6.3.3. Role of Glial Cells in Neuroprotection and Repair

Glial cells play a pivotal role in the central nervous system (CNS) processes of neuroprotection and repair, being more than mere support neurons. Non-neuronal glial cells, such as astrocytes, microglia, and oligodendrocytes, not only actively contribute to homeostatic maintenance by providing metabolic support and modulating communication between neural networks, but also become reactive after injury. Reactivity is critical in inhibiting secondary damage and making recovery possible. For example, astrocytes help to form a glial scar that gives a physical barrier for not allowing any further injury to the neurons while also secreting neurotrophic factors to promote neuronal growth and survival.

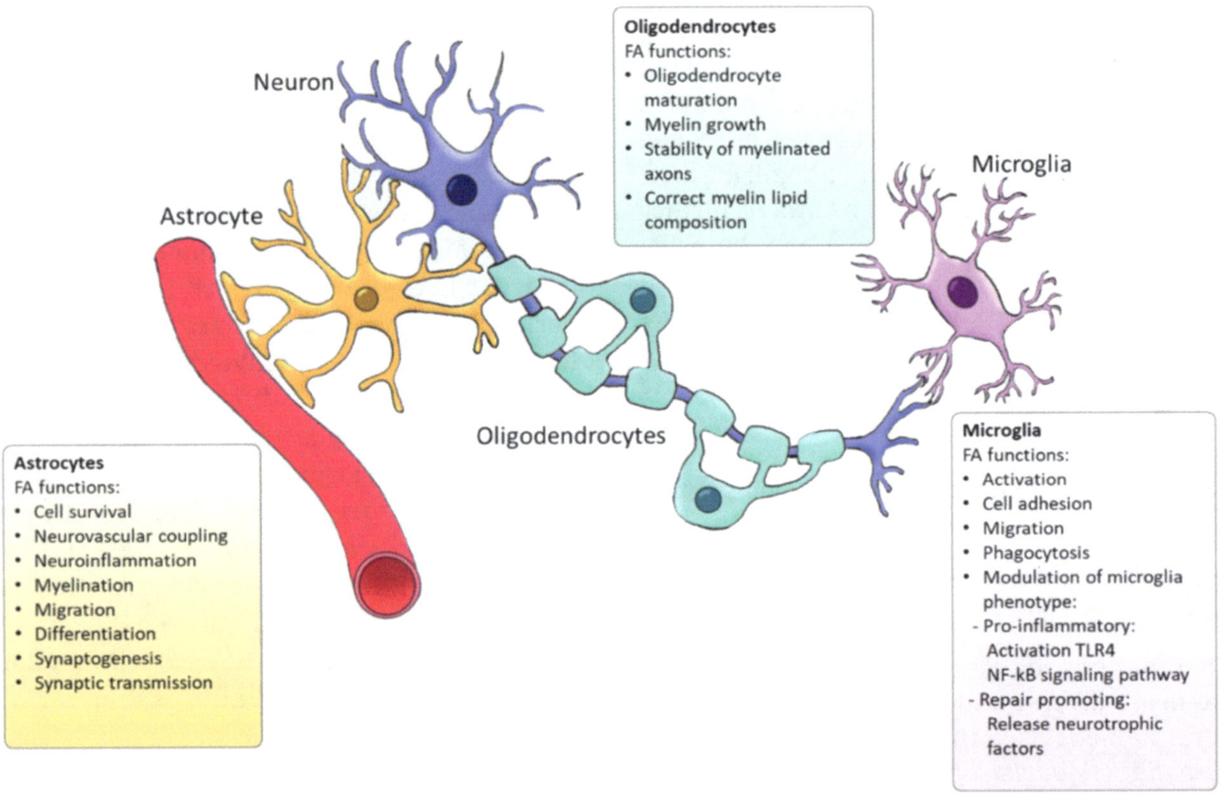

Figure 6.8. Role of glial cells in neuroprotection and repair.

Source: https://www.mdpi.com/ijms/ijms-22-08159/article_deploy/html/images/ijms-22-08159-g002.png.

This dual function emphasizes their importance both in the acute response to CNS damage and in the longer-term repair mechanisms needed for recovery in disorders such as multiple sclerosis, where endogenous repair mechanisms are often insufficient (Aigner, L. & Rivera, F.

J., 2012). Microglia, the resident immune cells of the CNS, have a key function in either promoting or suppressing neuroinflammation, with consequent direct implications for repair mechanisms. When the CNS is injured, microglia are triggered, transitioning from a resting to an active state. Activation results in the release and production of pro-inflammatory cytokines, which can remove cellular debris and infections. Excessive activation of microglia, however, exacerbates neuroinflammatory disorders, highlighting how closely microglia tread this tightrope in neuroprotection. Microglia further assist in synaptic pruning, essential for remodeling neural circuits during recovery. By their sensitivity to environmental change and capacity for response, microglia thus create a subtle game that dictates the outcome of neuroprotection and tissue repair (Gredilla et al., 2017). This balance highlights that glial cells are not merely passive witnesses but active participants in the dynamic nervous system environment. The oligodendrocytes, which are the myelinating cells of the CNS, are pivotal in the repair mechanism for myelin sheaths that are injured in neuroinjury, and they play a key part in regaining the efficacy of electrical signal conduction. In conditions like multiple sclerosis, in which demyelination occurs, oligodendrocyte precursor cells (OPCs) are recruited to damage sites to facilitate remyelination. The process's efficiency, however, can deteriorate due to aging or chronic trauma and needs to be explored for therapeutic interventions toward augmenting oligodendrogenesis. In recent research, it has been indicated that mesenchymal stem cells (MSCs) are able to improve oligodendrocyte maturation and myelin repair, and that they may offer new therapeutic strategies (Aigner, L. & Rivera, F. J., 2012). Elucidation of the complex functions of oligodendrocytes not only illuminates mechanisms of neuroprotection but also provides insight into therapeutic regimens that promote CNS repair and functional outcomes in patients with demyelinating diseases (Figure 6.8).

6.4. Histological Techniques for Studying Nervous Tissue

Histological techniques are essential for the examination of nervous tissue morphology and the elucidation of cellular architecture, interactions, and functional characteristics of the nervous system. Various staining methods, including the Nissl and Golgi stains, allow the demonstration of neuronal perikarya and the very highly branched dendritic patterns that play key roles in synaptic communication. Nissl staining, which colors ribosomal RNA within the rough endoplasmic reticulum, easily delineates the neuron and glial cell distribution with easily discernible cellular density and organization. Nevertheless, Golgi staining particularly labels entire neurons, making it possible for scientists to track particular neuronal arboreal structures and understand their interconnectivity with other cells. By applying these histological techniques, researchers can determine the complexities of neural circuit development, particularly in developmental processes, regeneration, and repair. In addition to traditional staining, advanced histological methods such as immunohistochemistry and *in situ* hybridization are progressively playing significant roles in the study of nervous tissue. These techniques allow for the identification and localization of specific proteins and mRNA transcripts in cells to give information on the molecular characteristics of neurons and glia. For instance, through the use of antibodies to neuropeptides such as orexin, scientists can chart the distribution of signal molecules in specific neural circuits and obtain insight into the neural function and communication. The use of immunohistochemical techniques in combination with histological methods enhances the resolution and specificity of neurotissue studies. The method makes it possible to investigate how changes in molecular expression relate to changes in morphology, providing a comprehensive view of neural dynamics between normal and pathological tissues, for instance, in studies on the structural organization of olfactory systems in various species (Dircksen et al., 2020). A detailed assessment of the morphological characteristics of nervous tissue is necessary to explain many neurological disorders. Histological techniques are not only utilized in examining normal tissue but are also a pivotal component of the examination of pathological changes as a component of conditions such as neurodegeneration, trauma, or developmental disorders. For example, histological examination can identify aberrant neuronal morphology or deranged glial function and serve as valuable markers of underlying pathophysiological processes. Techniques such as silver impregnation and other specialized stains can uncover unique features of neurodegeneration, including the presence of plaques or tangles characteristic of disease states like Alzheimer's. By controlled application of these histological techniques, researchers are able to correlate morphological characteristics with clinical presentations, a stepping stone toward potential therapeutic approaches. This interdisciplinarity emphasizes the degree to which evolved morphological research can be used to advance our understanding of nervous tissue integrity and inform future orientations in neuroscience (Fraser, S. E., Shih, J., 1996).

6.4.1. Staining Methods (Nissl Stain, Immunohistochemistry)

The exploration of staining methods is the focus of nervous tissue morphology because these procedures enable researchers to locate and distinguish the structures of cells in the brain. The Nissl stain is one of the most common procedures employed. It binds specifically to ribosomal RNA found in the rough endoplasmic reticulum of neurons. This stain enables discrimination of neuronal cell bodies and overall morphology, with clear separation between neuronal and glial cells. Through the illustration of Nissl body distribution, researchers can estimate neuronal density, which is critical in comparative studies in neuroanatomy. Notably, Nissl staining combined with immunohistochemical procedures can enhance the specificity of neuron identification, enabling adequate analysis of tissue morphology between various regions of the brain. Immunohistochemistry (IHC) is also a significant staining procedure that provides further information on the profiles of protein expression of nervous tissue. This method applies antibodies to identify particular antigens within the tissue in order to research cellular interactions and functions within the nervous system. For instance, a recent study conducted by IHC showed expression of the CD6 antigen in the human brain, showing that it is not only activated during the immune response but is also used in neurodevelopmental processes (Funke et al., 1990). By employing a panel of monoclonal antibodies, scientists can visualize cell types with unique antigen-expression patterns and thereby develop a comprehensive picture of cell diversity and organization. This discrimination is of major importance in identifying pathologies such as neurodegenerative diseases, wherein altered expression profiles may be able to reveal key disease mechanisms and therapeutic targets. The combination of Nissl staining and immunohistochemistry enhances the resolution of neuroanatomical examination, particularly in visualizing the morphology of various cell types of neurons and glia. The conventional Nissl staining enables a general cellular structure to be seen, while IHC enables specificity in protein expression (Zikopoulos et al., 2016). This two-approach strategy leverages the advantages of each method, enabling a thorough evaluation of intricate associations among different cell types in the cerebral cortex. Furthermore, the precise use of these staining methods makes it possible to establish valid criteria for the identification of cells, hence quantitative estimations of neuron populations and their glial counterparts. Lastly, such rigorous techniques enable us to move further towards increased knowledge of nervous tissue morphology and its contribution to health and illness.

6.4.2. Microscopy Techniques (Light Microscopy, Electron Microscopy)

Microscopy is a basis for the research of nervous tissue morphology, and light and electron microscopy are the most frequently used methods. Light microscopy, often the initial instrument to be applied to the examination of biological specimens, allows the observation of cellular detail in stained sections of tissue. Using various staining techniques, such as immunohistochemistry, researchers can visualize specific proteins and cell components, thereby enabling the establishment of neuronal circuits and synaptic relationships. However, light microscopy resolution can be restrictive with respect to observing delicate cellular characteristics, requiring more sophisticated means when a difficult structure in nervous tissue is involved. Here, electron microscopy plays its role by providing the increased resolution needed for an accurate appreciation of synaptic structure and intracellular designs and thus becomes an invaluable tool in neurobiology studies. Electron microscopy, particularly transmission electron microscopy (TEM) and scanning electron microscopy (SEM), yields information on the ultra-structural organization of nervous tissue that is unmatchable. TEM enables scientists to examine cellular components at higher resolution and to visualize organelles and synaptic junctions that are inaccessible to light microscopy. The precision achieved by electron microscopy is particularly evident in studies of synaptic connectivity and plasticity, wherein the refined morphology of dendritic spines or terminal axons can uncover functional meaning in neural circuitry. Specialized techniques, such as volume electron microscopy (vEM), further enhance this study by enabling reconstruction of complete neural networks and creation of a connectome, as seen in studies of insects such as *Caenorhabditis elegans* (Chisholm et al., 2018). Such techniques are necessary to understand the nuances of nervous system development and function. With neuroscience heading towards grander goals, such as simulating whole brains, the use of microscopy is still crucial. While the creation of exact models of human neural organization with current data and computation capacity is an uninspiring challenge, imitation of insect brains (IBE) is a more desirable intermediate target (Collins, 2018).

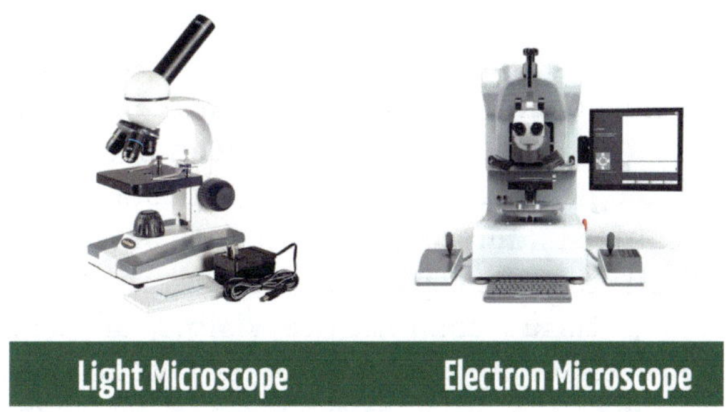

Figure 6.9. Microscopy techniques (light microscopy, electron microscopy).

Source: https://opticsmag.com/wp-content/uploads/2019/06/light-vs-electron-microscope-1024x586.jpg.

With advanced microscopy, researchers are able to produce biologically realistic simulations of entire insect nervous systems, which can, in turn, inform efforts to simulate mammalian and human brains. Such endeavors would not only enhance our understanding of cognitive function but also enable applications in robotics and artificial intelligence. The broad range of potential applications of microscopy here highlights the essential function of bridging the foundational knowledge of neural morphology with leading-edge technological innovation (Figure 6.9).

6.4.3. Challenges in Visualizing Nervous Tissue

Some of the challenges in visualizing nervous tissue stem from the need to clearly understand its complex morphology. One of the major challenges is the organization of neuronal networks that are kind of always big and interrelated arrays. Neurons are very branched and have synaptic associations, making it impossible to visualize and differentiate individual structures in what could be overwhelming networks. In addition, some classical staining methods do not explain all correlations because they mask important details or fail to highlight significant elements of the nervous system. Scientists, therefore, face the Herculean task of developing new imaging modalities that can come with improved resolution and clarity without compromising the biological integrity of nervous tissue. These difficulties underscore the necessity of creating methods that are capable of properly rendering nervous tissue complexities visible, allowing for greater comprehension of its function and structure. In addition to the internal structural complexities of the nervous tissue, technological limitations in existing imaging methods pose dominant challenges. Conventional microscopy is generally constrained by resolution limits that restrict visualization of delicate details in neurons, such as dendritic spines or synaptic interfaces. Thus, researchers are increasingly setting their sights on advanced imaging technologies, such as high-resolution fluorescence microscopy and 3D electron microscopy, to overcome these hurdles. However, these more advanced strategies have their drawbacks; the steps are time-consuming, costly, and require access to highly trained expertise that is perhaps not available in every research lab. Moreover, their integration into routine laboratory procedures requires a significant investment in training and equipment, ultimately impacting the availability of these methods for application across the neuroscience community. Closing the gap in neuroanatomical circuitry information is necessary, as advocated in recent calls for methodical experimental mapping at a mesoscopic level to fill existing gaps in our understanding of nervous tissue organization. By taking advantage of new methods such as tracer injections or viral vector approaches, scientists can offer more comprehensive, brain-wide coverage of neural circuits. This ambitious undertaking requires a commitment to the development of standardized, automated protocols and the building of a centralized, open-access data repository that will be a wealth of information for the scientific community. Attempts to these ends are essential to overcoming challenges to the visualization of complex nervous tissue and enhancing our understanding of its morphology and function. While scientists take this path, such activities as those discussed in recent research can create convergence and innovation, ultimately leading to understanding in how we perceive and comprehend nervous tissue structure, as seen in the suggestions for brain emulations within insects, which can further shed light on modeling and comprehending neural networks (MacKenzie-Graham et al., 2009; Collins., 2018).

6.5. Morphological Variations in Nervous Tissue

The extremely specialized morphology of nervous tissue is crucial to its function and varies significantly between various regions of the central nervous system. Within the brain, individual structures exhibit morphological features that are specific to their functional roles. The hippocampus, for instance, which is involved in the formation of memory, contains a layered organization of distinct types of neurons and synaptic structures. The mechanical characteristics of such a tissue play a significant role in neurodevelopment, and recent research has shown that the mechanical stiffness is different across varying morphological layers of the hippocampus.

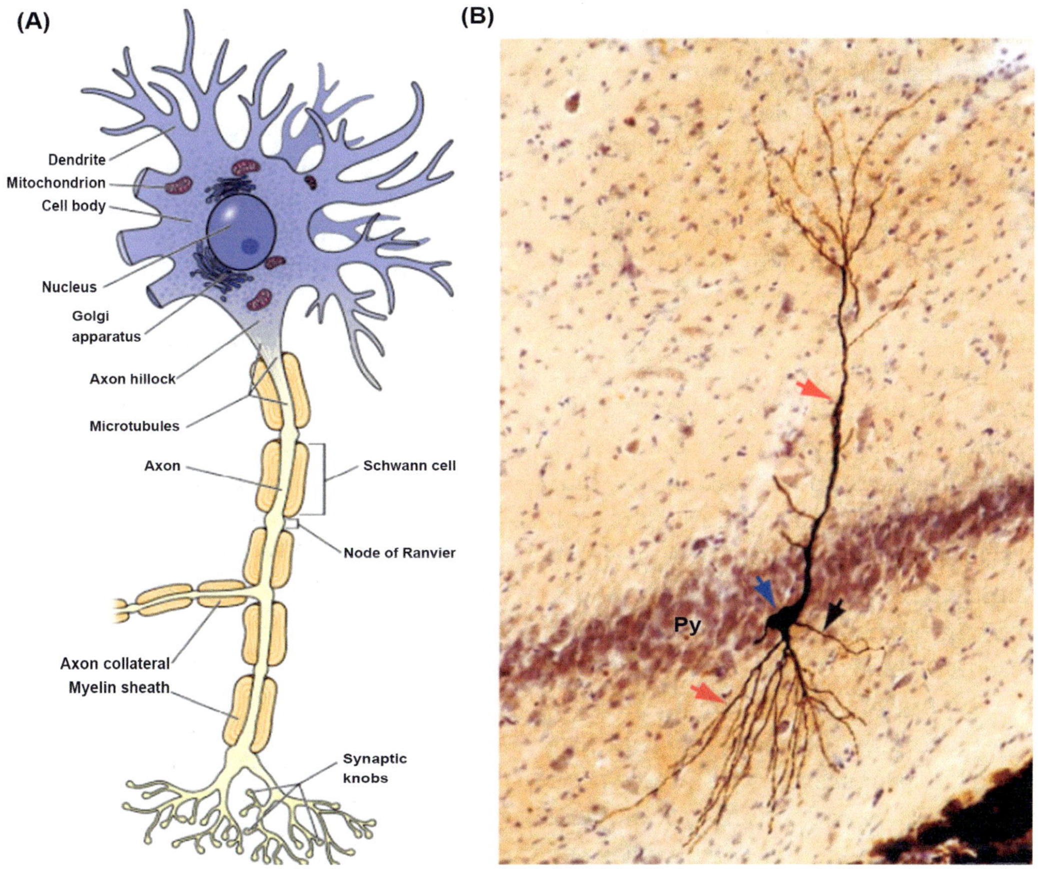

Figure 6.10. Morphological variations in nervous tissue.

Source: https://ars.els-cdn.com/content/image/3-s2.0-B9780128042540000028-f02-26-9780128042540.jpg.

The differences not only impact the biomechanical response of the tissue but also correlate with its cell composition, where denser cellular populations are typically found to have greater stiffness. Understanding such morphological variation aids in elucidating how structural differences render certain regions vulnerable to neurological disease, thereby affecting treatment strategies (Antonovaite et al., 2018). Aside from the central nervous system's morphological nuances, peripheral nervous tissue is also characterized by enormous morphological diversity. Morphology of sensory neurons, for example, is illustrated through their different shapes and sizes that align with their function. Morphological variations include patterns of myelination of axons, which may influence conduction velocity and efficiency in the transmission of neural impulses. Variation in cellular constituents of ganglia, including the presence of satellite cells, also contributes to the richness in complexity in peripheral nervous system architecture. Not only are these variations adaptive, but they also demonstrate the relationship between morphology and biological function. These precise observations of these intricate differences in morphology illuminate our understanding of many neuropathologies, as structural abnormalities have a tendency to lay the groundwork for dysfunction (Bácsy et al., 2005). Additionally, the morphology of pituitary adenoma cells presents us with an interesting window into another facet of the architecture of nervous tissue. Under microscopic examination, these cells exhibit key morphological differences that correspond to their functional activity when cultured *in vitro*. The study of viable monolayer cultures of pituitary adenomas has shown that the histological appearance under light and electron microscopy could reflect the underlying pathophysiologic states of these neoplasms. Of particular importance is the retention of the physiological characteristics in a range of adenoma types, suggesting an underlying morphology-endocrine function correlation. As this research progresses, the integration of morphological data with histopathological observations will enhance diagnostic accuracy and enable deeper understanding of the neuroendocrinological significance of pituitary tumors, underscoring the importance of morphological distinctions within nervous tissue (Bácsy et al., 2005) (Figure 6.10).

6.5.1. Differences Between Gray and White Matter

Nervous tissue is essentially composed of two primary forms: gray matter and white matter, both with different functions in the central nervous system (CNS). Gray matter is primarily made up of neuronal cell bodies, dendrites, unmyelinated axons, and glial cells. Its prominent location on the surfaces of brains, particularly the cerebral cortex, enhances its function in information integration and processing. White matter, in contrast, is composed mostly of myelinated axons that form the routes of communication between different gray matter regions. Myelin sheath, which gives white matter its color, facilitates rapid conduction of signals and thus plays a pivotal role in the general effectiveness of the nervous system. These structural differences are important to recognize in understanding how neural communication occurs and influences cognitive and motor functions. Gray and white matter's connections and distribution are fundamental to the brain's functionality. Gray matter is typically found in the cerebellum and cerebrum, where it is tasked with processing sensory information and coordinating motor responses. White matter, however, makes up the bulk of deeper brain structures and is required to convey signals from area to area of the brain. Such differentiation is particularly important in the field of neurodevelopment and neurodegenerative disease, where white matter damage can disrupt the pathways required for effective communication between neurons. Studies have established varied conditions involving alterations in white matter integrity, underscoring its critical role in maintaining cognitive operations and overall brain integrity, like (Atkinson et al., 2018), which elucidates TREX1 expression by microglia that engage with white matter structures during ischemia. Further, the interaction between gray matter and white matter plays a critical role in forming complex neural networks. Gray matter areas, which are rich in dense synaptic activity, serve as places of sensory input processing, whereas white matter pathways enable the integration of sensory input from various areas and coordinate appropriate responses. Recent research has also highlighted the function of cytoplasmic signaling adaptors like Cas proteins in axonal guidance and fasciculation in the development of neural circuits, as noted in the peripheral somatosensory system (Estep et al., 2018). These pathways represent the intricate interplay between white and gray matter, in which the former supports local synaptic interactions and the latter provides a mechanism for communication to be carried efficiently over extended distances. A comprehension of the interaction between these two tissue types can thus elucidate neural ontogeny and the pathophysiology of many neurological disorders.

6.5.2. Structural Adaptations in Response to Injury

When injury occurs to the nervous system, several structural adaptations occur, which are primarily aimed at preserving function and facilitating repair. Following nerve injury, a phenomenon known as neuroplasticity is set in motion, whereby morphological changes are performed in the nervous tissue. This involves the reorganization of neurons' connections and activation of glial cells, which are crucial for neuronal survival and growth. For instance, astrocytes, which are a type of glial cell, develop and form a glial scar upon injury. Although this glial scar might be able to inhibit the regeneration of neurons by physically hindering them, it ultimately serves to reinforce the site of damage and prevent other regions of tissue from further degenerating. Thus, neuroplasticity demonstrates how the nervous system responds structurally to pathological conditions, demonstrating both the resilience and complexity of nervous tissue morphology. As healing takes place, some proteins and genes are involved in mediating such structural changes. Among the key players in the human genome are proteins such as CHRFAM7A, a gene whose function seems to influence the immune response following injury. Research has established that CHRFAM7A is able to influence the hematopoietic stem cell reservoir of the bone marrow and induce differentiation towards the monocyte lineage. These changes might facilitate increased mobilization of immune cells necessary to combat inflammation and facilitate tissue repair after injury. These findings are consistent with the hypothesis that genes which are found only in humans, like CHRFAM7A, are involved in differences in resiliency and risk of complications during recovery, emphasizing the significance of genetic factors in the structural changes which occur in nervous tissue after injury (Baird et al., 2019). This places a multi-modal response in which both cellular activity and genetic predispositions play central roles in the recovery process. In addition to genetic considerations, environmental forces and even the nature of the injury itself play a dominant role in the structural changes taking place in nervous tissue. The extent of the damage, the overall health of the organism, and even variations in inflammatory responses, for example, can dictate the effectiveness and nature of the recovery process. When the inflammatory reaction is vigorous but well regulated, structural remodeling can yield positive outcomes, such as the regeneration of neuronal tracts and functional recovery. However, hyper-reactive inflammation will disrupt recovery with subsequent maladaptive changes that degrade tissue integrity. This complexity accentuates the fine balance between injury response and recovery processes and necessitates more research on how these structural changes play off various internal and external factors (Chan, 2005). This understanding is important in designing specific therapeutic strategies to optimize recovery in injuries of nervous tissue.

6.5.3. Variations Across Different Species

The morphology of nervous tissue across species exhibits pronounced variation that reflects adaptations to distinct ecological niches and behaviors. In the amphibian species *Xenopus laevis*, for instance, an African clawed frog, the nervous system has unique features compared with that of more common anurans. Contrast-enhanced computed tomography has yielded a high-resolution three-dimensional picture of the skeletal and nervous systems of X. laevis. This new approach not only supplements previous anatomical studies but also offers insights into the specific morphological features that allow it to be a model organism in biological science (Ahn et al., 2017). Such morphological findings explore how nervous tissue adaptations optimize sensory and motor functions and, consequently, affect survival and reproductive fitness across various environments. Invertebrate animals, particularly gastropods, possess another fascinating aspect of nervous tissue variability. Cephalic sensory organs (CSOs) in gastropods are important for interacting with the environment, and their innervation is precisely controlled by specialized cerebral nerves. Recent research employing nickel-lysine axonal tracing has demonstrated the somatic patterns of innervation of these nerves and testified to the morphological conservation of such patterns between different gastropod species. All the nerves found are associated with individual somatic clusters, reinforcing the evolutionary significance of the complexes. The findings are consistent with hypotheses of nerve homology and suggest that nervous tissue morphology disparity between species is not haphazard but rather governed by the requirement for functional efficiency in diverse environments (Croll et al., 2013). Thus, this type of study teaches us how the organization of the nervous system could possibly influence behavior and adaptation within various ecosystems. The variations in morphology in nervous tissues are not merely anatomical differences; they are at the heart of the evolutionary plans of species. Looking at the many structures in the nervous system found in invertebrates and vertebrates enables scientists to understand the selective pressures that evolved these systems. Thus, for instance, the ability to visualize and comprehend the intricate interconnectivity of nervous tissue in organisms such as X. laevis represents a significant advance for comparative anatomy, enabling a more complete understanding of evolutionary biology. The homologization of gastropod nerves also underlines the influence of structural consistency within the wider perspective of evolutionary divergence. With continued research defining such morphological differences, it is clear that the morphology of nervous tissue lies at the core of understanding the complexities of functional adaptations across species (Croll et al., 2013; Ahn et al., 2017)

6.6. Implications of Nervous Tissue Morphology

The morphology of nervous tissue is central to determining cellular function and nervous system health. Modifications of the neuronal architecture have the potential to influence synaptic connectivity, signal transmission speed, and the efficacy of neurotransmission. For instance, vulnerability of dopaminergic and cholinergic neurons to neurodegeneration with aging demonstrates how morphological characteristics influence neural resistance. The basal forebrain cholinergic system, linked to learning and memory, experiences significant atrophy in aging and in neurodegenerative diseases such as AD. Awareness of these morphological effects calls for therapeutic potential in the reprogramming of such vulnerable cell types, as technology in induced pluripotent stem cells has demonstrated. This research not only talks of cellular vulnerability but also encourages enhanced insight into how morphological features render specific neurons vulnerable to age-related disease and creates the prospect of individualized interventions (Goya et al., 2014). In addition to identification of neural vulnerability, research on nervous tissue morphology can offer insights regarding the neuroinflammatory processes driving such conditions as multiple sclerosis (MS). The MS pathological lesions are the result of chronic inflammatory responses that damage myelin. Research on oligodendrocyte progenitor cells illustrates the cellular structure-neuroprotection balance. The results showing that composite drugs, such as ultramicronized palmitoylethanolamide and luteolin (PEALut), elevate the expression of myelin proteins illustrate the relevance of morphological determinants in repairing damaged neural components. PEALut's ability to regulate inflammatory markers and support myelin repair reinforces the point that morphology is not a fixed trait; it is tightly linked to functional outcomes and plasticity in the context of degeneration.

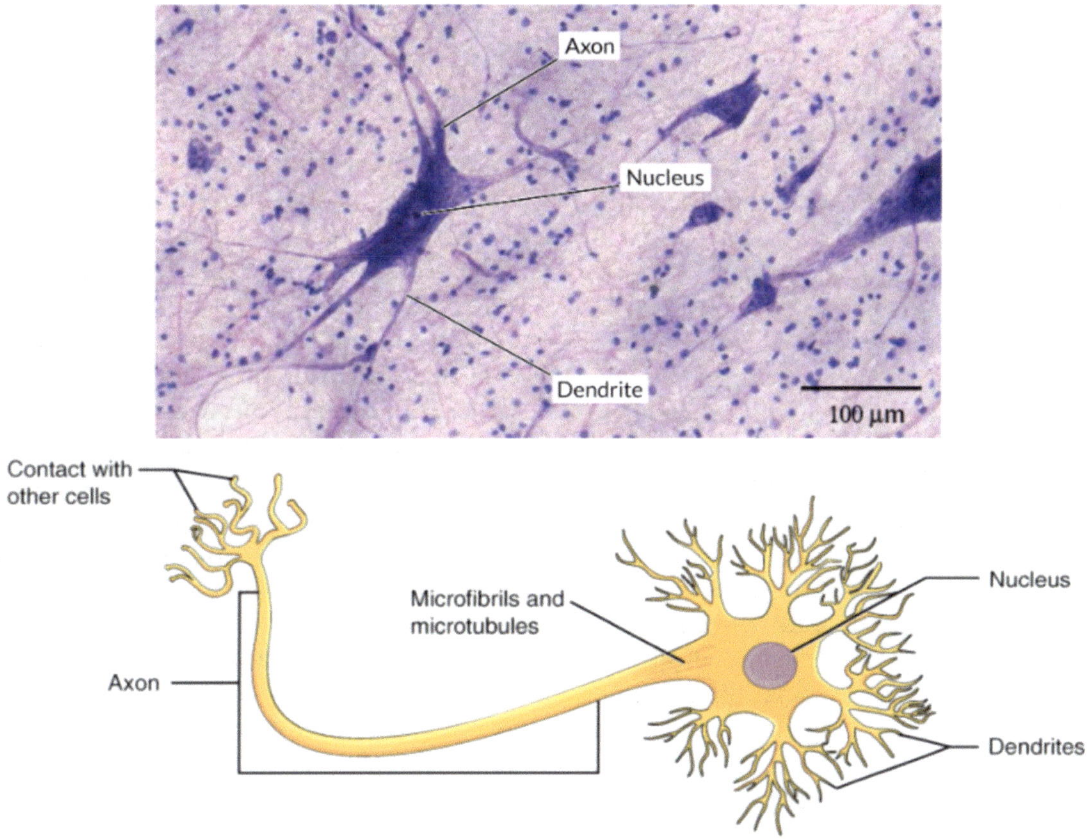

Figure 6.11. Implications of nervous tissue morphology.

Source: https://ubalt.pressbooks.pub/app/uploads/sites/67/2023/03/chapter04-26_1c.png.

This kind of knowledge is a reminder that treatments based on pharmacological modulation of nervous tissue morphology might be able to minimize neuroinflammatory damage in MS (Barbierato et al., 2019). Last, the implications of nervous tissue morphology extend to therapeutic intervention, underscored by the potential for innovative treatments from a firm understanding of cellular function and form. With ongoing research, a number of lineage or direct reprogramming strategies promise the ability to substitute missing or damaged neuronal groups. Such findings may hold the solution to resolving disease conditions following cell type loss, such as Parkinson's disease. Selective manipulation and targeting of neuronal morphology can open new avenues in regenerative medicine, with the potential to enable effective treatment of neurodegenerative disorders. With increasing understanding of nervous tissue morphology, integration of this knowledge with emerging technologies is a pathway to potentially revolutionize clinical practice and benefit the welfare of those suffering from such disabling disorders (Goya et al., 2014; Barbierato et al., 2019).

6.6.1. Relationship Between Morphology and Function

The relationship of morphology to function in nervous tissue is intricate, as it reflects the dynamic relationship between structural components and their functions in neurophysiology. Neurons possess diverse morphological characteristics, including variations in dendritic arbors and axonal projections, which directly impact their functional capabilities. For instance, the complexity of the dendrites' branching enhances a neuron's ability to integrate synaptic input, enabling the handling of vast amounts of information. Consequently, understanding such morphological distinctions is critical for elucidating how changes in neuronal structure can lead to defects or enhanced function, particularly in neurodevelopment and neuroplasticity. Such association is further highlighted through technological advances that allow one to make quantitative measures of neuronal morphology, thereby illuminating the fundamental principles of neural function and adaptation to environmental need. Furthermore, the cellular constituents of nervous tissue beyond neurons play a pivotal part in establishing the functional map of the nervous system. Glial cells, such as astrocytes and microglia, not only serve to support structure but also exert a broad influence on the activity and health of neurons. Modulation of glial morphology can be correlated with synaptic health, particularly in the framework of stress and aging. For example, research has shown that glial morphology is not altered under stress, but in aging, pronounced changes occur, which may influence the functioning of neuronal networks. These morphological transformations might hinder synaptic contacts so that information processing takes place abnormally and cognitive functions get impaired. Thus, the investigation of the morphology-function correlation within glial populations is critical to the understanding of their role in the overall dynamics of neural circuits and their implications in neurodegenerative diseases. Function and morphology are also linked to the extent that pathological mechanisms within the nervous system are covered, where structural alteration in neurons may even anticipate loss of function. The possibility of growing primary neuronal cultures has given scientists an experimental system for investigating specific morphological alterations resulting in specific neurodegenerative illnesses, e.g., those of Human Immunodeficiency Virus (HIV). Such systems allow investigation into how specific morphological alterations in neurons correspond specifically to dysfunction. For instance, alterations in synaptic structure and viability can tell us directly about HIV-associated neurocognitive disorders. As the topic unfolds, specifying the morphological alterations that are linked to functional impairments will enable us to improve work on the development of tailored treatments and therapies for a range of neurological conditions and thus emphasize the significance of the morphology-function correlation in nervous tissue function and disease (Saunders., 2009; McEwen et al., 2018).

6.6.2. Impact on Neurological Diseases

Nervous tissue morphology and the complexity of neurological disease underscore the role of structural and functional changes in the nervous system in disease progression. Alzheimer's disease and Parkinson's disease, as neurological disorders, describe how some neuron populations are particularly vulnerable to degeneration from intrinsic and extrinsic factors. For instance, the basal forebrain cholinergic system atrophies in

Alzheimer's, as cognitive performance degrades. Similarly, nigrostriatal dopaminergic neuron degeneration is the hallmark of Parkinson's disease, with a definite association between nervous tissue morphology and presentation of these debilitating diseases. Clarification of these interactions not only contributes to the disease pathophysiology but also to the development of targeted treatments in an effort to minimize the burden of neurodegeneration and re-establish neuronal integrity, which are significant challenges for neuroscience and regenerative medicine (Goya et al., 2014). Microglia, the resident immune cells of the brain, are pivotal in the pathogenesis of neurological disorders. These cells have complex morphological and phenotypic responses after injury or disease, which can cause or prevent neurodegeneration. Microglial activation phenotypes of pro-inflammatory (M1) and anti-inflammatory (M2) bifunctionality exemplify their multifaceted function in neurological diseases. While M1 microglia cause secondary neuronal injury through the release of pro-inflammatory cytokines and oxidative stress, M2 microglia can ensure recovery by promoting tissue remodeling and the release of growth factors. This balance of states of activation is of paramount significance; therefore, understanding and control of microglial function provide entry points for potential therapy in the instance of ischemic stroke. Sustained efforts at the pharmacological modulation of microglial activation could map onto increased neurogenesis and functional restitution, demonstrating the role that nervous tissue morphology has in influencing neurological health outcomes (Chen et al., 2020). Over the past few years, advances in cellular reprogramming techniques have given new hope in treating the neuronal loss that is a feature of most neurological disorders. Induced pluripotent stem cells (iPSCs) can be generated from adult somatic cells, offering a chance to replace lost or injured neurons by differentiating them into specific subtypes of neurons. This new method has significant promise, especially for conditions such as Alzheimer's and Parkinson's, in which replacement of the lost cholinergic or dopaminergic neurons is desperately needed. However, concerns including tumorigenicity caused by undifferentiated iPSCs and the complexity of lineage reprogramming remain hurdles to therapeutic application. Further exploration of direct reprogramming paths aims to generate specific types of neural cells directly from existing somatic cells, hopefully minimizing dangers and optimizing therapeutic performance. This dynamic setting is used to highlight the imperative interaction between the morphology of nervous tissue and new therapies for neurological diseases (Goya et al., 2014) (Figure 6.12).

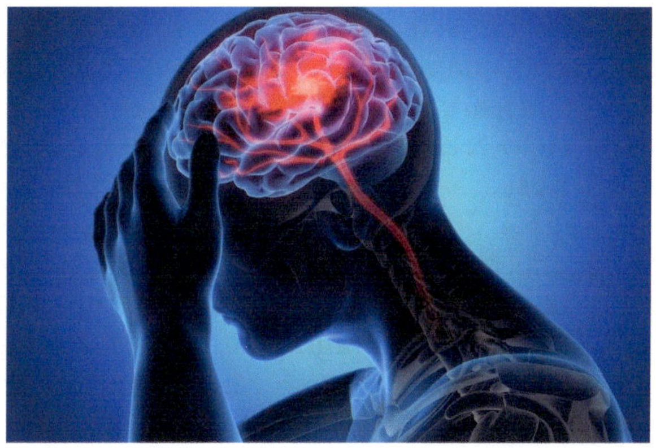

Figure 6.12. Impact on neurological diseases.

Source: https://www.godigit.com/content/dam/godigit/directportal/en/contenthm/neuro-disorder.jpg.

6.6.3. Advances in Research and Potential Therapies

The latest developments in nervous tissue morphology understanding have provided new platforms for innovative treatment avenues, particularly through stem cell technology. The development of induced pluripotent stem cells (iPSCs) has enabled scientists to reprogram somatic cells into the pluripotent state, thereby opening up enormous possibilities for treating neurodegenerative diseases. As noted, "cell reprogramming has new therapeutic potential for the cure of these incurable diseases." By effectively bypassing the disadvantages placed by traditional stem cell therapies, lineage reprogramming and direct reprogramming technologies enable one to reprogram one type of adult cell to another. These methods hold great promise for the goal of rebuilding lost neurons in neurodegenerative diseases such as Alzheimer's disease and Parkinson's disease, which are characterized by degeneration of specific neuronal populations. Treatment of neurodegenerative diseases could be drastically optimized in the coming years using these new techniques. Moreover, tremendous advances in stem cell replacement therapies have provided optimism towards the cure of diseases like multiple sclerosis (MS), a disease that significantly impacts nervous tissue integrity. Current research emphasizes the potential of neural stem cells and mesenchymal stem cells, which possess superior immunomodulatory and neurotrophic properties that facilitate the regeneration of injured neural tissue. The transplantation of iPSC-derived neural cells has produced encouraging results, including enhanced mobility and remyelination in demyelination models. "Significant enhancement of mobility and robust remyelination have been shown after transplantation of neural cells derived from iPSCs into demyelinated models. These findings point to the importance of continued research aimed at maximizing iPSC technologies, with a focus on gains in efficiency while eliminating potential side effects to gain widespread clinical relevance." These developments can result in significant advances in management and even the reversal of the course of several neurodegenerative conditions. The integration of new research tools into the clinic can potentially herald a paradigm shift in the design of nervous tissue morphology and therapy. The attempt at direct reprogramming of somatic cells into induced neural stem cells (iNSCs) offers a thrilling pathway to the realization of cell-based therapies. Not only do these procedures bypass the requirement of cells reverting back to a pluripotent state, but they are also tailored to make up for certain deficiencies in cell type in the nervous system. With continued advancements in such protocols in the pipeline, the generation of rejuvenated multipotent progenitor cells that can give rise to required neural populations is an intriguing area in regenerative medicine. The research presents the possibility of developing patient-specific treatments that may repair damaged functions and enhance the quality of life for neurodegenerative disease patients. The results of these advances have far-reaching implications, with the potential to dramatically transform the field of neurological treatments (Figure 6.13).

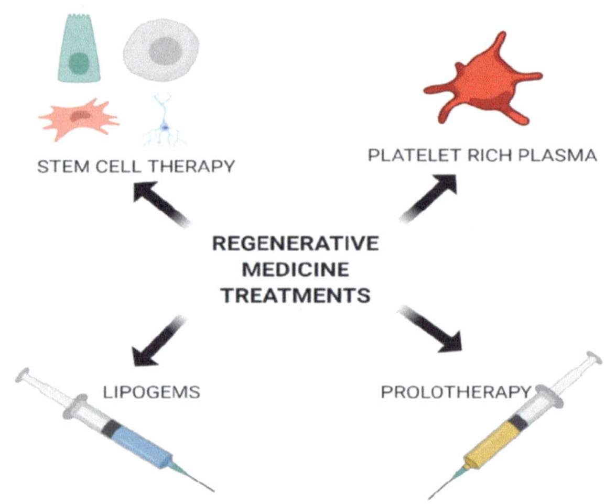

Figure 6.13. Advances in research and potential therapies.

Source: https://www.researchgate.net/publication/348139334/figure/fig1/AS:11431281425421566@1746574413602/Various-therapies-employed-in-regenerative-medicine-Currently-therapies-utilizing.tif.

SUMMARY

In cataloging the history of nervous tissue morphology discussion, one should reflect back on the incredible advances in the determination of neuron structure and dynamic changes with varying physiological and pathological conditions. In this regard, the discovery of primary neuronal cultures has been a revolutionary technique, allowing for an effective single neuron dissection and investigation. This method has enhanced the accuracy with which scientists can quantify morphological change, as demonstrated in research that has examined neurodegenerative processes caused by such diseases as human immunodeficiency virus (HIV) infection. The ability to identify these cellular changes not only enhances our fundamental comprehension of neuronal behavior but also provides a basis in therapeutic research directed towards reversing or blocking damage in nervous tissue (Saunders., 2009). The intricate interactions between different cell types in the nervous tissue also emphasize the nervous tissue's morphological complexity. Astrocyte observations, for instance, have shown their active participation in myelination, with morphological changes that facilitate interactions with axons and oligodendrocytes. These processes, as indicated by astrocyte membrane blebbing, highlight the fundamental role of glial cells in maintaining neuronal integrity and function (Anderson et al., 2014). As studies continue to reveal these interactions, increased knowledge of how many cells have roles in nervous tissue disease and health will be achieved, ultimately guiding future treatment and therapeutic interventions. Finally, continued research on nervous tissue morphology is essential in uncovering the complexities of the central nervous system. Through the use of combined advanced techniques and methodologies along with analytical tools, scientists can better comprehend the viability of cells, the development of synapses, and the implications of morphological changes on neurodegenerative diseases. As the research progresses, it is essential to define glial and neuronal populations, as such data are essential for identifying specific treatments. Through an integration of studies on many investigations, the interconnectedness of nervous tissue structures and functions shall be illuminated, which will impart greater knowledge and innovative solutions in managing neurological diseases.

Nervous tissue morphology is a wide-ranging group of cellular and structural characteristics essential for studying the central nervous system (CNS). One standout characteristic concerns the role of neural stem cells, which can differentiate into several different cell types, such as neurons, astrocytes, and oligodendrocytes. The processes that govern these differentiation events are multifaceted, especially concerning calcium signaling pathways. Low-frequency calcium transients were demonstrated in studies to play a critical role in the initial differentiation of neural precursors. Spontaneous calcium signaling influences neurite extension and neurotransmitter phenotype formation, an important convergence of cellular morphology and functional neurobiology (Berridge et al., 2003). This finding underscores dynamic neural developmental processes and reliance on precise intracellular signaling pathways that, in turn, govern the cellular morphology of nervous tissue. Nervous tissue structure is also governed by external factors and pathological processes. For instance, Ataxia telangiectasia (ATA) is a good example in which ATM kinase deficiency results in systemic effects, including morphological alterations in the skeletal muscle, which indirectly affect neuro-muscular interaction. Research on Atm-knockout models reveals dramatic myofiber size and composition changes with shifts in oxidative and glycolytic fiber types. This reveals not just that neuronal morphology is a requirement but also that muscle-nerve tissue interaction is necessary for the whole to function. Emerging complexity in neuromuscular junctions suggests that peripheral nervous system adaptations may reflect underlying neurodegenerative disease and other pathological processes (Aguanno et al., 2019). This relationship helps to explain why nervous tissue morphology must be explored in more integrated biological contexts. Overall, the morphological complexity of nervous tissue is controlled by both intrinsic cellular mechanisms and extrinsic environmental factors. The paradigm of neural stem cell differentiation and regulation through research gives us clues about the complexities of neuronal development. Furthermore, the concern about systemic diseases such as Ataxia-Telangiectasia underscores the interdependence of the nervous and muscular systems and illustrates how morphological changes in one can adversely affect the other. The consideration of these diverse dimensions not only broadens our understanding of the morphology of nervous tissue but also positions the field for future research to generate targeted therapeutic strategies aimed at countering a wide range of neuropathological disorders. The exploration of cellular dynamics and systemic interactions significantly contributes to the field's ongoing evolution, highlighting the essential merit of a multidisciplinary approach in neuroscience research.

A LOOK TO THE FUTURE:

BLOOD-BRAIN BARRIER (BBB):

The blood-brain barrier (BBB) is a highly specialised and dynamic physiological interface that protects the brain by regulating the movement of substances between the bloodstream and the central nervous system (CNS). Unlike capillaries in most other tissues, the microvasculature of the brain is characterised by tight junctions between endothelial cells, supported by pericytes and astrocyte end-feet, that create an extraordinarily selective and semipermeable barrier. This structure allows essential nutrients and metabolic substrates to reach neural tissues while restricting entry of potentially harmful pathogens, toxins, and immune cells that could disrupt neuronal function.

Physiologically, the BBB is vital for maintaining a stable chemical environment necessary for proper neural activity. Neurons are particularly sensitive to fluctuations in ionic concentrations, pH, and metabolic waste products, and even subtle imbalances can impair brain function or lead to neurological dysfunction. The barrier's selective transport systems—such as glucose transporters, ion pumps, and carrier proteins—ensure that required substrates like glucose, amino acids, and hormones are actively transported into the brain while waste products and excess ions are removed.

Structurally, the BBB is more than a single physical boundary. It is part of the neurovascular unit, which includes endothelial cells, astrocytes, pericytes, neurons, and extracellular matrix components that work together to regulate vascular permeability and maintain homeostasis. This complex interplay ensures coordinated responses to changing physiological conditions, such as alterations in blood flow, metabolic demand, or systemic inflammation.

The BBB also plays a crucial role in immune privilege of the CNS by limiting the entry of peripheral immune cells and large antibodies. While this protects the brain from unnecessary inflammatory responses, it also presents challenges for delivering therapeutics to treat neurological diseases, as most small-molecule drugs and virtually all large-molecule agents cannot cross the intact BBB at therapeutically relevant levels.

Under pathological conditions, disruption of BBB integrity is implicated in many neurological disorders. For example, breakdown of the tight junctions and loss of endothelial cohesion can contribute to neuroinflammation, stroke, multiple sclerosis, Alzheimer's disease, and other degenerative conditions. Researchers are actively investigating the mechanobiology of the BBB, including how mechanical forces, ageing, and disease processes influence barrier function, with the goal of identifying new therapeutic strategies to preserve or restore BBB integrity.

REFERENCES

1. Tassinari, V., De Gennaro, V., La Sala, G., Marazziti, D., Bolasco, G., Aguanno, S., De Angelis, L., Naro, F., & Pellegrini, M. (2019b). Atrophy, oxidative switching and ultrastructural defects in skeletal muscle of Ataxia Telangiectasia mouse model. *Journal of Cell Science, 132*(5). https://doi.org/10.1242/jcs.223008Ahn, M., Burgess, C., Burggren, W., Cannatella, D., Clemente, C., Cline, T., et al. (2017). Digital dissection of the model organism *Xenopus laevis* using contrast-enhanced computed tomography. https://core.ac.uk/download/96600364.pdf (accessed on 6th August 2025).
2. Aigner, L. & Rivera, F. J. (2012). Adult mesenchymal stem cell therapy for myelin repair in multiple sclerosis. https://core.ac.uk/download/30437095.pdf (accessed on 6th August 2025).
3. Amandusson, Å., Anderson, L. E., Balazs, M., Berkley, K. J., Blanchet, C., Blanco, F. C., Blok, B. F. M., et al. (2012). Nuclear expression of PG-21, SRC-1, and pCREB in regions of the lumbosacral spinal cord involved in pelvic innervation in young adult and aged rats. https://core.ac.uk/download/9991565.pdf (accessed on 6th August 2025).
4. Anderson, K. I., Barnett, S. C., Edgar, J. M., Ioannidou, K., et al. (2014). Astroglial-axonal interactions during early stages of myelination in mixed cultures using in vitro and ex vivo imaging techniques. https://core.ac.uk/download/20480212.pdf (accessed on 6th August 2025).
5. Antonovaite, N., Beekmans, S. V., Hol, E. M., Iannuzzi, D., et al. (2018). Structure-stiffness relation of live mouse brain tissue determined by depth-controlled indentation mapping. http://arxiv.org/abs/1802.02245 (accessed on 6th August 2025).
6. Atkinson, J. P., Bertram, P., Hajj-Ali, R., Jen, J., et al. (2018). TREX1 is expressed by microglia in normal human brain and increases in regions affected by ischemia. https://core.ac.uk/download/231816728.pdf (accessed on 6th August 2025).
7. Bácsy, E., Bálint, K., Fazekas, I., Hegedűs, K., et al. (2005). Characterization of human pituitary adenomas in cell cultures by light and electron microscopic morphology and immunolabeling. https://core.ac.uk/download/11856052.pdf (accessed on 6th August 2025).
8. Baird, A., Chan, T. W., Cohen, O., Costantini, F., et al. (2019). Uniquely human *CHRFAM7A* gene increases the hematopoietic stem cell reservoir in mice and amplifies their inflammatory response. https://core.ac.uk/download/323065430.pdf (accessed on 6th August 2025).
9. Barbierato, M., Contarini, G., Facci, L., Franceschini, D., et al. (2019). A co-ultramicronized palmitoylethanolamide/luteolin composite mitigates clinical score and disease-relevant molecular markers in a mouse model of experimental autoimmune encephalomyelitis. https://core.ac.uk/download/220684684.pdf (accessed on 6th August 2025).
10. Barnes, V. A., Crawford, M. W., Harden, K., Ravinder, A., et al. (2014). Widespread depolarization during expiration: A source of respiratory drive? https://core.ac.uk/download/131210052.pdf (accessed on 6th August 2025).
11. Becker, M.-B., Begemann, G., Meyer, A., Sanetra, M., et al. (2005). Conservation and co-option in developmental programmes: The importance of homology relationships. https://core.ac.uk/download/pdf/3800618.pdf (accessed on 6th August 2025).

12. Berridge, M. J., Bootman, M. D., Ciccolini, F., Collins, T. J., et al. (2003). Local and global spontaneous calcium events regulate neurite outgrowth and onset of GABAergic phenotype during neural precursor differentiation. https://core.ac.uk/download/16505471.pdf (accessed on 6th August 2025).

13. Boehm, B. O., Brenner, R., Fiedler, J., Gastl, G., et al. (2004). Efficient generation of neural stem cell-like cells from adult human bone marrow stromal cells. https://core.ac.uk/download/4890600.pdf (accessed on 6th August 2025).

14. Brockes, J. P., Fryxell, K. J., Lemke, G. E. (1981). Studies on cultured Schwann cells: The induction of myelin synthesis, and the control of their proliferation by a new growth factor. https://core.ac.uk/download/9124049.pdf (accessed on 6th August 2025).

15. Broide, R. S., Chen, Y., Leslie, F. M., Winzer-Serhan, U. H., et al. (2019). Distribution of α7 nicotinic acetylcholine receptor subunit mRNA in the developing mouse. https://core.ac.uk/download/323075429.pdf (accessed on 6th August 2025).

16. Brust, V., Creeley, C., Feldman, D., Grandjean, P., Herken, E., Panzica, G., Parent, M., et al. (2014). Neurotoxicity. https://core.ac.uk/download/286729125.pdf (accessed on 6th August 2025).

17. Buchner, E., Heisenberg, M. (2009). *Neurofly 2008 abstracts: The 12th European Drosophila neurobiology conference*, 6–10 September 2008, Würzburg, Germany. https://core.ac.uk/download/4881258.pdf (accessed on 6th August 2025).

18. Canillas, M., Chinnaro, E., Moreno, B., Rajnicek, A., et al. (2017). TiO_2 surfaces support neuron growth during electric field stimulation. https://core.ac.uk/download/156637162.pdf (accessed on 6th August 2025).

19. Chan, C. (2005). Influence of fetal tissue transplant on the morphology of the neuromuscular junctions of *tibialis anterior* and *medial gastrocnemius* following spinal transection in the rat. https://core.ac.uk/download/151556883.pdf (accessed on 6th August 2025).

20. Chen, R., Dallas, M. L., Jenkins, S., Rawlinson, S. C. F., et al. (2020). Post-ischaemic immunological response in the brain: Targeting microglia in ischaemic stroke therapy. https://core.ac.uk/download/305108884.pdf (accessed on 6th August 2025).

21. Chisholm, A. D., Holmyard, D., Meirovitch, Y., Mitchell, A. S., et al. (2018). A pipeline for volume electron microscopy of the *Caenorhabditis elegans* nervous system. https://core.ac.uk/download/323065107.pdf (accessed on 6th August 2025).

22. Collins, L. T. (2018). The case for emulating insect brains using anatomical “wiring diagrams” equipped with biophysical models of neuronal activity. http://arxiv.org/abs/1812.09362 (accessed on 6th August 2025).

23. Colombi, M., Frei, I. C., Hall, M. N., Heusermann, W., et al. (2022). Adipose mTORC2 is essential for arborization of sensory neurons in white adipose tissue and whole-body energy homeostasis. https://core.ac.uk/download/511532509.pdf (accessed on 6th August 2025).

24. Croll, R. P., Klussmann-Kolb, A., Staubach, S. (2013). Use of axonal projection patterns for the homologisation of cerebral nerves in *Opisthobranchia*, *Mollusca* and *Gastropoda*. https://core.ac.uk/download/14529220.pdf (accessed on 6th August 2025).

25. Díaz-Lucena, D., García, A., Gutierrez-Mecinas, M., Martínez-Sánchez, M., et al. (2018). Mechanisms involved in the remyelinating effect of sildenafil. https://core.ac.uk/download/96881851.pdf (accessed on 6th August 2025).

26. Dircksen, H., Hansson, B., Harzsch, S., Kirchhoff, C., et al. (2020). Functional morphology of the primary olfactory centers in the brain of the hermit crab *Coenobita clypeatus* (*Anomala, Coenobitidae*).

27. Ehrlich, S., Frank, G. K. W., King, J. A., Thompson, P. M., et al. (2018). Structural neuroimaging of anorexia nervosa: Future directions in the quest for mechanisms underlying dynamic alterations. https://core.ac.uk/download/288432964.pdf (accessed on 6th August 2025).

28. Estep, J. A., Riccomagno, M. M., Rosette, K. A., Rutlin, M., et al. (2018). Cas adaptor proteins coordinate sensory axon fasciculation. https://core.ac.uk/download/323067842.pdf (accessed on 6th August 2025).

29. Fraser, S. E., Shih, J. (1996). Characterizing the zebrafish organizer: Microsurgical analysis at the early-shield stage. https://core.ac.uk/download/4893784.pdf (accessed on 6th August 2025).

30. Funke, I., Mayer, B., Riethmüller, G., Seed, B., et al. (1990). Expression of the CD6 T lymphocyte differentiation antigen in normal human brain. https://core.ac.uk/download/12163958.pdf (accessed on 6th August 2025).

31. Giulivi, C., Napoli, E., Galuppini, F., Orso, G., Marsilio, I., Lante, I., et al. (2017). Toll-like receptor 4 modulates small intestine neuromuscular function through nitrergic and purinergic pathways. https://core.ac.uk/download/84923513.pdf (accessed on 6th August 2025).

32. Goya, R. G., Hereñú, C. B., López León, M., Reggiani, M., et al. (2014). Regenerative medicine for the aging brain. https://core.ac.uk/download/159285279.pdf (accessed on 6th August 2025).

33. Gredilla, R., Stevnsner, T., Zárate, S. C. (2017). Role of estrogen and other sex hormones in brain aging: Neuroprotection and DNA repair. https://core.ac.uk/download/159300108.pdf (accessed on 6th August 2025).

34. Guan, Y.-T., Liu, Y.-Q., Xie, C., Zhang, L., et al. (2016). Induced stem cells as a novel multiple sclerosis therapy. https://core.ac.uk/download/46975671.pdf (accessed on 6th August 2025).

35. Harden, S. (2009). Microscopic analysis of sympathetic and parasympathetic distribution, terminal morphology, and interaction in whole-mount atria. https://core.ac.uk/download/236316292.pdf (accessed on 6th August 2025).

36. Heller, J. P. & Rusakov, D. A. (2015). Morphological plasticity of astroglia: Understanding synaptic microenvironment. https://core.ac.uk/download/29412340.pdf (accessed on 6th August 2025).

37. Joseph, B., Stratoulias, V., Tremblay, M.-È., Venero Recio, C., et al. (2019). Microglial subtypes: Diversity within the microglial community. https://core.ac.uk/download/286564488.pdf (accessed on 6th August 2025).

38. MacKenzie-Graham, A., Reiner, A., Vercelli, A., Visel, A., Jones, A., Hattox, A. M., Toga, A. W., et al. (2009). A proposal for a coordinated effort for the determination of brainwide neuroanatomical connectivity in model organisms at a mesoscopic scale. https://core.ac.uk/download/4881776.pdf (accessed on 6th August 2025).

39. McEwen, B. S., Dumitriu, D., Bloss, E. B., Morrison, J. H., Chan, T. E., Lou, W., et al. (2018). Cell-type specific changes in glial morphology and glucocorticoid expression during stress and aging in the medial prefrontal cortex. https://core.ac.uk/download/323070965.pdf (accessed on 6th August 2025).

40. Saunders, J. J. (2009). Analysis of quantification methods used for cell viability, cell morphology, and synaptic formation in modeling HIV associated dementia in primary neuronal cultures. https://core.ac.uk/download/12208909.pdf (accessed on 6th August 2025).

41. Zikopoulos, B., Barbas, H., García-Cabezas, M. Á., John, Y. J. (2016). Distinction of neurons, glia and endothelial cells in the cerebral cortex: An algorithm based on cytological features. https://core.ac.uk/download/pdf/82862268.pdf (accessed on 6th August 2025).

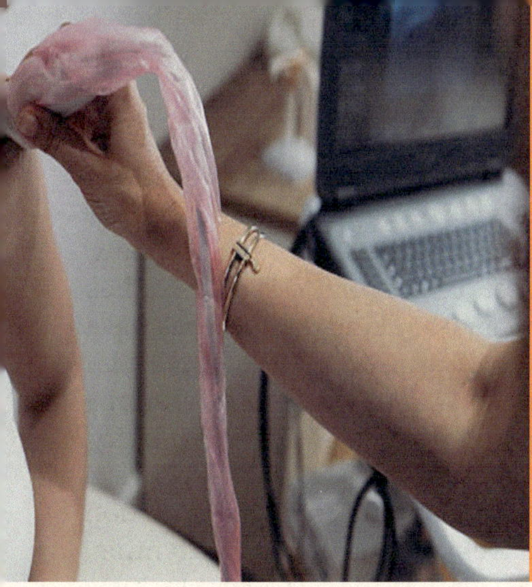

Chapter 7

VASCULAR AND LYMPHATIC TISSUE ANALYSIS

Contents

Introduction

The complex interdependence of vascular and lymphatic tissues is fundamental to many physiological and pathological processes. Vascular tissues, which are mainly responsible for blood transport, regulate the exchange of nutrients, the elimination of wastes, and the passage of immune cells. The lymphatic system, on the other hand, is essential for fluid homeostasis, immune protection, and absorption of fats. Both systems interact in close conjunction, and their failure can induce severe health implications like chronic inflammation and metastasis of cancer. Knowing the structure, function, and regulatory mechanisms of these tissues is crucial in order to create new therapeutic strategies and interventions. The following chapter will explain various characteristics of vascular and lymphatic tissue that exhibit their complications and involvement in human health, thereby creating a platform for further examination against the disease process. The role of neovascularization, or new vessel development, plays a particularly significant role in inflammatory conditions, including rheumatoid arthritis (RA). Neovascularization has been demonstrated through experiments to play a causative role in persistent synovial inflammation in early RA patients, affecting overall disease and patient prognosis. Ultrasound imaging techniques are now being employed to measure synovial blood flow, offering an indirect analysis of synovitis. Strong correlations between ultrasound Doppler studies and histological quantification of vascular dimensions and pro-inflammatory cytokine profiles have been established. The findings serve to emphasize the potential of ultrasound as a valuable tool in clinical as well as research settings to measure synovial inflammation and vascular alterations objectively, ultimately determining treatment options for RA. This interplay between vascularity, inflammation, and synovial tissue in RA is of paramount importance in deciding the pathways along which vascular and lymphatic dynamics play a role in disease. In cancer, the interaction between lymphatic function and metastasis of tumors has witnessed tremendous research attention, particularly in breast cancer. The role of CLEVER-1 in modulating lymph node (LN) metastasis came into focus, revealing the protein expression in lymphatic vessels and blood vessels in human breast cancer. Notably, high CLEVER-1 expression in lymphatic vessels was associated with an increased risk of LN metastasis, suggesting a crucial role in the metastatic cascade. Moreover, the correlation of CLEVER-1 expression with the invasion of macrophages points toward the involvement of inflammatory cytokines in manipulating the tumor's behavior. These findings accentuate the importance of investigating vascular and lymphatic interactions in cancer biology, particularly how alterations in these systems facilitate metastasis. (Figure 7.1).

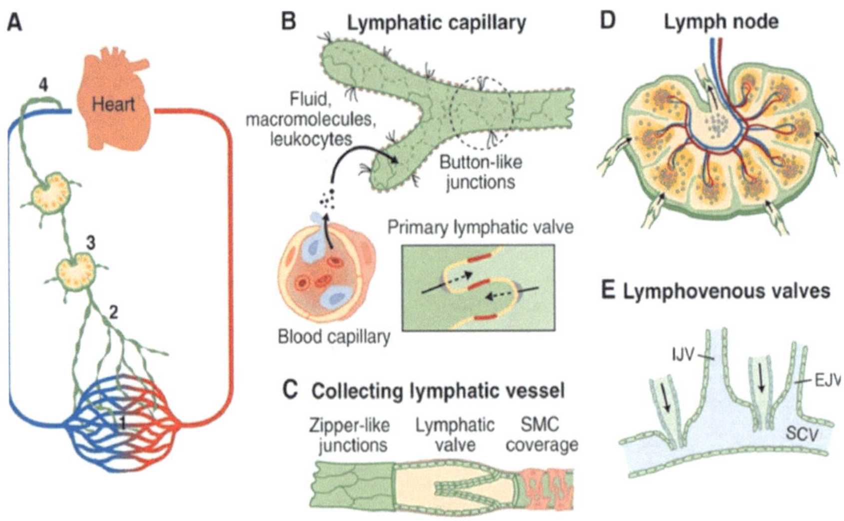

Figure 7.1. Vascular and lymphatic tissue analysis.

Source: https://www.researchgate.net/publication/349974171/figure/fig1/AS:1013621077327884@1618677505986/Anatomy-of-lymphatic-vascular-system-A-Lymphatic-vascular-system-consists-of-1.png.

Definition of Vascular and Lymphatic Tissues

The classification of vascular and lymphatic tissues is fundamental to understanding their roles within the body's complex biological systems. The vascular tissues primarily comprise the components of the circulatory system, including arteries, veins, and capillaries, that make it possible for the circulation of blood, oxygen, nutrients, and waste materials. These tissues consist of specialized cell types such as endothelial cells, smooth muscle cells, and connective tissue, which coordinate to produce a dynamic network responsible for homeostasis. Lymphatic tissues, such as lymphatic vessels and lymph nodes, however, represent a significant adjunct to the vascular system. They are crucial in maintaining fluid balance and as part of the immune response through the transportation of lymph, a fluid with white blood cells and other immune components. This disparity is used to illustrate the interdependent relationship between vascular and lymphatic systems in maintaining physiological balance and aiding in some of the body's functions. When learning about vascular and lymphatic tissues, an appreciation of their histological morphology and the way such tissues relate to their physiological function is important. Vascular tissue histology reveals a varied layering of tissues—tunica intima, tunica media, and tunica externa—that varies depending on the vessel type and function. For instance, arteries possess a robust tunica media in order to withstand high pressure, while veins possess valves to facilitate unidirectional blood flow. Lymph tissues, such as lymph nodes, possess structures called lymphatic sinuses, which enable filtration of lymph. The tissues also possess immune cells such as lymphocytes and macrophages, which are important in mounting immunity against causative organisms of disease. By studying these histological characteristics, researchers can gain valuable insights into the health and function of the vascular and lymphatic systems. This interaction between vascular and lymphatic tissues can also be seen in many diseases, and this informs us about the disease mechanisms as well as possible therapeutic approaches. For example, in cancer metastasis, cancer cells take advantage of these tissues' pathways to disperse in the body and thus become difficult to treat. Since this has lately been highlighted in a study, the interactive dynamics between invading cancer cells and the microenvironment influence the metastatic process significantly, and hence, more research on this topic is needed (Fares J et al., 2020). Furthermore, advances in drug delivery systems, such as lipid-based carriers, are illustrated by how understanding of vascular and lymphatic processes can be used to enhance the efficacy of therapeutic interventions by targeting specific tissue types (Danaei et al., 2018). Hence, it is important to understand at length the definition and function of vascular and lymphatic tissues to create new healthcare solutions and improve patient outcomes in an array of diseases.

Importance of Studying These Tissues

The importance of vascular and lymphatic tissue research extends beyond anatomical importance, strongly entrenched in clinical importance and etiology of diseases. Vascular tissues, such as arteries, veins, and capillaries, ensure homeostasis through blood supply regulation, transport of oxygen, and the delivery of nutrients to every part of the body. Knowledge of these tissues at the molecular level deciphers mechanisms for cardiovascular disorders like hypertension and atherosclerosis. Such pathologies usually follow from structural and functional changes of vascular tissue. From the exploration of remodeling responses of these tissues, investigators are also able to recognize biomarkers and therapeutic targets, ultimately determining fruitful treatment regimens. These observations not only better inform us as to the nature of normal physiology but also enlighten us as to the process of pathology, giving us avenues for new approaches to medical intervention as well as improving patient outcomes in vascular health. Concurrent with this is the appreciation of lymphoid tissues as essential to understanding the complexity of the immune system and their role in disease development, particularly cancer. Lymphatic pathways allow for immune cells to migrate, and their interaction with tumor microenvironments is a key feature in the metastasis and dissemination of tumors. The behavior of lymphatic tissue dynamics is capable of providing information on the behavior of tumor-associated macrophages (TAMs) that have been found to play a role in modifying the immune contexture of tumors. Analysis of TAM subpopulations indicates bidirectional functions—antitumor M1-like versus pro-tumor M2-like—within lymphatic tissues, which are likely to affect therapeutic outcomes in cancer patients. Hence, the systematic analysis of the lymphatic structures will significantly impact immunotherapy and tumor-targeting interventions by pinpointing the central function of the tissue in immune protection and tumor development (Wu et al., 2020).

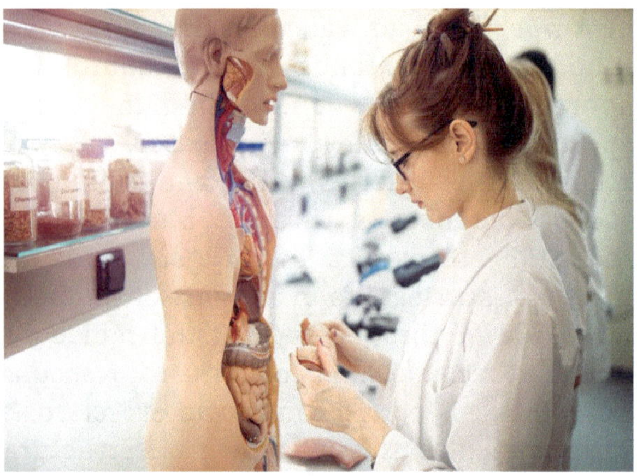

Figure 7.2. Importance of studying these tissues.

Source: https://iprocess.net/wp-content/uploads/2022/08/Study-of-Tissues-1024x683.jpg.

Furthermore, the coincidence of vascular and lymphatic tissues in pathology, particularly in tumorigenesis and metastasis, underlines the use of multidisciplinary methods while studying these systems. Tumor cells have a tendency to exploit vascular and lymphatic pathways to establish metastatic sites, allowing for cancer spread to secondary organs. This active interaction means that not only must the treatment target the cancer cells, but it should also target restoring balance in the vascular and lymphatic microenvironments that are implicated in tumor growth and metastasis. A detailed understanding of the remodeling of the microenvironment by tumor-associated stromal cells encompasses mechanisms that create a conducive metastatic microenvironment (Winkler et al., 2020). An integrated view of the understanding of both vascular and lymphatic tissue can pave the way for new therapies that shatter these pathways, ultimately resulting in better therapeutic efficacy against cancer and other diseases (Figure 7.2).

7.1. Anatomy of Vascular Tissue

The anatomy of vascular tissue underpins its diverse roles in circulatory and immune functions. Vascular tissue is comprised mainly of blood vessels that transport nutrients, oxygen, and waste products throughout the body. The tissue is made up of endothelial cells, smooth muscle cells, and connective tissue, and is layered, with each layer performing specific functions. For instance, the most inward layer, the tunica intima, provides unhindered blood flow, while the tunica media regulates vessel size and blood pressure. The complexity of this system also extends to the microscopic level, where structures like capillaries form interstices for gas and metabolite exchange. Hence, disruption of such elaborate anatomy can lead to numerous diseases, and this underscores the extreme importance of maintaining vascular integrity throughout life. When studying vascular and lymphatic tissues, particular attention needs to be given to lymphatic vessels since they play a role in immune defense and fluid balance. Unlike the role of blood vessels, lymphatic vessels are responsible for draining excess interstitial fluid and transporting immune cells such as lymphocytes from peripheral tissues to lymph nodes. This is reflected in their anatomical structure: lymphatic capillaries are more permeable than blood capillaries, which allows them to absorb larger molecules and pathogens. Detailed observations of these structures confirm that their packing and alignment can vary significantly between tissues, reflecting the different functional demands that they are exposed to. Hence, the lymphatic system's unique anatomical features mirror its vital role in maintaining the body's defense and fluid equilibrium. Studies on the anatomical development of vascular tissue during pregnancy increasingly make us aware of its intricacy. Studies on structures such as the spleen reveal distinct phases of maturity with significant implications for developmental biology and for clinical practice.

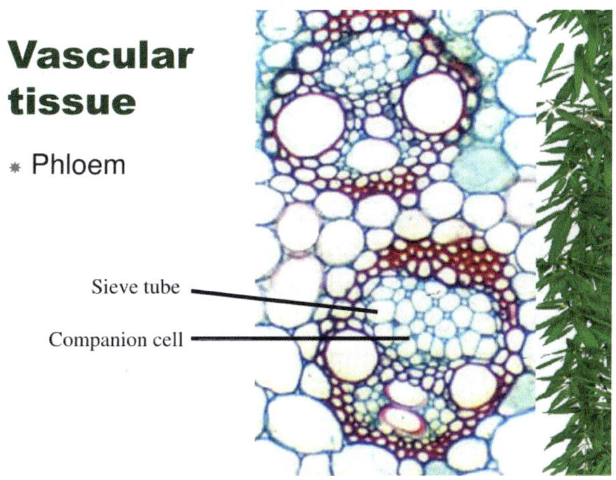

Figure 7.3. Anatomy of vascular tissue.

Source: https://png.pngtree.com/background/20230519/original/pngtree-the-human-vascular-system-picture-image_2656861.jpg.

For example, foetal spleen's high vascularity occurs between the 10th and 40th weeks of gestation, which emphasizes its core role in haematopoiesis and immune ontogeny. Progressive lymphocyte maturation and lymphoid clumping within the splenic architecture with advancing gestation suggest a crucial period in immune development, as established by studies. These results not only augment our knowledge of normal anatomical variation but also assist physicians and pathologists in diagnosing and treating vascular and lymph tissue-related disorders (Bala et al., 2024; Madhumalar et al., 2025) (Figure 7.3).

7.1.1. Components of Blood Vessels

The structure of blood vessels is responsible for the integrity and functioning of the circulatory system. The three major layers of blood vessels are the tunica intima, tunica media, and tunica externa (adventitia). The tunica intima is the inner layer that is made up of endothelial cells that ensure that there is a smooth surface to reduce friction as blood moves through the lumen. The middle layer, tunica media, is composed of elastic fibers and smooth muscle, significant in the regulation of blood pressure and blood flow modulation by vasoconstriction and vasodilation. Finally, the tunica externa is a connective tissue layer providing structural support and fixing the vessels to the surrounding tissues. This multilevel architecture allows blood vessels to be flexible and change according to varying physiological demands, thus providing proper circulation within the body; it clearly indicates the complexity of vascular structures in human anatomy. A most imperative process for vascular systems' growth and maintenance is angiogenesis, which is the formation of new blood vessels from pre-existing ones. This is a physiological process involving the growth and migration of endothelial cells, which leads to the formation of capillary beds required for the transport of nutrients and the elimination of waste products. Hypoxia and various growth factors, such as vascular endothelial growth factor (VEGF), are some of the strong inducers of this process. Conversely, vasculogenesis refers to the de novo formation of blood vessels during embryonic development when clusters of embryonic cells differentiate into endothelial cells to form primitive vascular structures. The understanding of the detailed mechanisms of angiogenesis and vasculogenesis is helpful in vascular biology as well as its applications in diseases like cancer and chronic inflammation, where inappropriate formation of blood vessels occurs (Bell et al., 2012). This relationship between tumor development and microvascular environment has been a focus of research interest, particularly the understanding of disease states such as medullary thyroid carcinoma (MTC). It was found that RET mutant tumors express higher levels of proangiogenic genes, which can lead to more aggressive vascular formation than wild-type counterparts. Specifically, studies indicate that RET-mutant tumors possess increased pericyte coverage of their microvessels, reflecting a higher level of vessel maturation and stabilization. This finding implies that RET-mutant MTCs may be more responsive to antiangiogenic therapies, demonstrating the clinical relevance of identifying blood vessel composition and dynamics during disease. The nuances of blood vessel reaction to mutations and therapy illustrate the essential relationship between vascular integrity and tumor advancement that needs to be explored within the context of vascular and lymphatic tissue analysis (Acquaviva et al., 2016).

7.1.2. Types of Blood Vessels: Arteries, Veins, and Capillaries

The circulatory system in humans has a vast network of vessels, which are categorized into arteries, veins, and capillaries, and all play a role in general homeostasis. Arteries transport oxygenated blood from the heart to other tissues of the body. They have thicker walls than veins under high-pressure conditions and consist of three layers, i.e., the tunica intima, tunica media, and tunica externa. This robust design enables arteries to withstand and manage blood pressure effectively, which is required for efficient oxygen and nutrient delivery. In addition, arterial wall elasticity, especially in the large vessels like the aorta, facilitates the adjustment to the pulsatile flow resulting from heart contractions, which is required for healthy circulation of the blood. Veins, on the contrary, have the crucial function of returning deoxygenated blood to the heart. Their thinner and less muscular walls than those of arteries reflect the lower pressure they carry. Veins have one-way valves preventing backflow of the blood, hence enabling effective circulation against gravity, particularly in the lower body. Muscular contraction over veins also helps venous return because skeletal muscles contract and press overlying veins during exercise. Identification of venous function is necessary, since compromised venous return can lead to circulatory disease in the manifestations of varicose veins or venous insufficiency. The interdependent functioning of arteries and veins is pivotal in cardiovascular dynamics, highlighting their complementary roles in sustaining blood flow. Capillaries, the most numerous and narrowest of the blood vessels, are where the primary exchange of gases, nutrients, and waste products occurs between the blood and tissues. Their wall is composed of one layer of endothelial cells, which facilitates diffusion and filtration to be exceedingly quick. This thin wall is significant for enabling oxygen and carbon dioxide to freely pass from blood into the surrounding cells and vice versa, in favor of cellular metabolism.

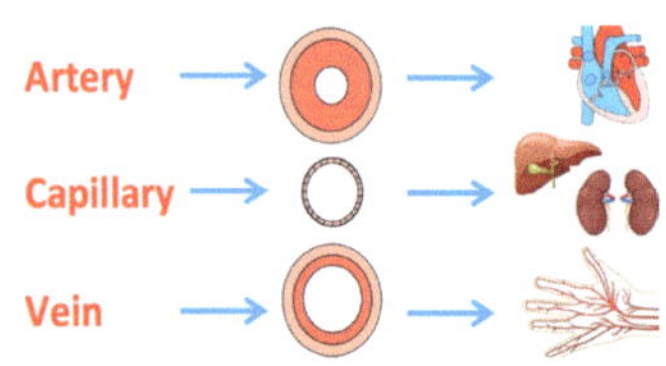

Figure 7.4. Types of blood vessels: arteries, veins, and capillaries.

Source: https://i.ytimg.com/vi/0q3Sbx08RB0/maxresdefault.jpg.

The extensive capillary network ensures that even the remotest cells are adequately oxygenated and fed simultaneously, as it removes metabolic waste products. As documented in reports of vascular malformations such as hemangiolymphangiomas and vascular malformations (VMs), every malfunction or structural defect in capillaries can have significant implications for the overall well-being of a system, highlighting the importance of intact vascular integrity towards maintaining homeostasis (Thomas et al., 2024; Gopishetty et al., 2024) (Figure 7.4).

7.1.3. Structural Differences Between Vessel Types

The vascular circulation contains a wide range of types of vessels, each having its own distinct structural characteristics that are essential to its specific physiological functions. Arteries, being pressure-bearing vessels for oxygenated blood, possess muscular walls that are thick and elastic, enabling them to resist and regulate blood pressure well. Veins, on the other hand, are low-pressure reservoirs with thin walls and wider lumens that permit the return to the heart of blood low in oxygen. The support structures of these vessels are indicated in their particular functions: arteries have to be able to withstand acute pressure changes within cardiac cycles, whereas veins employ valves to prevent backflow and allow unidirectional blood movement. Understanding these structural differences is important to understanding fully how vascular disease can ensue from vessel morphology change and impact cardiovascular health as a whole, and result in complications through varicose veins or atherosclerosis. In addition to arteries and veins, the microcirculation is comprised of capillaries and lymphatic vessels, which also have characteristic structural specializations. Thin capillary walls are key to capillary function for the delivery of oxygen and removal of waste, highlighting structure-function relationships in vascular biology. Lymphatic vessels, by contrast, are permeable tubes that receive interstitial fluid and proteins from tissues and are essential to fluid balance and immune function. The presence of valves and a thickened endothelial layer in lymphatic vessels helps to promote unidirectional flow of lymph against gravity, which helps to amplify the diverse structural variations of vessel types towards maximizing their functional efficiency in various physiological conditions. Recent research into the structure of various types of vessels has provided data concerning their dynamic adaptation responses to extrinsic stimuli, such as exercise. An example of this can be seen in studies that discuss the effect of exercise on vascular wall structure. Current meta-analyses indicate that prolonged aerobic exercise significantly reduces the thickness of large-vessel walls, suggesting adaptations that enhance vascular compliance and efficiency (Hamza et al., 2024). This finding highlights the significance of research on the influence of lifestyle on the structural characteristics of vessels, potentially avoiding the risk of vascular diseases. Additionally, structural differences between microvessels and large vessels, as observed in dermal studies, suggest that changes in vessel diameter and wall composition likely indicate their specialized functional roles within the circulatory and lymphatic systems (Rui et al., 2025). These observations increase our understanding of vascular biology and provide the potential for targeted therapeutic interventions in cardiovascular health.

7.2. Function of Vascular Tissue

Vascular tissue plays a critical role in the circulatory system, transporting nutrients, gases, and wastes throughout the body. Composed primarily of differentiated cells, including endothelial cells, smooth muscle cells, and pericytes, vascular tissue is organized hierarchically into arteries, veins, and capillaries. Arteries are responsible for transporting oxygenated blood away from the heart, whereas veins transport deoxygenated blood back to the heart. Capillaries, as microvessels, facilitate the exchange of nutrients and waste products between blood and tissues to maintain cellular homeostasis. The interplay of these factors is essential to the precarious balance of perfusion and oxygenation that ensures tissue viability, highlighting the importance of vascular tissue in the maintenance of physiological homeostasis. In addition to its transport functions, vascular tissue also has a vital function in the control of blood pressure and flow dynamics. Vascular smooth muscle cells within the vessel wall shorten and relax to vary the vessel diameter based on physiological requirements. Vasomotor function is critical in the process of homeostasis, as blood supply to tissues is controlled based on metabolic requirements. Dysfunction of vascular smooth muscle can lead to diseases such as hypertension and atherosclerosis. Growing research suggests a wealth of signaling pathways for these occurrences, demonstrating the manner in which vascular tissue reacts to disease and health states. This responsiveness depicts the complex interaction among cellular components and signifies that the preservation of vascular integrity is key to global cardiovascular well-being, as well as disclosing the prevailing role of vascular tissue in metabolism. The lymphatic network, traditionally considered a secondary system parallel to the vascular system, is also essential for fluid balance, defense against infection, and fat absorption. Lymph vessels transport excess interstitial fluid into the bloodstream, thereby preventing edema and maintaining plasma volume. Furthermore, lymphatic endothelial cells (LECs) exhibit specific gene expression patterns that contribute to antigen presentation and immune surveillance. As discovered in recent studies, there are certain subsets of LECs involved in various immune responses, and an intricate network of cellular niches in lymph nodes (Xiang et al., 2020). Moreover, the lymphatic architecture framework is critical to proper immunity since it has effects on lymphocyte and other immune cells' traffic. Thus, it is important to understand the complexity of vascular and lymphatic tissues in grasping how these systems work together to ensure immunological and physiological homeostasis (Patel et al., 2020) (Figure 7.5).

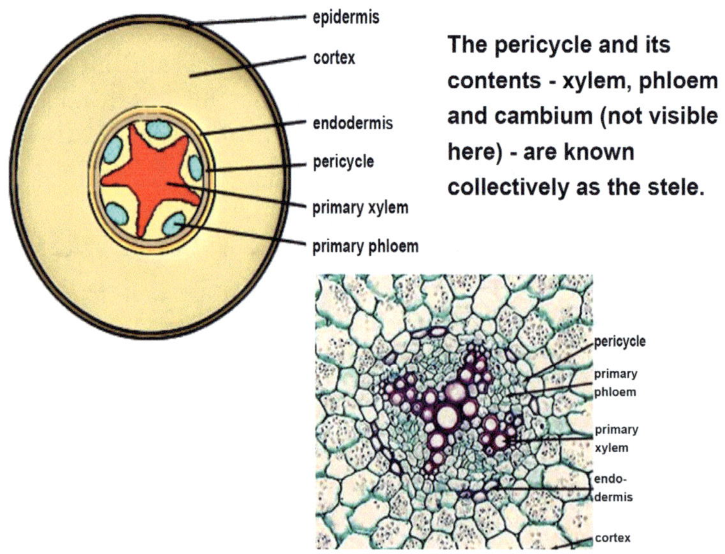

Figure 7.5. Function of vascular tissue.

Source: https://image1.slideserve.com/1931619/vascular-tissue-in-roots-l.jpg.

7.2.1. Role in Transportation of Nutrients and Oxygen

The circulatory system is responsible for transporting nutrients and oxygen throughout the body. Heart-perfused blood is a dynamic medium that delivers required molecules to cells while also collecting metabolic waste for removal. Oxygen bound to hemoglobin in red blood cells is a good example of this mode of transport, in which inhaled air is converted into energy beneficial to the tissues in the process of cellular respiration. The structure of the arteries, veins, and capillaries within the system enables efficient nutrient exchange; the capillary beds possess an immense surface area that facilitates the diffusion of oxygen and glucose directly into tissues and preserves cellular function and homeostasis. This intricate interaction underscores the significance of the vascular network as facilitating life processes and emphasizes that efficient nutrient transport is fundamental to general organismal health. In contrast, the lymphatic system supplements the vascular system by supporting the transport of lymph, which is essential in the immune response and fat absorption. Lymphatic vessels, spread throughout the body, gather excess interstitial fluid and return it into the bloodstream, maintaining fluid balance and avoiding edema. Furthermore, lymphatic transport is also essential in absorbing dietary lipids from the digestive tract, in addition to the nutrient supply for cells. This process occurs nearly entirely through lacteals, specialized small lymphatic capillaries of the intestinal villi that are used to capture lipid droplets. The interface between the vascular and lymphatic systems is critical not only for nutrition but also for immune defense, as lymphocytes travel along lymphatic pathways. Thus, determining the integrated functions of these systems provides valuable information on the intricacies of nutrient and oxygen transport within the human body. Experiments have also elucidated the pathologic effects of disease on the vascular and lymphatic systems, showing how disruptions in oxygen and nutrient transport can lead to adverse health outcomes. For instance, cancer growth is prone to promote abnormal angiogenesis, new blood vessel formation that can enhance nutrient supply to cancer cells while disrupting systemic oxygen delivery to normal tissues. This process is inextricably linked to the activity of various pro- and anti-angiogenic factors that can affect the efficacy of nutrient transport, as described by studies on angiogenic therapy for cancer management (Liu, 2023). Furthermore, recent advances in nanotechnology offer promising avenues for improving the molecular targeting of nutrient delivery or oxygenation to sites of disease, with the potential to expand therapeutic intervention (Chehelgerdi et al., 2023). This new area of research in lymph and blood vessel science highlights the critical need for continued study to inform clinical methods for optimizing nutrient and oxygen delivery in both physiological and disease states. (Figure 7.6).

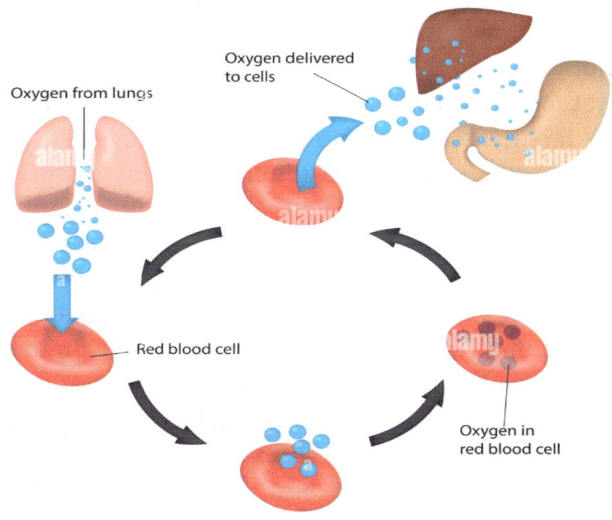

Figure 7.6. Role in the transportation of nutrients and oxygen.

Source: https://c8.alamy.com/comp/E1RBR7/oxygen-transport-cycle-from-lungs-to-organs-labeled-E1RBR7.jpg.

7.2.2. Regulation of Blood Pressure and Flow

Regulation of blood pressure and flow is a complex interplay of physiological mechanisms that optimize perfusion of the body's tissues. Central to this regulation is the vascular system, which is founded on an adaptive network of arteries, veins, and capillaries. Smooth muscle contraction and relaxation in the walls of the vessels primarily regulate the vascular tone, influenced by hormones, nervous impulses, and local biochemical mechanisms. For instance, vasodilators such as nitric oxide play an important function in decreasing vascular resistance and blood flow. Besides, flexibility to different physiological requirements is attested to by processes such as vasculogenesis and angiogenesis, which facilitate vessel development and remodeling to guarantee that increased metabolic requirements are provided for, as has been shown with respect to Bell et al. (2012). Another essential aspect of blood pressure regulation is the role of the lymphatic system, particularly in immune responses and fluid homeostasis. The role of lymphatic vessels is not only to drain excess interstitial fluid but also to facilitate the transport of larger molecules and immune cells. In situations where lymphatic drainage is impaired, such as during certain operations or familial disease states, regulation of interstitial fluid may be severely hindered, resulting in edema and altered tissue function. Additionally, there has been recent focus on the significance of lymphatic transport in processes like reverse cholesterol transport (RCT), in which cholesterol is mobilized from peripheral tissues into the circulation to eventually allow cholesterol balance and cardiovascular homeostasis. Studying lymphatic function has the ability to expand our understanding of systemic blood pressure regulation and flow, as shown in Tall et al. (2013). Coordination of vascular and lymphatic function highlights how these systems contribute to overall cardiovascular health. The regulatory mechanisms of blood pressure and flow are intrinsic and extrinsic factors that influence one another to meet the physiological and metabolic requirements of the body. For instance, systemic responses to stress or exercise are a consequence of immediate adjustment in blood pressure via neural and hormonal mechanisms, while long-term adjustment is based on structural changes in the vessels of blood and lymph. Understanding these mechanisms of regulation, including the roles of angiogenesis and lymphangiogenesis, is central to the management of disease with dysregulation, including hypertension and chronic heart failure. Continued research in vascular and lymphatic biology will continue to unravel the complexity of these interactions, paving the way for novel therapeutic approaches to cardiovascular and metabolic diseases.

7.2.3. Involvement in Thermoregulation

Lymphatic and vascular tissues play a critical role in homeostasis within the human body. The circulatory system, comprising arterioles, capillaries, and veins, plays a role in heat loss through the regulation of blood flow. When the temperature of the environment rises, vascular structures, particularly arterioles, are vasodilated to provide increased perfusion to the skin surface. This enhanced perfusion plays a role in heat loss by convection and radiation for the cooling of the body. Conversely, when temperatures are low, vasoconstriction diverts blood from the periphery, thereby maintaining body warmth. This dynamic engagement between vasoconstriction and vasodilation underscores the sophisticated mechanisms vascular tissues utilize upon encounter with heat stimuli to ensure optimal physiological process. In addition to the vasculature, lymphatic tissues contribute to temperature regulation by supporting fluid homeostasis. The lymphatic system regulates interstitial fluid volumes, efficiently managing edema as well as minimizing excessive tissue heat retention. It is especially crucial when there is an inflammatory reaction, where temperatures in the inflamed area rise. Through lymphatic vessels that drive away excess fluid from the inflamed area, they help dissipate heat in addition to expelling products of metabolism formed during tissue repair. This functional overlap highlights the mutual dependence between the vascular and lymphatic systems, as both are essential for regulating thermal dynamics and maintaining optimal tissue function under varying physiological conditions. The skin itself performs vascular and lymphatic coordination in order to regulate body temperature optimally. Its rich vascular system supports rapid heat exchange, and lymphatic drainage prevents fluid buildup that can interfere with thermoregulation. Specifically, skin thermoregulation is also closely related to the immune response since inflammatory processes can locally increase temperatures through enhanced blood perfusion and cellular activity. As a result, the presence of conditions such as skin failure, in which the capacity to thermoregulate is impaired, can contribute to severe health threats. Such health effects are also evident in conditions such as pressure injuries, where impaired vascular perfusion exacerbates thermal dysregulation. With these complexities, it is crucial to be well aware of how vascular and lymphatic tissues interact in understanding skin thermoregulation and its implications for overall health (Levine et al., 2022; Dudley, A. C., & Griffioen, A. W., 2023).

7.3. Anatomy of Lymphatic Tissue

The organization of lymphatic tissue is important for understanding how it functions in the immune system and in circulatory regulation within the body. Lymphatic tissue is well organized and can be divided into primary and secondary lymphoid tissues. Primary lymphoid tissues, such as the bone marrow and thymus, are responsible for the production and development of lymphocytes. In contrast, secondary lymphoid organs such as lymph nodes and the spleen are where these immune cells are activated and proliferate upon exposure to pathogens. The organizational structure of lymphatic tissue comprises an interconnected network of lymphatic vessels, lymph nodes, and associated cells, including lymphocytes, macrophages, and dendritic cells. Understanding of this anatomy is significant in describing how immune responses are enabled through lymphatic tissues and homeostasis in the vascular body environment. Proteins found in lymphatic tissues, such as keratin 10 (Krt10), have been studied and were found to contain meaningful information regarding cell interaction and structural organization. Recent studies have revealed that Krt10 not only occurs in primo-vascular tissues postulated to be related to acupuncture meridians but also within vascular and lymphatic tissues. Observations indicate that Krt10 has a diffuse distribution in the extracellular matrix, suggesting that it may function as a regulatory factor in the development and organization of lymphatic and blood vessels. The heterogeneous expression pattern here indicates divergent physiological roles of Krt10 in lymphoid organs compared to blood vessels, highlighting the specialization and complexity of lymphatic organization in facilitating cardiovascular and immune function within the organism (Kim et al., 2011). Developmental aspects of the lymphatic system also highlight its role in organ function, that of the pancreas in this case. Experiments have suggested that, during human embryogenesis, lymphatic vessels, defined by LYVE1 and PDPN expression, arise simultaneously with blood vessels, indicating concomitant development of these vascular networks. Blood vessels are already quite early in the pregnancy, while lymphatic vessels are comparatively restricted in early formation and only invade the surrounding tissues later. This gradual emergence underscores the lymphatic system's key function in complementing nutrient supply and immune control within the pancreas—an essential organ for endocrine secretion. The intricate relationship between the lymphatic and blood vascular systems throughout development is essential for identifying both typical physiological functions and potential treatment modalities, particularly in regenerative medicine (Carlotti et al., 2014) (Figure 7.7).

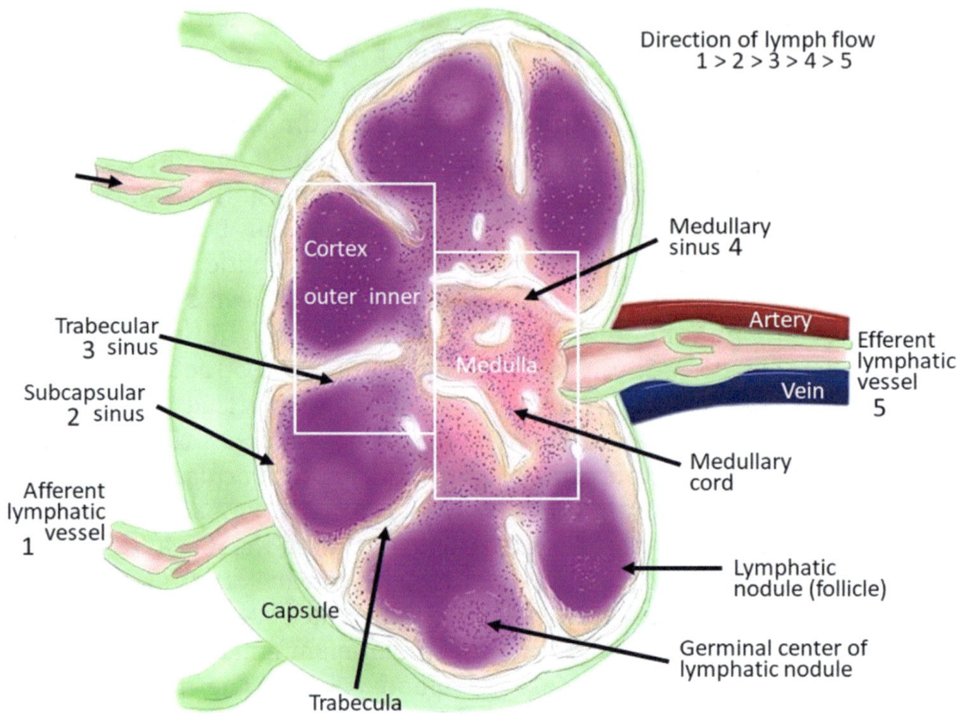

Figure 7.7. Anatomy of lymphatic tissue.

Source: https://uw.pressbooks.pub/app/uploads/sites/331/2020/09/Lymphatic_immune_system_lymph_node5-CROPPED-scaled.jpg.

7.3.1. Structure of Lymphatic Vessels

The development of lymphatic vessels is important for their function in fluid homeostasis and immunity. The lymphatic vessels consist of a unique arrangement of endothelial cells and are distinct from blood vessels both in form and function. Most importantly, the vessels have a thin-walled architecture, allowing them to be more permeable to absorb interstitial fluid, proteins, and immune cells effectively. Unlike blood vessels, lymphatic vessels contain one-way valves that allow unidirectional flow of lymph—essential for preventing backflow and directing lymph towards lymph nodes, where filtration and immune responses can be initiated. Such a special structure is essential for the lymphatic system's function in fluid control and immunosurveillance, and it emphasizes the importance of understanding vessel structure in the context of vascular and lymphatic tissue analysis. In addition to their basic building blocks, lymphatic vessels exhibit anatomical variation depending on the location and environment of the surrounding tissue. Studies have established that lymphatic vessels may be classified into primary lymphatics, which are blind-ending and in tissues, and larger collecting lymphatics, which transport lymph to primary lymphatic ducts. The initial lymphatics possess specialized anchoring filaments, which get fixed on the tissue matrix and provide a means for the intake of interstitial fluid. Collecting vessels, however, possess smooth muscle layers that help in peristaltic contractions, thus aiding in the propulsion of the lymph fluid. The relationship between function and structure in lymphatic vessels also underlines the significance of these vessels to health and lymphatic pathology, e.g., in lymphangiomatosis and lymphedema, where structural abnormalities may lead to significant compromise of health (Butz et al., 2017). Emergent technological advancements in imaging methods, for example, volume information-based histopathological analysis by 3D reconstruction and data extraction (VIPAR), have yielded additional insights into the anatomy of lymphatic vessels in disease conditions. This novel technique enables accurate visualization and description of blood and lymphatic vessels in tissue biopsies. VIPAR analysis has shown marked alterations in lymphatic vessel architecture, particularly in conditions such as lymphedema, where vessel disruption and reduced connectivity are evident. Notably, in lymphedematous skin, lymphatic segment length and linearity decrease, suggesting significant structural alterations that hinder normal lymph flow. Furthermore, these techniques pave the way for more accurate diagnostic and therapeutic intervention for lymphatic disorders by promoting an understanding of the delicate interface between vascular structure and disease manifestation, furthering our knowledge of the lymphatic system's role in overall well-being (Kim et al., 2011).

7.3.2. Key Lymphatic Organs: Lymph Nodes, Spleen, and Thymus

The lymph system is an essential component of the human immune response, with the primary organs such as lymph nodes, spleen, and the thymus serving as where the immune cells mature and become activated. Lymph nodes serve as the most important points of purification in the network of lymph, with a place for antigen presentation to T and B lymphocytes. When pathogens invade the body, lymph vessels transport these antigens to the local lymph nodes, where they induce an adaptive immune response (Luther et al., 2002). The organization of lymph nodes, with specific compartments such as the cortex and medulla, facilitates the structure and interaction of various immune cells, thereby ensuring more effective immune responses. Consequently, lymph node function is crucial to understanding how the body organizes defenses against infection and disease, including autoimmunity, in which dysregulation leads to inappropriate immune responses. The spleen, which has sometimes been referred to as the body's lymphatic filter, also plays a significant role both in immune surveillance and in the removal of old or damaged red blood cells. Located in the superior left abdomen, the spleen processes blood rather than lymph, cleansing pathogens and foreign matter by its heavy focus of white pulp and red pulp (Gonzalez et al., 2010). Immune response occurs in the white pulp, consisting of lymphocytes that react to blood-borne antigens. Furthermore, the spleen serves as a reservoir for various immune cells, e.g., T and B cells, which go to sites of infection in case of systemic challenge. The intricate interdependence of the spleen and the other lymphoid organs, such as lymph nodes, illustrates the integrated nature of the immune system, showing the need for an integrated knowledge of the organs in health and disease. The thymus, a specialized organ located in the thoracic cavity, plays a critical role in the development and maturation of T lymphocytes, which are essential components of the adaptive immune response (Gonzalez et al., 2010). There are different numbers of progenitor cells early in life that are migrating out of the bone marrow into the thymus, where they undergo strict selection processes to permit only self-tolerant, functional T cells to be exported into the circulation. This is particularly critical because disruption of T cell development can lead to lethal immunodeficiency or autoimmune disease. The thymus's unique function as the primary location of T cell development highlights the significance of the organ in the establishment of an effective immune defense mechanism. Knowledge of the regulation of thymic function not only improves our comprehension of immune system integrity but also has implications in the treatment approaches of immunological disorders (Figure 7.8).

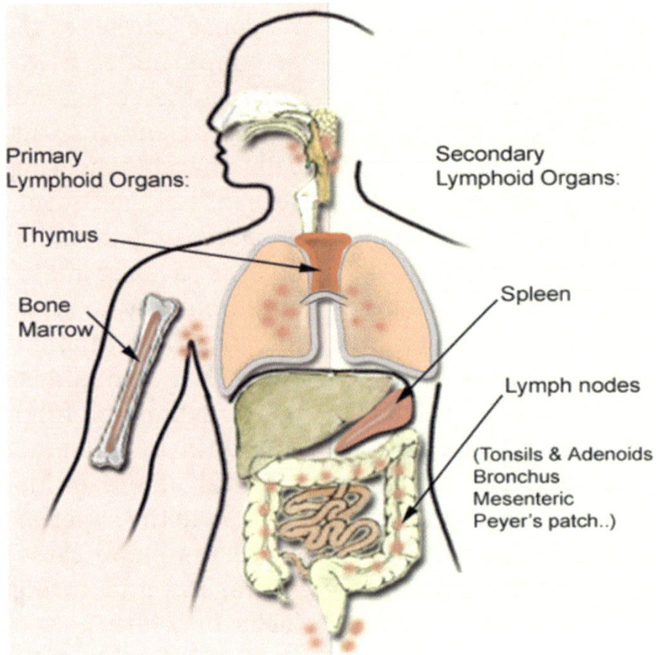

Figure 7.8. Key lymphatic organs: lymph nodes, spleen, and thymus.

Source: https://www.medicine.mcgill.ca/physio/vlab/immun/images/Lymph_org500.jpg.

7.3.3. Relationship Between Lymphatic and Circulatory Systems

The circulatory and lymphatic systems have a dependent relationship for the upkeep of homeostasis and normal immune function. The two systems work together to control fluid, transport nutrients, and assist in the removal of waste from the tissue. The circulatory system, made up primarily of veins and arteries, supplies oxygenated blood to various parts of the body and returns deoxygenated blood to the heart. Conversely, the lymphatic system collects excess interstitial fluid, proteins, and cellular debris, which are returned to the bloodstream. This subtle relationship is important, as deviations can lead to pathological conditions of edema or weakened immunity, further emphasizing the interdependence of these two vascular systems. The lymphatic system also plays a part in immune surveillance, communicating with lymphocytes and other immune cells to recognize and destroy infection. For instance, lymph nodes are gateways through which lymphatic fluid is filtered for foreign substances, enabling a rapid immune response. Interaction between the circulatory and lymphatic vessels is underscored by the signaling by cytokines and other messenger molecules. This interaction is also underscored in diseases, such as in obesity, where impaired lymphatic function has been implicated in increased cardiovascular risks. Explanation of these interactions is pivotal to the treatment of conditions that result from dysfunctional lymphatic or circulatory systems because it lays open potential avenues for therapeutic interventions, like perivascular adipose tissue (PVAT) interventions, which influence vascular contractility and hemodynamics (Pankova, 2024). Cancer cell metastasis through the lymphatics has been recently explained as well, which suggests an intricate interaction between lymphatics and vascular dynamics. For example, in esophageal squamous cell carcinoma, exosomal microRNAs have been shown to control tumor growth and lymphangiogenesis, revealing a novel mechanism by which cancer cells communicate with lymphatic endothelial cells. This not only captures the role of the lymphatic system in disease resistance but also its exploitation by disease states. The implications of such interactions can be substantial, with potential new therapeutic targets to interfere with these pathways in cancer treatment and to reduce lymphatic metastasis (Xiao et al., 2023). As a driving force, an interdisciplinary review of interactions between the circulatory and lymphatic systems is vital to advancing our understanding of vascular and lymphatic health and disease (Figure 7.9).

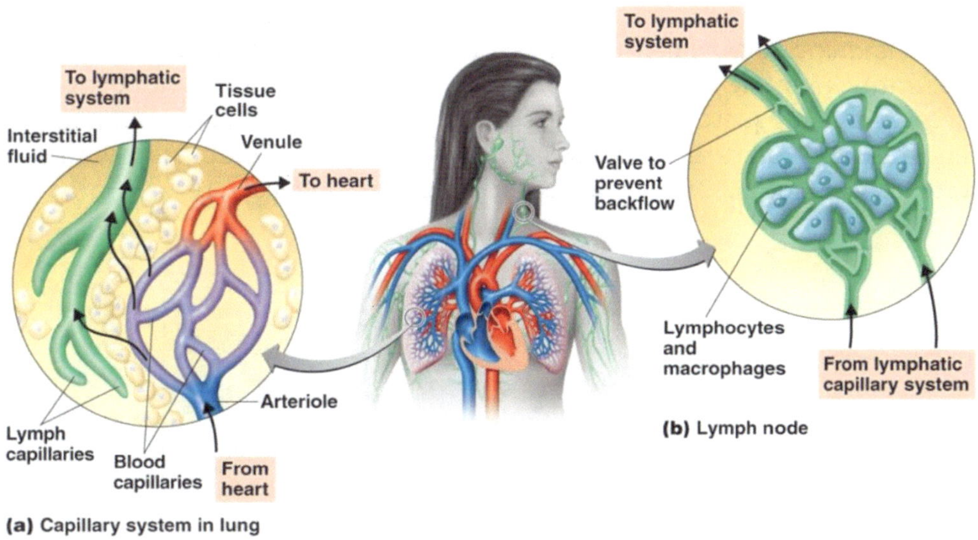

Figure 7.9. Relationship between the lymphatic and circulatory systems.

Source: https://image1.slideserve.com/2682115/cardiovascular-lymphatic-systems1-l.jpg.

7.4. Function of Lymphatic Tissue

Lymphoid tissue plays a critical role in maintaining homeostasis in the human body by facilitating fluid balance, immune responses, and dietary fat absorption. Through its role as a drainage system, lymphatic vessels resist the undue accumulation of interstitial fluid, and hence edema, and maintain the extracellular environment conducive to cellular function. Lymphoid tissue comprises lymph nodes, lymphatic vessels, and organized organs such as the spleen and thymus, all of which are involved in lymph filtration and the activation of immunocompetent cells. Embedded within each lymph node is lymphoid tissue having high densities of lymphocytes and other immune cells that monitor interstitial fluid, then react to infection or tumor cells. This interaction is essential to the initial recognition of infection and thus to successful immediate and adaptive immune responses. Lymphoid tissue plays an essential role in the intestinal absorption of fat-soluble vitamins and lipids. These are specialized structures known as lacteals, lymphatic capillaries located within the intestinal villi, which take up digested fats and deliver them to the lymphatic system. This pathway allows for efficient transport of glycerides and fatty acids into the bloodstream, circumventing initial hepatic metabolism. The role of lymphoid tissue in nutrient uptake underscores the coordinated interaction between the digestive and lymphatic systems and highlights how these tissues contribute to overall metabolic health. Furthermore, this role emphasizes the importance of the integrity of lymphatics, since compromise results in malabsorption syndromes, and all the associated nutritional deficiencies, which can spread throughout the body. The immune property of lymphoid tissue is also too important to be underestimated, acting as an immediate defense against infection. Lymphocytes, T cells, and B cells are produced and developed in lymphoid organs such as the bone marrow and thymus and are subsequently distributed throughout the circulatory system. Not only does lymphoid tissue support the maturation of immune cells, but it also enables their strategic localization within lymph nodes, where the cells encounter antigens and proliferate upon activation. This immune surveillance at the systemic level accentuates the lymphatic system's vital role in orchestrating immune responses in various states of physiology. Abnormalities in lymphatic tissue may result in inadequate immune responses, as observed in some immunodeficiency states, underscoring the need for further research into its complex relationship with the immune and vascular systems (Ding et al., 2017; Madsen et al., 2018) (Figure 7.10).

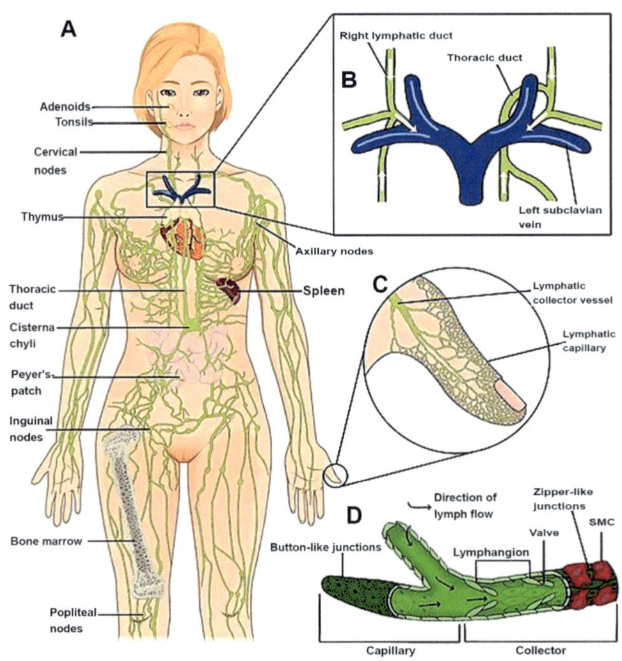

Figure 7.10. Function of lymphatic tissue.

Source: https://www.pharmacareers.in/wp-content/uploads/2024/06/lymphatic-system.jpg.

7.4.1. Role in Immune Response and Pathogen Filtration

The lymphatic and vascular systems are responsible for regulating immune processes and pathogen filtration. This interaction allows the body to achieve homeostasis and fight off infection. The vascular system, composed of veins, arteries, and capillaries, carries immune cells that are instrumental in immune response and surveillance. For instance, circulating lymphocytes infiltrate tissues, where they are likely to encounter pathogens. Parallel to this, the lymphatic system is used as a channel for lymph—a white blood cell-rich, protein- and waste product-enriched fluid that drains interstitial fluid from tissues in the body. In addition to aiding the filtration out of pathogens, this fluid also presents antigens to lymphoid tissue to enhance the adaptive immune response. Due to this constant interchange between vascular and lymphatic tissue, the body is able to successfully react against invading pathogens and maintain the internal environment in homeostasis. In the context of pathogen filtration, the lymphatic system possesses specialized features such as lymph nodes, serving as immunological checkpoints en route. Lymph nodes strain lymph fluid and hold pathogens in place so that immune cells, such as T cells and B cells, may be stimulated to orchestrate an optimal immune response. The lymph node structure is conducive to the interaction between antigen-presenting cells and lymphocytes, resulting in the production of an adaptive defense. This is much like the complex system of security, wherein lymph nodes serve as checkpoints that decide how the immune response should be mounted in the presence of pathogens. Furthermore, the vascular system's role in delivering and removing immune cells from these focal sites underscores the coordination of both systems in immune combat, thereby advancing our understanding of immune dynamics. Recent advances in biomedical science have given new insight into the potential for employing engineered tissue, such as organ-on-a-chip systems, to further investigate interactions of the vascular and lymphatic systems in immune response. These microfluidic devices simulate physiological conditions to enable closer examination of immune cell migration across tissues and response to infectious agents. They are important in the study of complex illnesses, including cancer, where immune evasion interactions and cancer cell filtration become critical. For example, nanomaterials are being investigated for cancer drugs delivered specifically to target sites in an effort to achieve maximal specificity and reduce toxicity, consistent with the lymphatic system's protective function in monitoring and controlling tumorigenic activity (Cheng et al., 2021). Understanding these interactions not only enhances knowledge in immune responses but also provides avenues for new therapeutic options in disease treatment that impacts the vascular and lymphatic tissues (Ingber, 2022) (Figure 7.11).

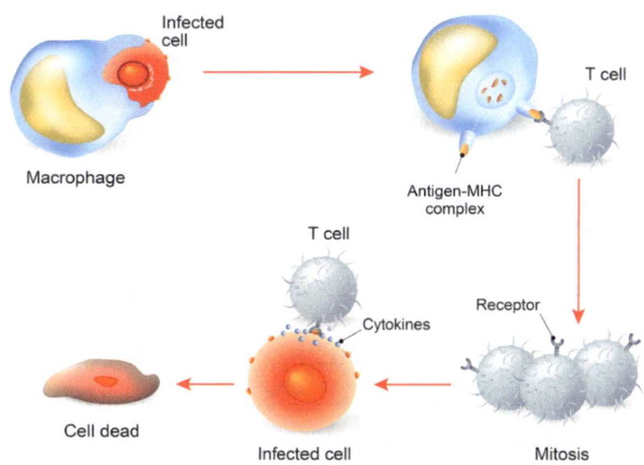

Figure 7.11. Role in immune response and pathogen filtration.

Source: https://www.immuneresponse.org/wp-content/uploads/2016/08/bigstock-127354466.jpg.

7.4.2. Maintenance of Fluid Balance in Tissues

Maintenance of tissue fluid balance is essentially linked to the process of the vascular and lymphatic systems. The vascular system, through a network of blood vessels, has the primary role of supplying oxygen and nutrients and eliminating waste products. This dynamic exchange relies on processes such as hydrostatic and osmotic pressures that govern the flow of fluids between blood and the surrounding interstitial tissue. By regulating these pressures, the vascular system sees to it that tissues are supplied with fluid to their needs for metabolic functions without permitting an overload of fluid that can lead to edema, a condition of swelling caused by fluid accumulation. Appreciation of these intricacies provides us with important insights into the physiological balance required for tissue health and function in a variety of biological contexts. At least as important as fluid balance is the lymphatic system, which helps to assist the vascular network by controlling interstitial fluid and returning excess fluid to the circulation.

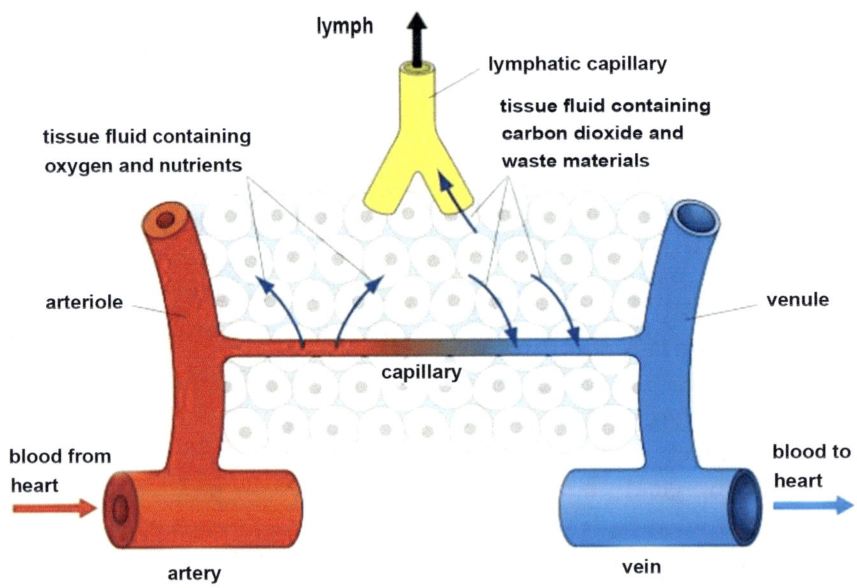

Figure 7.12. Maintenance of fluid balance in tissues.

Source: https://quizizz.com/_media/quizzes/7f059572-825f-42a1-9fcc-2c90603c9fc1.

Lymph vessels transport lymph, a fluid responsible for immune response and removal of waste, and thus tissue homeostasis. The capacity of lymphatic networks to regulate fluid flow is not static, but instead operates actively in reaction to physiological alterations, such as inflammation or infection, by modulating the permeability of the lymphatic vessels. Such sensitivity is particularly vital during immune responses because lymphatics deliver immune cells to sites of infection and return excess interstitial fluid to the circulation. These interactions highlight the lymphatic system's critical role in sustaining not only fluid homeostasis, but also global immune surveillance, and suggest its involvement in more generalized physiological processes. Recent research illuminates the intricate interaction between lymphatic function and divergent pathophysiological states, particularly during inflammation and cancer. The lymphatic system has also emerged as an essential regulator of immune modulation, influencing the progression and resolution of inflammatory diseases. For example, in the context of chronic inflammation, lymphatic dysfunction can trap immune mediators and potentiate local tissue responses. Moreover, the role of lymphatics in tumor metastasis underscores their importance in fluid balance; they offer openings for the spread of cancer cells and serve as routes for the migration of immune cells. This dual role places the lymphatic system at center stage in tissue homeostasis under health and disease, revealing broader implications for therapeutic strategies towards lymphatic and vascular function (Bell et al., 2012; Lund, A., & Swartz, M., 2018) (Figure 7.12).

7.4.3. Absorption of Dietary Fats Through Lacteals

The ingestion of dietary lipids by lacteals is a crucial function in the lymphatic and vascular system, greatly contributing to nutrient transport and immune defense of the gut. Lacteals are specialized lymph capillary vessels in the villi of the small intestine and are a critical factor in lipid absorption. These are the vessels through which the entry of large lipid molecules, such as chylomicrons, which are too large to enter the blood capillaries directly, is facilitated. Dietary lipids are instead emulsified and absorbed by enterocytes, which package them into chylomicrons and transport them in lacteals. This unique pathway is important for efficient lipid absorption and underscores the integration of the lymphatic system with digestive processes, which is fundamental for maintaining metabolic homeostasis in the organism. Apart from their function in the absorption of fats, lacteals are also very important in contributing to immune function in the gut. They not only transport absorbed lipids, but they are also a vehicle for immune cells and molecules, and hence fortify the local immune protection against invading pathogens via the gut. Lacteals can take up not just dietary fats but also microbial origin antigens, and so facilitate interaction between dietary intake and immune response. The lymph content of these vessels can be influenced by a variety of factors, including diet and the health status of intestinal microbiota. The new study has emphasized the significance of lacteal-microbiota interaction with a healthy microbiome, said to regulate lacteal function and enhance lipid absorption, once more emphasizing their dual role as absorptive and immune structures in the intestinal microenvironment (Marcozzi et al., 2021). Molecular processes governing lacteal function include continuous regeneration, which is necessary for optimal fat absorption. Research has indicated that the Notch signaling pathway is vital for preserving the structural and functional integrity of lacteals. Specifically, lacteal expression of the Notch ligand delta-like 4 (DLL4) is essential for regenerative capacity, enabling these vessels to withstand the mechanical stress imposed by constant dietary lipid intake. Genetic mutations that downregulate DLL4 expression induce regression of lacteals, resulting in impaired uptake of dietary fats and suggesting that a unique mechanism of slow lymphatic regeneration must exist in the gastrointestinal context (Barker et al., 2015). Such an understanding of lacteal biology serves to underscore the complexity of the lymphatic system, illustrating how a specialized response to dietary demand is critical to both nutrient uptake and immune function.

7.5. Pathologies of Vascular Tissue

The vascular tissue pathologies are a significant field of study, particularly for common diseases such as cardiovascular diseases. Obesity has been a significant determining factor for such diseases and has emerged as a major risk factor for most cardiovascular diseases. With increasing cases of obesity across the globe, it becomes crucial to learn about the direct role played by obesity on vascular tissues. Recent studies have highlighted the perivascular adipose tissue (PVAT) modulatory influence on vascular contractile function. This tissue typically releases anti-contractile signals for the maintenance of vascular homeostasis, but the absence of such protective functions in obese patients leads to enhanced vasoconstriction. Therefore, the elucidation of interactions between PVAT and vascular function can unveil opportunities for new therapeutic interventions on the prevention of obesity-induced vascular disturbances (Pankova, 2024). No less important in vascular pathology debates is the complex interaction between the nervous system and vascular and lymphatic tissues, particularly with respect to their roles in skeletal physiology. Type H blood vessels, which are characterized by specific markers, are the ones that are responsible for combining osteogenesis with angiogenesis and thereby provide proper delivery of nutrients and removal of waste products in bone and joint tissues. Deficiency in the vascular networks can lead to a cascade of pathological processes, including ischemia and arthritis. Recent research has elucidated the significance of lymphatic vessels in even the skeletal system, demonstrating their function to transport immune cells and tissue repair through lymphangiocrine signaling. This growing recognition of lymphatic circulation underscores the new perspective that such networks are key to comprehending skeletal homeostasis and disease (Huang et al., 2024). Moreover, the interaction between vascular and lymphatic tissues plays a crucial role in regulating inflammatory processes that often underlie most diseases. Failure to regulate the two systems will lead to chronic inflammation, which further accelerates the progression of diseases such as rheumatoid arthritis. Analyses of the structural and functional dynamics of vascular networks assist scientists in determining the mechanisms of inflammation and their subsequent effects on tissue health. Pathologic alterations in these networks highlight their paramount roles in conditions like ischemia, which can result from dysfunctional blood flow and repair processes. As interactions are increasingly understood, this may enable the development of therapies specifically designed to restore vascular integrity and lymphatic function, offering new hope for successful disease management and improved overall vascular health (Huang et al., 2024; Pankova, 2024) (Figure 7.13).

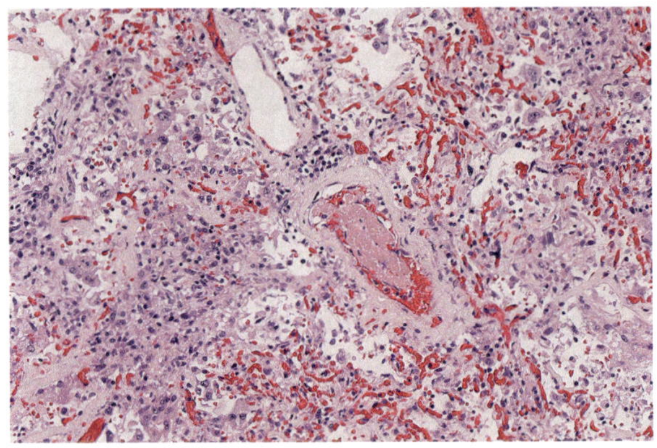

Figure 7.13. Pathologies of vascular tissue.

Source: https://external-content.duckduckgo.com/iu/?u=https%3A%2F%2Fwww.ccjm.org%2Fcontent%2Fccjom%2Fearly%2F2020%2F09%2F18%2Fccjm.87a.ccc063%2FF2.large.jpg%3Fdownload%3Dtrue&f=1&nofb=1&ipt=9e4db9e42344ee75f20643760005f9d680b87db7897b5d26f136576affb450a5.

7.5.1. Common Vascular Diseases: Atherosclerosis and Hypertension

Atherosclerosis, a common vascular disease, is the accumulation of lipids, inflammatory cells, and fibrous tissue in the walls of arteries and is the cause of plaque formation. This chronic disease significantly narrows down the arteries, leading to reduced blood flow and ultimately resulting in severe cardiovascular events such as myocardial infarctions and strokes. The pathophysiologic progression of atherosclerosis is complex and involves endothelial injury, inflammation, and smooth muscle cell proliferation. The pathologic impact of atherosclerosis on vascular tissue architecture is significant, as it disrupts normal function and leads to arterial wall hardening, a contributing factor to the progression of hypertension, another prevalent vascular disease. Thus, understanding the interaction of atherosclerosis with other vascular conditions is critical to creating effective treatment strategies to reduce their impact on public health. Unnaturally elevated blood pressure is referred to as hypertension, and it is a significant risk factor for the development of atherosclerosis and other cardiovascular diseases. The relationship between hypertension and vascular health is a bidirectional one; while hypertension can lead to vascular remodeling and increased arterial stiffness, atherosclerosis will also further elevate blood pressure. Systemic blood pressure increases the mechanical load on the vascular endothelium, thereby activating inflammation and further weakening arterial structure. The resulting arterial injury forms a rich substrate for plaque growth, creating a vicious cycle in which each condition exacerbates the other. Furthermore, obesity, lifestyle, and diet are all major contributors to the causes and exacerbation of hypertension, and therefore lifestyle changes are imperative to managing this disorder and, more generally, the broader category of vascular disease.

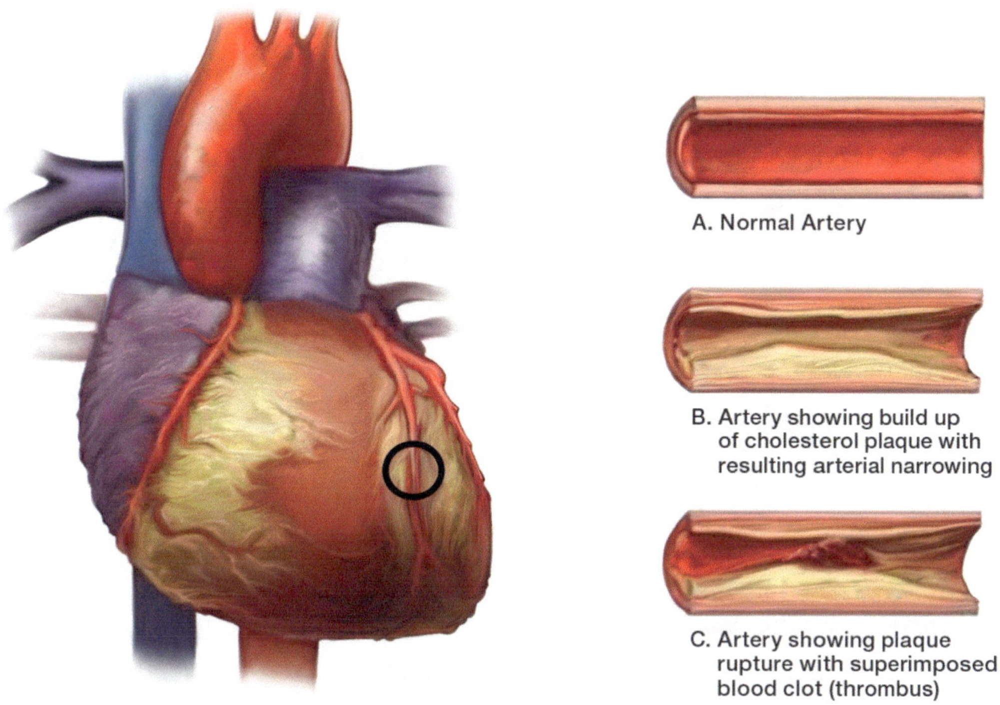

Figure 7.14. Common vascular diseases: atherosclerosis and hypertension.

Source: https://www.melbourneheartcare.com.au/wp-content/uploads/2011/07/MEL0011-Illustration-Captions4.jpg.

More recent research into the molecular control of these vascular diseases has emphasized the pivotal position of matrix metalloproteinases (MMPs) and tissue inhibitors of metalloproteinases (TIMPs). MMPs, with their pivotal function in extracellular matrix remodeling, are significant in the structural remodeling of atherosclerotic plaques. MMP dysregulation can lead to excessive degradation of the extracellular matrix, destabilizing the stability of arterial plaques and adding to the risk of thrombosis (Cabral-Pacheco et al., 2020). Furthermore, the balance between MMPs and TIMPs is crucial because a state of imbalance leads to both the development of atherosclerosis and the worsening of hypertension, driven by intensified vascular remodeling and inflammation. By intervening in these molecular pathways with pharmacological treatment, scientists seek to develop new therapies that can reverse or prevent the deleterious effects of these diseases, thereby improving the prognosis of patients with common vascular diseases (Lyon et al., 2022) (Figure 7.14).

7.5.2. Impact of Lifestyle Factors on Vascular Health

The intricate relationship between lifestyle and vascular health cannot be overstated, as many lifestyle behaviors directly affect vascular function and overall circulatory health. Physical inactivity is one of the leading causes of the development of vascular disease, and inactivity raises the risk for obesity, hypertension, and dyslipidemia.

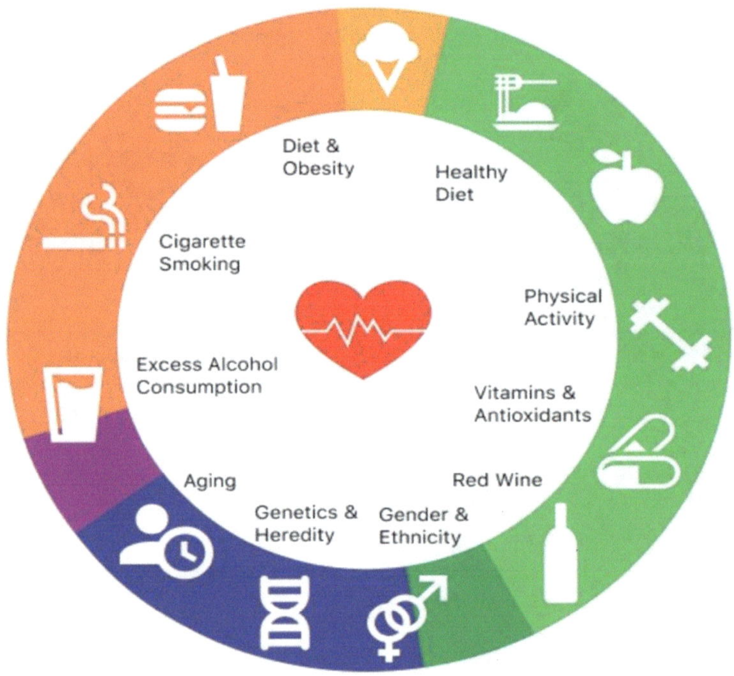

Figure 7.15. Impact of lifestyle factors on vascular health.

Source: https://www.drugwatch.com/wp-content/uploads/Heart-Health-Risk-Factors-640x0-c-default.jpg.

Exercise regularly enhances endothelial function and arterial compliance, both of which are essential for vascular health. Moreover, lifestyle factors such as an unhealthy diet high in saturated fat, sugar, and processed foods exacerbate these risks. As with a shift in dietary habits, awareness of the long-term vascular implications, particularly among young individuals, becomes increasingly important. With this knowledge, public health initiatives can effectively address vascular disease prevention by educating people about healthier lifestyle choices and encouraging greater physical activity in communities. Vascular health can also be affected by aging changes, as the aging process affects the structure and function of the vascular and lymphatic system. Chronic oedema (CO) and lymphoedema (LO) are the perfect examples of how age-related disorders worsen vascular health. Vascular compromise, along with low healing rates and compromised cardiovascular function, often demands individualized management strategies (Baumann et al., 2018). Such methods tend to emphasize important factors such as skin care, exercise, and compression therapy. Complications arising from age can compromise the effectiveness of such interventions, underscoring the delicate balance between lifestyle factors and aging. Hence, recognition of the role of such interactions is highly significant for the design of effective treatment regimens and for ensuring appropriate care for older patients to improve their vascular health outcomes. In addition, incorporating physiotherapy into lifestyle management is a viable strategy for managing peripheral vascular diseases. Research suggests that a systematic approach to exercise programs based on a person's condition has the ability to influence rehabilitation and overall vascular function (Cieślar et al., 2020). Physiotherapy not only benefits circulation but also helps improve mobility and optimizes quality of life for patients with vascular dysfunction. Since peripheral vascular disease continues to be a significant health issue, maintaining regular exercise and the incorporation of physiotherapeutic interventions will continue to be pivotal in reversing risks from such conditions. In establishing a foundation for understanding how lifestyle behaviors, such as exercise, influence vascular health, healthcare professionals can encourage patients to make informed choices that benefit their health and longevity (Figure 7.15).

7.5.3. Diagnostic Methods for Vascular Conditions

The assessment of vascular diseases relies heavily on a range of diagnostic imaging modalities that provide information about the underlying disease. Non-invasive imaging techniques such as ultrasonography have also gained a greater share based on their ability to visualize blood flow and vascular morphology in real-time. Doppler ultrasound is especially well adapted to evaluate blood flow dynamics and detect abnormalities such as stenosis or occlusions within the vascular bed. In addition, magnetic resonance angiography (MRA) delineates blood vessels better without the use of ionizing radiation and thus is suitable for repeated examination of patients. These modalities not only aid diagnosis but also disease monitoring and therapeutic response, enabling clinicians to make informed decisions based on evidence from sound data. Histological analysis is another important component in the diagnostic scheme for vascular disease. Techniques such as immunohistochemistry can detect biomarkers associated with vascular pathology. For instance, CLEVER-1, or common lymphatic endothelial and vascular endothelial receptor-1, can be indicative of metastatic activity in conditions such as breast cancer. Here, staining experiments reveal distinct patterns of CLEVER-1 distribution in blood and lymphatic vessels, suggesting that it may mediate tumor cell spread (Ammar et al., 2011). Moreover, immune cell infiltration by dendritic cells and macrophages can provide details on the inflammatory status of the vascular tissue, which again can guide therapeutic strategies. Thus, histological techniques not only support diagnosis but also provide greater insight into complex interactions within the vasculature. Recent technological advancements have revolutionized the evaluation of vascular conditions in the past few years. Among these, molecular imaging has been a powerful diagnostic tool for the detection of early pathological changes in vascular tissue.

Techniques such as positron emission tomography (PET) enable imaging of cellular metabolism, identifying subtle changes that may precede clinical manifestations. Furthermore, the pairing of artificial intelligence with imaging technology has shown the promise of improving diagnostic precision and productivity by offering automated interpretation of imaging results. Such innovation demarcates the evolving nature of diagnostic methods towards vascular diseases. With research advancing, tremendous potential exists for these technologies to make a difference in patient outcomes by ensuring earlier diagnosis and more precise monitoring of vascular and lymphatic tissue disorders (Assaad et al., 2018) (Figure 7.16).

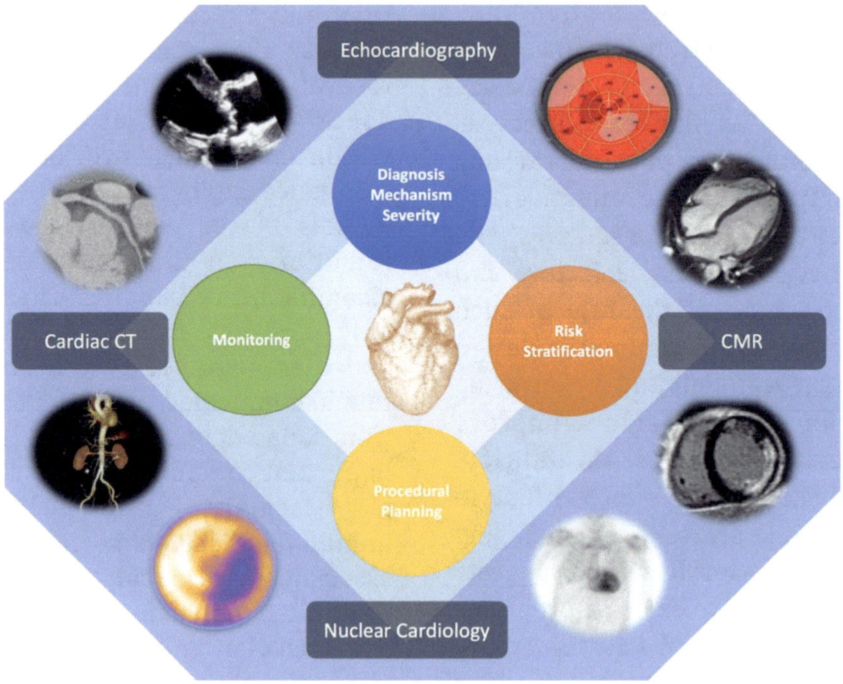

Figure 7.16. Diagnostic methods for vascular conditions.

Source: https://heart.bmj.com/content/heartjnl/108/21/e7/F1.large.jpg.

7.6. Pathologies of Lymphatic Tissue

Lymphatic tissue pathologies significantly impact many of the body's physiological processes and cause a range of diseases. Lymphangiogenesis, or the formation of new lymphatic vessels, is particularly significant because it plays a crucial role in both health and disease. Dysregulation of this process contributes to metastatic spread, graft rejection, and inflammatory diseases. It is presented in recent research that toluquinol, a molecule that has potent inhibitory effects on proliferation and migration of lymphatic endothelial cells, shows pharmacological potential. Molecule inhibition might lead to the inhibition of lymphatic tissue hyperplasia, ultimately impacting disease process progress and development related to pathological lymphatic function (Blacher et al., 2016). Through research on lymphatic pathologies, there is also the possibility of site-specific therapeutics that might alleviate the workload imposed upon such diseases as lymphedema and lymphatic malignancies. The therapeutic potential for targeting lymphatic pathologies is well-supported. In particular, the use of toluquinol has been shown to cause LEC apoptosis and block key signals in lymphangiogenesis, which include VEGF-C and VEGFR-3. This mechanism of action suggests a multi-dimensional approach to reversing the disease-causative effects of pathological lymphatic growth, reinforcing the notion that new treatments would significantly influence disease mechanisms. Additionally, the mechanisms by which toluquinol operates, such as the inhibition of Akt and ERK1/2 pathway activation, offer new avenues for exploring the molecular origin of lymphatic disease. Through exploration of these possibilities, investigators are able to prospectively identify additional targets for therapeutic intervention, setting the stage for future advances in the therapy for lymphatic disease (Blacher et al., 2016). Furthermore, understanding the nature of lymphatic dysfunction allows for the best possible clinical management of those disorders. For instance, pulmonary edema—a disorder related to increased pulmonary capillary permeability—may have etiologies rooted in lymphatic pathology. The identification of early signs of lymphatic failure or dysfunction may be a spur to enhanced diagnostic care and prevention in healthcare. Furthermore, it is worth exploring elementary diagnostic techniques and devices for the early diagnosis of lymphatic-related diseases. Fluid imaging and analysis could augment the sensitivity and specificity of diagnoses, enabling healthcare professionals to discriminate among various etiologies of edema. Ultimately, incorporating lymphatic tissue examination into overall vascular evaluations may enhance our ability to treat numerous diseases and improve outcomes for patients across many medical specialties (Figure 7.17).

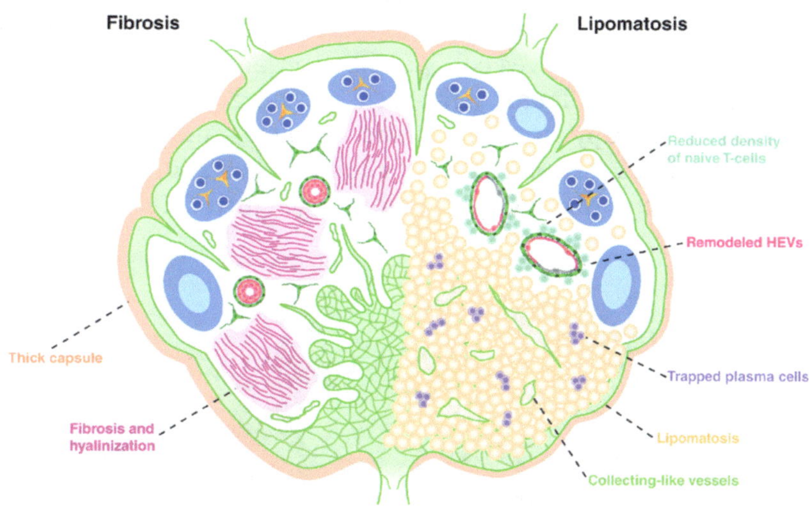

Figure 7.17. Pathologies of lymphatic tissue.

Source: https://www.researchgate.net/publication/370339264/figure/fig2/AS:11431281154761270@1683010253117/Aging-pathologies-of-the-human-lymph-node-LN-The-2-main-aging-pathologies-of-the-human.png.

7.6.1. Lymphedema and Its Causes

Lymphedema is a condition of abnormal retention of lymphatic fluid within the body tissues, which can be clinically troublesome, affecting mobility and quality of life. It is an acquired condition due to multiple etiologies, which can be broadly classified as primary and secondary lymphedema. Primary lymphedema develops due to congenital maldevelopment or genetic predisposition that influences the formation of the lymphatic vessels, resulting in inadequate lymph drainage. Secondary lymphedema is even more prevalent and occurs as a consequence of extrinsic causes, such as surgery, infection, or trauma, that inhibit the functioning of the lymph systems. Identifying these causes is critical, as it provides a basis for effective management and intervention to correct fluid accumulation and reinstitute lymphatic flow. The most common cause of secondary lymphedema is surgical complications, particularly after oncologic operations or lymphatic dissections. Impaired lymphatic drainage pathways from the excision of lymph nodes during surgery, such as mastectomy for breast cancer, result in lymphedema. The disruption of lymphatic drainage pathways is characterized by interstitial fluid overload, resulting not only in swelling but also changes in tissue content and metabolic derangement. New diagnostic techniques, such as bioimpedance spectroscopy (BIS), have been shown to accurately assess the severity of lymphedema by quantifying fluid distribution and composition within the affected limbs. Through this technology, healthcare providers are in a position to tailor treatment protocols, enabling early interventions against future complications of lymphedema, according to new evidence of the benefits of early diagnosis and treatment (Cavezzi et al., 2024). Moreover, the management of lymphedema is now challenged by regenerative medicine, particularly by the identification of adipose-derived stem cells (ADSCs). Research has proven that transplantation of ADSC can be very effective in minimizing lymphedema by triggering proliferation of lymphatic endothelial cells and by initiating new lymphatic vessels through mechanisms like intussusceptive lymphangiogenesis. This new approach not only alleviates the symptomatology of lymphedema but also its etiology by triggering lymphatic regeneration. Histological analyses have shown that treatment with ADSCs improves collagen fiber organization and reduces fibrosis, thereby restoring functional capacity in the affected lymphatic system. Such promising findings underscore the need to include cellular therapy in comprehensive management protocols for patients with lymphedema (Kikuchi et al., 2022). Exploration of such therapies is the key to more effective and sustainable methods of managing this complex disorder (Figure 7.18).

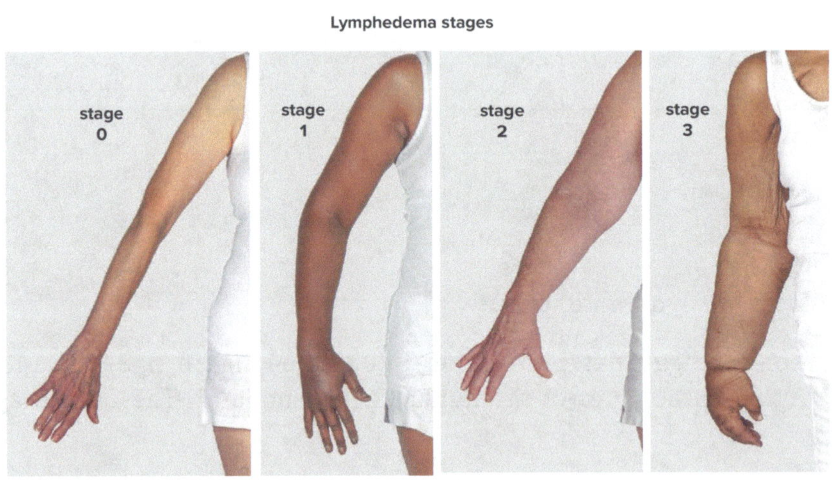

Figure 7.18. Lymphedema and its causes.

Source: https://www.blessinghealth.org/sites/default/files/2023-09/Lymphedema%20stages%20pic.jpg.

7.6.2. Lymphoma and Other Lymphatic Cancers

Lymphomas are a complex group of hematologic neoplasms originating from lymphoid tissue and are representative of the intricate interactions between immunity and the pathogenesis of malignancy. Predominantly made up of the proliferation of lymphocytes, which can further be divided into Hodgkin and non-Hodgkin lymphoma, these neoplasms are representative of the central role played by lymphoid tissues in both immune responses and malignancy. The incidence and prevalence of lymphomas globally have increased, and thus, it is essential to unravel their underlying mechanisms. Recent data from genomic studies indicate that specific molecular alterations are frequently the root cause of such neoplasms, thereby enabling targeted treatment. By applying next-generation sequencing, researchers can identify oncogenic mutations in non-malignant disease entities, suggesting potential molecular similarity across heterogeneous diseases (Adashek et al., 2020). Such an understanding is able to re-model therapeutic strategies and enhance predictive modeling for lymphoma prognosis. Lymphatic cancers' interaction with other cancers also contributes to the clinical scenario complexity, especially with respect to co-morbidities such as glomerulonephritis. Reports indicate that some glomerular disorders are associated with increased frequencies of non-Hodgkin lymphoma, suggesting a correlation between immune dysregulation and tumorigenesis (Birkeland et al., 2003). This correlating finding infers a two-pronged possible pathway: one that chronic inflammation leads to secondary malignancies, and the other where occult neoplasms cause inflammatory mechanisms that lead to renal morbidities. These findings are sufficiently persuasive to warrant close patient monitoring given the broad-ranging implications of treatment regimens. Since lymphatic cancers are heavily influenced by immune system dynamics, understanding the dynamics underlying their interaction with other diseases is critical to the development of integrative care plans and the optimization of patient outcomes. The therapeutic revolution over the last decade has transformed lymphatic cancer care paradigms through the development of targeted and immunotherapies. These emerging treatments exploit growing knowledge of the molecular biology of lymphomas and their interactions within lymphatic tissues. For instance, the development of monoclonal antibodies has enabled more effective targeting of cancerous lymphocytes while sparing collateral damage to non-cancerous cells. As noted, genetic alterations in lymphomas sometimes mirror those in underlying benign disease states; thus, established drugs are repurposed to treat non-cancerous diseases (Adashek et al., 2020). This therapeutic repositioning of drugs as a strategic maneuver not only broadens treatment choice against lymphatic cancer but also highlights the necessity of integrative models of treatment that account for the many interlocking relationships among pathological states. Consequently, the evolution of targeted therapies continues to open up the promise of personalized treatment, paving the way for fundamental breakthroughs in patient prognosis.

7.6.3. Infections Affecting Lymphatic Tissue, Such as Lymphangitis

Infections involving lymph tissue can lead to severe health complications, with the most significant one being lymphangitis. It results from inflammation of lymphatic vessels, typically caused by bacterial infections. The ensuing edema and pain can compromise lymphatic drainage and lead to further complications like chronic lymphoedema and advancing skin changes. The primary cause of lymphangitis is generally a skin wound through which bacteria enter, thereby perpetuating the inflammatory cycle. Interestingly, recurrent adenolymphangitis attacks, a concomitant disorder, may progress to severe forms such as elephantiasis if left untreated. Early treatment of these infections is essential to reduce their long-term impact on patient morbidity and overall quality of life because the impact is not only physically disabling but also socially stigmatizing (Rajasekaran, 2016). The treatment of lymphangitis and associated infections is complex and involves a multimodal intervention. Physical treatment protocols like manual lymph drainage and compression modalities have been inconsistently effective. While other studies highlight the benefits of these interventions towards volume reduction in the limb and patient comfort improvement, outcomes are usually inconclusive due to methodological errors. Design weaknesses and the small sample size of existing randomized trials limit knowledge regarding the best methods for managing lymphatic infection, such as lymphangitis. Adherence of patients to treatment protocols and also the psychological burden of living with chronic lymphoedema make the outcome of treatment difficult. As a result, concentrated research is necessary to develop evidence-based guidelines for efficient management practice (Ahmed et al., 2008). In addition to the therapeutic challenge of lymphangitis, sociocultural issues are significant in patient outcomes and management. Lymphatic infection patients are not only exposed to physical misery but also socially isolated and economically disadvantaged. Diseases such as lymphoedema and complications from such diseases can affect the capacity of individuals to work, interact socially, or carry out normal activities, leading to feelings of loneliness and distress. Healthcare professionals must recognize these psychosocial determinants and implement comprehensive care approaches that address both the medical and emotional needs of involved individuals. Greater awareness and targeted interventions are needed to improve the quality of life for patients with lymphatic tissue infection (Rajasekaran, 2016).

SUMMARY

In the intricate vascular and lymphatic tissues, a notable role is that of vascular endothelial cells in maintaining blood circulation homeostasis. These cells are a selective barrier that regulates the exchange of substances between the blood and surrounding tissues and thus has a profound impact on disease and health. Key points highlight the role of these cells in the inflammatory process, whereby their activity can regulate leukocyte trafficking and edema formation. The physiological behavior of these endothelial cells is the key to therapeutic intervention in disorders characterized by vascular dysfunction, e.g., chronic myeloid leukaemia (CML). The interconnection between the vascular system and the disease processes underscores the need for continued research into endothelial biology as it could yield significant intervention and treatment opportunities (Lyon et al., 2022). Another consideration in the analysis of vascular and lymphatic tissues is the role of the lymphatic system in immune protection and fluid regulation. This process is essential to the transport of lymph, which returns immune cells, waste products, and excess interstitial fluid to the blood. The lymphatic vessels, with their unique structure and permeability properties, can facilitate these processes effectively. Key points of importance note ways in which diseases such as pulmonary hypertension can prevent these processes and lead to severe health consequences. The novel guidelines for the management of pulmonary hypertension provide critical frameworks that incorporate such disruptions while attempting to improve patient outcomes. The insights gained from the interplay between lymphatic health and systemic disease highlight the complexity and necessity of a functioning lymphatic system, thereby shifting the debate on targeted therapies that account for these issues (Humbert et al., 2022). Lastly, the introduction of vascular and lymphatic analysis into the clinical environment involves the recognition of the multifaceted interaction between the two systems during disease conditions. Studies demonstrate the interdependence of the integrity of the vascular system and the function of the lymphatic system, where dysfunction of one would most often result in implications for the other. Comprehensive reviews of ongoing clinical trials suggest some avenues for the development of therapies intended to enhance the function of these systems. Interdisciplinary studies that integrate findings from vascular biology, immunology, and cardiology are increasingly important for designing holistic treatment protocols. As more studies are conducted, personalized medicine and targeted therapies will be able to elucidate new pathways in disease treatment that target both vascular and lymphatic tissues. This continuous debate is essential in designing effective healthcare strategies to address the challenges posed by these intricate biological systems.

A LOOK TO THE FUTURE:

REGULATE BLOOD PRESSURE:

The regulation of blood pressure is a foundational element of cardiovascular physiology and systemic homeostasis, reflecting the body's ability to adjust to both internal demands and external challenges. Blood pressure—the force exerted by circulating blood against the walls of blood vessels—is essential for ensuring that oxygen, nutrients, and hormones are delivered to tissues while waste products are efficiently removed. Maintaining this pressure within a relatively narrow range is vital: too low, and critical organs may be under-perfused; too high, and blood vessels and the heart are subjected to damaging stress. As a result, the human body has evolved multiple overlapping mechanisms that operate across different timescales to sustain blood pressure stability and meet changing physiological needs. At the most immediate level, neural reflexes provide short-term adjustments that respond within seconds to minutes. Central to this rapid response is the baroreceptor reflex, a negative-feedback mechanism in which stretch-sensitive receptors located in the carotid sinuses and aortic arch detect changes in arterial pressure. When blood pressure rises, these baroreceptors increase their firing rate and signal the cardiovascular control centers in the brainstem, leading to reduced heart rate, decreased cardiac contractility, and vasodilation—all of which lower blood pressure. Conversely, when pressure falls, decreased baroreceptor firing triggers increased sympathetic outflow to raise heart rate and constrict blood vessels.

Beyond rapid neural control, hormonal systems regulate blood pressure over intermediate and long-term periods. A key example is the renin-angiotensin-aldosterone system (RAAS), which is activated when renal perfusion pressure drops or when sodium levels are low. The kidneys release renin, initiating a cascade that produces angiotensin II—a potent vasoconstrictor that increases vascular resistance—and stimulates aldosterone secretion, promoting renal sodium and water retention. Together, this increases blood volume and sustained arterial pressure. The kidneys themselves play a crucial role in long-term blood pressure control by adjusting fluid balance and blood volume. Through modulation of sodium and water excretion, the renal system influences the volume of circulating blood; increased retention raises blood pressure, while increased excretion lowers it. This balance is central to long-term hemodynamic stability and interacts with hormonal regulators such as antidiuretic hormone and atrial natriuretic peptide.

Moreover, vascular adjustments through endothelial-derived factors like nitric oxide and endothelin help fine-tune resistance within the arterial network. Vasodilation decreases peripheral resistance and reduces pressure, while vasoconstriction increases resistance and raises it as needed.

Together, these systems—neural reflexes, hormonal feedback loops, renal fluid regulation, and vascular tone modulation—work in concert to maintain blood pressure within optimal bounds, safeguarding tissue perfusion and preserving cardiovascular health.

REFERENCES

1. Verrienti, A., Tallini, G., Colato, C., Boichard, A., Checquolo, S., Pecce, V., Sponziello, M., Rosignolo, F., De Biase, D., Rhoden, K., Casadei, G. P., Russo, D., Visani, M., Acquaviva, G., Ferdeghini, M., Filetti, S., & Durante, C. (2016). RET mutation and increased angiogenesis in medullary thyroid carcinomas. *Endocrine Related Cancer, 23*(8), 665–676. https://doi.org/10.1530/erc-16-0132Adashek, J. J., Kato, S., Kurzrock, R., Lippman, S. M., et al. (2020). The paradox of cancer genes in non-malignant conditions: Implications for precision medicine. https://core.ac.uk/download/323064613.pdf (accessed on 6th August 2025).
2. Ahmed, S., Andersen, J., Badger, C., Bergan, J., Bertelli, M., Carroll, C., et al. (2008). Physical therapies for reducing and controlling lymphoedema of the limbs. https://core.ac.uk/download/68433.pdf (accessed on 6th August 2025).
3. Ammar, A., Ellis, I. O., Martin, S. G., Mohammed, R. A., et al. (2011). Lymphatic expression of CLEVER-1 in breast cancer and its relationship with lymph node metastasis. https://core.ac.uk/download/161514767.pdf (accessed on 6th August 2025).
4. Assaad, S., Friedman, M. B., Kratzert, W. B., Perrino, A. C., et al. (2018). Assessment of pulmonary edema: Principles and practice. https://core.ac.uk/download/145643671.pdf (accessed on 6th August 2025).
5. Bala, N., Kaur, K., Kullar, J. S., & Ipshita. (2024). Morphological and morphometric variations of spleen: A cadaveric study in North Indian population. *Asian Journal of Pharmaceutical and Clinical Research*. https://www.semanticscholar.org/paper/3c5625238152c1ca30eb58d492e7fc0e2774a336 (accessed on 6th August 2025).
6. Barker, B., Cansaran Saygili Demir, C., Cisarovsky, C., Radtke, F., Humphrey, J., Bernier-Latmani, J., et al. (2015). DLL4 promotes continuous adult intestinal lacteal regeneration and dietary fat transport. https://core.ac.uk/download/77158378.pdf (accessed on 6th August 2025).
7. Baumann, F., British Dermatological Nursing Group, Cooper, G., Davies, A., Farage, M. A., Ferrari, A. U., James, S., et al. (2018). Chronic oedema and the older person: The effects of ageing upon treatment outcomes. https://core.ac.uk/download/196185642.pdf (accessed on 6th August 2025).
8. Bell, C. G., Preziosi, L., & Scianna, M. (2012). A review of mathematical models for the formation of vascular networks. https://core.ac.uk/download/pdf/9695546.pdf (accessed on 6th August 2025).
9. Bianchi, A., Painter, K. J., & Sherratt, J. A. (2015). A mathematical model for lymphangiogenesis in normal and diabetic wounds. http://arxiv.org/abs/1501.00421 (accessed on 6th August 2025).
10. Birkeland, S. A., & Storm, H. H. (2003). Glomerulonephritis and malignancy: A population-based analysis. https://core.ac.uk/download/pdf/81169032.pdf (accessed on 6th August 2025).
11. Blacher, S., García-Caballero, M., Medina, M. Á., Noël, A., et al. (2016). Novel application assigned to toluquinol: Inhibition of lymphangiogenesis by interfering with VEGF-C/VEGFR-3 signalling pathway. https://core.ac.uk/download/214834432.pdf (accessed on 6th August 2025).
12. Butz, S., Dierkes, C., Drees, D., Goerge, T., et al. (2017). VIPAR, a quantitative approach to 3D histopathology applied to lymphatic malformations. https://core.ac.uk/download/96566811.pdf (accessed on 6th August 2025).

13. Cabral-Pacheco, G. A., Garza-Veloz, I., Castruita-De la Rosa, C., Ramirez-Acuña, J. M., Perez-Romero, B. A., Guerrero-Rodriguez, J. F., Martínez-Avila, N., et al. (2020). The roles of matrix metalloproteinases and their inhibitors in human diseases. *International Journal of Molecular Sciences, 21*, 9739. https://doi.org/10.3390/ijms21249739 (accessed on 6th August 2025).

14. Carlotti, F., Chuva de Sousa Lopes, S. M., de Koning, E. J. P., de Melo Bernardo, A., et al. (2014). Lymphangiogenesis and angiogenesis during human fetal pancreas development. https://core.ac.uk/download/55800083.pdf (accessed on 6th August 2025).

15. Cavezzi, A., Colucci, R., Cavezzi, S., & Paccasassi, S. (2024). Phlebolymphedema and bioimpedance: General concepts and personal experience. *Journal of Theoretical and Applied Vascular Research*. https://www.semanticscholar.org/paper/95a2e08be3420b37c054a2db85dffb44617436fc (accessed on 6th August 2025).

16. Chehelgerdi, M., Chehelgerdi, M., Allela, O. Q. B., Pecho, R. D. C., Narayanan, J., Rao, D. P., Thamaraikani, T., et al. (2023). Progressing nanotechnology to improve targeted cancer treatment: Overcoming hurdles in its clinical implementation. *Molecular Cancer, 22*. https://doi.org/10.1186/s12943-023-01865-0 (accessed on 6th August 2025).

17. Cheng, Z., Li, M., Dey, R., & Chen, Y. (2021). Nanomaterials for cancer therapy: Current progress and perspectives. *Journal of Hematology & Oncology, 14*. https://doi.org/10.1186/s13045-021-01096-0 (accessed on 6th August 2025).

18. Cieślar, G., Pasek, J., & Stanek, A. (2020). The role of physical activity in prevention and treatment of peripheral vascular disorders. https://core.ac.uk/download/328109330.pdf (accessed on 6th August 2025).

19. Danaei, M., Dehghankhold, M., Ataei, S., Hasanzadeh Davarani, F., Javanmard, R., Dokhani, A., Khorasani, S., et al. (2018). Impact of particle size and polydispersity index on the clinical applications of lipidic nanocarrier systems. *Pharmaceutics, 10*, 57. https://doi.org/10.3390/pharmaceutics10020057 (accessed on 6th August 2025).

20. Ding, X., Cheng, Z., & Qian, Q. (2017). Intravenous fluids and acute kidney injury. *Blood Purification, 43*, 163–172. https://doi.org/10.1159/000452702 (accessed on 6th August 2025).

21. Donald, E. I. (2022). Human organs-on-chips for disease modelling, drug development and personalized medicine. *Nature Reviews Genetics, 23*, 467–491. https://doi.org/10.1038/s41576-022-00466-9 (accessed on 6th August 2025).

22. Dudley, A. C., & Griffioen, A. W. (2023). Pathological angiogenesis: Mechanisms and therapeutic strategies. *Angiogenesis, 26*, 313–347. https://doi.org/10.1007/s10456-023-09876-7 (accessed on 6th August 2025).

23. Fares, J., Fares, M. Y., Khachfe, H. H., Salhab, H. A., & Fares, Y. (2020). Molecular principles of metastasis: A hallmark of cancer revisited. *Signal Transduction and Targeted Therapy, 5*. https://doi.org/10.1038/s41392-020-0134-x (accessed on 6th August 2025).

24. Gopishetty, A., Amarnath, K., Uma Magesh, D. P., & Saichand, G. (2024). Successful treatment of low-flow vascular malformation in the lip using intralesional bleomycin: A case report. *Cureus, 16*. https://www.semanticscholar.org/paper/94c492182d11f35b51406ddd146a87016c5fbab7 (accessed on 6th August 2025).

25. Hamza, F., Shah, S., Khan, A. A., Farooqui, S., & Borges, K. J. J. (2024). Effects of aerobic exercise on vascular wall thickness: A meta-analysis of pre-clinical trials on rat model. *Journal*

of the College of Physicians and Surgeons–Pakistan: JCPSP, 34(10), 1216–1220. https://www.semanticscholar.org/paper/f77555daac7b518b0c981a7a62be056374aad700 (accessed on 6th August 2025).

26. Harding, J., Ritter, A., Rayasam, A., Fábry, Z., & Sándor, M. (2015). Lymphangiogenesis is induced by mycobacterial granulomas via vascular endothelial growth factor receptor-3 and supports systemic T-cell responses against mycobacterial antigen. *American Journal of Pathology, 185*, 432–445. https://doi.org/10.1016/j.ajpath.2014.09.020 (accessed on 6th August 2025).

27. Huang, J., Liao, C., Yang, J., & Zhang, L. (2024). The role of vascular and lymphatic networks in bone and joint homeostasis and pathology. *Frontiers in Endocrinology, 15*. https://www.semanticscholar.org/paper/54169d9deb1c02b634782afbdf8ce6573b407f04 (accessed on 6th August 2025).

28. Humbert, M., Kovács, G., Hoeper, M. M., Badagliacca, R., Berger, R. M. F., Brida, M., Carlsen, J., et al. (2022). 2022 ESC/ERS guidelines for the diagnosis and treatment of pulmonary hypertension. *European Respiratory Journal, 61*, 2200879. https://doi.org/10.1183/13993003.00879-2022 (accessed on 6th August 2025).

29. Kikuchi, H., Haneda, R., Soneda, W., Kawata, S., Murakami, T., Booka, E., Matsumoto, T., et al. (2022). 51st Annual Meeting of the Japanese Society for Wound Healing. *Wound Repair and Regeneration, 30*. https://www.semanticscholar.org/paper/6a004534c305b8bdc6e8d11e1dd4b97b7b5fd976 (accessed on 6th August 2025).

30. Kim, S. R., Lee, S. K., Jang, S. H., Choi, Y., et al. (2011). Expression of keratin 10 in rat organ surface primo-vascular tissues. https://core.ac.uk/download/pdf/82044703.pdf (accessed on 6th August 2025).

31. Koch, A. E., Marrelli, A., Mahto, A., Mould, A. W., Pitzalis, C., Pyne, D., et al. (2015). Angiogenic gene expression and vascular density are reflected in ultrasonographic features of synovitis in early rheumatoid arthritis: An observational study. https://core.ac.uk/download/30697659.pdf (accessed on 6th August 2025).

32. Levine, J. M., Delmore, B., & Cox, J. (2022). Skin failure: Concept review and proposed model. *Advances in Skin & Wound Care, 35*, 139–148. https://doi.org/10.1097/01.asw.0000818572.31307.7b (accessed on 6th August 2025).

33. Liu, Z., Chen, H., Zheng, L., Sun, L.-P., & Shi, L. (2023). Angiogenic signaling pathways and anti-angiogenic therapy for cancer. *Signal Transduction and Targeted Therapy, 8*. https://doi.org/10.1038/s41392-023-01460-1 (accessed on 6th August 2025).

34. Lund, A., & Swartz, M. (2018). Role of lymphatic vessels in tumor immunity: Passive conduits or active participants? https://core.ac.uk/download/159154967.pdf (accessed on 6th August 2025).

35. Lyon, A. R., López-Fernández, T., Couch, L. S., Asteggiano, R., Aznar, M. C., Bergler-Klein, J., Boriani, G., et al. (2022). 2022 ESC guidelines on cardio-oncology developed in collaboration with the European Hematology Association (EHA), the European Society for Therapeutic Radiology and Oncology (ESTRO) and the International Cardio-Oncology Society (IC-OS). *European Heart Journal, 43*, 4229–4361. https://doi.org/10.1093/eurheartj/ehac244 (accessed on 6th August 2025).

36. Madhumalar, S., Thenmozhi, A., Mythily, N., Sruthi, M. A., & Anand, K. (2025). Histogenesis of white pulp of the human foetal spleen at different gestational age groups: A cross-sectional

study. *International Journal of Anatomy Radiology and Surgery*. https://www.semanticscholar.org/paper/8a3b8205ebc2d32543a93334ad943146a0b1e6bb (accessed on 6th August 2025).

37. Madsen, R. R., Vanhaesebroeck, B., & Semple, R. K. (2018). Cancer-associated PIK3CA mutations in overgrowth disorders. *Trends in Molecular Medicine, 24*, 856–870. https://doi.org/10.1016/j.molmed.2018.08.003 (accessed on 6th August 2025).
38. Marcozzi, C., Moriondo, A., Negrini, D., Solari, L., et al. (2021). Interplay between gut lymphatic vessels and microbiota. https://core.ac.uk/download/480433213.pdf (accessed on 6th August 2025).
39. Mueller, S. N., Gebhardt, T., Carbone, F., & Heath, W. R. (2012). Memory T cell subsets, migration patterns, and tissue residence. *Annual Review of Immunology, 31*, 137–161. https://doi.org/10.1146/annurev-immunol-032712-095954 (accessed on 6th August 2025).
40. Pankova, M. N. (2024). Obesity and anticontractile effects of adipose tissue in the regulation of aortic tone. *Timiryazev Biological Journal*. https://www.semanticscholar.org/paper/10fdaf6269b719d5e668dcb3404c707be7214f0d (accessed on 6th August 2025).
41. Patel, G., Fury, W., Yang, H., Gomez-Caraballo, M., Bai, Y., Yang, T., Adler, C., et al. (2020). Molecular taxonomy of human ocular outflow tissues defined by single-cell transcriptomics. *Proceedings of the National Academy of Sciences, 117*, 12856–12867. https://doi.org/10.1073/pnas.2001896117 (accessed on 6th August 2025).
42. Rajasekaran, S. (2016). Clinical, immunological and therapeutic aspects of lymphatic filariasis. https://core.ac.uk/download/270241668.pdf (accessed on 6th August 2025).
43. Rui, S., Cao, Z., Wang, Y., & Liu, L. (2025). Characterization of microvessels in the human forehead dermis using intravascular dual perfusion and immunofluorescence staining. *Scientific Reports, 15*. https://www.semanticscholar.org/paper/cb7d88b9bcde0ea54f238d501de07d6047d1d178 (accessed on 6th August 2025).
44. Tall, A. R., Platt, A. M., Fulp, B., Martel, C., Kreisel, D., Gautier, E. L., Randolph, G. J., et al. (2013). Lymphatic vasculature mediates macrophage reverse cholesterol transport in mice. https://core.ac.uk/download/16457327.pdf (accessed on 6th August 2025).
45. Thomas, E. T. S., Pattanshetty, G., Prakash, P., & R, P. C. (2024). Mesenteric hemangiolymphangioma: A rare entity with unusual location. *IP Archives of Cytology and Histopathology Research*. https://www.semanticscholar.org/paper/00f83deac5d98354a9cc1d71bfa665058210949b (accessed on 6th August 2025).
46. Winkler, J., Abisoye-Ogunniyan, A., Metcalf, K. J., & Werb, Z. (2020). Concepts of extracellular matrix remodelling in tumour progression and metastasis. *Nature Communications, 11*. https://doi.org/10.1038/s41467-020-18794-x (accessed on 6th August 2025).
47. Wu, K., Lin, K., Li, X., Yuan, X., Xu, P., Ni, P., Xu, D. (2020). Redefining tumor-associated macrophage subpopulations and functions in the tumor microenvironment. *Frontiers in Immunology, 11*. https://doi.org/10.3389/fimmu.2020.01731 (accessed on 6th August 2025).
48. Xiang, M., Grosso, R. A., Takeda, A., Pan, J., Bekkhus, T., Brulois, K., Đermadi, D., et al. (2020). A single-cell transcriptional roadmap of the mouse and human lymph node lymphatic vasculature. *Frontiers in Cardiovascular Medicine, 7*. https://doi.org/10.3389/fcvm.2020.00052 (accessed on 6th August 2025).

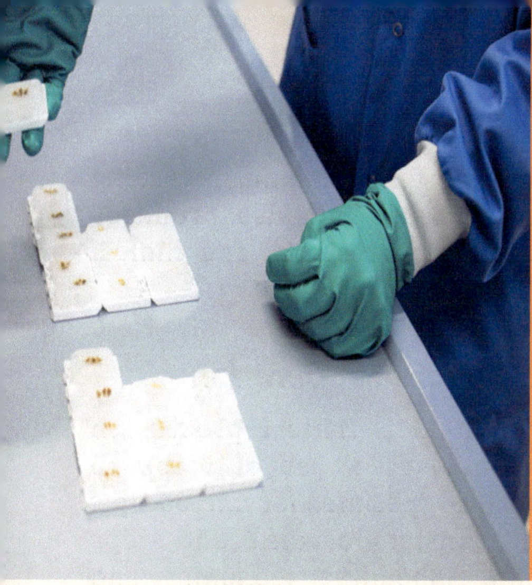

Chapter 8

TISSUE PREPARATION AND SECTIONING

Contents

Introduction

Sectioning and tissue preparation are important steps in histological analysis that are needed for both experimental and diagnostic use. It is a tissue handling process of gentle care of biological material to preserve cellular structure while permitting microscopic examination of the architecture of the tissue. Traditional methods such as paraffin embedding followed by microtomy have been the cornerstones of histopathological techniques. However, these techniques do not effectively portray the complex three-dimensional interactions within living tissues. Therefore, researchers and clinicians are increasingly aware of the limitations created by standard thin-section histology, which does not accurately reflect the complete repertoire of tissue physiology and pathology. The resolution of these constraints is important to continue gaining insight into many diseases, leading to improved diagnosis and treatment plans. Advanced imaging techniques are a key landmark in sectioning and tissue preparation. For instance, serial optical coherence microscopy (SOCM) is a breakthrough in the form of label-free imaging of large volumes of tissue as a whole organ, hence preserving the native three-dimensional architecture. This approach is feasible for contrast agent-free quantitative regional volume analysis, which carries the risk of altering tissue properties (Azaripour et al., 2020). The ability to examine tissues in their original state has significant implications for disease investigation and therapeutic design. With high-throughput analysis blended with top-of-the-line imaging tools, scientists can determine information regarding tissue dynamics previously obscured by traditional histological approaches.

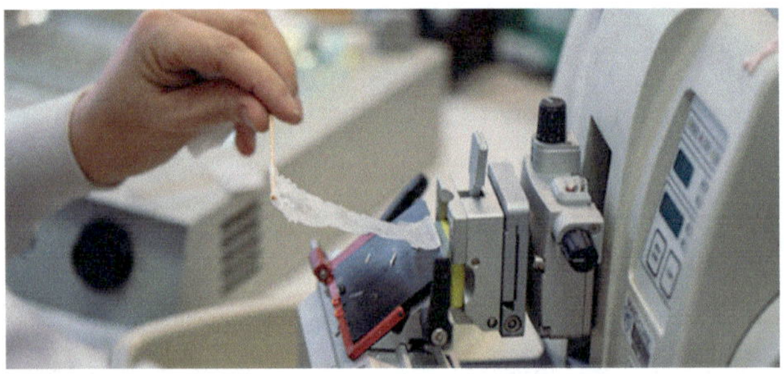

Figure 8.1. Tissue preparation and sectioning.

Source: https://www.mayo.edu/-/media/kcms/gbs/research/images/2019/04/25/14/58/prc-biospecimen-3406805-0095-8col.png.

In addition, research into intact tissue methods underscores the value of alternative methods in histopathology. Hydrogel-based biphasic methods enable the study of soft and heterogeneous tissue that would otherwise be challenging to examine with conventional histological methods. These advancements allow for tissue structures to be measured in a representative manner of the complexity of biological systems, particularly in studying developmental and pathologies within tissues (Arda et al., 2017). The promise of such approaches underscores the ongoing evolution of histological techniques, with the aim of enhancing diagnostic accuracy and research applications. Therefore, the introduction of novel techniques in tissue preparation and sectioning not only simplifies our understanding regarding the properties of tissues but also promises new horizons in medical research and clinical applications (Figure 8.1).

Definition of Tissue Preparation

Tissue preparation is a critical process in histology that involves a set of steps to prepare the biological specimen for microscopic examination. It consists of different steps including fixation, embedding, sectioning, and staining. Fixation is purposed to preserve the tissue architecture and minimize autolytic changes, usually performed by chemical agents such as formaldehyde. Following fixation, embedding in a hard substance like paraffin or resin provides mechanical support, allowing the thin sections to be sliced for microscopy. The quality of these sections is crucial in histological studies, as they should preserve important morphological details for accurate interpretation. Tissue preparation is thus an accurate technique whose impact directly influences the validity of subsequent diagnoses, whether research laboratory or clinical diagnostics. The sectioning phase of tissue preparation is critical, as it requires technical proficiency and precision to produce thin sections that enable the easy observation of cellular structure. Traditionally, it has been accomplished using microtomes, but technological advancements have introduced methods such as femtosecond laser microtomy that significantly reduce tissue deformation during sectioning. State-of-the-art techniques, such as 3D virtual histology, harness innovative imaging technologies, e.g., x-ray microCT, to visualize tissue in three dimensions, allowing for accurate quantitative assessments and mitigating the challenges inherent in traditional methods. These advances not only provide better anatomical perception but also improve the precision of pinpointing regions of interest in the tissue. Thus, the evolution of sectioning methods is a direct concern of histology, enhancing researchers' and practitioners' capabilities. Recent research has, for instance, used histological procedures to validate the possibility of the use of histology in forensic examination, particularly when examining burnt and unburnt bones. The experiments have shown that, even after exposure to high temperatures, the histomorphological characteristics of the cranial bones remain intact en masse, thereby preserving vital details for analysis. Decision tree classification based on a number of histological features has been shown to yield high accuracy in distinguishing human and non-human samples, as a demonstration of the potential of high-quality tissue sections. Furthermore, qualitative analysis shows significant differences between tissue subtypes regardless of species and extrinsic conditions, further highlighting the importance of proper tissue preparation. The ability to utilize histology as a powerful means in forensic contexts emphasizes its fundamental role in creating scientific understanding and pragmatic uses within the discipline (Crawley et al., 2016; Albers et al., 2018).

Importance in Histology and Pathology

Histology and pathology are closely interconnected disciplines that depend on the pivotal process of tissue preparation and sectioning, which in turn determines the accuracy and reliability of diagnostic findings. Histological techniques allow for careful microscopic examination of tissue architecture so as to reveal essential information regarding cellular organization and disease. By utilizing proper techniques in fixing, embedding, and sectioning tissue, pathologists are better placed to identify abnormalities typical of diseases such as cancer or infections. Proper preparation of tissue samples not only preserves morphological integrity but also enhances visibility of specific cellular components after staining, thereby enabling accurate diagnoses and informed clinical decisions. This fundamental text in histology emphasizes the significance of stringent quality control of tissue processing and accordingly becomes of paramount importance in effective patient management in health care. Recent advances in tissue preparation methods further illustrate their vital importance in histology and pathology. Standard thin-section histology, despite its widespread use, is not always able to preserve the three-dimensional tissue architecture, which conceals significant physiological relationships and pathological details. In response to these constraints, novel techniques, such as biphasic hydrogel techniques, are being created that provide more comprehensive analysis of complex tissues. This new method has made it possible to perform high-throughput, quantitative analysis of spatially asymmetrical tissues commonly encountered in clinical practice, which brings significant improvements over conventional techniques. More significantly, the ability to analyze soft, heterogeneous tissue enhances diagnostic accuracy, particularly in heterogeneous clinical specimens. These developments underpin the argument that tissue preparation not only enhances research but can also transform pathology diagnostics. Additionally, the importance of tissue preparation extends into real-time application with some instances being techniques like nonlinear microscopy (NLM). Intraoperative assessment of unprocessed fresh surgical specimens can be achieved using this technique without the usual need for fixation and embedding. The use of NLM allows for rapid evaluation of benign and malignant conditions and is particularly important in the situation of breast cancer re-excisions, where rapid decisions about re-excision can significantly impact patient outcomes. The use of advanced imaging technologies, coupled with traditional histological methods, represents an emerging paradigm in pathology, with a focus on speed and diagnostic effectiveness. With a sensitivity and specificity rate of almost 95%, NLM describes the potential for novel approaches to revolutionize tissue evaluation, consequently enhancing the overall efficiency of pathologic examination in modern medicine, as shown in Ahsen et al. (2014) (Figure 8.2).

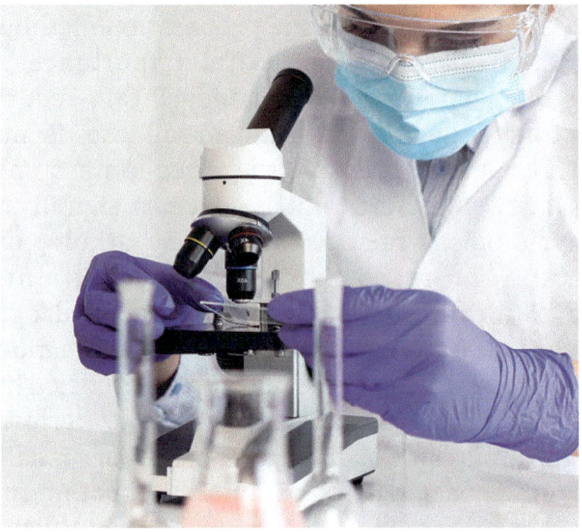

Figure 8.2. Importance in histology and pathology.

Source: https://www.cncpathlab.com/assets/uploads/122_1682060793blog-histopathology-biopsy-perform.jpg.

8.1. Types of Tissue Samples

Tissue specimen division in histology is essential for effective diagnosis and research. Fresh, frozen, and fixed are the general classifications of tissue specimens. Fresh tissues are usually taken to preserve cellular structure and are usually examined in real time to obtain immediate information on cellular morphology. Frozen tissues enable rapid sectioning followed by immediate examination without complex processing, making them highly valuable in critical cases. Simultaneously, fixed tissues are fixed, generally by formalin fixation, to maintain cell structure and permit long-term storage. Each sample type has characteristic strengths and potential drawbacks that dictate subsequent steps in tissue preparation and sectioning, which are modified to meet the requirements of different diagnostic protocols. In the case of small tissue samples, as with biopsies, the preparation technique used influences observed pathology in a highly important manner. A recent study demonstrated that staining small tissue and organ samples with various dyes may enhance their visibility prior to preparation, indicating that employing different dyes can improve the colorimetric contrast of small samples such as the breast, lung, and intestine (Benjakul et al., 2019). This enhancement is important for ensuring that pathologists can accurately identify and diagnose pathological processes that may be encountered in the small tissue sample at hand. Second, the suitability of hematoxylin as a marking stain over other dyes is a testament to the worth of intentional choice to enhance tissue visibility with minimal toxicity. These remarks concerning the selection of dyes find broader application to standard pathological slide analysis and underscore the importance of proper handling of tissue samples. Furthermore, higher-order tissue categories, such as tissues derived from ancient samples, pose particular challenges for extraction methods and downstream analysis. Fragile and sheared DNA typically complicate the analysis of past tissues, necessitating expert methodological approaches to maximize extraction yield and quality. In a comparative analysis of tissue types (bone, teeth, and soft tissue), homogenization significantly improved DNA extraction success (Hayter, 2007). Studies indicated that some methods, i.e., applying Proteinase K and Guanidinium Thiocyanate, yielded the best results. These findings not only highlight the importance of tissue type but also the requirement for specifically adopted extraction methods that consider the particular challenges involved in processing ancient or preserved specimens. The choice of tissue type and preparation method is pivotal, as it directly influences subsequent sectioning procedures and the reliability of histopathological investigation (Figure 8.3).

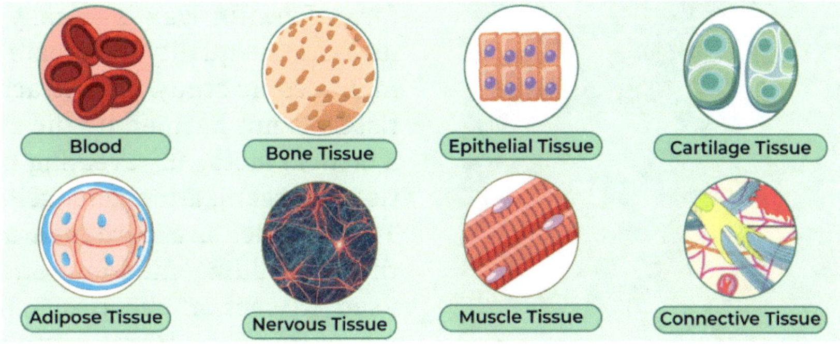

Figure 8.3. Types of tissue samples.

Source: https://media.geeksforgeeks.org/wp-content/uploads/20231116171441/Animal-Tissue.png.

8.1.1. Fresh Tissue Samples

Analysis of a fresh tissue sample plays a core function in the field of histology, providing information regarding both disease and normal physiology. The advantage of fresh samples lies in the preservation of native cellular architecture and biochemical characteristics, which are often lost during processing and fixation. Preservation enables investigators and clinicians to have a precise analysis of cellular morphology, tissue architecture, and ultrastructure. The urgency of conducting experiments on freshly acquired samples also benefits methods such as live-cell imaging and functional assays, providing a clearer understanding of tissue dynamics in varying conditions The immediate use of fresh samples enhances the accuracy of diagnostic and research results, leading to improved patient outcomes and scientific knowledge. Preparation of freshly excised tissue samples for histological examination involves several crucial steps in an attempt to present the optimum preservation and visualization. The tissues must first be obtained emergently and handled with care in an attempt to minimize degradation while structural integrity is maintained. Minimization of delay between excision and preparation is sometimes required, in that air conditions may lead to cellular artifacts. Immediately upon collection of samples, samples could frequently be frozen or embedded in optimal cutting temperature (OCT) media for sectioning of such tissue. MUSE-the microscopy with ultraviolet surface excitation-has recently made it possible to work on fresh samples without undergoing many of the conventional preparation challenges. It is a rapid technique that yields high-resolution images resembling conventional histology, with no loss of essential cellular and tissue morphology, thereby expanding the versatility of methods for analyzing fresh samples (Bishop et al., 2017). Also, the advancement of imaging devices has significantly enhanced the capability of fresh tissue analysis. For instance, serial optical coherence microscopy (SOCM) is an imaging method that is non-destructive and allows visualization at large scales of intact samples, like complex 3D structures typical of whole organs. It provides rapid imaging and information that traditional sectioning methods might miss due to spatial constraints and depth limits. Furthermore, SOCM's lack of necessity for contrast agents reduces potential artifacts inherent in staining processes (Azaripour et al., 2020). Subsequently, *in vitro* tissue specimens are not only important in themselves for immediate histopathological observation but also present a canvas for new imaging methods that transform research methods and diagnostic precision in contemporary biomedical science (Figure 8.4).

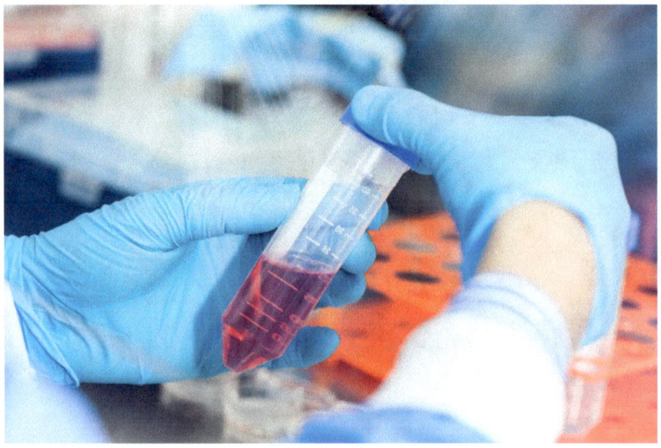

Figure 8.4. Fresh tissue samples.

Source: https://audubonbio.com/wp-content/uploads/2021/09/iStock-869796118-1-scaled.jpg.

8.1.2. Fixed Tissue Samples

The fixation of tissue samples is an essential histological procedure that transforms biological samples into a form suitable for microscopic examination. Fixation is necessary since it preserves the morphological integrity of cellular structures, preventing degradation and morphological changes that could hamper diagnosis. This process typically involves chemical solutions like formaldehyde or paraformaldehyde, which cross-link proteins and stabilize cell structures. Its success has a direct bearing on the procedures to be followed in tissue preparation, i.e., dehydration, embedding, and sectioning, where the goal is to maintain true-to-life snapshots of the architecture of the tissue. Advanced methods, like those brought to the fore by MUSE, achieve rapid histological imaging, allowing high-resolution assessments that reflect conventional methods but shorten preparation time (Bishop et al., 2017). Thus, the meticulous fixation process forms the foundation for accurate histopathological study and has significant implications in research and clinical diagnoses. Once fixed, the second significant step is embedding the tissue sample into a stabilizing and supporting medium that preserves its form. Paraffin wax is usually employed due to its optimal quality to create thin sections for microscopic study. This is achieved so that the tissue is not harmed by the sectioning process, a critical factor in revealing minute patterns of tissue organization and cellular orientations. The samples are hardened and chilled within the embedding medium, and microtomes are used to section the tissue into thin sections measuring 3 to 10 micrometers in thickness.

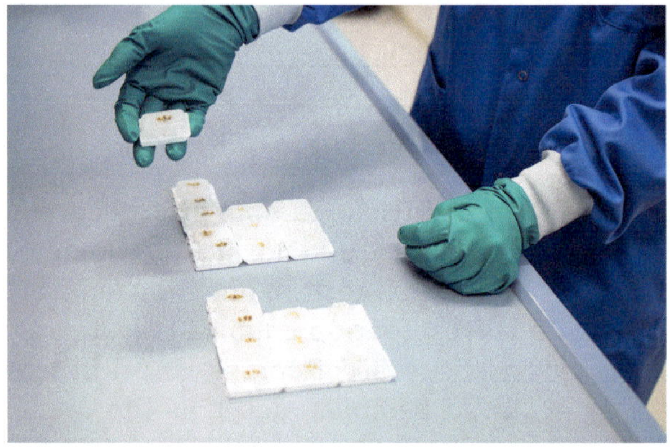

Figure 8.5. Fixed tissue samples.

Source: https://www.lexogen.com/wp-content/uploads/2024/03/02-Figure_FFPE-Blog_Scientist-holding-an-FFPE-sample-block.png.

The quality of such sections may impact the histological assessment quite considerably because poor cutting procedures may cause artifacts, which misrepresent the tissue morphology. While traditional methods are effective, techniques like MUSE substantially enhance the efficiency and precision of fixed tissue sample observation. (Bishop et al., 2017). Fixed tissue sample analysis not only supports diagnostic pathology but also forensic applications, attesting to the broad applicability of histological techniques. For instance, research has confirmed that fixed cranial bone samples, burnt or otherwise, are able to retain histological characteristics that distinguish between human and non-human specimens. The importance of histomorphology in forensic science and the ability to classify samples effectively using established classification systems are highlighted in this critical appraisal. Identification of specific tissue types provides greater insight into the biological and pathological context in which the samples arose, thereby improving accuracy. With advancing techniques, particularly those introduced within MUSE, comes the prospect of rapid and reliable histopathological analyses, thereby resecuring the fixed tissue sample in both medical and forensic contexts (Figure 8.5).

8.1.3. Frozen Tissue Samples

Freezing tissue samples is a critical step in histological analysis, preserving cellular morphology and the integrity of biomolecules. The procedure is typically performed using a freezing medium, such as an Optimal Cutting Temperature (OCT) compound, to facilitate tissue cutting in a cryostat. Importantly, freezing must be controlled well enough to avoid ice-crystal formation that compromises cellular structure and histological slide integrity. Differences in the freezing protocols used can yield different results, which necessitate careful consideration of the selected method for optimal outcomes in tissue preparation. Literature comparing freezing methods has shown that some methods yield better morphological preservation of tissues than others, thereby influencing the histological analysis and interpretation of results in subsequent experiments (Hughes, 2018). In addition to physical freezing techniques, researchers are increasingly studying the effects of different embedding media on tissue sample quality. Even though OCT is well-liked, there are instances when other compounds may prove to be better for the protection of injured tissues or for particular applications. For example, some studies have reported that paraffin embedding is a better structural preservative than OCT under certain conditions. Still, freezing remains a viable option for rapid histology because it avoids fixation, allowing specimens to be examined immediately in fresh tissue. This approach, in addition to expediting workflows, ensures the preservation of biochemical and morphological integrity of samples; thus, frozen tissue preparation is becoming a technique of choice in most laboratory environments (Hughes, 2018). Moreover, the advancement in imaging technologies as well as data analysis is highly enhancing the potential of frozen tissue sample assessment. Techniques such as volume electron microscopy (vEM) have transformed how researchers view and understand the complex architecture of tissue at the microstructural level. vEM enables high-resolution mapping of connectivity and cellular interactions across various tissues, thereby enabling investigations of developmental and disease processes at new levels of resolution. This shift towards high-throughput imaging techniques requires corresponding accurate sample preparation protocols to not destroy frozen tissues during processing. As researchers continually refine their methodologies, familiarity with the techniques and consequences of frozen tissue preparation will remain indispensable for obtaining reliable, reproducible histological results.

8.2. Fixation Techniques

The position of fixation procedures in tissue preparation cannot be overemphasized since they are the foundation for successful histological examination. Fixatives such as formaldehyde and glutaraldehyde modify cellular structures to preserve tissue morphology, thereby enabling objective assessment of pathological conditions. Stabilization of cellular lipids and proteins and interruption of enzymatic processes leading to autolytic degradation are the primary objectives of fixation. Fixatives of varying types are applied for specific purposes; formaldehyde, for instance, is applied due to its penetration characteristic and its compatibility with a variety of staining methods. This cautious selection of fixative is necessary because it ultimately determines the credibility of cellular information obtained through microscopic observation. It is therefore essential to understand the finer points relating to fixation procedures so that researchers and clinicians can achieve consistent and reliable histopathological observations. Furthermore, the application of new fixation methods also contributes to the overall efficiency in tissue preparation, particularly compared to traditional methods. By way of example, innovation in applying a technique such as microscopy with ultraviolet surface excitation (MUSE) signifies a significant advancement in histology. MUSE supports the acquisition of images quickly and with histological integrity without the time-consuming temporal gaps involved in conventional sectioning processes. This non-destructive approach highlights the potential for rapid acquisition of high-resolution diagnostic imaging, an approach that can transform clinical practice when timely decision-making is critical. With these developments illustrating that effective fixation is no longer followed by lengthy procedures, such advancements ensure fundamental research as well as clinical application can benefit from improved workflow efficiency and diagnostic accuracy (Bishop et al., 2017). In addition, fixation techniques are evolving to be compatible with new imaging technologies to widen the scope of tissue research. Serial optical coherence microscopy (SOCM) illustrates how combined fixation and advanced imaging can yield rich 3D images of tissue structure. SOCM, for instance, enables whole-organ visualization in ex vivo samples, providing informative information about native tissue architecture without the burden of conventional embedding and sectioning. This new technique avoids delay in histological examination while preserving the complex spatial interactions between cells. Such fixation innovations not only optimize diagnostic accuracy but also open up new possibilities for research. Thus, ongoing improvements in fixation techniques will be central to optimizing tissue preparation and sectioning for diagnostic purposes in an era of accelerating technological advancement (Azaripour et al., 2020) (Figure 8.6).

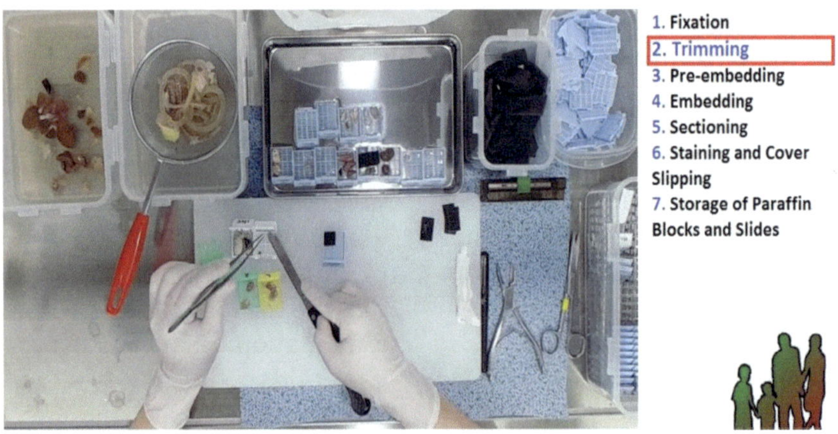

Figure 8.6. Fixation techniques.

Source: https://www.labtestsguide.com/wp-content/uploads/2021/01/Trimming-1024x576.jpg.

8.2.1. Chemical Fixation Methods

The chemical fixation process is a critical step in the process of tissue preparation and sectioning because it preserves the morphology of biological samples for future study. The process involves the use of fixatives that stabilize tissue and cell morphology by cross-linking proteins and nucleic acids. Fixation halts autolysis and putrefaction, thereby allowing accurate observation by microscopy. Various fixatives such as formaldehyde, glutaraldehyde, and alcohols are applied according to the downstream applications, e.g., transmission electron microscopy (TEM). Fixation stabilizes the structural components, allowing the sample to be used for investigating. (Dumančić et al., 2023). Tissue preservation quality also strongly depends on the type of fixative. For instance, formaldehyde is typically employed because it is effective in stabilizing protein structures and is less harsh than other fixatives such as glutaraldehyde. However, fixation time, fixative concentration, and temperature applied for fixation can influence the outcome. The use of rapid fixation methods, such as cryo-fixation via rapid freezing, prevents artifacts resulting from prolonged exposure to fixatives. These methods make it possible to preserve fine cellular details deemed crucial for immunolabeling and imaging procedures. This caution during the fixation stage forms the foundation for proper sectioning, where, during the acquisition of slices, these could be representative and true to the original tissue topology (Dumančić et al., 2023). The significance of chemical fixation lies beyond mere preservation, as it also enhances the morphological clarity of the sample throughout the process of sectioning. Tissue fixed in the correct way allows for more precise sectioning by ultramicrotomes, which is essential for high-resolution imaging techniques like volume electron microscopy (vEM). The evolution of fixation methods still conforms to the demands of newer imaging, allowing researchers to study complex biological questions, such as those regarding synaptic connections in neural tissues. As techniques improve, a better understanding of the role of chemical fixation in sample preparation for microscopy can inform best practices across studies, generating new insights into cellular functions and interactions within systems. This linking of fixation protocols and subsequent analytical techniques highlights the importance of proper tissue processing to produce consistent and reproducible results (Figure 8.7).

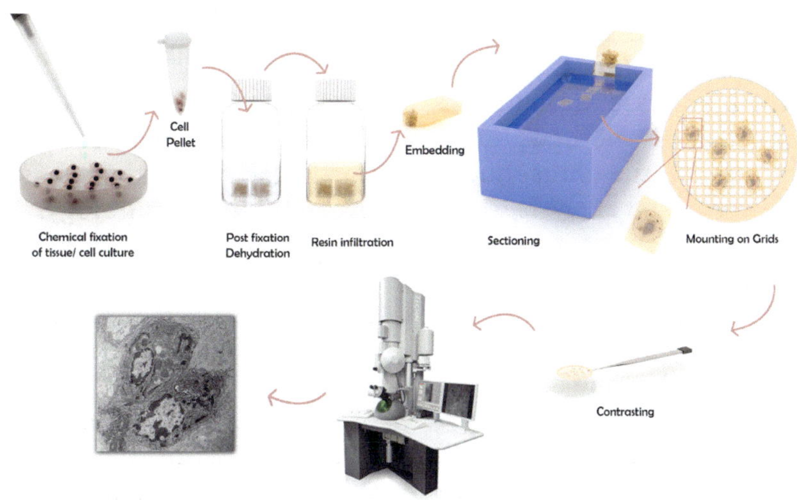

Figure 8.7. Chemical fixation methods.

Source: https://www.weizmann.ac.il/ChemicalResearchSupport/sites/ChemicalResearchSupport/files/2023-03/ChemicalFixationSteps%20inside_1.jpg.

8.2.2. Physical Fixation Methods

The importance of the physical fixation methods for tissue preparation and sectioning cannot be overstated. These methods help to retain structural integrity and biochemical characteristics of biological tissues, which are of primary importance in ensuring that microscopic observation is accurate. Physical fixation is usually performed using heat fixation and cryofixation methods, which have their advantages. Heat fixation, for example, quickly coagulates proteins within tissue and thus fixes cellular architecture, while at the same time destroying possible contamination. The technique is of great use in laboratory conditions where immediate analysis is necessary. Cryofixation, on the other hand, consists of snap freezing tissues, which is useful for maintenance of antigenicity and the fragile protein structure, thus being useful for immunohistological investigations. With the application of effective physical fixation methodologies, researchers are in a position to ensure maximum fixation of tissue samples prior to subsequent processing, consequently resulting in better overall sample quality for histological analysis. In addition to selecting the appropriate fixation process, its application can be crucial for determining sample compatibility with downstream analysis. For instance, both heat fixation and cryofixation offer tactical advantages in the molecular fixation of proteins and nucleic acids, which are essential in some assays. The physical fixation methods must be selected depending on the subsequent techniques to be used for tissue analysis, since the quality of imaging and sectioning depends directly on the fixation process. Based on this, new techniques like microscopy with ultraviolet surface excitation (MUSE) hold promising capabilities that can reduce the time of fixation without losing sample integrity. Unlike investing in the commitment of classical bright-field microscopy, which is founded on long tissue sectioning, MUSE produces rapid, high-resolution images that appear like common histology. The advent of such technologies is indicative of the dynamic state of tissue fixation and the interface of technology and histopathologic assessment (Bishop et al., 2017). Furthermore, the use of physical means of fixation bears real implications for the diagnostic potential in clinical and research environments. As depicted in existing studies, effective preservation techniques advance efficient processes in histopathology by shortening tissue processing time. For instance, serial optical coherence microscopy (SOCM) is a significant advance in that it makes possible the visualization of three-dimensional tissue structures without requiring enormous sectioning. The non-destructive imaging procedure has been found to provide high-resolution histopathological information regarding the intact tissue structures of the brain and kidneys (Azaripour et al., 2020). By applying modern physical fixation methods alongside new imaging technologies, researchers and clinicians can enhance diagnostic precision with reduced turnaround time for traditional histology protocols. Ultimately, the continued advancement of fixation methods is key to advancing tissue preparation technology, thereby enhancing a wide range of applications in patient care and biomedical research.

8.2.3. Importance of Fixation in Preserving Tissue Morphology

Fixation of biological tissues is a highly critical step in the tissue preparation process, particularly when one is assuring preservation of cellular morphology. Fixation stabilizes structural components of tissues by cross-linking proteins, which prevents autolysis and degradation that otherwise alter cellular architecture. This stabilization is necessary because even minor morphological changes would lead to misinterpretation in subsequent analyses. For instance, the regularity of shape and size of cells is central to impacting diagnostic outcomes in pathology. As such, effective fixation is imperative to showing well-quality images that actually reflect the tissues' *in vivo* condition so that researchers and clinicians can base sound conclusions regarding the concerned biological processes. Also critical is the type of fixative used and the fixation period to ensure the integrity of molecular markers within the tissue. Molecular markers are required for understanding tissue pathology and biology, particularly in cancer and other diseases, where accurate assessment can have a profound effect on treatment. For instance, it is demonstrated that average fixation time for breast cancer biopsies is important; over 90% of BU report fixation times between 6 and 24 hours, but there is high variability in adherence to best practice (Bargiacchi et al., 2021). The variation indicates the potential for suboptimal tissue morphology, which may cause a challenge in preserving key diagnostic information. Thus, standardization of fixation protocols remains essential to enhance the reproducibility of pathological findings. Moreover, techniques such as light-sheet fluorescence microscopy (LSFM) underscore the importance of fixation in current research. LSFM provides accurate three-dimensional reconstructions of biological specimens, which aid in explaining the complex dynamics of tissues. Successful preservation of intricate structures, acquired from adequate fixation procedures, is essential to successful imaging and analysis, particularly for the study of complex systems such as the human urogenital system (Baskin et al., 2020). Such a range of imaging technologies necessitates stringent fixation protocols in order to enable resultant data to be accurate and informative. Therefore, a quest for precision in fixation processes not only helps maintain morphology but also contributes significantly towards the development of biomedical research (Figure 8.8).

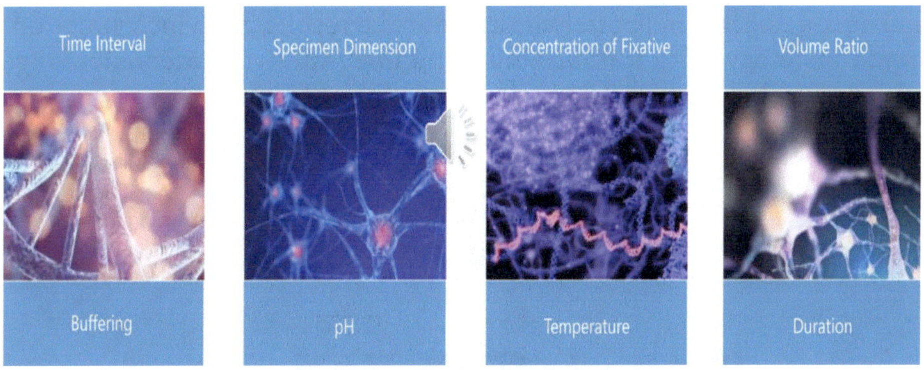

Figure 8.8. Importance of fixation in preserving tissue morphology.

Source: https://image.slidesharecdn.com/abriefguidetotissuefixation-240723020548-8a68ce77/75/A-Brief-Guide-to-Tissue-Fixation-and-Its-Importance-in-Pathology-Analysis-4-2048.jpg.

8.3. Dehydration Process

Dehydration is a critical process in preparing tissue specimens for sectioning and subsequent microscopic analysis. In this process, water in biological tissues must be effectively removed to enable more efficient infiltration of embedding media, such as paraffin. This is done through a gradual series of alcoholic solutions in increasing concentration levels, commonly beginning at 70% and ending at 100% ethanol. The gradual increase in alcohol concentration minimizes the cellular shrinkage and distortion, thereby ensuring the preservation of the morphological characteristics of the tissue. The tissue is then embedded in paraffin or resin media following dehydration to allow accurate sectioning necessary for histopathological studies. Efficiency and effectiveness of dehydration are paramount as they form the foundation for all the succeeding imaging and diagnostic maneuvers that are based on tissue architecture integrity. The advances in dehydration techniques have significantly contributed to the overall quality of tissue sectioning and tissue preservation in histopathology. Modern-day techniques give a high emphasis on the preservation of spatial relationships in tissues, particularly during the transition from dehydration to embedding. Dehydration in a careful manner preserves cellular details as well as tissue structure, which is most important for accurate diagnosis. Furthermore, new imaging technologies, as demonstrated in recent studies, bring insight into serial sectioning approaches that optimize three-dimensional tissue sample reconstructions. For instance, spectral optical coherence microscopy (SOCM) enables high-resolution, label-free imaging and can image complex tissue structures without compromising their integrity during dehydration and preparation procedures (Azaripour et al., 2020). These sophisticated methods are leading to more precise histopathological evaluations. Together with traditional dehydration methods, new methods are enlarging the scope of tissue preparation by combining high-precision processes. One such method is microgrinding, which has been modified to preserve delicate spatial relationships within soft tissues and bone. This systematic approach effectively enables the creation of accurate three-dimensional models through minimizing distortion in dehydration (Majdani et al., 2013). By using precise measurement procedures during grinding, researchers can achieve high accuracy and support successful imaging and assessment. Thus, dehydration techniques keep improving and shape the terrain of tissue preparation, enabling enhanced diagnostic capabilities and better clinical practice results. Such incorporation is a significant point of triumph in histology, with it underlining the imperative for adequate dehydration during tissue specimen preparation (Figure 8.9).

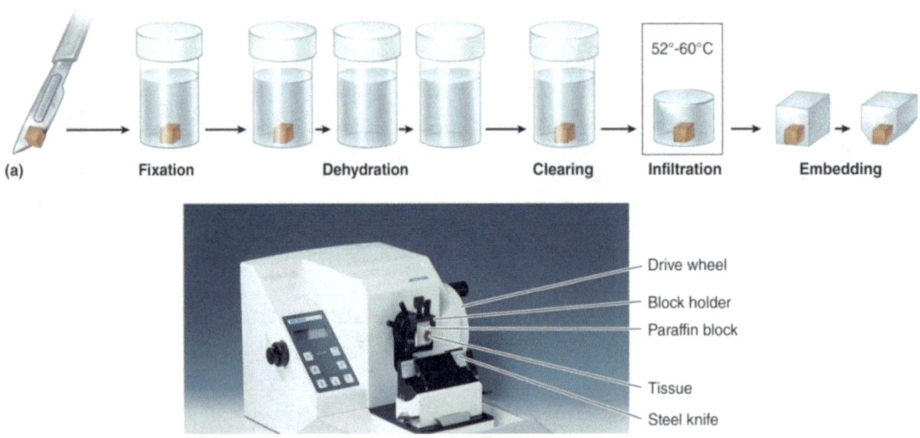

Figure 8.9. Dehydration process.

Source: https://medicallabscientist.org/wp-content/uploads/2018/12/Tissue-Processing-1024x539.jpg.

8.3.1. Role of Dehydration in Tissue Preparation

The step of dehydration during tissue processing is of primary significance in maintaining structural characteristics and biochemical composition of biological specimens. Water is evaporated during dehydration of the tissues to allow impregnation of embedding media, such as paraffin or resin. It is a critical step because water will interfere with infiltration, leading to tissue architecture collapse or distortion. A study has mentioned that diffusible ions, i.e., potassium (K^+) and sodium (Na^+), are typically lost upon dehydration, which could impact the credibility of the following analytical procedures. Due to this, techniques that minimize ion loss in terms of dehydration, like the application of cryo-sectioning with freeze drying, have been developed. This technique preserves cell properties and natural ion content, yielding higher quality histological sections and simpler use of accurate imaging techniques in plant pathology and physiology studies (Aarts et al., 2016). The development of accurate dehydration techniques also greatly enhances the discipline of histology, enabling improved imaging of soft and hard tissues. Tissue preparation techniques, such as microgrinding, aid in preserving spatial relationships and improve cross-sectional image resolution. Besides offering accurate three-dimensional reconstruction of tissue structures, these technologies highlight the importance of appropriate dehydration procedures within the overall tissue preparation process. By embedding the sample in materials such as epoxy resin, researchers can prevent loss of informative morphological detail during dehydration, resulting in high-contrast images. These advances bear witness to the need for methodical approaches that maintain sample integrity while providing sound histological data for clinical applications, especially for anatomically intricate structures (Majdani et al., 2013). Lastly, the role of dehydration in tissue preparation is multifaceted and affects both structural preservation and analytical potential of histological samples. Dehydration is not merely a step in processing; it is actually required to maintain tissue integrity during processing so the findings of subsequent analyses are true. With the help of sophisticated methods that buffer against the detrimental effects of dehydration, researchers are able to boost the integrity of histologic interpretation and ensure better experimental outcomes. The integration of novel methods, such as maintaining ion composition during conventional dehydration, will further advance the science of tissue preparation toward greater biomedical research and diagnostic use. The continuous refinement of these techniques is sure to advance understanding of complex tissue structure and biochemical behaviors in both health and disease states (Majdani et al., 2013; Aarts et al., 2016).

8.3.2. Common Dehydration Agents

In sectioning and tissue preparation, standard dehydration reagents are critical in the preparation of the tissue specimens for microscopic examination. Dehydration is essential for the maintenance of cellular structure, facilitating the removal of water from biological tissues that would otherwise interfere with subsequent procedures. The most frequent dehydration reagents are ethanol, methanol, and isopropanol. Ethanol, for instance, is widely used due to its capacity not only to dehydrate tissues but also to maintain cellular morphology. Alcohol-induced dehydration leads to a tissue state that is conducive to infiltration with embedding media, thereby enhancing the quality of resultant histological sections. Choice of dehydration agent, particularly its concentration and duration of exposure, can significantly influence sample structural integrity and plays a critical role in the resolution of sectioning-induced images. Following initial dehydration, consideration should be given to the impact that these agents can exert on subsequent processing procedures, i.e., staining and imaging. For instance, variations in ethanol content in the dehydration process could influence penetration of histological dyes into the tissue and their capacity to bind effectively with the target molecules. With the progress made in imaging technologies, the choice of dehydration agents becomes more applicable. Studies involving microcomputed tomography (microCT) illustrate the significance of dehydration agents in enhancing contrast and visualization of tissue specimens. Specifically, the use of proper contrast agents in addition to successful dehydration will greatly improve imaging in tissue structures, allowing for better definition of pathological change, such as ischemic lesions, as in studies on brain samples (Bouajjani et al., 2001). The application of improved contrast-enhancing methods also holds significant promise in increasing the use of dehydration agents for future studies. For instance, certain X-ray contrast materials, if blended with common dehydrating agents, would potentially enhance the quality of imaging, such as in infected lung tissues caused by diseases like tuberculosis (Arjona et al., 2019). This new technique not only helps in the visualization of tissue architecture's fine details but also addresses the mounting demand for sophisticated methods in histopathological analysis. Understanding of the relationship between dehydrating agents and imaging techniques is crucial for researchers and pathologists, as it has the potential to enhance the completeness and accuracy of our explorations into tissue pathologies and their corresponding histological presentations.

8.3.3. Steps Involved in the Dehydration Process

Dehydration is a critical phase of tissue preparation, allowing the cell structure to be preserved for subsequent microscopic examination and assessment. It starts with the removal of water from the tissue sample since water could interfere with the infiltration of the embedding agents, such as paraffin. Dehydration typically uses a series of ethanol solutions with increasing concentration, starting from a minimal ratio (usually around 50%) and finishing with absolute ethanol (100%). The process in stages avoids cellular components from being damaged due to the osmotic pressure adjustments that may happen too rapidly, thus preserving the tissue architecture. This organized dehydration must be carried out to prevent tissue distortion and maintain structural properties when sections are eventually prepared for histological study, which is important for making accurate diagnoses and conducting research. Following treatment of the tissue with the ethanol series, clearing is the next step. In this process, the dehydrated tissue must be treated with an organic solvent, typically xylene or toluene. The main purpose of clearing is to drive out the ethanol in order to allow subsequent infiltration of the embedding media. The solvents used are low-viscosity and high-refractive-index to facilitate smoother embedding when adding paraffin. The procedure also enhances the transparency of the tissue to facilitate viewing with the microscope. Notably, the clearing agent should be completely removed prior to paraffin embedding since leftover solvents will taint the histological sections. Clearing, therefore, is a crucial component of dehydration, eventually leading to proper tissue sectioning and histopathological diagnoses. During the last phases of dehydration, paraffin infiltration is achieved by soaking the dehydrated and washed tissue samples in warm paraffin wax. Infiltration is crucial because it imparts a solidifying substrate to the clearing agent upon cooling, facilitating thin sectioning. The tissue remains in the paraffin bath for a number of hours or overnight to ensure good penetration, which is often several hours to overnight, depending on the density and size of the specimen. Tissue embedded in paraffin is then sectioned into thin slices for microscopy. This process enhances visualization of tissue structure and pathology, enabling clinicians and researchers to make more accurate diagnoses of most conditions, including neoplasms, as documented in recent studies (Bishop et al., 2017). These advances in tissue preparation highlight the importance of effective dehydration processes in histology.

8.4. Clearing Agents

In histology, clearing agents are central to the process of preparing tissue samples for microscopic analysis. They are usually organic solvents and are employed in the removal of embedding media like paraffin or resin without compromising the structural integrity of the tissues. The effectiveness of clearing agents relies on the ability of the clearing agent to reduce the refractive index contrast between the tissue and the mounting medium, enhancing optical clarity upon microscopic viewing. The most commonly utilized clearing agents, such as xylene and toluene, possess different chemical properties that influence the clearing process and cellular architecture maintenance. The visibility of fine details in the tissue sections is at the heart of accurate diagnosis and inquiry, and therefore, there is a requirement to select appropriate clearing agents on the basis of the precise requirements of the specific histological study in question. In addition, novel imaging technologies such as serial optical coherence microscopy (SOCM) illustrate the insufficiency inherent to traditional slide-based microscopy, an approach that relies heavily on successful clearing agents. Traditional microscopy will not capture larger-scale tissue structures due to the need for thin sections and the physical limitation of optical imaging depth. As detailed in recent research, SOCM enables 3D organ architecture imaging without traditional contrast agents, thereby exhibiting unique strengths in histopathology (Azaripour et al., 2020). This paradigm shift underscores the necessity of clearing agents, as they remain vital reagents in tissue preparation for conventional and cutting-edge imaging techniques. Their utility goes beyond the enhancement of optical performance to the opening up of our eyes to complex biological constructs, guiding more informed diagnosis and treatment regimens. Histological preparation of marine animals, bivalve mollusks, and crustaceans represents one more instance of the specialized application of clearing agents in diverse biological contexts. Histological processing according to current guidelines for marine biology entails some adjustments of classical procedures due to differences in tissue structure and composition (Howard et al., 2004). The use of specially engineered clearing agents becomes a necessity since these chemicals are to effectively dehydrate sensitive marine tissues without compromising structural integrity. This delicate process of tissue preparation allows scientists to study the pathological status of marine organisms with precision, further highlighting the need to learn how to select and apply clearing agents proficiently. With greater histopathological investigation of marine animals, the continued improvement and development of clearing agents will remain significant, resulting in increased understanding and assessment of marine animal health (Figure 8.10).

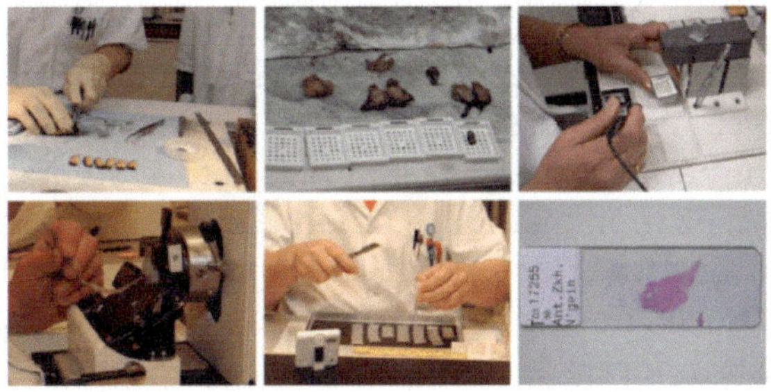

Figure 8.10. Clearing agents.

Source: https://s2.studylib.net/store/data/010274034_1-c887f33216327ff914fecc6e06c0eccf-768x994.png.

8.4.1. Purpose of Clearing in Tissue Preparation

Tissue clearing is a technique central to histology, aimed solely at enhancing the clarity of tissue structures during microscopic examination. During tissue preparation, clearing agents are incorporated after dehydration to equalize the tissue's refractive index with that of the embedding medium, typically paraffin. This critical step minimizes light scattering that occurs due to differences in refractive indices, thereby maximizing the optical resolution and clarity of processed tissue sections. The effectiveness of the process of clearing directly impacts the quality of histological staining and imaging techniques, such that the choice of clearing agent is crucial in achieving high-resolution and contrasting observations in subsequent examinations, particularly in complex specimens like those encountered in operations and research studies. Effective clearing processes rely on the specific characteristics of the tissue of interest being processed. For example, using a good, clear agent like xylene not only speeds up the paraffin infiltration but also preserves important morphological information that is key to accurate analysis and diagnosis. In a study of fish embryos, the method through a series of ethanol solutions culminating in xylene highlighted the importance of correct dehydrating and clearing procedures for achieving maximum histological details following sectioning. Clearing is a transition corridor for going from one solution to the next, e.g., from fixatives to embedding media, preserving tissue integrity and spatial relationships en route. Clearing, then, is not merely a first step; it is a crucial function in preserving histological morphology and enabling precise image acquisition. Furthermore, the introduction of advanced clearing protocols, such as those using epoxy resin, has expanded the possibilities for histological analysis, enabling increased spatial resolution and accuracy in three-dimensional reconstructions of tissues. This carries significant implications for computer-assisted surgery, in which the need for precise anatomical modeling is increasingly being appreciated. Techniques like systematic microgrinding, in combination with computerized visualization methods, underscore the powerful role of clearing in reproducing replicates of complex anatomical shapes that are spatially accurate. These methods not only enhance the clarity of tissue sections but also provide new opportunities, illustrating the key position held by clearing in contemporary histological techniques and its impact on surgical planning and evaluation processes (Majdani et al., 2013; Kurniawati et al., 2017) (Figure 8.11).

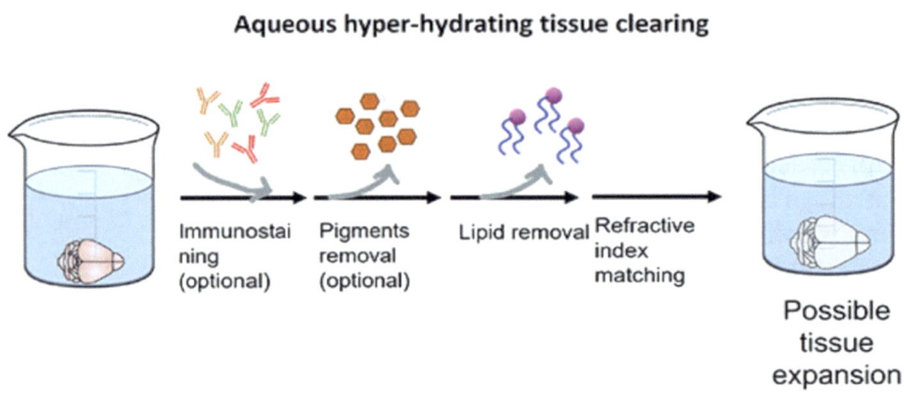

Figure 8.11. Clearing agents.

Source: https://www.oxinst.com/learning/uploads/inline-images/figure4-resized-20221103133548.jpg.

8.4.2. Types of Clearing Agents Used

In sectioning and tissue preparation, the most important step in rendering biological samples visible for microscopic observation is the choice of clearing agents. Several clearing agents have been developed for this purpose, and each agent possesses specific attributes and applications. One of the most widely used clearing agents is organic solvents such as xylene and toluene, which effectively strip tissue samples of lipids and hydrophobic compounds. These agents allow maximum penetration of embedding agents like paraffin, hence the Fine structure of tissues can be well preserved during sectioning. Additionally, the use of clearing agents offers better optical characteristics in histological examination, which is an essential prerequisite for accurate diagnosis in pathology. Hence, the selection of a good clearing agent is of utmost significance to acquire high-quality tissue preparations that ensure the successful evaluation of biological samples (Cinci et al., 2023). In newer trends, alternatives for traditional organic solvents have been investigated with a focus on reducing toxicity as well as environmental load. These newer chemicals, such as aqueous solutions containing glycerol or mixtures of ethanol, have proved to be promising in making tissues optically clearer and decreasing the punitive effects traditionally attributed to organic solvents. For instance, studies have shown that a mixture of glycerol and ethanol could enhance the spectral transmittance of muscle tissues to a great extent, even penetrating more impermeable areas of light (Clemente et al., 2010). This advancement is particularly important in three-dimensional histological applications. As the technology advances towards less traumatic and more efficient methods of clearing tissues, it still remains crucial for pathologists and researchers to learn about the performance and limitations of these alternatives. In general, the flexibility of clearing agents is a testimony to the intricacy and precision required in tissue sectioning and preparation. As we consider the forms of clearing agents, it is apparent that the selection process depends on several tissue attributes, the intended analysis, and safety considerations. Continuous evolution of these agents not only affects histological section appearance and quality but also allows for advanced imaging techniques, such as three-dimensional fluorescence microscopy. With new techniques reconstructing the field, a robust understanding of the operation and coordination of different clearing agents and their coordination with the biological tissues will be necessary. By further developing the approaches, researchers can extend the limits of tissue investigation, leading to game-changing uses in clinical pathology and beyond (Cinci et al., 2023).

8.4.3. Impact of Clearing on Tissue Transparency

Tissue clearing has revolutionized the field of histology by offering an unprecedented degree of insight into the three-dimensional structure of biological tissues. Traditional histological methods, based on thin sectioning, are generally unable to reveal the sophisticated interactions present in intact tissue. This deficiency is most clearly seen in soft and inhomogeneous tissues, where context is paramount in interpreting physiological and pathological status. Clearing techniques enhance transparency by reducing light scattering and refractive index discontinuities in tissues, enabling high-resolution imaging. By enabling visualization of tissue architecture in its native state, the techniques create opportunities for studying developmental and disease processes more comprehensively, exposing the necessity of advanced clearing techniques in research and in the clinic (Arda et al., 2017). The evolution of tissue clearing methods has also increased the opportunities for studying tissues further and led to better imaging modalities. Techniques such as hydrogel embedding provide a biphasic environment that enhances transparency without sacrificing spatial integrity—a basic issue of traditional histology. High-throughput volumetric interrogation techniques allow researchers to quantitatively analyze spatially nonuniform tissues that are otherwise difficult to assess. This combined approach not only improves tissue transparency but also the precision of three-dimensional reconstructions inherent in clinical diagnosis and therapy planning. An example from research on pancreatic innervation and development shows that the improvements in tissue clearing technologies bring key information on disease cause and progression and are therefore essential to whole tissue analysis (Arda et al., 2017). The impacts of tissue clearing extend beyond mere research applications, and there are significant implications for clinical applications, especially surgical planning and intervention. Enhanced visibility facilitates enhanced pre-surgical assessment and intraoperative navigation, particularly in complex anatomical regions such as the temporal bone. By providing high-contrast and high-definition visualization of both soft tissues and bones, clearing techniques facilitate improved intraoperative decision-making. In addition, the ability to generate and analyze three-dimensional anatomical structures from cleared tissue sections enables enhanced image-based segmentation and finite element analysis for simulation in surgery. Thus, tissue clearing technology significantly advances our understanding and handling of biological tissues, culminating in clinical advances and patient safety (Figure 8.12).

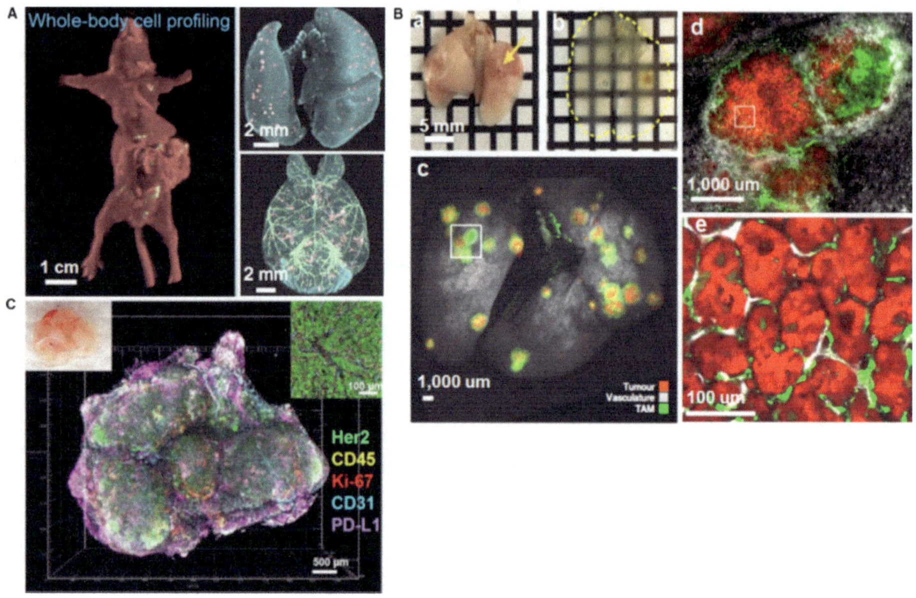

Figure 8.12. Impact of clearing on tissue transparency.

Source: https://onlinelibrary.wiley.com/cms/asset/9c3687eb-2b58-4a7e-ac05-a2b0daf6cdab/joa13309-fig-0008-m.jpg.

8.5. Embedding Techniques

One of the most important steps of sectioning and preparation of tissue is the embedding methods that are employed to preserve the integrity of biological samples for microscopic examination. Various embedding methods exhibit various merits and drawbacks based on the effect on subsequent analysis. Paraffin embedding, for example, is one of the most widely employed methods due to providing excellent tissue support and allowing finely adjustable cutting. This method involves drying out the tissue and subsequently embedding it with melted paraffin wax to form a solid block that can be readily sectioned into thin samples. In contrast to frozen embedding, frozen embedding employs such media as Optimal Cutting Temperature (OCT) compound to allow fast processing of the tissues without fixation, thus retaining some original structural features. However, methods such as these need to be exercised with care in embedding so as to limit artifacts that can jeopardize the quality of histopathological observations. Choosing an embedding method has a significant effect on the outcome of histological examination since it influences the visualization and interpretation of tissue morphology. For instance, whereas frozen embedding of tissue conserves enzyme activity and antigenicity, the process is not problem-free. The formation of ice crystals during freezing can induce cellular damage, potentially compromising the results of immunohistochemical staining protocols and histological evaluations. Moreover, components inherent in the freezing process, including the particular methods used and the temperatures used, have the potential to introduce heterogeneity in tissue quality. Comparative studies among different methods have consistently shown that paraffin-embedded specimens preserve morphology and staining quality better than frozen specimens and score highest in image definition and inter-rater reliability in quality assessments of murine colonic tissue sections (Hughes, 2018). This is an indication that protocols of embedding must be validated rigorously to satisfy the specific requirements of histological studies. Besides, rapid progress in imaging modalities is revolutionizing the tissue embedding and sectioning paradigms into new research directions. Serial optical coherence microscopy (SOCM) is one such novel optical technique that has the major advantage of enabling label-free imaging of voluminous tissues without the need for traditional embedding processes (Azaripour et al., 2020). This technology is capable of three-dimensional morphological reconstructions of structure, including a complete impression of tissue architecture, and eliminating issues with section artifact introduction. The integration of such imaging technologies with traditional approaches holds a promising future for histopathology because they have the potential to increase the fidelity of applications in diagnosis and research. As researchers continue to improve embedding techniques and adopt complementary technologies, the quest for improved methodology is key to enhancing the resolution and precision of histological investigations in different biological situations (Figure 8.13).

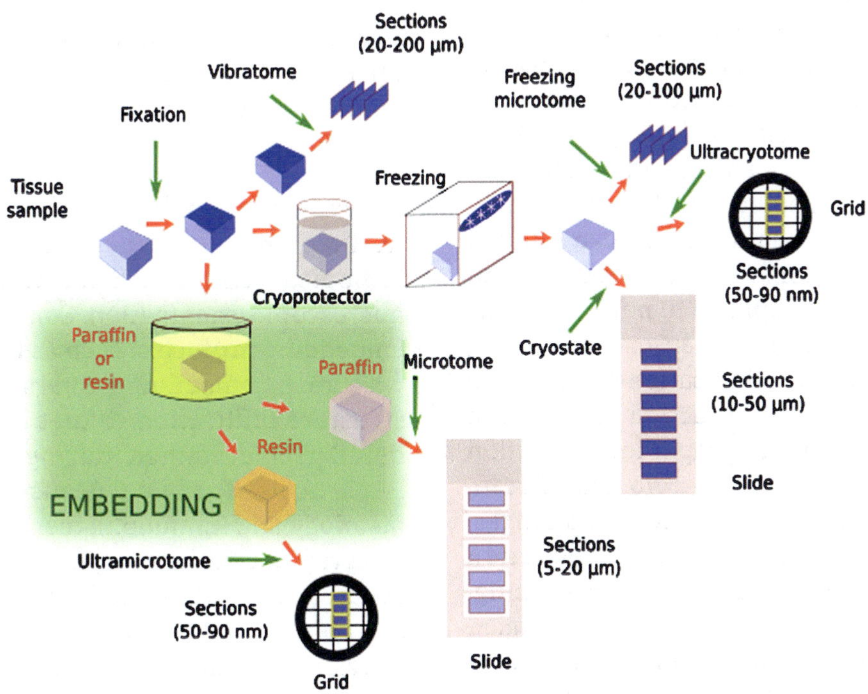

Figure 8.13. Embedding techniques.

Source: https://mmegias.webs.uvigo.es/02-english/6-tecnicas/imagenes/3-inclusion.png.

8.5.1. Paraffin Embedding

Paraffin embedding is a crucial step in tissue preparation required for the generation of high-quality histological sections suitable for study under microscopic examination. It's a technique where fixed tissue samples are impregnated with melted paraffin wax, which solidifies on cooling, thereby precisely retaining the cell architecture. The procedure of embedding is initiated after tissue fixation, usually with formalin, which cross-links proteins and fixes the tissue structure. The unique properties of paraffin, the fact that it can provide support throughout sectioning and also hold morphology intact after cutting, render paraffin a very valuable medium to handle in histological processes. Paraffin embedding, therefore, allows for the production of thin sections that are easy to mount on slides and stain, facilitating effective histopathological analysis. Relative to other embedding approaches, paraffin embedding has particular merits that make overall histological specimen quality. Notably, it facilitates preservation of fine cellular details and allows long-term storage of biological samples without loss of integrity. This is particularly critical in research where tissue integrity must be preserved. As indicated, paraffin embedding received the highest quality rating in a blinded test that compared some of these freezing and embedding techniques applied to murine colonic samples, demonstrating its efficacy (Hughes, 2018). Also, paraffin's solidification in a uniform manner allows for uniform section thickness in a way that is important for proper interpretation and quantitation of the histological detail. Paraffin embedding is not without challenges, however, one of which is the introduction of artifacts in the course of embedding, particularly when the tissue was not well fixed or dehydrated before infiltration. Paraffin also tends to obscure certain antigens, complicating immunohistochemistry. Still, ongoing progress in the integration of protocols and innovation into paraffin formulations continues to improve the overall outcomes of this method. Paraffin embedding issues demonstrate the importance of precise technique and highlight the reason why histological examination remains a dynamic specialty, strongly reliant upon precise preparation techniques to yield significant evidence of tissue pathology (Allen et al., 2009) (Figure 8.14).

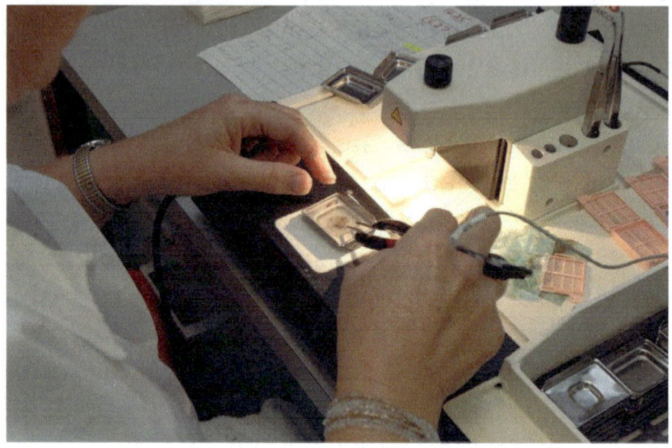

Figure 8.14. Paraffin embedding.

Source: https://paraffinwaxco.com/wp-content/uploads/2017/10/Tissue_processing_-_Embedding_station.jpg.

8.5.2. Resin Embedding

Resin embedding is a critical technique in biological tissue preparation for accurate microscopic examination. Compared to standard embedding protocols, such as the use of paraffin wax, resin embedding offers increased tissue structure infiltration so that important cellular detail is maintained during sectioning. This is particularly advantageous in fields such as histology and immunohistochemistry, where the integrity of cellular morphology is critical. Using synthetic resins like epoxy or acrylic, researchers are able to make extremely strong blocks that provide extremely thin sections appropriate for analysis by transmission electron microscopy (TEM). The stability and support provided by the resin to fragile tissues in the prevention of damage minimizes the susceptibility to injury, hence enhancing the microscopic images obtained. It is a basic method, particularly in biomedical research, where precise visualization is all-important in understanding complex biological processes. Insofar as it has several advantages, resin embedding does come with some complications that need to be approached cautiously. The process of resin embedding polymerization generates a lot of heat, which can adversely affect delicate tissue components if not properly controlled. Embedding medium selection may also affect the quality of tissue preservation altogether. For example, varying resins can produce varying effects on tissue breakdown or alteration of fine structures. It is essential to obtain precise protocols for resin infiltration and curing to minimize artifacts that may compromise ensuing examination. In addition, resin-embedded tissues produce more information-dense images but can be more difficult to manipulate due to brittleness, necessitating specialized equipment and cutting methods. These requirements underscore the importance of simplifying resin embedding procedures to balance preparation time against histological information quality. Furthermore, advances in resin embedding protocols are revealing the potential for improved histological analysis in research and clinical diagnostics. New methods are being designed to incorporate molecular markers and visualize specific cellular components more effectively in resin-embedded tissues. For instance, the integration of resin embedding with imaging modalities such as X-ray computed tomography (CT) has been explored to achieve more precise anatomical images of target regions, as highlighted in current studies (Albers et al., 2018). Such advancements broaden the use of resin embedding beyond what can be achieved using standard techniques and can transform pathologists' and investigators' perceptions of tissue morphology. In addition, new forms of embedding resin are being developed to increase contrast and reduce the risk of artifacts during sectioning, thereby addressing most of the previous issues with the technique (Hughes, 2018). Collectively, these advances look toward an active future for resin embedding, continuing to keep it around and still viable for the preparation of tissues and sectioning (Figure 8.15).

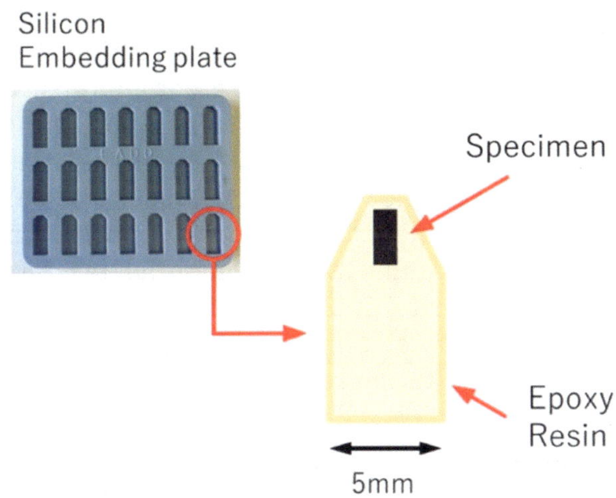

Figure 8.15. Resin embedding.

Source: https://www.jeol.com/words/assets/images/7cc39a617211a62097f0e2176af687ddbeae27c9.jpg.

8.5.3. Importance of Embedding for Sectioning

Embedding of the tissues is a critical histological preparation procedure with profound effects on the quality and accuracy of the resulting sectioning. During embedding, the specimens are infused with a suitable medium, such as paraffin or epoxy resin, which encapsulates the tissue in a rigid support that cannot be altered when cut. Through stabilization, thin, consistent sections can be obtained, and this is vital for microscopic examination. Without proper references during the embedding process, the fragile tissue structures can be destroyed, encouraging artifacts that obstruct the interpretation of histological features. The significance of the procedure is divulged in advanced methodologies, where spatial relationships and three-dimensional structures need to be preserved to effectively image and analyze, as demonstrated by studies that enhance histological preparations with optimized embedding techniques (Majdani et al., 2013). Besides, choosing the embedding medium has a major role in the solution of sections achieved in the sectioning process. Different materials may affect the hardness and additional slicing characteristics of embedded tissues, and ultimately, histological outcomes. For instance, epoxy resins allow more delicate detailing of small and sensitive tissue structures to be mapped well, which is essential when examining complex tissues in clinical settings, such as in the human inner ear. The ability to create detailed three-dimensional reconstructions from well-sectioned samples has revolutionary potential in areas such as and finite element analysis. This adaptability serves not only for visualization but also for evaluating surgical techniques and treatments, pointing out the greater significance of blending approaches toward creating medical practices (Majdani et al., 2013). Lastly, embedding as a process is not only an antecedent; it enhances the potential for other analytical techniques, such as immunohistochemistry. By providing a firm matrix for tissues, embedding facilitates accurate sectioning that is essential in staining and labeling procedures. For example, studies using Technovit 7200 VCR demonstrate that proper embedding enhances immunohistochemical labeling of proteins in bone tissue samples, thereby enhancing the scope for analyzing cellular behavior and tissue response under various conditions. This union of embedding and sectioning not only explains cellular mechanisms but also benefits diagnostics and treatment evaluation. As the practice of histology becomes more sophisticated, the significance of embedding remains a part of successful tissue preparation that reaffirms its use in advancing research as well as clinical practice (Figure 8.16).

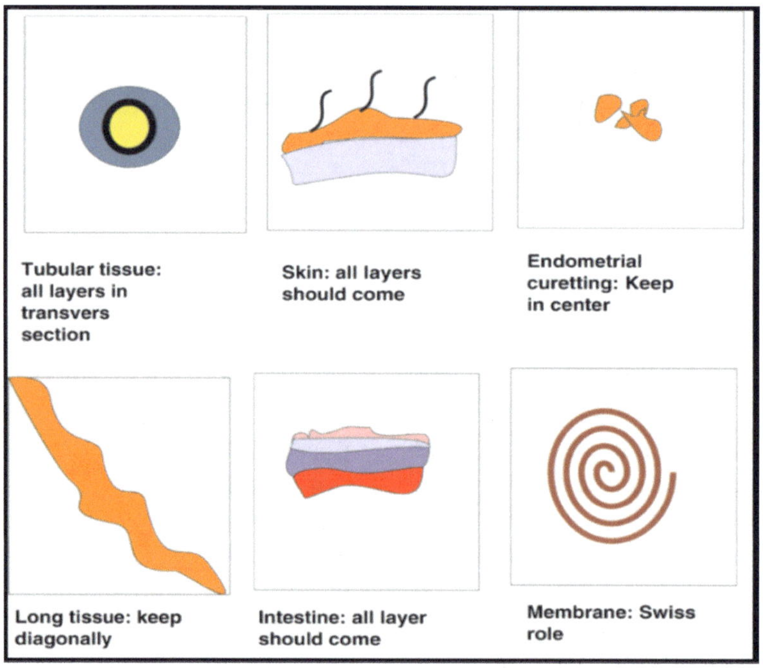

Figure 8.16. Importance of embedding for sectioning.

Source: https://media.springernature.com/lw685/springer-static/image/chp%3A10.1007%2F978-981-19-6616-3_3/MediaObjects/456657_2_En_3_Fig6_HTML.png.

8.6. Sectioning Methods

Sectioning methods are the cornerstone of tissue sample studies, enabling researchers and clinicians to examine histopathological features with precision. Traditional methods such as paraffin embedding have been employed widely, generating thin, homogeneous sections important for microscopic examination. However, these precise cutting methods have inherent limitations, such as the potential loss of three-dimensional structural details and sample distortion. As an antidote to these constraints, innovations in sectioning techniques have been established, some of which protect tissue architecture. These innovations have had an essential role to play in yielding more discernible and improved-quality histological images from biopsies or surgically resected specimens, ultimately leading to more accurate diagnoses as well as a greater insight into disease mechanisms. This innovation in methods indicates the ongoing need for improvement and advancement in tissue sectioning to deal with the complexities of biological materials. Advances in imaging technology have just begun to facilitate normal sectioning methods, thereby broadening the horizons of tissue analysis. Techniques such as serial optical coherence microscopy (SOCM) allow label-free, high-throughput, and large-volume imaging of *ex vivo* organ structure, importantly in soft tissue that has long been difficult to study. The SOCM method has been very effective in untangling the three-dimensional anatomy of organs such as the mouse brain and kidney, imaging intricate blood vessel networks not achievable by standard sectioning techniques. These advances do not only enhance the visualization of endogenous structures but also allow quantitative assessment of tissue motion without contrast agents, thus preserving sample integrity. This integration of imaging technology with sectioning methods is a significant step toward a more comprehensive means of tissue evaluation, resulting in improved insight into pathological conditions (Azaripour et al., 2020). Besides, the development of intact-tissue techniques has revolutionized the investigation of complex tissue architecture. Traditional thin-section histology is often incapable of visualizing the complex three-dimensional topology in tissues, particularly in samples with irregular or heterogeneous morphology. The biphasic hydrogel technique is an advancement that facilitates high-throughput quantitative volumetric imaging of spatially irregular tissues, enabling in-depth studies of normal and pathological conditions alike. For instance, in research on pancreatic innervation and development, this technique offers particular advantages over standard procedures, as it enables observation of dynamic tissue changes that are critical to understanding disease progression. As more researchers turn towards these new cutting techniques, opportunities for actual applications to clinical studies and diagnostics increase, demonstrating the need for continuous improvement of biological sample preparation processes (Arda et al., 2017).

8.6.1. Microtomy Techniques

Microtomy techniques are a crucial component of the process of tissue processing because they play a major role in preparing thin sections for microscopic examination. Techniques involved in microtomy involve slicing formally prepared tissue samples into ultra-thin sections, either between 3 and 10 micrometers thick. Care in the selection of the proper microtome is essential, since the specific model—rotary, sliding, or cryostat microtomes—is a function of the tissue type sectioned. Soft tissues, for instance, are generally more compliant when sectioned, whereas harder tissues, such as bone, require a special technique for successful maintenance of structural integrity. Good microtomy also relies on the skill of the operator because it is essential that even and constant thickness be achieved for subsequent analysis, e.g., histochemistry or immunohistochemistry, in a way that the process becomes not only technical but an art in histological investigation. Microtomy procedures in hard tissues need additional considerations so that the samples can be processed well without causing any damage. Density and mineral content make hard tissues such as bones and teeth harder to cut naturally. These samples are typically prepared by putting them through decalcification to relax the tissue before cutting, where this is done using acidic solutions such as formic acid or chelating agents such as EDTA. To this end, such treatments stand the risk of destroying tissue structures inadvertently, highlighting the delicacy of work required from histologists. Techniques like the Technovit 9100 embedding method are now in vogue to minimize such damage and enable the preparation of good-quality sections for various histological applications, including enzyme histochemistry and *in situ* hybridization. Thus, the preparation of microtomy techniques ensures the proper preparation of hard tissues for detailed study and makes a significant contribution to research in fields like dental and musculoskeletal. Under current histological protocols, new imaging modalities are enhancing traditional microtomy, particularly for optical imaging. Photoacoustic tomography (PAT) is a prime example of such enhancement, as it provides depth-resolved tissue imaging without extensive sample preparation that deforms cellular architecture. Such a technique takes advantage of the light absorption feature, which predisposes it to be sensitive to biomolecules such as hemoglobin, thus achieving histology-like images from unprocessed samples. As evidenced in recent studies, using methods like UV-PAM, histologists are able to provide multicolored photographs with valuable cellular data required for diagnostic purposes, including surgical margin assessment in oncology. Such technologies not only enhance the microtomy technique itself but also broaden the areas of applications of histological analysis in the clinic, giving us a glimpse of future imaging in which image quality and efficiency are significantly increased, which is key to speeding up biomedical research and clinical diagnosis (Figure 8.17).

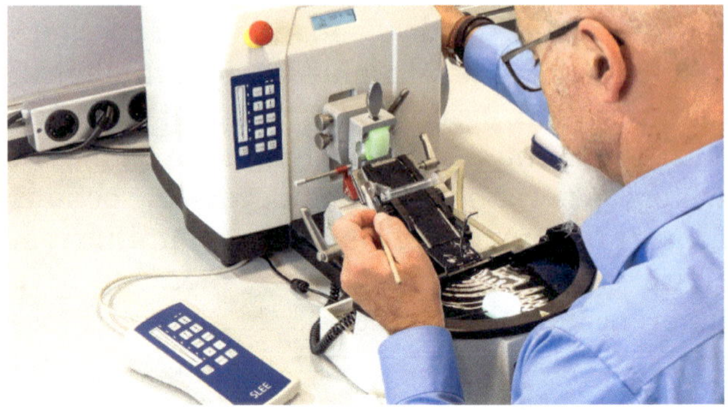

Figure 8.17. Microtomy techniques.

Source: https://www.solmedialtd.com/wp-content/uploads/2021/04/auqatec_detail2.jpg.

8.6.2. Cryosectioning Techniques

Cryosectioning is an important histological method in which tissue samples are rapidly frozen to enable high-quality sectioning without chemical fixation. This method is particularly advantageous when dealing with delicate or antigen-sensitive tissues because it preserves the native architecture of the sample. The cryostat, which is essential to this process, makes the precise cutting of frozen tissue into extremely thin sections that are stainable and observable by microscope possible. Compared to traditional paraffin embedding, which requires longer preparation time and could break down the natural states of certain biomolecules, cryosectioning retains the proteins' natural states, thereby enabling credible immunohistochemical studies. However, issues such as the formation of ice crystals when freezing must be addressed to enhance the quality of histological slides generated, as implied by studies comparing the effectiveness of different modes of freezing on murine colonic tissue (Hughes, 2018). Among the determinants of cryosectioning success is the choice of embedding medium. The

Optimal Cutting Temperature (OCT) medium is commonly used to maintain specimen stability during sectioning, but its selection is also important for ensuring tissue quality. The effectiveness of various freezing processes, i.e., snap freezing and piezoelectric freezing, can deliver alternative results on the structural and cellular information in the resultant sections. In comparative studies, multiple freezing protocols have been used in murine colonic tissues and showed that paraffin embedding gave the optimal quality sections but OCT embedding was not very bad, particularly when stored at sub-zero temperatures (Hughes, 2018). The findings emphasize the importance of optimizing cryosectioning protocols for specific research needs and preserving histological features that are important for proper diagnosis and research. The combining of cryosectioning techniques is not only for general tissue preparation; it also emphasizes the relevance of methodological advances in histopathologic diagnostics and research. Studies have found that morphometric examinations performed on cryosectioned tissue have been able to detect fine features that do not register when other embedding methods are utilized. A demonstration was the use of cryosectioning to examine claw conformations in dairy cows, enabling detailed analysis of vascular changes in hoof anatomy. These analyses enhance not only the understanding of pathological conditions but also agricultural breeding and management. The advances, thus, in the techniques of cryosectioning reflect their applicability and utility in various fields, ranging from veterinary medicine to cancer research, finally linking laboratory findings and clinical applications in tissue analysis and diagnosis.

8.6.3. Factors Influencing Section Thickness

The selection of section thickness during tissue preparation is governed by a combination of interrelated factors, all vital to ensuring the accuracy of the eventual histological images. Of primary consideration is what tissue is being prepared; various tissues possess unique mechanical properties and cellular architectures. For instance, fibrous tissues can require thicker sections to allow for their structural integrity, while softer gelatinous tissues can generally be sectioned thinly without compromising morphology. Additionally, the inherent characteristics of the microtome, such as blade sharpness and angulation, play a significant role in achieving equal thickness. Similarly, as with studies of myocardial infarct morphology, tissue anisotropy at the microscopic scale has a large impact on section quality, and operator expertise and calibration are essential to obtain optimal results (Bluemke et al., 2017). Physical parameters during preparation are also significant to consider, as they can lead to thickness inconsistencies across sections. For instance, the viscosity of embedding mediums will influence tissue behavior with sectioning cutting blades. A medium of higher viscosity may require thicker sections, whereas a lower viscosity may permit finer sectioning. Additionally, the microtome and embedding medium temperatures can cause the tissue to become harder, again influencing sectioning results. The inflammatory response present in other materials, such as poly(L-lactic acid) films, means that similar responses could be initiated during tissue preparation, altering the microstructure and consequently cutting accuracy (Baier et al., 1995). Appropriate environmental condition control is therefore paramount to attain even section thickness. Finally, the interrelationship between section thickness and subsequent histological procedures cannot be emphasized enough. Thinner sections support more effective penetration by the staining solutions, with resultant improved visualization of extracellular and cellular structures. However, excessively thin sections can result in loss of structural detail, particularly in recalcitrant tissues. A compromise must thus be struck that optimizes both analytical utility and histological integrity. The ability to assess tissue orientation and microstructural changes is crucial to understanding disease states, as evidenced by research on myocardial infarction, in which section thickness has been shown to be associated with remodeling in the heart across three dimensions (Bluemke et al., 2017). Ultimately, interaction between the inherent characteristics of the tissue, the strategies for preparation, and the expected analytical requirements guides the best decisions regarding section thickness in the process of tissue preparation and sectioning (Figure 8.18).

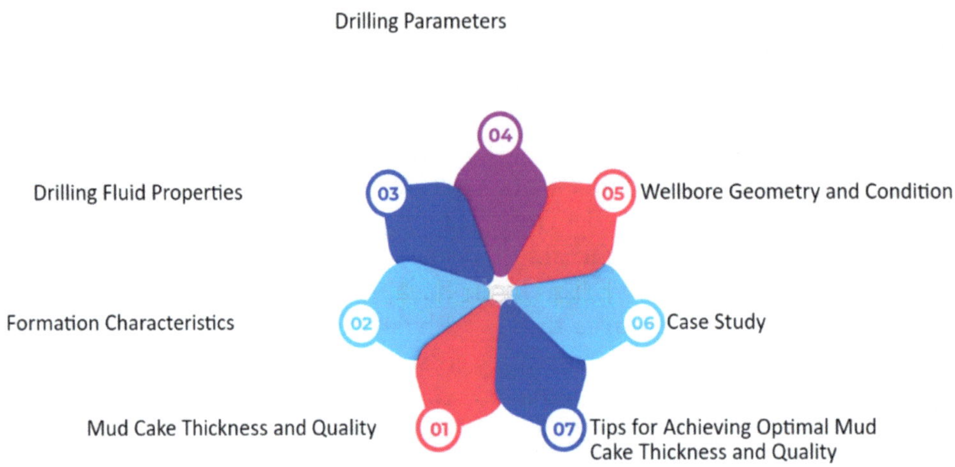

Figure 8.18. Factors influencing section thickness.

Source: https://fastercapital.co/i/Mud-cake-formation--A-Shield-Against-Formation-Damage--Factors-Influencing-Mud-Cake-Thickness-and-Quality.webp.

SUMMARY

Lastly, the intricacies of tissue sectioning and preparation are of utmost importance in expanding the discipline of histology and imparting a lasting effect on diagnostic and research applications. Optimal practices in this regard enable the production of superior-quality sections with morphological and molecular integrity. Attentiveness in the use of precise methodologies not only minimizes artifacts but also maximizes the reproducibility of results between studies. In addition, understanding the limitations and obstacles of various sectioning methods is essential for researchers to confidently and correctly interpret their data. As mentioned, critical thinking in preparation of tissues determines subsequent analysis, such as imaging and molecular methodologies, ultimately leading to better comprehension of complex biological systems. Moreover, the embrace of emerging technologies, such as imaging mass spectrometry (IMS), demonstrates the potential to complement traditional histological techniques. IMS facilitates spatial visualization of tissue section molecular composition and provides insights into diseased and healthy tissue biochemical terrain. Lipid and other biomolecule direct analysis from sections highlights the necessity of preserving sample integrity throughout preparation. Robust protocols that are resistant to degradation are thus essential, especially in multi-institutional collaborative studies, where sample integrity is compromised. The need to develop standardized protocols that consider these variables cannot be overstressed, since it is their role to provide reproducible and credible data under diverse research settings (Allen et al., 2009; Patterson, 2016). Furthermore, as the area of research in tissue preparation continues to advance, the need for continuing education and training of laboratory personnel comes to the forefront. Effective utilization of sophisticated methods is closely related to the performance skills of researchers performing these processes. Training courses to instruct researchers on the nuances of tissue preparation will guarantee that optimal results are achieved. As we conditions, continue to elucidate disease processes through improved histopathological techniques, scientific collaboration, and experience sharing will be essential. Ultimately, the ongoing development of tissue preparation and sectioning techniques has the potential to profoundly improve our capacity to diagnose and study complicated conditions, ultimately narrowing the gap between basic research and clinical practice.

Tissue sectioning and preparation are core procedures of histological studies because it significantly influences the quality of the outcome data. The initial process frequently involves fixation, which preserves cellular integrity and prevents autolysis. Fixatives such as formaldehyde or paraformaldehyde are penetrating agents that stabilize proteins by cross-linking them, making them suitable for detailed microscopic investigation. Inclusion of later in a medium, typically paraffin wax or resin, fixes the tissue and permits the production of ultra-thin sections. Such sections, usually five to ten micrometers thick, are necessary to observe cellular structures at high resolution, thereby enhancing the detectability of alterations that are pathological. The precision during this early stage of tissue preparation cannot be overstressed since minor variations can lead to misinterpretation of histological data, which in turn affects the conclusions of research investigations. Secondly, developments in imaging technology complement traditional sectioning methods, providing greater dimensions to tissue analysis. Techniques such as optical sectioning have changed the landscape of microscopic research by enabling scientists to obtain three-dimensional images without the need for major sectioning. The use of multiphoton microscopy, grounded in diffuser-based temporal focusing, is just one solution to how emerging technologies can facilitate enhanced spatial resolution while maintaining frame rate within reason and being biocompatible with live tissue. These methods preserve the native condition of cellular microenvironments, as well as enabling dynamic observation in real-time, adding richness to histological investigations. The integration of conventional preparation techniques with new imaging modalities indicates a holistic perception of tissue structure, complementing comparative analysis among specimens. With a combination of these effective practices in tissue preparation and cutting, the utility of standard protocols is maximized. For example, the development of a new stereotaxic device providing stunning accuracy for brain placement shows how necessary precision is in performing anatomical studies. By integrating experimental measurements of skull profiles with brains, scientists can be sure that researchers' neurophysiological recordings are correctly pinned to specific brain structures. This device is not species-specific, showing its adaptability for experimental animals. Such developments in stereotaxic procedures in tandem with stringent neuroanatomical processing are reflective of the need for standardized processes as they enable collation and comparability of histological data, thus enhancing rigor and reproducibility of results across studies (Andres et al., 1986; Blake et al., 2011).

A LOOK TO THE FUTURE:

COMPUTER-ASSISTED SURGERY:

Computer-assisted surgery (CAS) represents a transformative shift in surgical practice, blending advanced computing, imaging, and robotic technologies to enhance how procedures are planned and executed. At its core, CAS uses computer systems to guide surgical actions, offering a level of precision and control far beyond traditional manual methods. This integration of technology has helped surgeons visualize complex anatomical structures in three dimensions, simulate procedures in virtual environments, and perform with improved accuracy, ultimately elevating patient outcomes and safety. The roots of CAS trace back to efforts to improve surgical accuracy through better imaging and planning. Early systems focused on diagnostic imaging — such as CT, MRI, and X-rays — to create detailed models of the patient's anatomy. Through data fusion techniques, multiple imaging modalities are combined to generate an integrated 3D dataset that accurately reflects both normal and pathological structures. Surgeons can then manipulate this virtual model to assess risks, optimize surgical paths, and rehearse key steps before entering the operating room.

During the procedure, computer assistance comes in several forms. Navigation systems track surgical instruments in real time and relate their position to the patient's virtual anatomy, similar to a GPS in a car that guides the surgeon along a precise route. Intraoperative imaging — including mobile CT or MRI — updates the surgeon on anatomical changes during surgery, maintaining accuracy even when tissues shift. Robotics can also augment human dexterity; robotic arms controlled by the surgeon execute fine movements with stability and repeatability that surpass human hand-eye coordination alone.

The advantages of computer-assisted surgery are compelling. Enhanced visualization and precise guidance significantly reduce the likelihood of intraoperative complications and improve the surgeon's ability to avoid damage to critical tissues. Minimally invasive techniques enabled by CAS result in smaller incisions, less blood loss, shorter operating times, reduced pain, and faster recoveries for patients. In fields such as orthopedics, neurosurgery, and ENT, CAS has become an indispensable tool, enabling surgeons to perform complex interventions with confidence.

Despite its promise, CAS also poses challenges. High initial costs for equipment and training remain barriers to universal adoption, and the complexity of integration requires significant investment in both infrastructure and personnel education. Yet as technology continues to advance — including augmented reality overlays and AI-assisted systems — computer-assisted surgery stands as a cornerstone of modern surgical innovation, pushing the boundaries of what is possible in patient care.

REFERENCES

1. Persson, D. P., Chen, A., Aarts, M. G., Salt, D. E., Schjoerring, J. K., & Husted, S. (2016). Multi-element bioimaging of Arabidopsis thaliana roots. *PLANT PHYSIOLOGY, 172*(2), pp.00770.2016. https://doi.org/10.1104/pp.16.00770Ahsen, O. O., Brooker, J. S., Cable, A. E., Connolly, J. L., et al. (2014). Assessment of breast pathologies using nonlinear microscopy. https://core.ac.uk/download/78062117.pdf (accessed on 6th August 2025).
2. Albers, J., Alves, F., Dullin, C., Markus, M. A., et al. (2018). X-ray based virtual histology allows guided sectioning of heavy ion stained murine lungs for histological analysis.
3. Allegrini Junior, S., Coelho, P. G., Konig Jr, B., Martins, G., et al. (2011). Identification of the nuclear factor kappa-beta (NF-kB) in cortical of mice Wistar using Technovit 7200 VCR. https://core.ac.uk/download/84751677.pdf (accessed on 6th August 2025).
4. Allen, B., Duignan, P., Graf, J., Gurevich, M., Hohn, A. A., et al. (2009). Comparison of two histological techniques for age determination in small cetaceans. https://core.ac.uk/download/2797176.pdf (accessed on 6th August 2025).
5. Andres, B., Bock, G., Bures, Z., De Valois, W., Schuller, G., Betz, M., et al. (1986). A stereotaxic method for small animals using experimentally determined reference profiles. https://core.ac.uk/download/12164086.pdf (accessed on 6th August 2025).
6. Arda, H. E., Burns, V. M., Chakravarthy, H., Charville, G. W., et al. (2017). Pathways to clinical CLARITY: Volumetric analysis of irregular, soft, and heterogeneous tissues in development and disease. https://core.ac.uk/download/129069108.pdf (accessed on 6th August 2025).
7. Auvinen, E. (2023). *Manual for hard tissue research laboratory: Hard tissue sectioning*. https://core.ac.uk/download/571678705.pdf (accessed on 6th August 2025).
8. Azaripour, A., Garcia-Sanz, A., Li, A., Eddy, A. A., Ucero, A. C., Schain, A. J., Gillett, C., et al. (2020). Serial optical coherence microscopy for label-free volumetric histopathology. https://core.ac.uk/download/323383992.pdf (accessed on 6th August 2025).
9. Baier, M., Barbe, C., Blaauw, B., Black, M. T., Busscher, H. J., Cameron, A. B., et al. (1995). The influence of surface morphology and wettability on the inflammatory response against poly(L-lactic acid): A semi-quantitative study with monoclonal antibodies. https://core.ac.uk/download/pdf/11474688.pdf (accessed on 6th August 2025).
10. Bargiacchi, L., Bortul, M., Burlizzi, S., Cataliotti, L., et al. (2021). Pre-analytics, a national survey of Senonetwork Italia breast centers: Much still to do ahead. https://core.ac.uk/download/566469359.pdf (accessed on 6th August 2025).
11. Baskin, L., Calvert, M., Cao, M., Cunha, G. R., et al. (2020). Imaging the developing human external and internal urogenital organs with light sheet fluorescence microscopy. https://core.ac.uk/download/323311359.pdf (accessed on 6th August 2025).
12. Benjakul, N., Nonsiri, P., Onkaew, S., Srivilai, W., et al. (2019). The effectiveness of using dye models for small tissue biopsies in the surgical pathology laboratory. https://core.ac.uk/download/568065794.pdf (accessed on 6th August 2025).
13. Bishop, J., Borowsky, A. D., Demos, S. G., Fereidouni, F., et al. (2017). Microscopy with ultraviolet surface excitation for rapid slide-free histology. https://core.ac.uk/download/323068262.pdf (accessed on 6th August 2025).

14. Blake, G. A., Chen, Y., Guo, C.-L., Holland, E. C., et al. (2011). Wide-field optical sectioning for live-tissue imaging by plane-projection multiphoton microscopy. https://core.ac.uk/download/4893263.pdf (accessed on 6th August 2025).

15. Bluemke, D. A., Gai, N., Halperin, H., Herzka, D. A., et al. (2017). Submillimeter diffusion tensor imaging and late gadolinium enhancement cardiovascular magnetic resonance of chronic myocardial infarction. https://core.ac.uk/download/323064815.pdf (accessed on 6th August 2025).

16. Bouajjani, A., Steffen, B., Emerson, E. A., Esparza, J., Burkart, O., et al. (2001). Computed microtomography visualization and quantification of mouse ischemic brain lesion by nonionic radio contrast agents. https://core.ac.uk/download/pdf/17339118.pdf (accessed on 6th August 2025).

17. Chisholm, A. D., Holmyard, D., Meirovitch, Y., Mitchell, K., et al. (2018). A pipeline for volume electron microscopy of the *Caenorhabditis elegans* nervous system. https://core.ac.uk/download/323065107.pdf (accessed on 6th August 2025).

18. Cinci, L., Costantini, I., Franceschini, A., Laurino, A., Mazzamuto, G., Montalbano, A., Nesi, G., et al. (2023). A guide to perform 3D histology of biological tissues with fluorescence microscopy. https://core.ac.uk/download/576923411.pdf (accessed on 6th August 2025).

19. Clemente, M. P., Lage, A., Oliveira, L., Tuchin, V. V., et al. (2010). Rat muscle opacity decrease due to the osmosis of a simple mixture. https://core.ac.uk/download/47142091.pdf (accessed on 6th August 2025).

20. Crawley, M., Forbes, G., Mulhern, D. M., Nelson, R., Stout, S. (2016). Decision tree analysis as a supplementary tool to enhance histomorphological differentiation when distinguishing human from non-human cranial bone in bothz burnt and unburnt states: A feasibility study. https://core.ac.uk/download/42137084.pdf (accessed on 6th August 2025).

21. Dumančić, E., Fulgosi, H., Vojta, L. (2023). Beginners guide to sample preparation techniques for transmission electron microscopy. https://core.ac.uk/download/590723716.pdf (accessed on 6th August 2025).

22. González Arjona, M., Muñoz Barrutia, M. A., Ortega Gil, A., Rullas, J., et al. (2019). X-ray-based virtual slicing of TB-infected lungs. https://corzze.ac.uk/download/288501927.pdf (accessed on 6th August 2025).

23. Hayter, S. M. (2007). *Improving genetic profiling techniques for low copy number DNA* (Master's thesis). https://core.ac.uk/download/84407188.pdf (accessed on 6th August 2025).

24. Howard, D. W., Keller, B. J., Lewis, E. J., Smith, S. A., et al. (2004). *Histological techniques for marine bivalve mollusks and crustaceans* (2nd ed.). https://core.ac.uk/download/19793342.pdf (accessed on 6th August 2025).

25. Hughes, J. (2018). Comparison of varying tissue freezing methods on murine colonic tissue. https://core.ac.uk/download/158200230.pdf (accessed on 6th August 2025).

26. Kurniawati, I. D., Setyawan, P., Wijayanti, G. E. (2017). A simple paraffin embedded protocol for fish egg, embryo, and larvae. https://core.ac.uk/download/268410666.pdf (accessed on 6th August 2025).

27. Laven, L. J. (2014). *Anatomical studies of claw conformation in New Zealand dairy cattle* (Doctoral dissertation, Massey University). https://core.ac.uk/download/162617331.pdf (accessed on 6th August 2025).

28. Majdani, O., Lenarz, T., Rau, T. S., Würfel, W. (2013). Three-dimensional histological specimen preparation for accurate imaging and spatial reconstruction of the middle and inner ear. https://core.ac.uk/download/pdf/81268781.pdf (accessed on 6th August 2025).
29. Patterson, N. H. (2016). *Development of imaging mass spectrometry analysis of lipids in biological and clinically relevant applications.* https://core.ac.uk/download/151555215.pdf (accessed on 6th August 2025).
30. Wong, T. W. (2018). *Developing photoacoustic tomography devices for translational medicine and basic science research.* https://core.ac.uk/download/233214849.pdf (accessed on 6th August 2025).

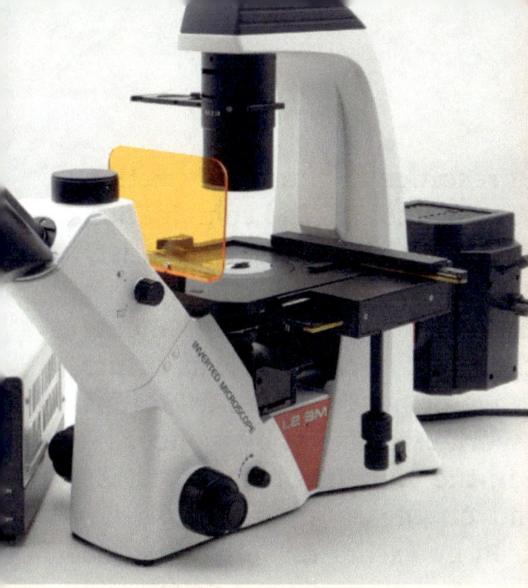

Chapter 9

HISTOCHEMICAL AND CYTOCHEMICAL TECHNIQUES

Contents

Introduction

Histochemistry and cytochemistry are critical techniques for investigating cellular structures and biochemical processes. They enable scientists to visualize and define cellular components at histological levels with information about normal physiology and also disease states. Histochemistry employs chemical staining techniques that enable the identification of specific molecules, i.e., proteins, lipids, and carbohydrates, in tissue samples. Concurrently, cytochemistry is even more specialized in the chemical content of cells, enabling the study of cellular components with the aid of a series of staining procedures. Combined, these methods constitute an effective set of instruments indispensable for cellular and molecular biology and make important contributions to the progress of diagnostics, therapeutics, and basic research. In this regard, new approaches have become eminent, utilizing molecular methods that improve the accuracy of cellular characterization. *In situ* DNA synthesis primed (PRINS), for instance, has emerged as a leading method of DNA sequence study at the chromosomal level. By detecting specific genetic elements, PRINS is complemented by standard fluorescence in situ hybridization (FISH) techniques, which are more specific and exhibit less nonspecific binding. The combination of such molecular processes with histochemical approaches has revolutionized the way scientists approach cell studies. For example, the detection and visualization of telomere sequences using the commercial PRINS kit not only underscores the importance of accurate genetic assessments but also the continuous development in the field of histochemistry and cytochemistry, as in the applications spanning disparate organisms. Moreover, the importance of historical contributions to these techniques cannot be raised high enough. The pioneering work established by pioneering researchers set the ground for the advanced methodologies used in the contemporary world. As the discipline progresses, as explicated, today's researchers stand on the shoulders of giants, leveraging the extensive literature and experimental methods devised by earlier researchers. This heritage establishes a scientific inquiry and progress culture, where new methods are developed from existing concepts. Moreover, journals such as Histochemistry and Cell Biology are significant in facilitating the high quality and integrity of such advancements. The interplay between history and modern approaches underscores the significance of continuous learning and integration of new approaches in histochemical and cytochemical research, eventually enhancing our understanding of cellular biology (Figure 9.1).

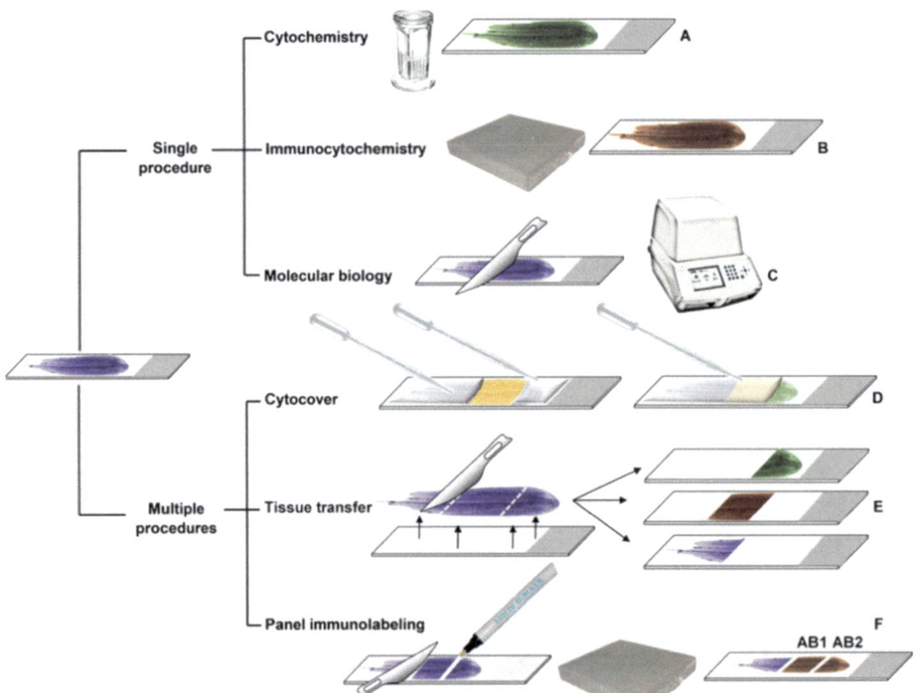

Figure 9.1. Histochemical and cytochemical techniques.

Source: https://www.researchgate.net/profile/Ricardo-Marcos/publication/361405301/figure/fig1/AS:11431281360881912@1744096204493/Schematic-overview-of-the-multiple-uses-of-a-cytologic-smear-Single-procedure-refers-to.png.

Definition of Histochemistry and Cytochemistry

Histochemistry and cytochemistry are allied disciplines that analyze the chemical composition of tissues and cells, respectively. Through the usage of chemical reactions in the identification and localization of various biological macromolecules within tissue sections, scientists can ascertain cellular composition and function on a molecular level. Conversely, cytochemistry is especially concerned with the chemical processes in cells, employing techniques that define specific constituents, such as enzymes and proteins. Through the application of different staining techniques and probes, scientists can see minute details of cellular structure and metabolism, and gain insight into physiological processes and disease conditions. Both fields end up giving essential information that aids in informing understanding of biological systems, enhancing our understanding of how cells operate in tissues and organisms. The relationship between histochemistry and cytochemistry is exemplified in the diverse methodological approaches, which allow for a comprehensive investigation of tissue and cell architecture.

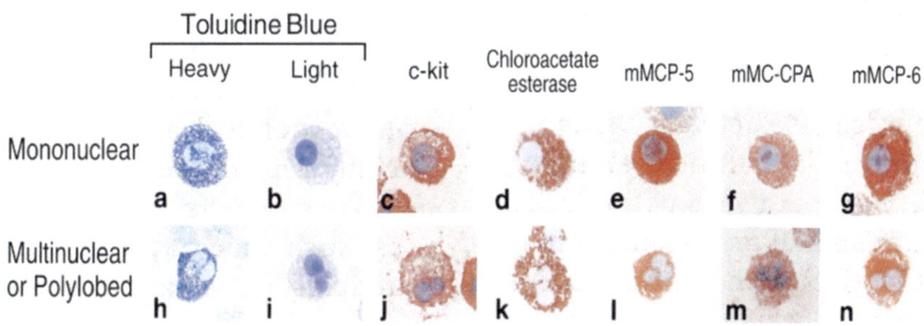

Figure 9.2. Histochemistry and cytochemistry.

Source: https://www.researchgate.net/profile/Richard-Stevens-12/publication/14010868/figure/fig1/AS:499915483566080@1496200547249/Histochemistry-enzyme-cytochemistry-and-immunohistochemistry-of-cells-in-4-week.png.

For instance, employing histochemical staining techniques, researchers can determine the presence and location of specific enzymes or substrates in cells. Techniques such as the use of naphthol AS D acetate for visualization of non-specific esterases fall into this category, since it gives us essential information about the activity and localization of the enzyme in tissues like roots of *Vicia faba* (James, 1974). Quantitatively, analysis from these staining techniques also helps us to know more about cellular dynamics, for example, measuring enzyme kinetic parameters in relation to specific stages in development during plant ripening. This juxtaposition of methodologies underscores the complementary role of both disciplines in describing the biochemical landscape of cells and tissues in health and disease. Methodological advances in histochemical and cytochemical techniques have greatly enhanced our understanding of cellular behavior, particularly when combined with imaging tools such as electron microscopy. A variety of electron microscopy methods, including scanning electron microscopy (SEM) and transmission electron microscopy (TEM), provide high-resolution images of cellular structures and their interactions at the molecular level. Such imaging augments histochemical analysis by allowing researchers to correlate biochemical findings with ultrastructural observations. For example, histochemical staining to uncover extractives during mechanical and kraft pulping of wood fibers demonstrates the value of integrating biochemical and structural information (Fernando., 2007). Integrative techniques such as these not only enhance our knowledge of plant biology but also facilitate easier exploration of applications in biotechnology and materials science, making the value of histochemistry and cytochemistry extend to other areas of research (Figure 9.2).

Importance of These Techniques in Biological Research

The significance of histochemical and cytochemical procedures in biological science is underscored by their ability to introduce fine information on cellular structures and functions. The procedures allow scientists to view specific macromolecules within the cellular matrix, which is significant in identifying intricate biological processes. For instance, histochemical stains can selectively visualize proteins, carbohydrates, and lipids, enabling one to chart biochemical pathways within cells. Furthermore, cellular spatial arrangement may demarcate structure-function relationships and therefore elucidate disease pathology and developmental biology. Such a level of specificity is very useful in fields like plant biology, in which differential characteristics of tissues may give critical information in terms of physiological processes and adaptation to survive in different environmental conditions. Also, the application of new histochemical dyes and cytochemical techniques further clarifies enzymatic activity in cells. Thus, for example, studies that have examined acid hydrolases involved in plant cell division and differentiation have applied these methods to yield information on their temporal and spatial distributions in developing tissues. Such results are one illustration of the potential of statistical treatment of histochemical information to elucidate significant enzymic roles in plant growth and development, for instance, the involvement of non-specific esterases in senescence and ripening of fruit (James, 1974). Such results not only contribute to fundamental biological knowledge but also have practical implications for agricultural treatments and the improvement of crop yields. By these techniques, researchers are able to measure enzymatic activity change, which may have implications for maximizing fruit quality and shelf life. The use of cytochemical analysis, that is, electron microscopic techniques, once again shows the importance of such methods in biological research. Techniques such as transmission and scanning electron microscopy provide high-resolution images of cellular ultrastructure, revealing the microscopic details of cell wall morphology, organelle morphology, and the distribution of components such as lignin and glucomannan in wood fibers (Fernando., 2007). Such structural information can be utilized to control industrial processes, particularly in pulp and paper manufacture, where fiber morphology integrity is critical. Therefore, the combined use of histochemical and cytochemical techniques not only deepens our knowledge of cell functions but also supports accelerating biotechnological uses, such that outcomes of research become practically relevant and applicable to both academia and industry.

9.1. Historical Background

The development of histochemical and cytochemical methods has deep roots in the history of cellular biology and microscopy. First, during the late 19th century, scientists began to use staining methods to distinguish cellular elements, resulting in the classification of different tissues on the basis of their biochemical characteristics. Techniques such as the *Feulgen* reaction set the stage for DNA quantification in cell nuclei, which would become significant in cell physiology and pathology. Such progress was demonstrated in studies like that on the effects of adrenocorticotropin (ACTH) on adrenal nuclear DNA content, where cytophotometry had shown significant increases in nuclear DNA after prolonged ACTH treatment, demonstrating the utility of histochemical techniques to expose cell physiological changes (Burns, 1957). Mid-20th-century enzyme histochemistry advancements were a landmark in the visualization and quantification of metabolic processes at the cellular level. These techniques enabled enzyme activity staining of tissues, and an enhanced understanding of cellular metabolism and disease ensued. A pioneering study compared skeletal muscle biopsies and enzyme characteristics of various organs' tissues and demonstrated how intricate the interactions were between enzyme activity and disease states.

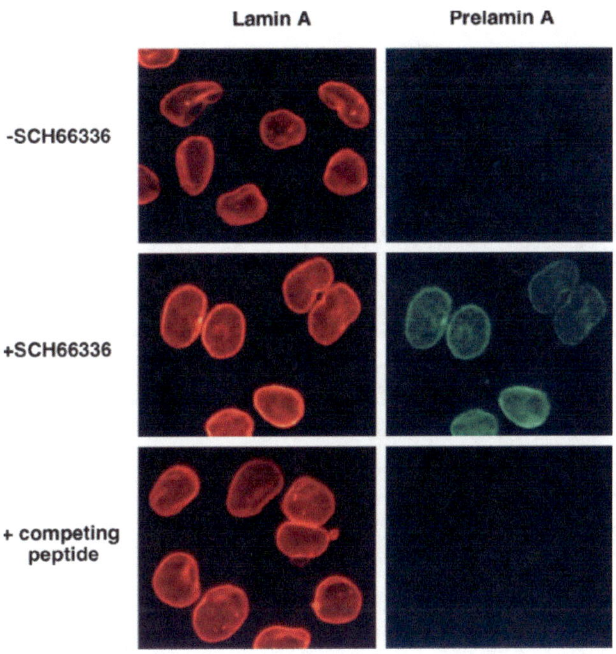

Figure 9.3. The development of histochemical and cytochemical techniques.

Source: https://duckduckgo.com/?q=development+of+histochemical+and+cytochemical+techniques+&t=h_&iar=images&iaf=size%3ALarge&iai=https%3A%2F%2Fwww.researchgate.net%2Fprofile%2FPaul-Kirschmeier%2Fpublication%2F12550721%2Ffigure%2Ffig3%2FAS%3A281710869663746%401444176513349%2FDevelopment-of-a-histochemical-assay-for-prelamin-A-A549-cells-treated-with-diluent.png.

By comparing enzyme activity across various tissues and health statuses, researchers were better placed to tackle metabolic diseases and the physiological roles of specific enzymes using enzyme histochemistry as a crucial analytical tool (Elias et al., 1988). These findings have profound implications both in basic research and in clinical diagnosis. The evolution of these techniques reflects not only advances in technology but also a growing understanding of the cellular environment. As an example, the correlation of enzyme activity with the histochemical investigation paves the way towards the investigation of pathologies in multidimensional terms that directly translates to directed therapeutic interventions. With continuous developments in contemporary histochemical techniques, more emphasis is now put upon the understanding of the interaction between cellular components, enzyme activity, and gene expression, paving the way for an era of precision medicine. Hence, the background to histochemical and cytochemical methods is proof of how they remain relevant and applicable to enhancing our understanding of biological processes and illness (Elias et al., 1988) (Figure 9.3).

9.1.1. Development of Histochemical Techniques

The development of histochemical techniques is a milestone in biological science, particularly in the investigation of cellular structure and function. Histochemistry, or the technique of localization of chemical components in tissues by specific staining or reactions, traces its beginnings to early cellular morphological investigations. Advancements in microscopy during the late 19th and early 20th centuries fueled this growth, enabling scientists to visualize cellular components at an unprecedented resolution. Early pioneers, such as Paul Ehrlich and Santiago Ramón y Cajal, developed staining methods that laid the groundwork for modern histochemistry. These foundational techniques facilitated the visualization of cells and tissues, establishing histochemistry as an indispensable tool for pathologists and researchers alike. With the advancement of science, the fusion of the older staining methods with novel technologies produced ever more sophisticated histochemical methodologies. The invention of fluorescence histochemistry allowed researchers to identify specific cellular structures with greater sensitivity and specificity. This was particularly important in cancer biology, in which discrimination of tumor from normal cells is still critical to diagnosis and treatment. For instance, fluorescence *in situ* hybridization (FISH) research has provided complex chromosomal aberrations in various cancers, underlining the importance of precise genetic material localization.

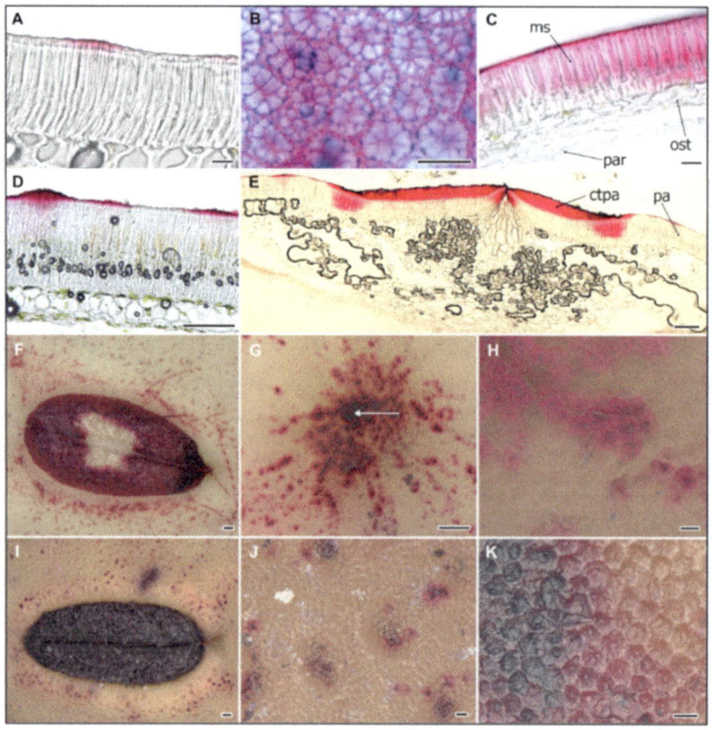

Figure 9.4. Development of histochemical techniques.

Source: https://www.mdpi.com/ijms/ijms-22-04602/article_deploy/html/images/ijms-22-04602-g005.png.

One notable thyroid cancer study, for instance, used fluorescence methods to assess karyotype abnormalities and identify unbalanced translocations, highlighting how histochemical advances have significantly contributed to our understanding of cancer biology and the genetic processes of tumorigenesis (Baumgartner et al., 2009). The ongoing development of histochemical procedures continues to push the boundaries of what is achievable in cellular and molecular biological research. Advanced technologies, such as multiplex staining techniques, are able to visualize several cellular markers simultaneously, thus providing a clearer view of the cellular landscape. These technologies play a crucial role in distinguishing complex biological processes and diseases because they enable researchers to investigate cell signaling pathways as well as their interactions with the tissue microenvironment. Moreover, histochemistry-derived methods increasingly find their application in clinical practice, enhancing the diagnostic potential, particularly in reproductive medicine, where preimplantation genetic diagnosis (PGD) can benefit from histochemical treatment. As attested by recent efforts to standardize DNA probe preparation for translocation carriers in IVF, the inclusion of histochemical techniques into clinical schemes offers promising avenues for patient treatment development (Baumgartner et al., 2009). Thus, the development of histochemical techniques not only deepens our understanding of cell dynamics but also paves the way for advances in medical diagnosis and therapy (Figure 9.4).

9.1.2. Key Figures in the Advancement of Cytochemistry

The development of cytochemistry has been influenced by several key figures whose contributions have shaped the field over time. Some of the most well-known researchers include Paul Ehrlich and Robert Koch, who contributed significantly to the early development of histochemical techniques, particularly through their use of staining techniques to examine cellular components. Ehrlich, being the originator of colored dye work, initiated the use of stains towards cell-type-specific differentiation, which served as a foundation for subsequent cytochemical developments later on. This pursuit of cellular identification has also led to contemporary techniques that facilitate detailed analysis of cellular structure and function. As cytochemistry evolved, advances in technology were incorporated, resulting in techniques that have enhanced the specificity and sensitivity of cellular studies. These foundational contributions from its early stages continue to influence current practices in histochemistry and cytochemistry. After the pioneering efforts, subsequent improvements in microscopy and staining techniques expanded the field of cytochemistry. Great scientists, such as George Palade, initiated the use of electron microscopy, through which cellular structures could be studied at unprecedented resolution levels. His work deciphered the minute morphology of cellular structures and organelle configurations, emphasizing the value of ultrastructural analysis in understanding cellular function. The introduction of innovative staining techniques, followed by laboratory automation, introduced further radical transformations into the field of cytochemical analysis. Such methods as fluorescent probes and multiplex staining methods, developed by other scientists, have enabled one to see more than one aspect of a cell simultaneously. These methods not only generate a greater understanding of cellular variety but also elevate the diagnostic potential of histological examination in the medical field, illustrating how their work advanced the science into the next stage of inquiry.

Furthermore, the development of correlative methods evidenced a significant breakthrough in the capabilities of cytochemical analysis. Among the major developments, for instance, those involving researchers employing correlative light-electron microscopy (CLEM), were the union of different imaging modalities for a comprehensive insight into cell processes. By combining immunostaining for specific biological molecules with ultrastructural imaging, CLEM has allowed investigators to study the same cells at both light and electron microscopy resolution, gaining a more nuanced understanding of cellular interactions and dynamics. Another major breakthrough within the field has been delivered by serial block-face imaging with scanning electron microscopy (SBF-SEM), which now allows large-scale 3D reconstruction of cellular anatomy. These methods not only enhance our understanding of basic cellular processes but also demonstrate the significant impact influential cytochemists have had on broadening the scope of histochemical methods to ultimately augment the scientific community's understanding of cellular biology and pathology, such as with advanced methods (Fernando., 2007; Saitoh, 2018) (Figure 9.5).

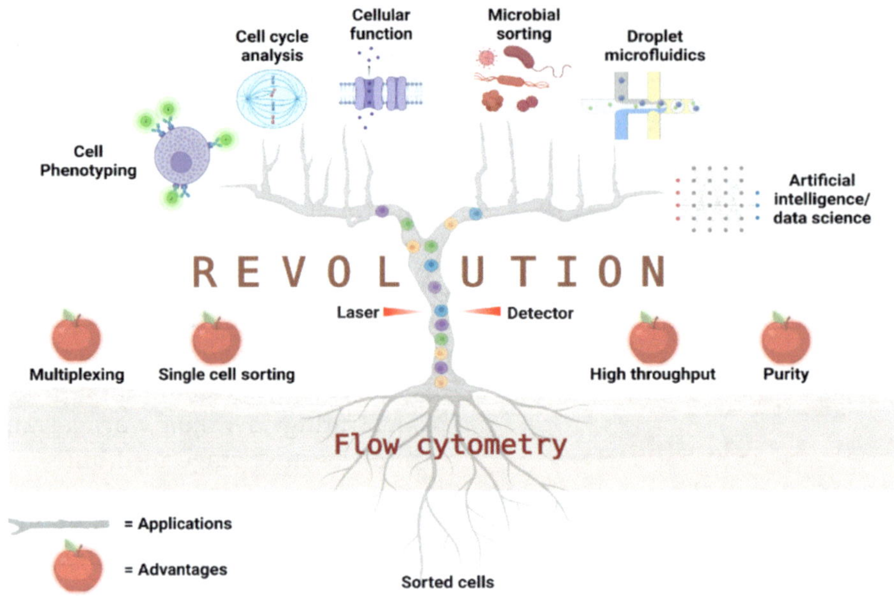

Figure 9.5. Key figures in the advancement of cytochemistry.

Source: https://pub.mdpi-res.com/cells/cells-12-01875/article_deploy/html/images/cells-12-01875-ag.png?1689648440.

9.1.3. Evolution of Methodologies Over Time

Methodological changes between histochemistry and cytochemistry mirror a broader trend of technological and conceptual evolution in the life sciences. Early techniques were based primarily on stain-based methods that allowed overall visual discrimination among cell components. Improved staining methods, coupled with evolving microscopy technology, increased the capacity to assess cell structure and function. This initial work paved the way for more sophisticated methodologies that would enable scientists to dissect cellular processes at the level of the molecule. When scientists tried to define the biochemical background of disease, the need for greater resolution and specificity was fulfilled and led to the development of methodologies encompassing immunocytochemistry and *in situ* hybridization. The invention of newer imaging technologies has revolutionized the field of histochemical and cytochemical techniques, paving the way for hitherto unprecedented insights into cellular dynamics. Scanning electron microscopy (SEM) has begun making inroads into histopathological investigation, providing three-dimensional views of tissue architecture not previously attainable with traditional instruments. Our own experience with the application of scanning electron microscopy in cardiology, gastroenterology, and ophthalmology is described. SEM has yet to contribute significantly to myocardium pathology. Nevertheless, in the short term, SEM could be a harmless means of supplementing information from alternative sources. In the case of atherosclerosis, SEM allowed us to have a better look at the initial stages of the disease; certain pathological details, not always disclosed by ordinary morphological studies, can be communicated (Laschi et al., 1987). In addition, the integration of molecular techniques with traditional histochemistry has enabled a comprehensive understanding of cell interactions and disease pathogenesis. The convergence of immunocytochemistry with SEM is another example of this widening, wherein certain cell populations and their functional state are being identified in hematologic disorders. With technology advancing further, interaction between imaging techniques and biochemical techniques provides a more integrated approach to pathological processes. Consistent and simultaneous correlations with other techniques for SEM are needed in fine-tuning our understanding of morphological research to ultimately enhance diagnostic specificity and therapeutic usefulness. Therefore, the development of the methodologies over the years is a collective endeavor to harness technological progress while addressing complex biological issues in histochemistry and cytochemistry.

9.2. Basic Principles of Histochemistry

Histochemistry is a fundamental technique that fills the gap between biochemical reactions and structural biology in cells. By using various techniques of staining, researchers are able to observe specific components of cells and be aware of their biochemical characteristics. The principles that are involved here are the selective binding of dyes to specific cellular constituents based on their chemical nature and spatial organization. For instance, different dyes stain proteins, nucleic acids, or carbohydrates, and then this provides information on cellular function and pathology. It is a targeted method that allows detailed examination of tissue samples to identify better histological features and the biochemical processes influencing cellular action in health and disease. In describing the chemical nature of tissue constituents, histochemistry is a very helpful tool in diagnostic and research laboratories when contrasting conditions. As the field of histochemistry has developed, there have been numerous techniques developed for enhancing the specificity and resolution of staining procedures. Histochemical techniques such as hematoxylin and eosin (H&E) are conventional ones, and they are rudimentary techniques that provide first-hand information about tissue architecture and cell morphology. More advanced techniques, however, such as immunohistochemistry, utilize antibodies to specifically bind to proteins of the cell milieu and thus offer exquisite specificity and sensitivity. Synergy with molecular techniques has further enhanced the development of histochemistry, enabling scientists to map the localization of biomarkers in tissues. In particular, studies employing electron microscopy have made ultrastructural data of paramount significance for the understanding of tissue morphology and function (Fernando., 2007). With further development of these methods, histochemists have improved capabilities to achieve increased diagnostic specificity and develop therapeutic approaches that are targeted against the individual cellular profiles. Historical context is of paramount significance in discussing the evolution of histochemical techniques. The early foundational work of trailblazing scientists provided the background for existing techniques and our knowledge of cellular biology today. As the historiographical account of the field points out, numerous contemporary methods rely on the successful collaborations and findings of previous researchers (Koji et al., 2019). Acknowledgment of the historiographical progression lineage not only respects these scientific predecessors but also highlights the cooperative nature of scientific advancement. In this way, contemporary histochemistry represents both the culmination of what has come before and the launchpad for what lies ahead. Having an understanding of histochemistry's past developments, current researchers are more likely to appreciate the complexities of histochemical analysis, in turn making them more efficient at employing these techniques in answering modern biological issues.

9.2.1. Types of Staining Techniques

Understanding the various staining methods is important in cytochemistry and histochemistry, since the methods facilitate the visibility of cell structures and components. One such widely used method is the hematoxylin and eosin (H&E) stain, which facilitates differentiation of cellular morphology. Hematoxylin stains nuclei deep blue, and eosin stains the cytoplasm pink, creating a dramatic contrast that allows for detailed examination of tissue architecture. These stains are vital in disease diagnosis, particularly for conditions like cancer, because they highlight specific cell structures. Some other staining techniques, including the methylene blue stain, can also be applied to nucleic acid and cell activity visualization, making detection by researchers and medical practitioners easier in pathological analysis. Another key category of staining techniques is immunohistochemistry (IHC), which involves the use of antibodies to identify specific antigens in cellular samples. IHC is particularly valuable in the medical sector for the detection of tumor markers, allowing for personalized therapeutic strategies in oncology. IHC employs chromogenic substrates that yield colorimetric responses in the tissue sections and, hence, allow for visualization of target antigens. In addition, fluorescent labeling is usually combined with IHC to offer a better insight into molecular interactions within cells. The application of these methods has increased with their integration, extending the use of histochemical techniques to provide insights into cellular processes and the effects of different treatments on tissue samples. Through the rich spatial context, IHC is an effective tool for studying disease mechanisms at the cellular level. Besides the common staining methods, newer staining procedures, such as electron microscopy staining, provide a more definitive view, which is necessary for viewing subcellular structures. Techniques such as transmission electron microscopy (TEM) use heavy metal stains to penetrate biological samples, yielding high-resolution images of macromolecules and organelles. This approach has been a key factor in the identification of ultrastructural differences between normal and disease tissues, particularly in cancer research, where the cell membranes and intracellular organelles may have altered structure. Electron cytochemical techniques, however, allow localization of enzymatic activities within cells, providing information regarding the functional state of cellular constituents. The employment of these newer staining techniques in histochemical and cytochemical studies improves our understanding of the cellular structure and function, ultimately culminating in the development of therapeutic regimes and diagnostic tools (Koshiba, 1968; Fernando., 2007) (Figure 9.6).

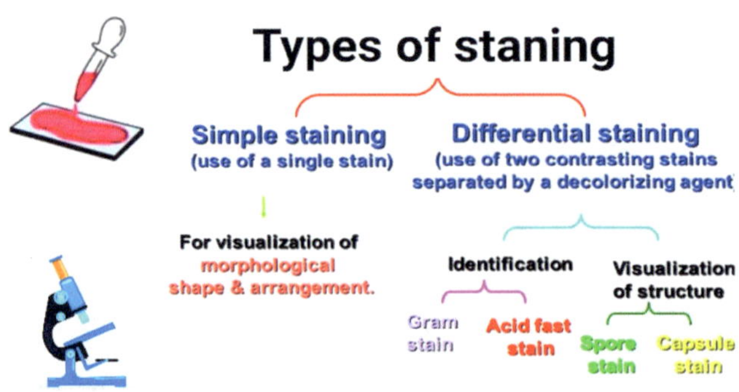

Figure 9.6. Types of staining techniques.

Source: https://i.ytimg.com/vi/85KBu1RLRxQ/maxresdefault.jpg.

9.2.2. Mechanisms of Chemical Reactions in Tissues

The intricate mechanisms of chemical reactions in living tissues form the essence of their functional nature and pathological condition. The reactions offer the required processes, such as cellular communication, metabolism, and tissue repair, which are attained through specific biochemical interactions and pathways. Histochemical and cytochemical techniques form crucial means of visualizing and exploring these reactions, allowing researchers to uncover the underlying molecular dynamics that govern tissue behavior. For instance, histochemical staining can identify particular proteins or metabolites that indicate cellular responses to stimuli, showing how chemical reactions can influence cell function and tissue integrity. It is important in achieving such knowledge for unravelling the processes of disease states, where misdirected chemical processes are the rule. Unraveling chemical interactions in tissues is also important in designing therapeutic interventions. The control of cytokine signaling by proteins such as suppressor of cytokine signaling 1 (SOCS1) is a classic case of the need for chemical mechanisms in disease and health. SOCS1 functions as a key controller of the TLR4-NFκB pathway that plays a role in immune responses and inflammatory processes. In the science of carcinogenesis, as has been studied with research in carcinoma of the larynx, the intersection of signaling pathways and tissue cell makeup is one such example of the complex nature of chemical reactions at the cellular level (Bryś et al., 2010). By utilizing cytochemical techniques to assess the expression of molecules of utmost importance within these signaling pathways, researchers are able to gain an understanding of tumor biology and microenvironment interaction that affects disease development. Besides, advancements in electron microscopy have demonstrated comprehensive information about the ultrastructure of various tissues and enlightened the physical aspect of chemical reactions. One such method is transmission electron microscopy (TEM), which enables researchers to investigate the morphology and topochemistry of cell components and comprehend how structural details affect chemical interactions between tissues. For example, studies on wood fibers in mechanical pulping processes revealed that structural changes, as seen by TEM, are found to be associated with fiber properties and performance (Fernando., 2007). This study points to the importance of understanding the physical and chemical environment in tissues, since the ultrastructural integrity correlates with the efficiency of biochemical reactions. Thus, the combination of histochemical and cytochemical procedures with electron microscopy enhances our knowledge of tissue function and the chemical processes underlying biological activity and enables us to devise more effective therapeutic measures (Figure 9.7).

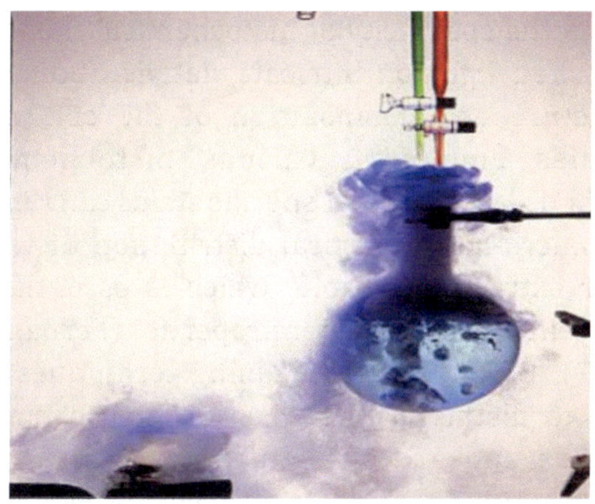

Figure 9.7. Mechanisms of chemical reactions in tissues.

Source: https://image2.slideserve.com/5118920/slide1-l.jpg.

9.2.3. Importance of Specificity in Histochemical Methods

Specificity of histochemical techniques plays a crucial role in ensuring meaningful and accurate outcomes in tissue examination. The methods entail specific interaction of biological molecules with reagents or stains that are meant to be visualized for the visualization of cellular components. The process is highly specific since background staining is minimized, thus allowing the structures of interest to stand out. For instance, impurities in contaminant contaminations within stain solutions may lead to nonspecific binding that compromises the interpretability of results. Processes using the Feulgen reaction, for example, require precision to detect differences in deoxyribonucleic acid (DNA) composition in nuclear cells, meaning specificity is necessary to provide accurate quantification.

Furthermore, specificity allows scientists to derive strong correlations between histochemical results and biological functions, hence obtaining better insights into tissue functions as well as pathologies. In the case of materials like wood, the specificity of histochemical methods can shed light on intricate details about the structure and composition of the cell wall. Studies employing various histochemical methods indicated that specific stains can render the micro-morphological distribution of wood fiber extractives visible, which is essential in assessing pulp and paper properties (Fernando., 2007). Better specific staining techniques are able to distinguish between existing chemical species and are of significant value in our understanding of their processing behavior and physical characteristics. Not only does such specificity aid in distinguishing among different wood species, but it also provides valuable knowledge regarding their processing behaviors. Better specificity of histochemical investigations, thus, encourages a more subtle and precise understanding of materials' physiological and biochemical properties. Furthermore, the specificity of histochemical procedures also plays a significant role in the implications for the reproducibility of results under varying experimental conditions. Variability in staining methods can result in great error if not kept under control, as seen in cytochemical investigations where comparison among various slides may yield erroneous conclusions (Burns, 1957). The only quality required is specificity, which ensures that the conclusions made from histochemical investigations are true and can be used as a basis for further research by scientists with added faith. Reproducibility is especially crucial in fields highly reliant on histochemical techniques for therapy evaluations or diagnostic purposes, where accurate cell-type identification and its respective status may influence treatment regimens. Lastly, specificity not only enhances the detail and accuracy of histochemical methods but also makes the foundation on which further research is conducted stronger (Figure 9.8).

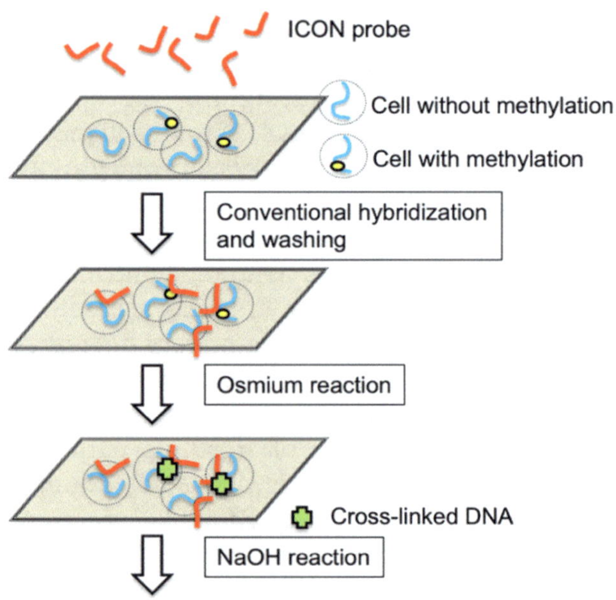

Figure 9.8. Importance of specificity in histochemical methods.

Source: https://www.researchgate.net/publication/365712688/figure/fig5/AS:11431281125975735@1678503630651/Illustrative-histochemical-procedure-for-sequence-specific-demonstration-of-single.png.

9.3. Basic Principles of Cytochemistry

The fundamental principles of cytochemistry provide the foundation for the knowledge required for the spatial organization and chemical makeup of cellular structures. The science necessitates the localization of certain biomolecules in the cell, and this is achievable with many staining methods employed to visualize structure and function at a cellular level. The cytochemical strategy tends to be dependent on antibodies specific to individual antigens, on which the immunohistochemical studies can be performed. For instance, the application of specific antibodies against chromogranin A in pancreatic tissues illustrates how cytochemistry shows the localization of varied hormones and enzymes in endocrine cells. In experiments that tested bovine pancreatic cells, computer-based techniques on the intensity of staining were more than 80% successful in demonstrating that immunoreactive chromogranin A was localized within B-cells, which illustrates the power of cytochemistry in the disclosure of cellular complexities and their physiological relevance (Ehrhart et al., 1988). Furthermore, techniques employed in cytochemistry are of great importance for advancing knowledge of biochemical processes and cellular behavior. Through the blending of the application of histochemical procedures and immunochemical techniques, researchers can make a detailed study of cellular milieus. For example, the uptake and metabolism of biomolecules can be traced by specific staining procedures, providing information regarding metabolic status or disease status. These procedures are not only routine, but they are also a heritage based on the achievements of origin scientists in the field. The range of the heritage underscores the interplay of historic context and contemporary techniques in cytochemistry. As the discussion of the legacy of leading researchers in cell biology and histochemistry has highlighted, subsequent research is helped by the procedures developed from earlier research, and therefore, a successive gradual establishment of analytical capabilities follows (Koji et al., 2019). Overall, basic principles of cytochemistry form a necessary guideline in cytochemical and histochemical methods.

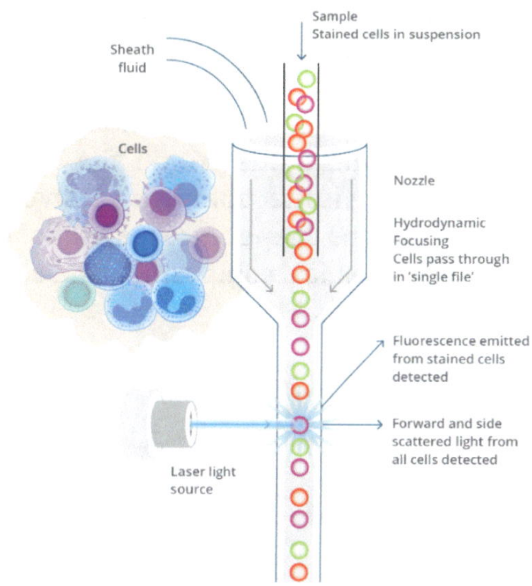

Figure 9.9. Basic principles of cytochemistry.

Source: https://www.streck.com/wp-content/uploads/2020/11/flow-cytometry-light-scatter-illustration.jpg.

The wise application of these principles enhances the accuracy and depth of biological investigations, allowing for the absolute determination of cell components. With researchers striving to unscramble the mysteries of cellular dynamics, the intersection of high-technology imaging techniques and robust staining procedures takes center stage. Ultimately, cytochemistry not only allows for the examination of the cellular blueprint but also helps uncover the interconnectedness of science through the ages. Hence, the field will continue to progress with the need for increased insight and creative strategies that respond to the evolving boundaries of cellular and molecular biology (Figure 9.9).

9.3.1. Differences Between Histochemistry and Cytochemistry

The distinction between histochemistry and cytochemistry is vital in understanding their function in the study of biology. Histochemistry is primarily focused on the localization of chemical constituents in tissues and employs methods that reveal cells' structures as well as the biomolecules associated with them through staining methods. Scientists can thereby ascertain the placement of substances such as proteins, carbohydrates, and lipids within the intricate architecture of tissue samples. Conversely, cytochemistry aims deeper into individual cells, such as on the chemical composition and cellular metabolic processes.

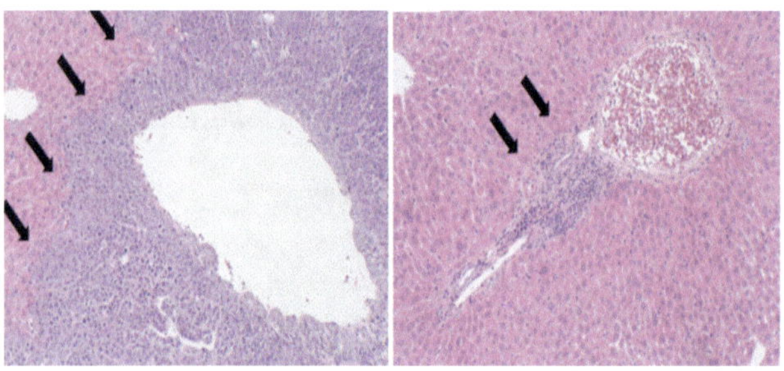

Figure 9.10. Differences between histochemistry and cytochemistry.

Source: https://journals.sagepub.com/pb-assets/cmscontent/jhc/Editor's%20choice%20Carousel/JHC_APRIL_2021_EDITORS_CHOICE_2020-00054R1_Fig_2.png.

By using specific staining methods, cytochemistry makes it possible to identify organelle components and biochemical sequences, resulting in an appreciation of the functions and interactions of cells. Both techniques are important, but with each serving a particular function in biological studies, histochemistry provides the general background of tissues and cytochemistry suggests cellular nuances. Techniques applied to histochemistry and cytochemistry also define their distinction. Histochemical techniques typically involve the use of multiple stains to seek reactions between enzymes and substrates in mounted sections of tissues, which allows for detailed morphological examinations. These techniques are able to explain the spatial arrangement of elements in tissue structure, as can be seen in studies researching wood pulp properties, whose cell morphologies were characterized based on histochemical staining to demarcate extractives and the way they affect paper quality (Fernando., 2007). The techniques in cytochemistry, however, usually include immunocytochemistry and fluorescence *in situ* hybridization, where researchers are able to explore the molecular elements. These methods can reveal the existence and localization of particular proteins or nucleic acids in individual cells so that one can get closer to understanding cellular behavior, as in the aberrant expression of receptor tyrosine kinases in thyroid cancers (Baumgartner et al., 2009).

The uses of these variations extend across most scientific disciplines. Histochemistry is also commonly utilized within developmental biology, pathology, and histopathology, wherein the determination of the location of specific biochemical entities within tissues can be applied to inform disease development and diagnosis. For example, within wood cell structure, histochemical processes have provided an insightful understanding of chemical and morphological differences in fibers across species that have direct consequences for processing techniques and product quality (Fernando., 2007). Cytochemistry is nevertheless critical in cell biology and cancer research, enabling the examination of cellular responses and signaling pathways that may inform therapeutic options. Visualization of chromosome aberrations, such as in studies of papillary thyroid carcinoma, illustrates the relevance of cytochemical procedures in the disclosure of disease mechanisms and treatments (Baumgartner et al., 2009). Thus, while histochemistry and cytochemistry are both important sources of information about biological systems, their very techniques and uses attest to their respective contributions to the understanding of life at tissue and cellular levels, respectively (Figure 9.10).

9.3.2. Techniques Used for Cellular Analysis

In cellular examination, histochemical techniques are important for identifying the biochemical properties of cells and tissues. These techniques are founded on the selective binding of chemical entities to cell components and offer insights into the various macromolecules, which involve proteins, nucleic acids, and carbohydrates. Techniques such as immunohistochemistry employ antibodies for the recognition and visualization of specific antigens and allow researchers to follow the localization of proteins within the cell. This technique is particularly valuable when studying cancer tissues, where aberrant protein expression may be a marker of cancer progression or response to therapy. By correlating histochemical findings with clinical findings, these techniques yield important information for personalized medicine that can be used to guide therapy and enhance patient treatment. Cytochemical techniques, on the other hand, are aimed at studying cell structures and cellular processes at the microscopic level.

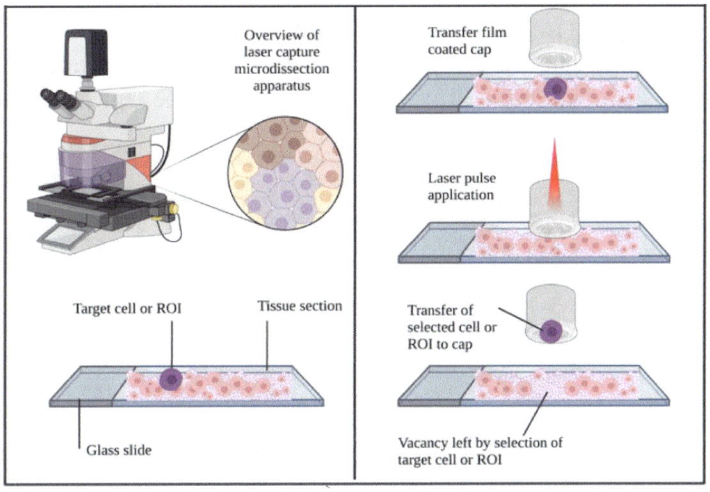

Figure 9.11. Techniques used for cellular analysis.

Source: https://api.intechopen.com/media/chapter/78769/media/F3.png.

By the use of different staining methods and enzyme histochemistry, cytochemical techniques can provide information regarding cellular constituents such as organelles and membranes, as well as on metabolic processes. For instance, through the use of specific dyes that have a binding affinity with metabolic enzymes, enzymatic activity as well as cells may be observed and quantified, and thus allow for the detection of physiological states or pathological processes. Furthermore, advanced techniques like FACS allow for the separation and study of individual cell populations based on their specific cytochemical characteristics. This aspect is invaluable to cancer research and immunology since the capability to interrogate cellular heterogeneity can reveal much regarding mechanisms of disease and therapeutic approaches. Cellular analysis has been further facilitated by developments in microscopy, notably electron microscopy and fluorescence techniques. By employing methods such as scanning electron microscopy (SEM) and transmission electron microscopy (TEM), researchers can generate high-resolution images of cellular organization, enhancing understanding of cellular morphology and ultrastructure. As an example, research into the fiber cells of wood tissue has uncovered how electron microscopy can be employed in order to analyze the topochemistry of cell walls under various treatments. The application of these techniques has rendered significant evidence about the chemical and structural wood fiber contents during the mechanical pulping processes, which reflects the importance of precise cellular analysis in plant science as well as industrial practice. Such observations illustrate the versatile usage of histochemical and cytochemical techniques in different fields of science (Fernando., 2007; Baumgartner et al., 2009) (Figure 9.11).

9.3.3. Role of Enzymes in Cytochemical Staining

Cytochemical staining techniques utilize the catalytic activity of enzymes for the visualization of cellular structures and biochemical processes. Enzymes play a critical role as indicators in such processes, as they produce a quantitative signal upon substrate conversion within the target cellular site. As an example, differential dehydrogenase activity, i.e., diphosphopyridine nucleotide diaphorase (DPNH-D) and triphosphopyridine nucleotide diaphorase (TPNH-D), can be observed in cancer cells with a highlighting factor of metabolic differences meaningful to tumor biology. These enzymes, which occur in large amounts in the cytoplasmic granules of cells, contain varying intensities of reaction, displaying information on the condition of the metabolism and proliferative stage of tumor cells, thus emphasizing enzymatic activity in cytochemical staining as a process of revealing cellular functions and disease states (Kawashima, T. & Ogata, T., 1963).

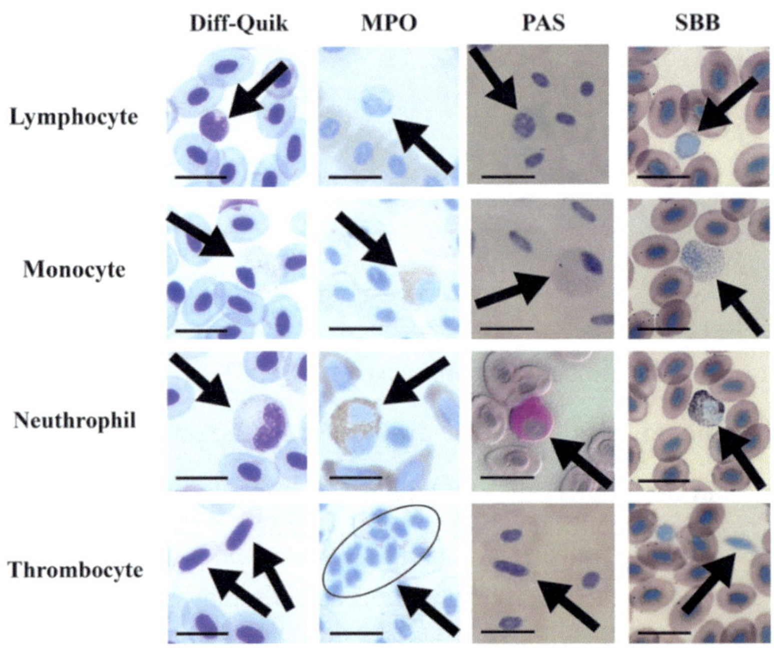

Figure 9.12. Role of enzymes in cytochemical staining.

Source: https://www.researchgate.net/profile/Andrea-Radalj/publication/371695198/figure/fig1/AS:11431281169071842@1687198691981/Cytochemical-staining-of-peripheral-blood-cells-in-the-Prussian-carp-Lymphocytes-were.ppm.

The role of enzymes is not restricted to straightforward detection because their localization and activities provide essential information regarding cellular organization and dynamics. Succinic dehydrogenase (SDH) and α-glycerophosphate dehydrogenase (α-GDH), for example, exhibit differential localization patterns and activities depending on the cell cycle stage. Such differentiation emphasizes the significant role of enzymes in catalyzing cytochemical reactions, signifying cellular processes as well as overall viability. Enzyme activities also offer comparative findings across different cell types, such as cancer cells and normal lymphocytes.

Cytochemical staining information, in this regard, not only facilitates the characterization of malignant cells but also helps in an understanding of global metabolic alterations that accompany cancer development (Koshiba., 1968). Moreover, cytochemical staining effectiveness relies on factors such as fixatives, which influence the activity and localization of enzymes. For instance, glutaraldehyde fixation may be inhibitory to certain enzyme activities, ultimately affecting staining outcomes. This poses a particular challenge for interpreting results and underscores the need for careful attention to experimental conditions when applying cytochemical techniques.

The conjunction of enzymatic assays and histochemical staining allows researchers to gain more precise information about cell structure and function. Thus, enzymes play the functions of facilitators and markers in cytochemical staining, bringing about the changeover from biochemical activity to histological appearance and further elucidating our understanding relating to cellular processes (Kawashima, T. & Ogata, T., 1963; Koshiba, 1968) (Figure 9.12).

9.4. Common Histochemical Techniques

Histochemical techniques are core techniques of the study of tissue and cellular composition, playing a key role in identifying biochemical properties of biological specimens. Periodic acid-Schiff (PAS) staining and Alcian blue staining are some common techniques employed that allow the detection of polysaccharides and glycoproteins within tissues. For instance, PAS staining permits the visualization of glycogen and other carbohydrate-containing structures, thus enabling researchers to identify the glycopatterns in specific cell types. Similarly, staining with Alcian blue facilitates discrimination among acidic and neutral mucopolysaccharides in tissue samples and thereby further supports understanding of their function and role in cellular architecture. Through these techniques, researchers can draw useful inferences from the biochemical composition of tissues, providing a foundation for further investigation in developmental pathology and biology. Lectin histochemistry increases the toolset available for investigating glycosylation patterns of biological tissues. Lectins are protein ligands with specificity toward specific glycan structures and thus can be very valuable in questioning glycopatterns in a cellular context. For example, the application of various lectins has served to distinguish the composition of glycan residues in the extracellular matrix, as seen in studies carried out on amphibian reproductive tissue (Moramarco et al., 2011). The application of a blend of various kinds of lectins in histochemical analyses enables scholars to enhance the sensitivity and specificity of their studies to detect minute differences in glycan expression. These techniques not only uncover important nuances in cellular behavior but also illuminate the physiological and disease states of glycosylation, showing how vital the presence of lectins is in today's histochemical technology. The linkage of histochemical techniques to advanced imaging technologies has sparked a revolution in cellular biology, with the capability for high-resolution imaging of histochemical staining. Techniques such as confocal or electron microscopy, when combined with traditional histochemical staining, can ascertain the spatial organization of cellular components with great precision. For example, through histochemical staining, morphology, and ultrastructural correlation at the nanometer scale, researchers can gain a better knowledge of cellular organization and interactions. This was typically demonstrated in studies of fertilization envelope and jelly layers of amphibian eggs, determining characteristic histochemical patterns of staining and their application to reproductive biology (Moramarco et al., 2011). Furthermore, advances in image analysis software complement these techniques by offering qualitative measurements and thus broadening the scope of studies of cellular differentiation and pathology across various organisms and conditions.

9.4.1. Hematoxylin and Eosin Staining

Hematoxylin and eosin (H&E) staining is one of the simplest techniques utilized in histology, providing valuable information about tissue morphology and disease. The hematoxylin component of the stain stains cell nuclei deep purple or blue, allowing for the determination of nuclear details and cell integrity. Eosin, however, stains the cytoplasm and extracellular matrix various pinks, which reveal the general tissue architecture of the test sample. This differential staining finds great utility in pathological diagnosis, where tissue sections examined under the microscope reveal disease process abnormalities such as tumors or inflammatory diseases. The widespread use of H&E staining across medical and research settings renders it an indispensable aid to histologists as well as pathologists in analyzing normal as well as diseased tissues with utmost diligence. In the pathology of neuromuscular disease, H&E staining is particularly useful, especially when used in conjunction with other histochemical methods. Muscle biopsies may be stained with H&E in an effort to observe morphological changes, like myofibrillar degeneration and inflammation, that can signify underlying conditions like muscular dystrophy or myasthenia gravis. Although this staining procedure can reveal non-specific features, it is a preliminary test that steers clinicians toward further testing. The combination of H&E with histochemical methods, as reported in the literature, allows for a better knowledge of the biochemistry of muscle fibers and facilitates an easier comprehension of disease mechanisms (Paciello, O. & Papparella, S., 2009).

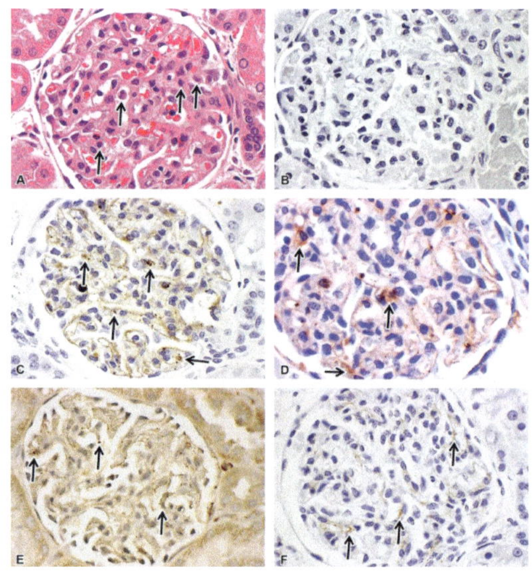

Figure 9.13. Hematoxylin and eosin staining.

Source: https://www.researchgate.net/profile/John-Lin-33/publication/260684361/figure/fig1/AS:601626096177186@1520450247859/A-Hematoxylin-and-eosin-staining-of-the-glomerular-changes-including-moderate.png.

This dual process enhances diagnostic value and enables classification of neuromuscular pathologies by histological pattern. The usefulness of H&E staining is not limited to its initial diagnostic use; it is an integral component of the research setting in order to study the influence of treatments on tissue function and integrity. Studies intended to analyze the cellular response to interventions, e.g., chemotherapy or regenerative therapies, will often employ H&E staining in order to assess the morphological alterations in tissues. Through the study of changes in cellular structure or of signs of tissue repair, investigators are able to determine the efficacy of therapeutic interventions. Furthermore, substrate and enzyme kinetics uncovered by adjunctive histochemical techniques provide additional interpretive value to H&E findings, increasing the appreciation of tissue performance under health and disease (Hirose, 1968). H&E staining itself is a central pillar supporting both diagnostic and investigative strategies in histochemical and cytochemical methods (Figure 9.13).

9.4.2. Immunohistochemistry

Immunohistochemistry (IHC) is a key histochemical and cytochemical method used to localize specific antigens in tissue sections. By this technique, protein distribution and localization are seen in the cellular milieu by utilizing the antigen-antibody reaction principle.

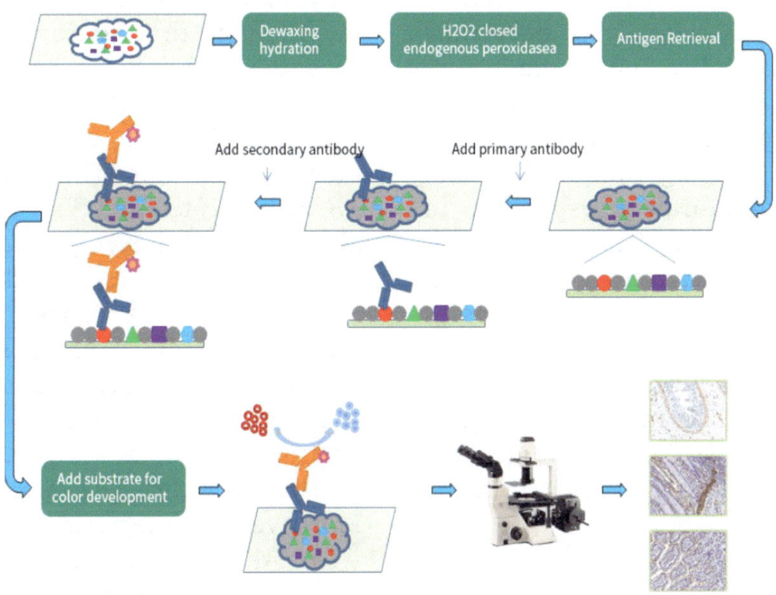

Figure 9.14. Immunohistochemistry.

Source: https://cdn1.sinobiological.com/styles/default/images/pdyimg/IHC/ihc_protocol/u12.jpg.

The need for robust automated methods is also underscored by their ability to enhance accuracy in tumor characterization and study of disease pathways at the genetic level. For example, state-of-the-art segmentation methods developed using unsupervised color class-clustering and morphological filtering have been found to excel by being able to accurately characterize cancer regions within tissue samples with less interference from background (Acquaviva et al., 2010). The use of these techniques not only streamlines workflow but also increases the validity of immunohistochemical analysis. As such, IHC continues to adapt by integrating conventional techniques with advanced technologies to enable more insightful studies of cellular behavior, thereby advancing personalized medicine and targeted treatment across malignancies (Figure 9.14).

IHC application is prevalent, from diagnostic pathology to research laboratories, where precise identification of protein expressions can define mechanisms of disease and direct treatment modalities. Technical improvements in IHC have also revolutionized cancer diagnosis, making it possible to characterize and classify neoplasms by tumor type. Improved characterization of these protein markers is of paramount significance as they correlate with tumor behavior, patient prognosis, and personalized therapeutic regimens. Recent developments in IHC techniques have bridged the traditional limitations by incorporating automated and semi-automated systems. The innovations improve staining efficiency and accuracy as well as analysis efficiency and accuracy. For instance, improvements in automated membrane segmentation techniques have significantly improved cellular examination through addressing imaging complexities and detecting cellular membranes, especially in complex tissue architectures (Acquaviva et al., 2011). Through the consistent identification of the morphology of cells, these technologies enable quantification of the expression of membrane proteins. They are not incremental technologies but a paradigm in histological sample treatment and analysis that will lead to improved research and clinical diagnostic outcomes.

9.4.3. In situ Hybridization

In situ hybridization (ISH) is a central technique within the domain of histochemical and cytochemical techniques that facilitates the localization of specific nucleic acid sequences in cells or fixed tissues. The method relies on the hybridization of labeled complementary DNA or RNA probes to the target sequences so that it is feasible for scientists to investigate patterns of gene expression at the subcellular and cellular levels. The versatility of ISH extends well beyond biological sciences to the study of developmental biology, cancer, and genetics. Perhaps more significantly, the selective potential for the targeting of sequences aids in the definition of aberrant chromosome configurations and gene rearrangements that are essential within such environments as tumor pathology. Thus, ISH is not just a diagnostic tool but an extremely useful tool in unraveling complex genetic interactions that contribute significantly to organismal development and disease progression. *In situ* hybridization possesses one of its most significant applications in the elucidation of the genetic etiology of a variety of diseases, particularly in the field of oncology research. For instance, structural chromosome aberrations have been established to be key players in tumorigenesis. Most significantly, in papillary thyroid carcinoma, activation of receptor tyrosine kinase oncogenes like RET and NTRK1, as evidenced by fluorescence *in situ* hybridization, has emerged as a major mechanism of tumor initiation and progression. Through ISH techniques, researchers have been able to chart karyotype changes in specific subtypes of tumors, e.g., those resulting from environmental exposures like the Chornobyl disaster. By discovering such chromosomal abnormalities, ISH not only enhances the understanding of tumor biology but also provides critical data that may impact therapeutic options and clinical care (Baumgartner et al., 2009). Moreover, the integration of *in situ* hybridization with other techniques enhances its value in diagnosis as well as in research, particularly within personalized medicine approaches. Use of patient-specific DNA probes for the detection of structural chromosomal aberrations is a major advancement that enhances the effectiveness of preimplantation genetic diagnosis (PGD) in *in vitro* fertilization. As recent studies have shown, hybridization techniques can optimize the selection of healthy embryos by accurately identifying genetic breakpoints implicated in conditions such as reciprocal balanced translocations in reproductive medicine applications. With their continued advancements, the use of standard rapid ISH protocols will be increasingly brought within reach, ultimately for various patient populations, and advance genomic medicine (Baumgartner et al., 2009) (Figure 9.15).

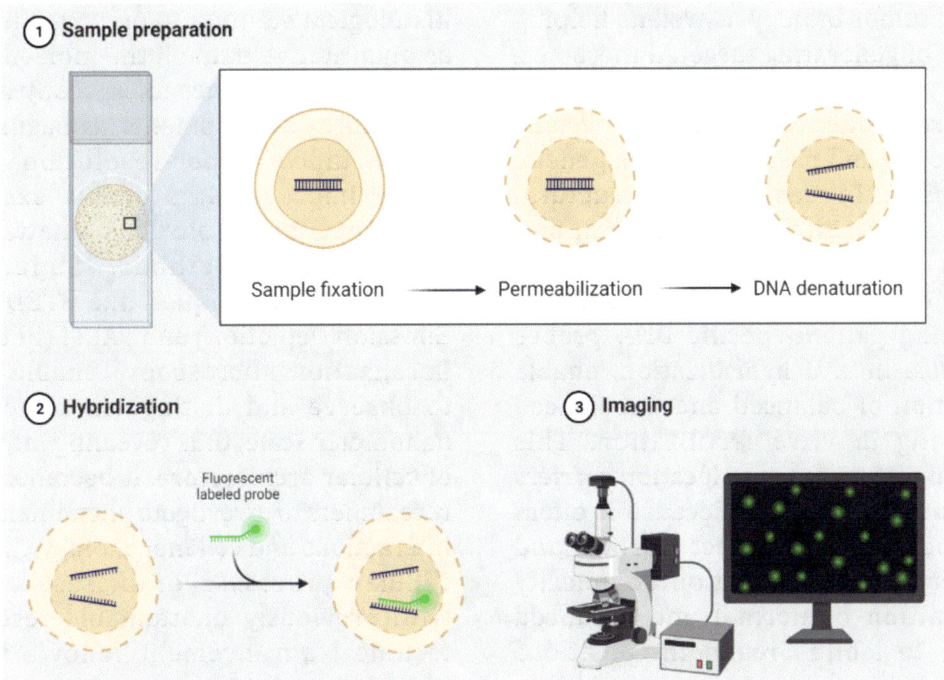

Figure 9.15. *In situ* hybridization.

Source: https://images.aatbio.com/universal/catalog/FISH/Fluorescence_In_Situ_Hybridization_(FISH).png.

9.5. Common Cytochemical Techniques

Cytochemical techniques are important tools for the analysis of cellular structure and function, enabling scientists to identify and localize molecules within cells. Cytochemical techniques utilize varied staining techniques that enable scientists to see cellular components based on their biochemical nature. Enzyme histochemistry, immunohistochemistry, and fluorescence *in situ* hybridization (FISH) are prevalent cytochemical techniques. All such methods are advantageous in nature; enzyme histochemistry, for instance, is aimed at certain enzymes for the assessment of metabolic processes, whereas immunohistochemistry employs antibodies to detect specific protein expressions. FISH has proven beneficial to identify chromosomal abnormalities and gene expressions, particularly in cancer research. Such cytochemical practice is becoming increasingly significant for clinical diagnostics, particularly in clinical oncology. Methods such as FISH have made it possible to change the way structural chromosome aberrations are diagnosed and play a crucial role in determining the nature of most tumors. For instance, studies have proven structural chromosome aberrations to be distinguishing characteristics of most solid tumors, including the papillary thyroid cancer (PTC). In this regard, fluorescent probes employed in cytochemical techniques allow insight into the genetic etiology of the disease, such as the activation of receptor tyrosine kinase (RTK) genes, which can be a result of complex chromosomal rearrangements. This shows the utility of cytochemical techniques in discovering tumor biology as well as helping in the process of generating targeted therapies. Additionally, cytochemical techniques are invaluable in reproductive medicine, especially genetic counseling and preimplantation genetic diagnosis (PGD). In cases with structural chromosomal abnormalities like translocations, the precision of examining genetic material is of critical concern. Advanced techniques, such as creating patient-specific DNA probes via fluorescence in situ hybridization, enable the identification of balanced and unbalanced embryos during in vitro fertilization. This capability is important for translocation carriers who have issues of infertility because it offers them an opportunity to select normal and balanced embryos for implantation. Complexity in the recognition of normal and balanced embryos due to labile breakpoint positions highlights the need for continuing innovations in cytochemical methods, as demonstrated by recent research attempts to improve PGD efficiency and availability (Baumgartner et al., 2009).

9.5.1. Fluorescence Microscopy

Fluorescence microscopy occupies a significant position in the world of histochemical and cytochemical techniques, primarily due to its ability to generate high-resolution images of biological samples without having to pre-treat the samples invasively. With the use of specific fluorophores that bind to cellular components, researchers can track various biological processes in real-time, thereby increasing our understanding of cellular dynamics. The technique enables one to consider the localization of nucleic acids, proteins, and other biomolecules in their native form. It is a feature that is invaluable, especially when studying disease or monitoring cellular response to certain stimuli, as it enables deeper insights into the mechanism of biological function and disease. This new technique illustrates how fluorescence microscopy expands the methods of conventional histological staining to offer qualitative as well as quantitative data on the molecular structure of cells. Fluorescence microscopy is made more powerful by developments in imaging technology, for instance, super-resolution microscopy. These improvements enable examination of structures at resolutions unattainable with conventional methods. Super-resolution microscopy techniques like STED (Stimulated Emission Depletion) and PALM (Photo-Activated Localization Microscopy) enable researchers to observe and distinguish structures at the nanometer scale, thus revealing intricate aspects of cellular architecture. It becomes possible for researchers to investigate phenomena like protein interactions and cell morphology changes during cellular processes or disease advancement with previously unattainable resolution. This technical advancement follows the goals of histochemical and cytochemical investigation, aiming to simplify the spatial and temporal relationships of cellular events, thereby making fluorescence microscopy an essential tool for modern biological investigation. Further, the use of fluorescence microscopy in conjunction with other cytochemical methods complements its applications, which enable one to have enhanced analysis of biological specimens. Techniques such as immunofluorescence enable direct protein labeling, and their distribution and concentration can be investigated in cells. Moreover, with the help of molecular probes for particular RNA or DNA sequences and fluorescence microscopy, the pattern of gene expression and the mechanism of control could be determined. This interdisciplinary approach is particularly useful in fields such as oncology, where understanding the molecular mechanism of tumorigenesis is crucial. With scientists extending the boundless directions opened by fluorescence microscopy and its coupling with other histochemical and cytochemical techniques, an even deeper, richer understanding of complex systems of biology will undoubtedly ensue, further directing treatment strategies and diagnostic tools (Figure 9.16).

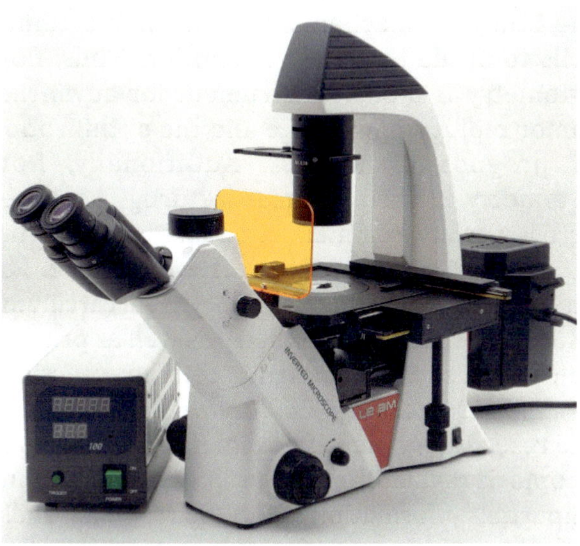

Figure 9.16. Fluorescence microscopy.

Source: https://www.deltapix.dk/wp-content/uploads/2020/07/45a-view.jpg.

9.5.2. Electron Microscopy

Of all the histochemical and cytochemical operations, electron microscopy (EM) is an essential facility that greatly enhances our understanding of cell structure and function at the microscopic scale. This high-level imaging method, particularly in its iterations known as transmission electron microscopy (TEM) and scanning electron microscopy (SEM), provides unparalleled resolution for viewing cellular organelles and their intricate structures within tissues. With the application of such methods, scientists can not only differentiate the cell morphology but also refine the fineness that is relevant to biochemical processes. Such a capability is essential for detecting and mapping the locations of single biomolecules, thereby enabling correlation of histochemical characteristics with cellular functions across various biological systems. One of the most effective applications of EM is shown in studies on wood fibers in mechanical pulping, where techniques like immuno-gold TEM have been used to examine their ultrastructural properties. Through this technique, the influence of lignin and glucomannan distribution on fiber behavior during processing can be closely examined. For instance, different pulping methods, such as thermomechanical pulping (TMP) and stoneground wood (SGW) processing, yield different results in terms of fiber morphology and structural stability. Ultrastructural studies on Norway spruce and Scots pine fibers reveal crucial differences in the way these trees respond when exposed to mechanical stress, essentially linking microscopic observations with macroscopic physical properties. Such findings highlight the value of electron microscopy in solving difficult problems in histochemistry and cytochemistry, providing a powerful platform for studying the interaction between chemical composition and structural features. Also, with the discovery of the backscattered electron imaging (BEI) mode of SEM, its application in cytochemical studies has been transformed. The technique permits intracellular structures and organelles to be seen in excellent resolution, enabling discrimination of various cell types within heterogeneous tissues. The potential for relating enzymatic activity to physical properties of cell surfaces has opened an extensive arena for cell biology investigations. Of special value is the fact that BEI studies have yielded important information on blood cell populations, revealing formerly obscure dynamics relating to their enzymatic activities and interactions. Due to the advancements in technology, the promise still exists for applications of electron microscopy in cytochemistry in the future that will illuminate new breakthroughs, which will bridge the structure-function gap at the cellular level and thus ultimately advance our understanding of biological processes (Figure 9.17).

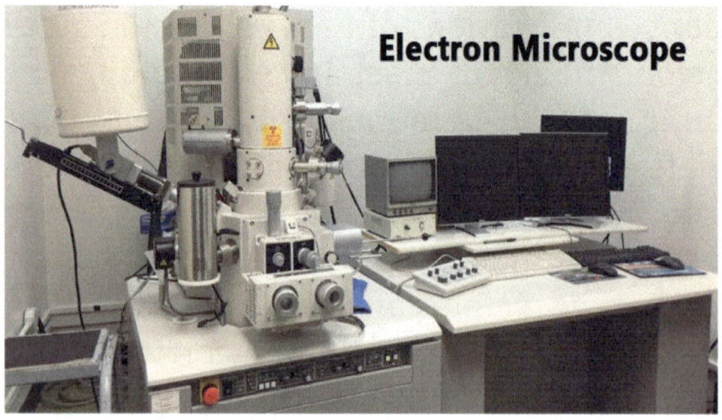

Figure 9.17. Electron microscopy.

Source: https://microbenotes.com/wp-content/uploads/2018/10/Electron-Microscope.jpg.

9.5.3. Flow Cytometry

Flow cytometry has immensely transformed the history of histochemical and cytochemical procedures with unparalleled potential for quantitative measurement of cellular attributes. The technology operates on the premise of hydrodynamic focusing, whereby single cells are caused to move along a laser beam, where they induce light scattering and fluorescence based on specific markers. The ability to examine multiple parameters at a single-cell level has made flow cytometry an essential instrument in numerous research disciplines, such as immunology, oncology, and cell biology. In cancer research, flow cytometry is applicable to detect specific protein expressions in cancer cells to investigate tumor immunology and patient prognosis. These results are of key importance in maximizing therapeutic interventions and maximizing patient management protocols in clinical practice. The integration of flow cytometry with molecular techniques has also enhanced its usage, particularly in disease state identification. For instance, studies have demonstrated the presence of HLA-G in B-cell chronic lymphocytic leukemia (B-CLL), demonstrating that flow cytometry can identify specific markers that define malignancies. As with the case of HLA-G research, a crucial molecule in immune evasion, flow cytometry analysis has demonstrated its capacity for detecting cellular response both at RNA and protein levels. By illustrating the presence of this non-conventional HLA class I molecule in B-CLL samples, researchers have underscored the significance of the method in the study of mechanisms that enable tumor cells to evade immune recognition. Thus, flow cytometry is a basic instrument for advancing tumor biology knowledge and the optimization of prognostic markers. Additionally, flow cytometry is used to measure drug responses across various treatment regimens, underscoring its applicability to personalized medicine. For instance, one study involving laryngeal carcinoma used laser scanning cytometry as well as primary cell cultures to investigate cellular reactions against cisplatin. By flow cytometric analysis, the researchers identified significant changes in apoptosis regulator protein expression, providing important information about the responsiveness of tumor cells to chemotherapeutic drugs. The relationship between P53 and BCL-2 protein expression, as reported in the work, not only indicates the significance of flow cytometry in drug efficacy research but also the power of this technology to define patients who would benefit from specific treatment regimens. With these advances, flow cytometry is now a standard technique in histochemical and cytochemical methods, pushing the limits of medical science and clinical practice.

9.6. Applications in Research and Medicine

Histochemical and cytochemical techniques are indispensable tools in the laboratory and clinical setting, permitting greater understanding of cellular structure and function. With these techniques, scientists are able to visualize cellular components with high specificity and obtain information that leads to advances in areas like oncology and immunology. For instance, localization of specific proteins in cells by means of immunohistochemistry has significantly advanced our understanding of tumor microenvironments. The demarcation of this distinction enables researchers to identify proper biomarkers for disease development, thereby advancing targeted therapeutics. Their incorporation into routine diagnostic practice also grants medicine professionals knowledge with which to effectively tailor treatment in a manner attesting to their utility in personalized medicine. Within materials science, histochemical methods have also been beyond essential. As an example, electron microscopy examination of wood fibre ultrastructure depicts the way that these technologies show mechanisms with mechanical processing detail. Compared to the influence of thermomechanical and stoneground wood treatment on fibre structure, the importance of histochemical examination in material property optimization becomes apparent. Particularly, determination of lignin and glucomannan distribution using these techniques provides fundamental fibre strength and resistance mechanisms essential to the paper industry.

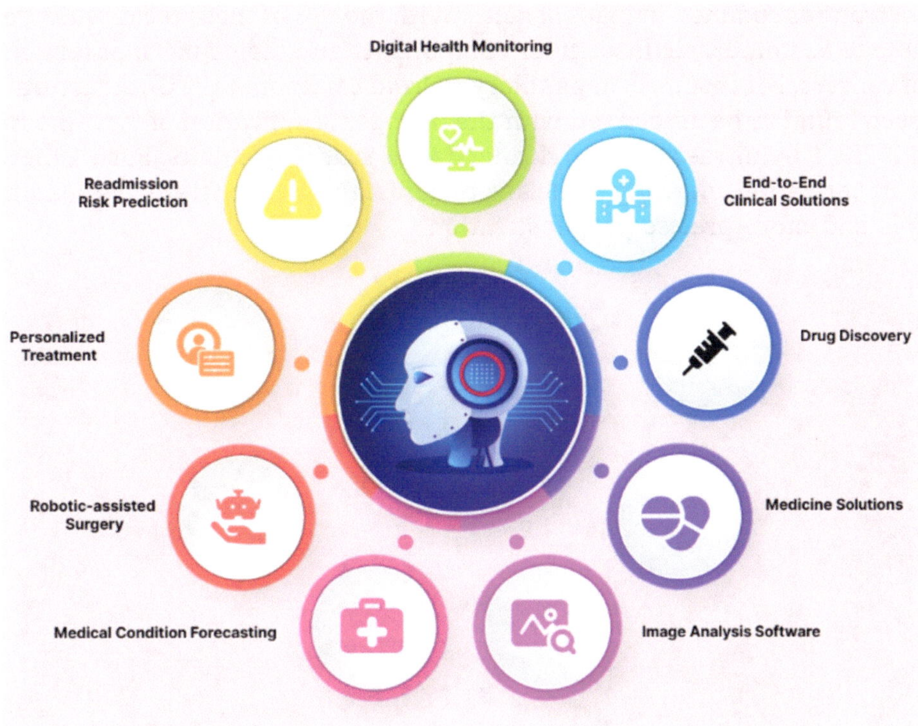

Figure 9.18. Applications in research and medicine.

Source: https://www.bacancytechnology.com/blog/wp-content/uploads/2024/03/Applications-of-AI-in-Healthcare.webp.

Secondly, histochemical studies enable detailed examination of the processing challenges of wood extractives, thereby informing best practices for improving end-product quality and supporting the broader application of these techniques in enhancing material performance. The advancement in image analysis software, and in particular when used in conjunction with immunohistochemistry, indicates a new direction that enhances the clinical and research performance. The trend towards computer-aided analysis and virtual slide imaging allows more uniform diagnostic interpretation to be achieved, thereby restricting subjective error. Software packages like Dako ACIS III and Aperio Image Analysis enhance quantitation of staining results, making high-throughput screening of tissue microarrays effective. These developments not only increase the reproducibility of research but also allow for large-scale research capable of deconstructing patterns of disease pathology. As fluorescence techniques pick up steam, as in studies employing multispectral imaging, the potential of multiplexed analysis holds tremendous promise for extensive biomarker exploration. This advancement in histochemical methods calls attention to the revolutionary impact of technology on clinical practice and research and its significance for improved patient outcomes (Fernando., 2007; Bueno et al., 2010) (Figure 9.18).

9.6.1. Role in Cancer Diagnosis and Treatment

The role of histochemical and cytochemical techniques in cancer diagnosis and therapy is fundamentally radical, particularly with the methods enabling the identification of structural chromosome aberrations common in malignancies. With the use of these techniques, researchers and clinicians are able to examine specific cellular components and molecular markers characteristic of various types of cancers. For instance, in papillary thyroid carcinoma (PTC), structural chromosomal changes have been found to be associated with the oncogenic activation of tyrosine kinase receptor genes RET and NTRK1 by intra- and interchromosomal rearrangements. Such genetic data enable precise tumor categorization, allowing clinicians to adjust treatment strategies, leading to improved patient outcomes and more precise prognostication.

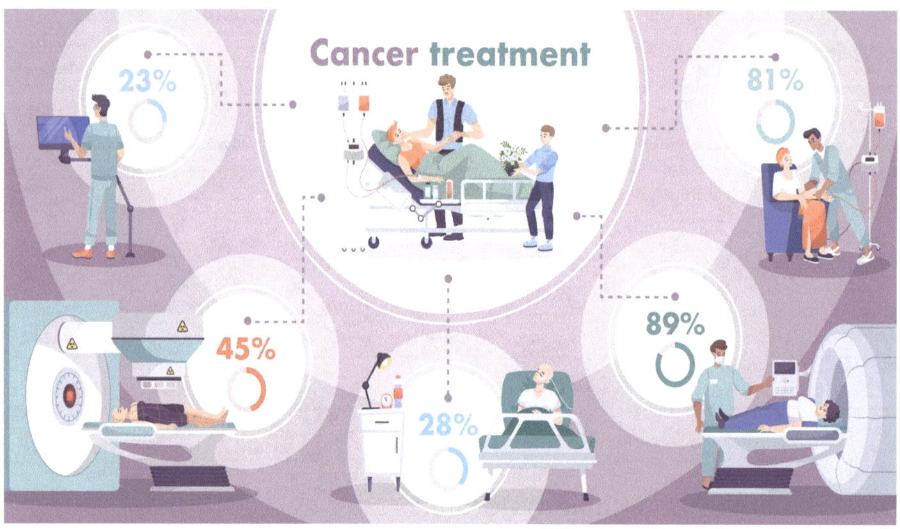

Figure 9.19. Role in cancer diagnosis and treatment.

Source: https://upload.wikimedia.org/wikipedia/commons/thumb/4/47/Stained_microscope_slide.jpg/330px-Stained_microscope_slide.jpg.

Also supporting the prospect of histochemical and cytochemical techniques extending cancer diagnostics is the introduction of fluorescence *in situ* hybridization (FISH) techniques. In studies of tumor karyotype alterations in children after the Chornobyl disaster, researchers have been able to identify complex chromosome aberrations characteristic of this PTC subcategory. With FISH-based techniques, high-speed visualization of chromosomal derangements allows for more advanced characterization of tumor pathology and behavior. This type of information can guide treatment strategies that are tailored to address the specific genetic environment of the tumor, illustrating the potential of histochemical techniques to influence therapeutic decision-making directly. As such, these strategies not only improve diagnostic accuracy but also play a major role in individualized therapy plans. Aside from aiding in diagnosis, application of histochemical and cytochemical techniques has revolutionized cancer treatment modalities, particularly in preimplantation genetic diagnosis (PGD) of *in vitro* fertilization (IVF) programs. For patients with structural chromosome abnormalities, such as reciprocal translocations, PGD may allow selection of embryos with preferable genetic characteristics and minimize the chance of transferring embryos with unbalanced chromosomal arrangements. Design of patient-specific DNA probes that can precisely map breakpoints in translocations demonstrates the manner in which enhanced cytochemistry can directly benefit such reproductive technologies. Even with some lingering challenges of separating balanced from unbalanced embryos, utilization of such rapid, optimized techniques holds out promise to render PGD more feasible and effective for translocation carriers, raising reproductive success. Through such uses, histochemical and cytochemical procedures illuminate their invaluable position in the therapeutic and diagnostic aspects of cancer treatment (Figure 9.19).

9.6.2. Use in Developmental Biology Studies

The application of histochemical and cytochemical approaches is extremely significant in developmental biology studies, particularly in identifying complex tissue differentiation processes and organogenesis. Applying various staining procedures, researchers can make individual cellular components, e.g., proteins, lipids, and carbohydrates, visible in developing animals. These discoveries provide valuable information on the distribution and timing of expression of molecules involved in developmental events. For instance, in studies of the ultrastructure of softwood fiber cell walls, histochemical methods have outlined mechanisms by which morphological changes during mechanical pulping correlate with fiber strength and light-scattering characteristics. This kind of information not only enhances organismal development knowledge but also completes knowledge gaps for species-specific development variations (Fernando., 2007). Along with these instruments, new techniques such as whole-mount immunohistochemistry have changed developmental biology research. Immunocytological examination can be performed using a freeze-cracking approach on embryos and sidesteps the intricacies of conventional egg handling techniques. The technique was tested successfully in a study involving the macrostomid flatworm *Macrostomum lignano*, where successful immunolocalization of critical developmental proteins was achieved. The simplification of the process reduces not only the time and resources required for experimental analysis but also preserves the developing embryo's intrinsic environment, thereby enabling improved interpretation of developmental cues. This innovation is the realization of histochemical techniques to render research processes more streamlined while enhancing the quality of data made available in embryonic research (Artois et al., 2009). The uses of these cytochemical and histochemical techniques extend beyond basic research and play a pivotal role in applied sciences such as developmental therapeutics and regenerative medicine. Awareness of spatial and temporal associations of cellular constituents can be utilized to guide tissue engineering and stem cell differentiation protocols. For example, data obtained from histochemical analyses can be utilized to create novel therapies for the treatment of congenital malformations or degeneration-related illnesses. By interpreting the molecular mechanism of developmental biology, researchers can design directed interventions that take advantage of the body's own repair mechanisms. Inclusion of such techniques into developmental work has far-reaching implications since it optimizes both the fundamental scientific knowledge and its translation into human well-being (Fernando., 2007; Artois et al., 2009Fernando., 2007).

9.6.3. Applications in Neurobiology and Pathology

The importance of histochemical and cytochemical techniques in neurobiology runs deep and is extensive, and yields priceless information concerning the cellular and molecular architecture of the nervous system. Such techniques can visualize and examine the localizations of specific biomolecules, e.g., neurotransmitters, receptors, and enzymes within neurons and glial cells. With the application of stains and markers for particular proteins, scientists can solve the intricate interactions between cell types, neural circuits, and their functional importance.

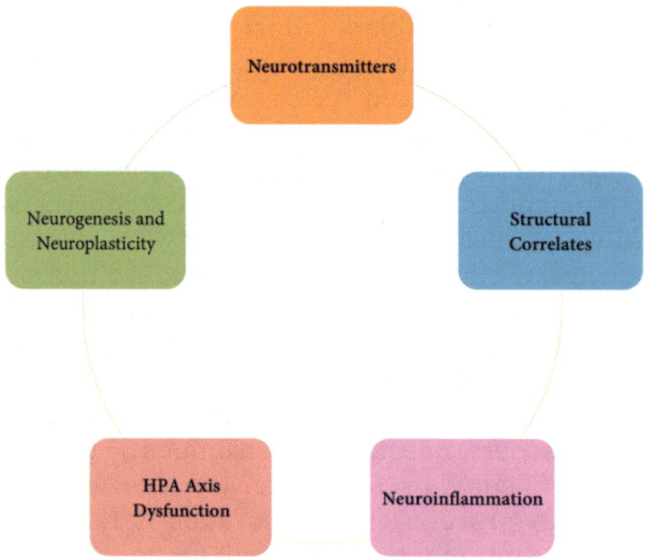

Figure 9.20. Applications in neurobiology and pathology.

Source: https://psychscenehub.com/wp-content/uploads/2022/02/Neurobiology-of-Depression-Main-Hypotheses-1024x587.png.

As (Pellicciari et al., 2010) suggests, histochemistry has created unparalleled opportunities for observing the structure and chemical composition of cells during normal and pathological conditions, and much more than ever before is known about how neurobiology functions. Besides, such approaches not only find use in basic research but also are of diagnostic significance, allowing one to identify pathological changes for neurodegenerative disorders as well as other neurological disorders. In pathology, the significance of histochemical and cytochemical approaches cannot be overestimated. Such approaches allow one to examine tissue samples with great care, and the detection of disease markers and insight into underlying mechanisms become easier. For instance, in cancers of the nervous system, histochemistry can reveal aberrant expression patterns of specific proteins and thereby aid in diagnosis and treatment. The ability to ascertain the topological organization of molecular components in tissue preparations also predisposes the inclusion of histochemical findings into clinical procedures with better prognostic and therapeutic outcomes. As Pellicciari (2010) indicate, the evolving applications of these methods point to their significance in veterinary and human pathology and biology and show the cross-disciplinary value of histochemistry in scientific studies and clinical medicine. The applications of histochemical techniques also extend to newer fields such as plant pathology, underscoring the flexibility of these methods for practical applications beyond traditional biomedical contexts. Through the examination of biochemical changes of plant tissues following infection by pathogens, researchers can advance disease control strategies and enhance crops. Techniques akin to those in neurobiology enable a way to understand plant cell reactions, which is applicable to the delineation of the molecular bases of resistance or susceptibility to various phytopathogens, as stated. This overlap of histochemical methods across different biological settings highlights both the flexibility of these methods and their essential role in informing our understanding of pathology in other organisms. These types of applications highlight the significant potential for interdisciplinary collaborations that are capable of generating scientific advances and solutions for application in both neurobiology and broader biological research fields (Figure 9.20).

SUMMARY

In summarizing observations and findings through the chapter on histochemical and cytochemical techniques, the fact remains that such techniques are at the forefront of diagnostics in a broad spectrum of biological and medical sciences. The central role these techniques play in revealing cellular and molecular data cannot be overestimated. From the discrimination of muscle fibers to the determination of specific cellular components, histochemical and cytochemical techniques enable one to better understand pathological processes. This is particularly true in the study of neuromuscular disorders, where histochemical staining reveals inconsistencies that inform diagnosis and treatment. Furthermore, the advancement of methods in relation to preimplantation genetic diagnosis (PGD) underscores the importance of precise cellular analysis in reproductive medicine, outlining the widespread application of these methods in other biological contexts. Furthermore, the issues that encompass the use of histochemical and cytochemical methods are outstanding. For instance, the variability of outcomes on account of the interpretative subjectivity of staining poses pertinent challenges to standardization and reproducibility. In neuromuscular disorders, histochemical investigation may, at times, lead to non-specific myopathological results, and hence, diagnosis would be challenging. A synergy of approaches has overcome some of these issues, such as the employment of immunohistochemistry along with traditional histological methods. However, the rigorous training and standardization of techniques are still the sole prerequisites to ensure consistent results. As the review of muscular dystrophies and other diseases has indicated, continuous evolution of these methods is the key to increased diagnostic accuracy and therapeutic strategies, and histochemical and cytochemical techniques are irreplaceable equipment in modern clinical laboratories. The future for histochemical and cytochemical techniques is promising, with innovative methodologies and technical developments able to supply more fertile biological data. The merging of molecular genetic studies further highlights the potential of these techniques with resultant early and accurate diagnoses of complex diseases. As an example, advanced preimplantation genetic diagnosis using highly developed DNA probes demonstrates the capacity of these methods to be tailored to specific clinical situations, thereby guaranteeing higher success rates of treatment, such as *in vitro* fertilization. As research continues to evolve, greater emphasis on individualized medicine will progressively augment the effectiveness of histochemical and cytochemical procedures. Ultimately, continued investment in education and research into these techniques will not only add to the corpus of knowledge on cellular pathology but will propel improved patient care strategies across a number of areas of health-related study, maintaining their grounding role in contemporary biomedical science.

A LOOK TO THE FUTURE:

MICRO-MORPHOLOGICAL DISTRIBUTION:

In the biological and earth sciences, the term *micro-morphological* refers to the study of very small structural features — often at microscopic or sub-microscopic levels — that reveal information about the shape, arrangement, and characteristics of tiny components in tissues, cells, soils, seeds, or particles. Micromorphology focuses on structures that are too small to be observed by the naked eye and typically requires specialized microscopes such as scanning electron microscopes or optical microscopes for detailed visualization.

The *distribution* of micro-morphological features refers to how these fine structural characteristics are arranged or vary across space, among different species, or within particular environments. This distribution may reflect biological, ecological, or geological patterns, and understanding it can help scientists interpret how organisms are adapted to their environments, how materials behave under stress, or how soils and sediments formed over time. For example, in plant taxonomy, micro-morphological traits like epidermal cell patterns or seed surface ornamentation are used to differentiate among closely related species — because their distribution across taxa often highlights evolutionary relationships that macro-features alone might obscure.

In ecological studies, the variation and spatial distribution of micro-morphological traits can inform researchers about how microscopic structures influence a species' interaction with its habitat. For instance, micro-morphological traits on leaf surfaces — such as hair density or stomatal arrangements — can affect how plants respond to environmental stressors like dust, pollution, or drought. Analyses of these distributions enable scientists to correlate structural patterns with ecological performance or environmental tolerance.

Micromorphological distribution is also an important concept in soil science and archeology. Soil micromorphology examines the very fine structure of soil samples to decipher past depositional environments or to investigate how soil particles are distributed through space, which may reveal clues about climate history, land use, or sedimentation processes. These distributions, mapped at microscopic scales, provide insights that complement field observations and large-scale geological data.

Across disciplines, advances in imaging techniques have expanded the ability to quantify and compare micro-morphological distributions rigorously. Quantitative distribution patterns — such as frequencies of cell types, size distributions of particles, or spatial variation in surface features — offer researchers powerful tools to test hypotheses about development, adaptation, and evolutionary history. As a result, micro-morphological distribution has become an essential concept for anyone seeking to understand the complex architecture of living systems and natural environments at their most fundamental levels.

REFERENCES

1. Di Cataldo, S., Ficarra, E., Acquaviva, A., & Macii, E. (2010b). Automated segmentation of tissue images for computerized IHC analysis. *Computer Methods and Programs in Biomedicine*, *100*(1), 1–15. https://doi.org/10.1016/j.cmpb.2010.02.002Acquaviva, A., Di Cataldo, S., Ficarra, E., Macii, E., et al. (2011). Automated segmentation of cells with IHC membrane staining. https://core.ac.uk/download/pdf/11419237.pdf (accessed on 6th August 2025).
2. Artois, T., Boone, M., Borgonie, G., Couvreur, M., et al. (2009). Use of freeze-cracking in ontogenetic research in *Macrostomum lignano* (Macrostomida, Rhabditophora). https://core.ac.uk/download/55789072.pdf (accessed on 6th August 2025).
3. Baumgartner, A., Escudero, T., Kwan, S., Johnson, L., Lu, Y., et al. (2009). Rapid mapping of chromosomal breakpoints: From blood to BAC in 20 days. https://core.ac.uk/download/4886407.pdf (accessed on 6th August 2025).
4. Bojarska-Junak, A., Dmoszyńska, A., Giannopoulos, K., Roliński, J., et al. (2009). Expression of HLA-G in patients with B-cell chronic lymphocytic leukemia (B-CLL). https://core.ac.uk/download/268436757.pdf (accessed on 6th August 2025).
5. Bryś, M., Forma, E., Krajewska, W. M., Lewy-Trenda, I., et al. (2010). The expression of SOCS1 and TLR4-NFκB pathway molecules in neoplastic cells as potential biomarkers for the aggressive tumor phenotype in laryngeal carcinoma. https://core.ac.uk/download/268436702.pdf (accessed on 6th August 2025).
6. Bueno, G., García Rojo, M., Słodkowska, J. (2010). Review of imaging solutions for integrated quantitative immunohistochemistry in the pathology daily practice. https://core.ac.uk/download/268436697.pdf (accessed on 6th August 2025).
7. Bugno, M., Słota, E., Wnuk, M. (2008). Application of primed in situ DNA synthesis (PRINS) with telomere human commercial kit in molecular cytogenetics of *Equus caballus* and *Sus scrofa scrofa*. https://core.ac.uk/download/268436813.pdf (accessed on 6th August 2025).
8. Burns, J. K. (1957). *The effect of adrenocorticotropin on the nucleic acids and histochemistry of the guinea-pig adrenal cortex*. https://core.ac.uk/download/287589682.pdf (accessed on 6th August 2025).
9. Cassens, R. G., Eddinger, T. J., Moss, R. L. (1985). Fiber number and type composition in extensor digitorum longus, soleus, and diaphragm muscles with aging in Fisher 344 rats. https://core.ac.uk/download/213063910.pdf (accessed on 6th August 2025).
10. de Harven, E., Lambertenghi-Deliliers, G., Nava, M. T., Polli, N., et al. (1985). Scanning electron microscope cytochemistry of blood cells. https://core.ac.uk/download/395017505.pdf (accessed on 6th August 2025).
11. Ehrhart, M., Gratzl, M., Grube, D., Jörns, A., et al. (1988). Cellular distribution and amount of chromogranin A in bovine endocrine pancreas. https://core.ac.uk/download/12168026.pdf (accessed on 6th August 2025).
12. Elias, E. A., van der Heul, R. O. (1988). The evaluation of the activity of glucose-6-phosphate dehydrogenase and 6-phosphogluconate dehydrogenase under different patho-physiological conditions: A combined enzyme histochemical and biochemical approach. https://core.ac.uk/download/20116516.pdf (accessed on 6th August 2025).

13. Fernando, D. (2007). *Ultrastructural characterization (morphological and topochemical) of wood pulp fibres*. https://core.ac.uk/download/11695137.pdf (accessed on 6th August 2025).

14. Hirose, M. (1968). Tissue culture of human thyroid cancer. https://core.ac.uk/download/12547140.pdf (accessed on 6th August 2025).

15. Huang, S.-P. (1980). Behavioral and developmental responses induced in *Caenorhabditis elegans* and in some plant-parasitic nematodes by 5-hydroxytryptophan and dopamine. https://core.ac.uk/download/359473004.pdf (accessed on 6th August 2025).

16. James, D. J. (1974). *A cytochemical and biochemical study of acid hydrolases in developing plant cells, with particular reference to non-specific esterases*. https://core.ac.uk/download/9658006.pdf (accessed on 6th August 2025).

17. Joshi, P. A. (1987). Ultrastructural histochemical localization of beta-glycerophosphatase and adenosine triphosphatase activity in developing cotton fiber *Gossypium hirsutum* L. cv. Hancock. https://core.ac.uk/download/555440001.pdf (accessed on 6th August 2025).

18. Kawashima, T. & Ogata, T. (1963). A cytochemical study of oxidative enzymes in Ehrlich ascites tumor cells. https://core.ac.uk/download/12547097.pdf (accessed on 6th August 2025).

19. Klatka, J., Kupisz, K., Paduch, R., Pietruszewska, W., et al. (2008). Application of primary cell cultures of laryngeal carcinoma and laser scanning cytometry in the evaluation of tumor reactivity to cisplatinum. https://core.ac.uk/download/268436795.pdf (accessed on 6th August 2025).

20. Koji, T., Roth, J., Schrader, M., Taatjes, D., et al. (2019). *Histochemistry and Cell Biology*: 61 years and not tired at all. https://core.ac.uk/download/224783901.pdf (accessed on 6th August 2025).

21. Koshiba, K. (1968). An electron cytochemical demonstration and biochemical analysis of adenosine triphosphatase activity in cancer cell plasma membrane. https://core.ac.uk/download/12547196.pdf (accessed on 6th August 2025).

22. Laschi, R., Pasquinelli, G., Versura, P. (1987). Scanning electron microscopy application in clinical research. https://core.ac.uk/download/395018237.pdf (accessed on 6th August 2025).

23. Moramarco, A. M., Scillitani, G., Mastrodonato, M., Rossi, R. (2011). Glycopattern analysis and structure of the egg extra-cellular matrix in the Apennine yellow-bellied toad, *Bombina pachypus* (Anura: Bombinatoridae). https://core.ac.uk/download/pdf/26921114.pdf (accessed on 6th August 2025).

24. Musumeci, G. (2015). The old and the new concepts of histochemistry. https://core.ac.uk/download/604620742.pdf (accessed on 6th August 2025).

25. Paciello, O. & Papparella, S. (2009). Histochemical and immunohistological approach to comparative neuromuscular diseases. https://core.ac.uk/download/268436712.pdf (accessed on 6th August 2025).

26. Pellicciari, C. (2010). Histochemistry through the years, browsing a long-established journal: Novelties in traditional subjects. https://core.ac.uk/download/pdf/8613128.pdf (accessed on 6th August 2025).

27. Saitoh, S. (2018). Correlative light-electron microscopy (CLEM) and 3D volume imaging of serial block-face scanning electron microscopy (SBF-SEM) of Langerhans islets. https://core.ac.uk/download/322439926.pdf (accessed on 6th August 2025).

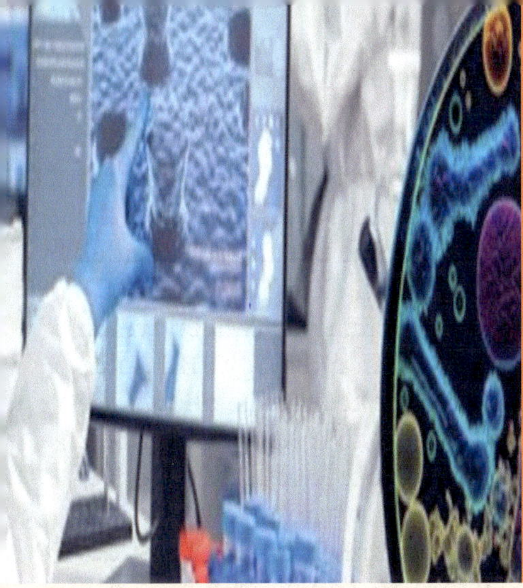

Chapter 10

IMMUNOHISTOCHEMISTRY (IHC)

Contents

Introduction

The field of immunohistochemistry (IHC) has significantly revolutionized histopathology, providing valuable insights into the cellular and molecular mechanisms of disease. The technique employs antibodies Detect antigens in tissue sections, enabling pathologists to visualize patterns of protein expression that inform diagnoses and prognoses. Based on antigen-antibody interaction, IHC allows for an advanced understanding of tissue architecture, segregating normal and diseased tissues. As a foundation of modern diagnostics, IHC has transformed the management of different malignancies, and the ability to properly classify tumors has been enhanced. patient outcomes and individualized therapeutic options. Utilization of IHC is particularly critical in evaluating breast cancer, especially in the assessment of HER2 status. Here, distinguishing between HER2 overexpression overexpression from gene amplification is paramount for treatment. Immunohistochemistry and fluorescence *in situ* hybridization (FISH) are complementary modalities to this diagnostic endeavor. The IHC methodology evaluates overexpression of the HER2 protein, while FISH provides evidence of gene amplification and, therefore, guides targeted therapies such as trastuzumab and pertuzumab. As discussed in the literature, the blending of the two approaches ensures a better diagnosis that ultimately decides on therapeutic decisions in accordance with a more tailored therapeutic plan (Kona et al., 2025). This comprehensive assessment reiterates the significance of precision medicine in cancer, which supports the central contribution of IHC to enhancing patient care. Apart from oncology, IHC holds promise in infectious diseases and neurodegenerative disease disorders. The technique allows the detection of targeted pathogens in tissue samples and thus is an important tool in the diagnosis of infections that might otherwise be hard to detect. Furthermore, IHC enables interrogation of protein expression changes in neurodegenerative disorders, such that their pathophysiology and therapeutic targets can be investigated. While its numerous advantages are present, potential limitations such as nonspecific staining and tissue artifacts are factors to consider, which can influence accuracy in interpretation. Pathologists should take these constraints into consideration for robust outcomes in utilizing IHC. With technology advancements, the integration of digital pathology may enhance the precision of IHC examinations, overcoming some of these limitations and expanding its application in the clinic (Yigzaw et al., 2024) (Figure 10.1).

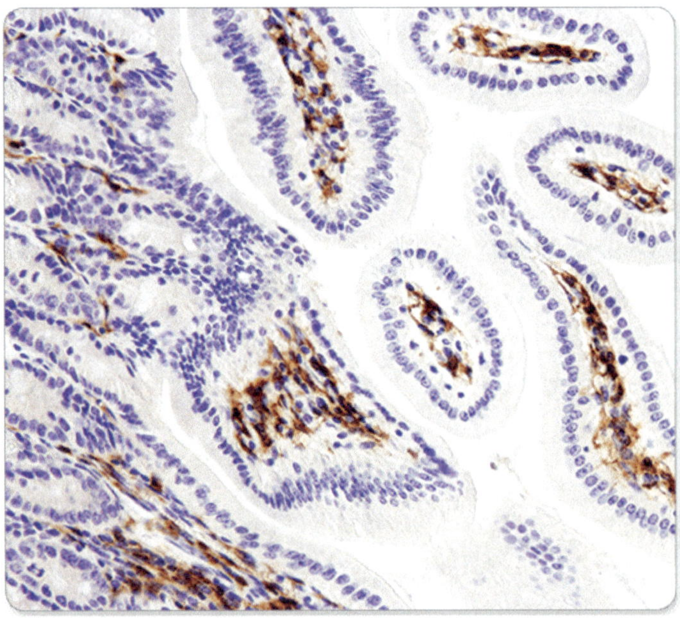

Figure 10.1. The field of immunohistochemistry (IHC).

Source: https://media.cellsignal.com/www/images/resources/applications/ihc/Immunohistochemistry-IHC-70076-intestine.png.

Definition and Significance of IHC

Immunohistochemistry (IHC) is a critical tool in the field of pathology that acts as an interface between clinical application and basic science. Quite simply, IHC is the technique that uses antibodies to detect particular antigens in tissue sections so that scientists and physicians can visualize the spatial relationship and localization of proteins in situ. It is a field of significance in the diagnosis and grouping of most cancers since this may provide tumor biology independent of histological analysis. It could emphasize significant biomarkers, hence influencing prognosis as well as treatment. Thus, IHC also plays a crucial role in personalizing cancer treatment by helping clinicians make informed decisions based on tumor molecular characteristics, thereby directly impacting patient care and outcomes. The utilization of IHC extends to diagnostic purposes alone; its implications are extensive in research for the field of oncology and personalized medicine as well. For example, the study of immune checkpoint proteins like PD-L1 via IHC has become standard in evaluating the efficacy of immunotherapies. Increased PD-L1 expression has been associated with improved responses to specific immunotherapeutic drugs, underscoring the role of IHC in determining treatment suitability. Similarly, examining multiple biomarkers simultaneously can provide an overall view of the microenvironment of a tumor, such as in IHC and genomic profiling combinations used to unveil significant molecular alterations. Multidimensional data from IHC can thus be utilized to guide treatment, thus positioning it as an invaluable asset in current oncology practice, as underscored by findings in large-scale studies conducted within clinics (Cantarella et al., 2024). Besides, IHC has a significant clinical role in tumor type identification, which is essential for effective treatment planning. For example, in triple-negative breast carcinoma (TNBC), a challenging cancer subtype to prognosticate and with limited treatment options, IHC defines the immune microenvironment and identify biomarkers to guide immunotherapy. Research demonstrating elevated PD-L1 expression in TNBC by IHC suggests that immunotherapy may improve patient outcomes (Seager et al., 2024). The ability of IHC to stratify also enables clinicians to individualize treatment protocols. Therefore, the use of IHC in clinical practices not only enhances diagnostic precision but also contributes to target therapies, rendering it even more crucial in cancer therapy.

Historical Development of IHC Techniques

The immunohistochemistry (IHC) techniques (IHC) techniques Has its origin in microscopy and an understanding of the immune system. The first identification of cellular constituents was carried out by using rudimentary staining methods. The breakthrough, however, came with the discovery of antibodies in tissue diagnosis. The 1940s and 1950s saw a surge in the production of polyclonal antibodies, allowing researchers and clinicians to target specific antigens in tissues. The technique enabled visualization of cellular structures and immune responses, thereby laying the foundation for IHC as an accepted technique. The invention of enzyme-linked antibodies, including horseradish peroxidase and alkaline phosphatase, also enhanced the sensitivity and specificity of antigen detection within various tissue types, further advancing IHC. Following the initial innovations in the 20th century, the 1970s and 1980s were pivotal in solidifying IHC as a norm within pathological research and diagnostic procedures. During this time, some of the key developments were the identification of monoclonal antibodies, which provided a reproducible and consistent approach to selectively targeting unique markers, thus making the diagnostic process easier. Therefore, IHC became an essential tool in the characterization of tumors, facilitating enhanced prognostication and therapy planning. Additionally, procedural refinements, such as the application of polymer-based detection systems, greatly improved the quality and readability of stained samples. This era of exploration largely expanded the horizon of IHC applications beyond oncology to immunology and histopathology, thus intertwining its development with more universal developments in biomedical research. The course of evolution of IHC techniques has, at the same time, followed, reflecting the growing complexity and sophistication of scientific study of cellular phenomena and disease mechanisms.

New technologies have integrated molecular biology innovation, such as the use of fluorescent markers and multiplex strategies, to enable the detection of multiple targets in the same tissue section. This indicates a continued striving for precision in disease diagnosis at increasingly finer levels. In addition, the use of high-throughput technologies and digital pathology has simplified the interpretation of IHC results and facilitated greater interdisciplinary collaboration in biomedical research. As emphasized in the historiography of immunology, the methodologies and information gathered from previous methods provide a solid basis for subsequent research, discovering the interrelatedness of immunohistochemistry to the broader institution of immunological research (Bommanavar, 2017; Gallo et al., 2022) (Figure 10.2).

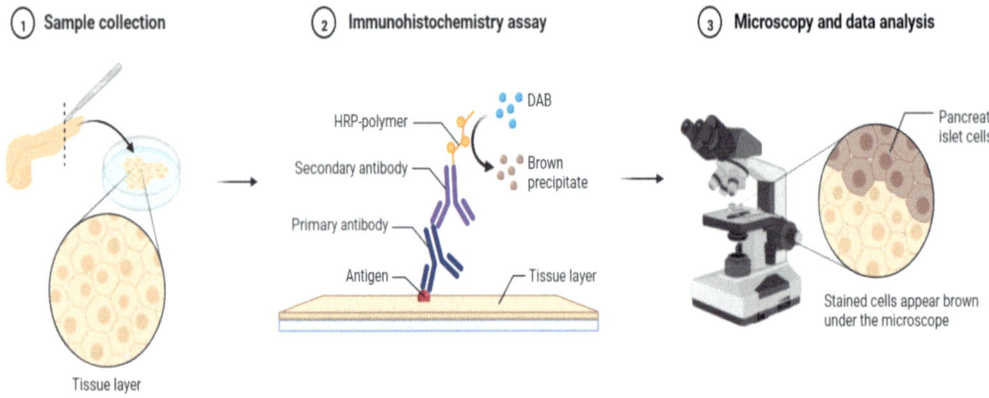

Figure 10.2. Development of IHC techniques.

Source: https://www.biomol.com/media/image/bd/22/8d/Principle_IHC_EN.png.

Overview of Applications in Research and Clinical Settings

The applications of immunohistochemistry (IHC) have significantly transformed research and clinical settings, particularly in oncology. IHC is an essential tool for the identification and definition of specific proteins in tissue specimens, thereby enabling the diagnosis of many cancers. Using this method, pathologists and researchers are able to differentiate cellular markers of cancer development, finally guiding treatment. In addition, the repeatability of IHC in producing images of protein expression facilitates patient stratification based on potential treatment responses. In this manner, immunohistochemistry, besides assisting diagnostics, contributes to the overall landscape of personalized medicine, thereby enhancing targeted treatment strategies for cancer patients. In the research field, IHC has facilitated paradigms like the exploration of cellular microenvironments as well as tumor heterogeneity. The technique allows researchers to ascertain protein localization and density, returning data on disease mechanisms at the cellular level. New technologies such as the Tissue Array Co-Occurrence Matrix Analysis (TACOMA) demonstrate the evolution of IHC in high-throughput applications. TACOMA makes it easier to analyze IHC images since cellular phenotypes are quantified from textural relationships among pixels. This algorithm is flexible, considerably reducing the time of evaluation and variability associated with traditional techniques. Through the use of the least data to train the algorithm, scientists are able to perform valid analyses, thus enhancing the potential of IHC as a research high-volume tool for oncology (Knudsen et al., 2011). The use of IHC in precision medicine illustrates its central function in improving patient management strategies. Individualized therapies according to molecular profiles, represented by various proteomics methods, have been shown to be able to yield better therapeutic outcomes. IHC represents part of these efforts through the precise characterization of protein biomarkers that can enhance therapy options and predict patients' responses to therapy. A good example of this is bladder cancer, in which IHC has been crucial for the characterization of specific markers with the aims of prognosis and therapy stratification. These uses emphasize the significance of IHC not only in diagnostic procedures but also in the continued quest for improved, individualized treatments in clinical oncology (Frantzi et al., 2017).

10.1. Principles of Immunohistochemistry

The principles of immunohistochemistry form the foundation to successful application of this technique in pathology. At its core, IHC relies on the antigen-antibody binding specificity. cellular content and activity. Key components of this process This specificity allows proteins to be visualized wherein monoclonal and polyclonal antibodies are both very significant. Monoclonal antibodies, produced by one clone of B lymphocytes, provide high specificity, while polyclonal antibodies, which are produced by numerous cell lines, allow for broad recognition of numerous different epitopes. The careful selection and verification of such antibodies are vital to gain accurate and reproducible results, reflecting the complexity and importance of IHC protocols in diagnostic tests and research investigations (Kohale et al., 2023). Apart from antibody selection, the process adopted within IHC encompasses some crucial steps, including tissue processing, antigen retrieval, and detection approaches. Tissue samples need to be carefully prepared, and in many instances, this requires formalin fixation and paraffin embedding to maintain morphology while permitting antigen preservation. Antigen retrieval is a crucial step since formalin fixation can obscure epitopes, requiring heat-induced or enzymatic retrieval treatments. Various detection techniques follow, ranging from chromogenic techniques that use enzyme-linked antibodies to produce a colored product to fluorescence techniques based on fluorescently labeled antibodies. Choice of detection methodologies has a far-reaching impact on specificity and sensitivity and must be consistent with the study objectives. Using standardized protocols and optimized conditions, investigators can maximize the validity of the IHC results (Binch et al., 2020).

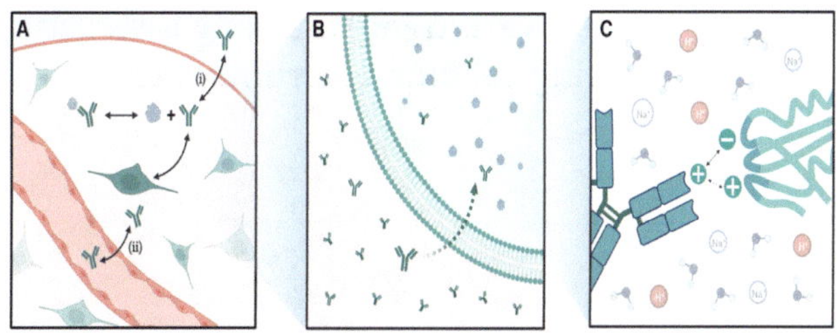

Figure 10.3. Principles of immunohistochemistry.

Source: https://www.cell.com/cms/attachment/9d47bb07-eb47-4fce-877a-a5749f5752f2/gr1_lrg.jpg.

The clinical and research uses of IHC are widespread and growing, reflecting the dynamic character of the technique. One of the particular uses of IHC is tumor characterisation and classification, where it allows the pathologist to classify tumor types, grade, and forecast prognosis accurately. IHC plays a significant role in the identification of biomarkers for several diseases so that targeted therapy and personalised medicine can be practiced. Beyond oncology, IHCs' flexibility extends into infectious disease and autoimmune disease research, where it enables the detection of infectious agents and the examination of immune responses. As methods and technology advance, merging multiplex IHC with digital pathology brings its diagnostic power to even greater heights. The continued development of IHC emphasizes its utility in facilitating both clinical and basic research, with enormous potential for impending advances in the biomedical sciences (Kohale et al., 2023) (Figure 10.3).

10.1.1. Antigen-Antibody Interactions

Antigen-antibody complexes are the backbone of the science of immunohistochemistry (IHC), enabling direct antigen detection in tissue samples. Antigen-antibody complexes arise due to antibodies binding uniquely to their cognate antigens This interaction is highly specific and is influenced by factors such as pH, temperature, and ionic strength. Conditions are optimized to enhance the specificity and sensitivity of antibody interaction, which is vital for achieving accurate experimental results. The specific binding allows cellular morphology to be visualized using various detection systems, including fluorescent and chromogenic substrates The reproducibility of this interaction is the basis for the importance of antibody specificity testing and is a central theme in IHC protocols. Therefore, all processes in the IHC process are obliged to methodically engage these interactions in order to induce effective staining and proper histological sample interpretation. Moreover, the capacity to observe antigen-antibody interaction by different methods has significantly contributed to understanding cellular environments.

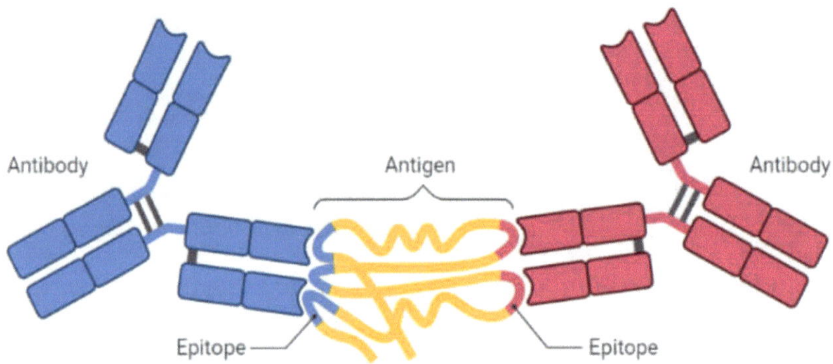

Figure 10.4. Antigen-antibody interactions.

Source: https://microbenotes.com/wp-content/uploads/2022/05/Antigen-Antibody-Ag-Ab-Interaction.jpeg.

For example, multiplex fluorescence immunohistochemistry allows simultaneous localization of more than one antigen in one tissue section and thus provides an understanding of complex cell-cell interactions as well as immune responses in different contexts. This method enhances the pheno-typing ability of immune cell subsets and tumor-associated markers, thereby facilitating prognostication and treatment decision-making in oncology. Because of the specialized requirements of antigen retrieval and optimal antibody levels, mastering these nuances is crucial for researchers and clinicians who aim to employ IHC for comprehensive examination. Lastly, the progress in antigen-antibody kinetic visualization not only validates the effectiveness of IHC but also opens the gates towards additional advancements in diagnostic and therapeutic use. In specific cases, for instance, the diagnosis of pigmented lesions, the antigen-antibody relationship nuances can present very particular challenges. The interfering factor of melanin, which obscures tissue morphology, directly prevents the visibility of specific antigens and hence complicates the diagnosis of diseases such as melanoma. Melanin's inherent pigmentation has the ability to inhibit antibody binding as well as interfere with chromogenic detection, hence ultimately inhibiting histopathological analysis. To counter this challenge, melanin bleaching is now a significantly useful procedure in IHC practice. By using agents such as hydrogen peroxide to bleach melanin without damaging antigenicity and tissue morphology, pathologists are able to optimize the clarity of antigen-antibody interactions. Hence, integration of these bleaching techniques not only supports accurate diagnosis but also serves as an example of ongoing progress in IHC protocols to overcome barriers in antigen detection and interpretation while following rigid standards in clinical practice (Yeh et al., 2024) (Figure 10.4).

10.1.2. Types of Antibodies Used in IHC

The success of immunohistochemistry (IHC) largely depends on the type of antibodies employed in staining. Antibodies are found in two broad types: polyclonal and monoclonal antibodies. Polyclonal antibodies are immunized from various clones of B-cells, resulting in a mixture of antibodies that will react with different epitopes within one antigen. Because this provides diversity that enhances sensitivity and may increase affinity within complex tissue environments, polyclonal antibodies are widely employed. Such heterogeneity, though, can lead to batch-to-batch variability and render inter-experiment comparison challenging.

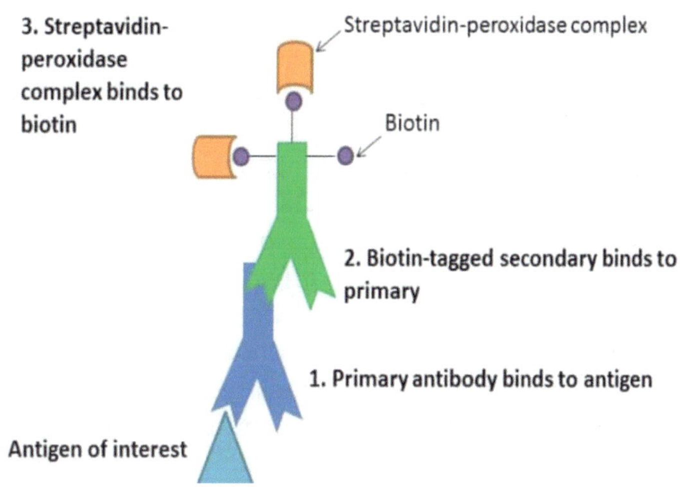

Figure 10.5. Types of antibodies used in IHC.

Source: https://bitesizebio.com/wp-content/uploads/2011/09/Immunohistochemistry.jpg.

Monoclonal antibodies, on the contrary, are derived from a single clone of B-cells and interact with a single defined epitope in a highly specific fashion. This attribute is well-suited for monoclonal antibodies for quantitative analysis and reproducibility, essential aspects for enhancing the reliability of IHC assays for clinical diagnosis or research applications. Specificity and cross-reactivity are significant factors in selecting antibodies for IHC. Highly specific antibodies bind uniquely to their individual target, reducing background noise and artefacts that could produce false conclusions. Often, conventional IHC protocols involve a high level of antibody validation through testing against known markers and controls. For example, immunohistochemical studies employing integrins have demonstrated their significance in cancer research, as they are involved in cellular signaling and migration (Arun et al., 2018). A strict selection process ensures that all antibodies employed are suitable for the type of tissue being studied, thereby maximally replicating the precision of antigen localization. In addition, the use of antibody validation techniques like western blotting and cross-contamination testing has an important part to play in determining whether antibodies are suitable prior to their use in IHC studies. The advances in production and antibody engineering technology have generated new forms of antibodies, such as recombinant antibodies and nanobodies. Recombinant antibodies that are generated through the use of genetic engineering technology can be designed for desirable binding characteristics and therefore offer new advantages for application in IHC. In addition, nanobodies—small single-domain camelid-derived antibodies—are more tissue-permeating and stable than regular antibodies and are therefore best suited for challenging tissues with limited epitope accessibility. Along with improving the quality of IHC imaging, these developments further expand the application area in research and diagnostics. There is a focus in current studies on the ease of such advanced antibodies for complex research, enabling intricate protein expression and localization studies, thereby enhancing our understanding of complex biological systems (Estep et al., 2015) (Figure 10.5).

10.1.3. Detection Methods in IHC

The methods of detection that are employed in immunohistochemistry (IHC) play a crucial role in detecting and visualizing specific antigens within tissue sections. The traditional approaches are enzyme-linked immunosorbent assays (ELISA), which detect proteins based on the antigen-antibody reaction. However, with the improvement in IHC over time, histochemical staining methods have been utilised that deliver higher specificity and sensitivity. Another such development is the use of automated staining platforms, which increase reproducibility and minimize errors due to human intervention during staining. Automated systems facilitate high-throughput analysis, which is essential in clinical and research settings where several samples must be analyzed at once, hence streamlining diagnostic procedures. A new application of detection methods in IHC is membrane segmentation techniques, which significantly enhance cellular component visibility. Accurate membrane segmentation is critical for cellular morphology characterization and the determination of the spatial distribution of some antigens in cancer and other pathologies. Use of automated membrane segmentation on stained tissue images has become more and more common, as shown in more recent studies.

By providing accurate quantification of target membrane proteins, such methods enable thorough morphological examination. Furthermore, this progress is imperative to the engineering of individualized therapy and cancer classification, exemplifying the importance of possessing strong detection methods for effective diagnostics and treatment planning in the realm of IHC (Acquaviva et al., 2011). In addition, other histochemical staining methods, such as the Solophenyl-Red 3 BL-method, illustrate the perils and specificity of traditional IHC methods. Applied to the visualisation of collagen type III in skin wound healing, for instance, contrast between IHC results and Solophenyl-Red staining serves to underscore the need for selection of detection methods based on contextual requirements.

While IHC definitively established high levels of collagen type III in skin wounds, Solophenyl-Red staining produced variable results, thus serving to establish its non-specificity in certain contexts (Nerlich et al., 1992). This difference underlines the necessity of using complementary detection methods in validating findings and arriving at firm conclusions, particularly in complex biological systems where accurate localization of specific proteins is imperative for valid conclusions in research and clinical practice (Figure 10.6).

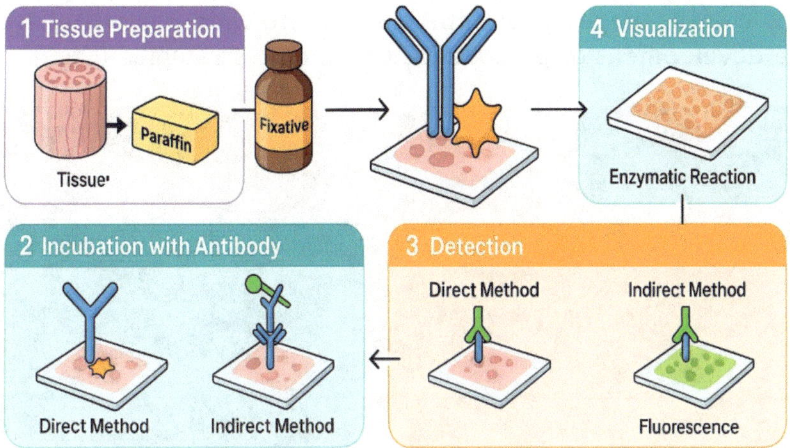

Figure 10.6. Detection methods in IHC.

Source: https://oncodaily.com/pub/uploads/2025/05/Immunohistochemistry_Process_Fixed_OncoDaily.jpg.

10.2. IHC Techniques and Protocols

Immunohistochemistry (IHC) is a fundamental research tool and clinical diagnostic method that allows the visualization and localization of target antigens in tissue sections. The IHC procedure typically begins with the processing of formalin-fixed, paraffin-embedded (FFPE) tissues, which are subsequently sectioned and mounted on slides. The choice of an appropriate primary antibody is crucial since it will determine the specificity and sensitivity of the staining. After antibody incubation, several detection systems, such as enzyme-linked or fluorochrome-based systems, these systems amplify the signal, allowing for the visualization of antibody-antigen complexes. For successful IHC, optimizing each phase is critical. For instance, antigen retrieval techniques are designed to maximize epitope access and suppress non-specific binding, which can lead to inaccurate results and interpretations IHC evolution has included the introduction of sophisticated methods to increase diagnostic specificity. For instance, biomarker advancement has allowed for more precise definitions of states of disease; measurement of certain tumor-related fusion proteins can be highly informative in terms of treatment. Techniques such as fluorescence *in situ* hybridization (FISH) and next-generation sequencing (NGS) have been coupled with IHC to get a comprehensive evaluation of tumor genetics. A prime example would be the detection of NTRK fusions in wild-type GISTs, where IHC methods such as Pan-TRK staining have revealed varying sensitivity and specificity compared to genomic methods (Cao et al., 2022). It is important to understand the pros and cons of these methods to adopt effective clinical protocols and obtain valid diagnostic findings. Furthermore, the role of IHC is not only antigen detection, but also serves as a tool to reveal the pathophysiologic mechanisms of diseases. Current studies have demonstrated the utility of immunohistochemical profiling for the assessment of treatment response and prognosis of disease. For instance, regucalcin (RGN) tissue expression has been used as a biomarker for illegal steroid use in agricultural practices, demonstrating IHC's value in a range of biological fields of study (Benedetto et al., 2021). In-depth information regarding IHC techniques, in addition to robust protocols, is important for ensuring reproducibility and reliability in diagnosis and research purposes. As science evolves, ongoing optimization of IHC methods will drive improvements in patient care and the development of personalized medicine strategies (Figure 10.7).

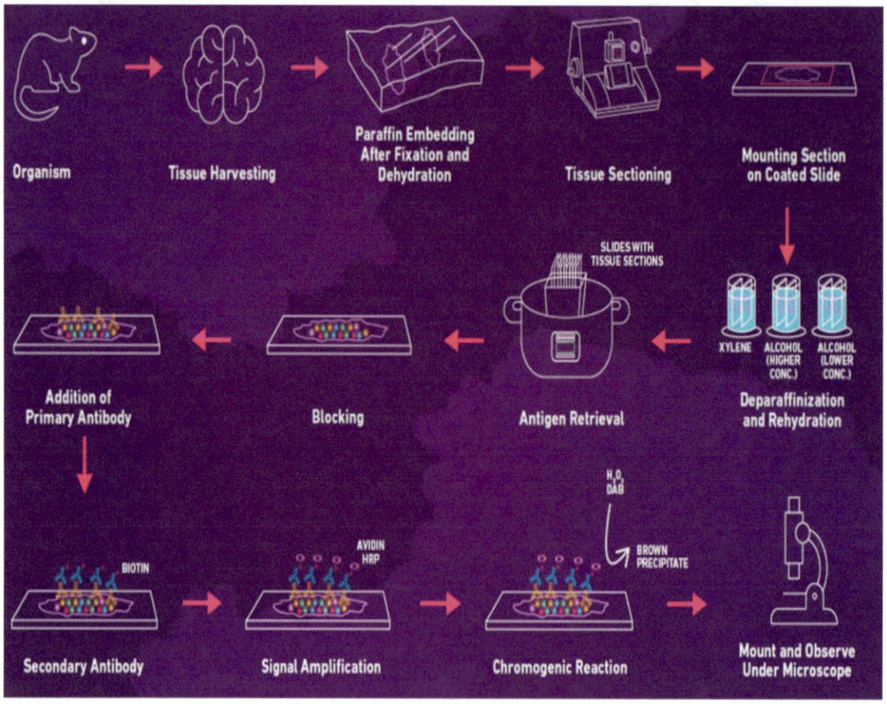

Figure 10.7. IHC techniques and protocols.

Source: https://cdn.technologynetworks.com/tn/images/body/immunohistochemistry-seo-article-fig-4-final_resized1657011723147.jpg.

10.2.1. Sample Preparation and Fixation

In immunohistochemistry (IHC), fixation and sample preparation are essential steps with a direct impact on interpretability and quality of diagnostic results. Fixation, as long as it is appropriate, guarantees that cellular morphology and antigenicity are preserved, which is most valuable in downstream antibody recognition. Chemicals such as formaldehyde and paraformaldehyde are most commonly used because they can cross-link proteins, thereby stabilizing tissue structure and preventing antigen degradation. However, the fixative employed, fixation duration, and temperature used to treat samples can strongly affect IHC assay results, and hence reproducing data and ensuring result reliability through proper regulations using predefined protocols is essential. Apart from simple fixation, complexities in sample handling also extend to the entire pre-analytical process and encompass tissue processing, embedding, and sectioning. This holds particularly in human brain tissue analysis, where post-mortem processing may greatly alter tissue integrity unless conducted with precision. Effective sample preparation may involve prolonged fixation of specimens, e.g., where specimens were fixed for years but are still viable for high-resolution analysis. Maintaining ultrastructural features and antigen access is crucial for modalities like electron microscopy, which can supplement IHC by providing accurate visualization of cellular components Thus, understanding the finesse of specimen handling is essential for successful IHC applications. The role of specimen fixation in quality assurance protocols cannot be emphasized enough, especially in clinical applications where biomarkers guide therapeutic management In the interpretation of programmed death ligand 1 (PD-L1) expression in non-small-cell lung cancer, for example, meticulous preparation of tissue samples plays a significant role in interpretative precision and clinical implications. Pre-analytical variables like fixation methods affect the display of antigens to the antibodies presented in IHC tests. Guidelines focusing on standardized fixation and processing protocols are therefore of importance to ensure maximum consistency of results among samples and laboratories. With strides in the field achieved through new diagnostic technologies, ongoing research and understanding of fixative strategies will be of prime importance to tackle tissue preparation-related issues and optimize diagnostic utility of IHC methods to bring about proper patient stratification and treatment regimens, as reiterated in current publications (Liu et al., 2014; Booton et al., 2016) (Figure 10.8).

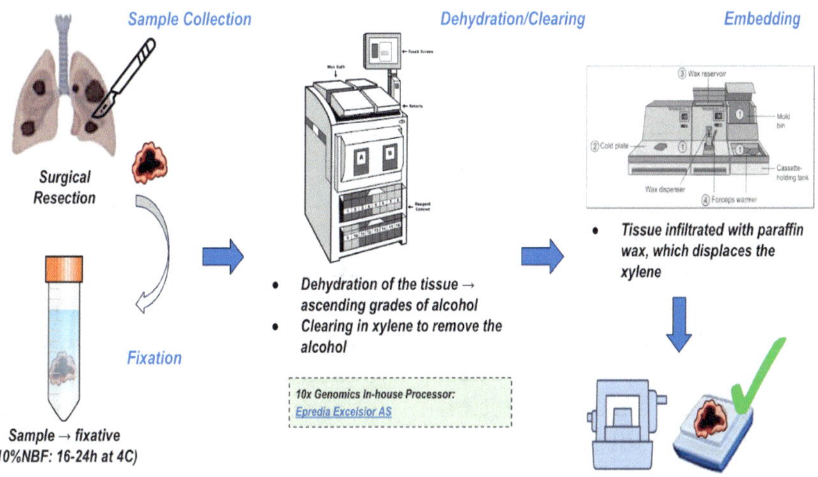

Figure 10.8. Sample preparation and fixation.

Source: https://lh6.googleusercontent.com/kIkjvQa_1evlsiJtJit89qhVqJq3ul8frR4myVPklEmgYDDkg74-E-Jz9ATuURXIhRl5p-qXmAfQpl1q2mHf13TSPtDY5SrNyxWyfy4fYFvRmbGeRpVCa6O8IJynxeLyuDZSxB0NITtjAGD_PiiJMsQ.

10.2.2. Staining Procedures and Protocols

Optimizing staining procedures in immunohistochemistry (IHC) is essential for achieving reproducible, consistent results. A crucial element to this process is the adjustment of antigen retrieval procedures, which aids in greater access to target antigens bound in formalin-fixed, paraffin-embedded (FFPE) tissue. A number of methods can influence the quality of staining, including heat-induced antigen retrieval or enzymatic digestion. For instance, Watson et al. (2025) point out that different protocols yield different outcomes based on the tumor type, as evidenced by their experiment involving FGFR2b expression in different cancers. This highlights the necessity for protocols tailored to specific histological types to ensure that the staining process accurately reflects the underlying tissue biology. The efficiency of these steps not only enhances diagnostic consistency but also aids in the identification of prognostic markers that are vital in treatment determination. Besides antigen retrieval, the procedures of primary antibody incubation are significant in efficient immunostaining. Heat, time, and dilutions of antibodies could have a tremendous impact on the interaction of antibodies with antigens, hence the intensity and specificity of the staining response. Optimization at this time can improve sensitivity, enabling one to pick up low-abundance antigens that would otherwise go undetected. The method highlighted by Gorris et al. (2023) provides insight into advanced multiplex IHC techniques, which enable the simultaneous visualization of multiple targets and therefore improve the information obtained from a single tissue section. Such methodological innovation allows examination of complex interactions between elements of the tumor microenvironment, such as immune and tumor cells, with a more seamless understanding of tumor biology. Finally, staining protocol assessment should not discount the importance of detection systems following the application of primary antibodies. The chosen detection system—chromogenic or fluorescent—can strongly influence the quality of the outcome. Chromogenic detection is typically preferred due to its simplicity and versatility with traditional tissue samples, whereas multiplex fluorescence techniques provide greater information by simultaneously identifying multiple antigens. Application of machine learning models for interpretation of multiplexed images, according to Gorris et al. (2023), represents a cutting-edge frontier of data interpretation that addresses the multifaceted nature of tumor tissue. This advancement not only simplifies the analysis but also enhances prognostic assessments by linking analyzed immune populations with spatial relevance. These advancements reinforce the significance of complete protocol optimization in IHC, which is essential for making cancer diagnostics and therapeutic advances possible.

10.2.3. Quality Control Measures in IHC

Quality control measurements for immunohistochemistry (IHC) are central to yielding accurate and reproducible results. The quality of the antibodies used, the reproducibility of staining protocols, and the histological fixation and preparation of the tissue samples are primarily responsible for the accuracy of IHC results. The utilization of control slides, including positive and negative controls, is mandatory to verify staining procedures. Employing control tissues, the laboratories are able to calculate the specificity and sensitivity of the antibody binding to ensure signals detected are as expected for specific histological features. Such control measures not only assist in troubleshooting but also enable standardization of protocols across labs, thus enhancing the overall quality and reliability of IHC as a diagnostic tool. Moreover, quantitative analysis in IHC requires meticulous attention during staining. Automated and computer-based methods have also been shown to be effective quality control methods with increased accuracy and reproducibility over manual techniques. Recent advances in automated tissue image segmentation demonstrate their applicability in reducing common human errors associated with subjective visual evaluation. For instance, unsupervised color clustering algorithms work to distinctly mark cancerous areas without incorporating non-targeted stroma in order to enhance the specificity of analyses. Additionally, developments in the segmentation of nuclear membranes ensure that protein expression quantification in cancer cells is reliable and consistent, which is critical for subsequent clinical uses and interpretations of pathology outcomes (Acquaviva et al., 2010). Most significantly, the integration of biomarker research into IHC procedures can further refine quality control measures. The identification of specific biomarker expression profiles can provide insights into patient response to treatment, thereby personalizing therapeutic strategies. For instance, in trials of head and neck cancer correlating DNA repair protein expression with response to therapy, specific biomarkers such as XPF and pMK2 predicted patient response to chemotherapy (Cohen et al., 2014). The utility of combining molecular diagnostics into IHC, ensuring the highest quality control by correlating laboratory findings with therapeutic response, is therefore established. With continued development, continued validation, and incorporation of these biomarker-based strategies will be the key to improving diagnostic specificity and oncology patient care (Figure 10.9).

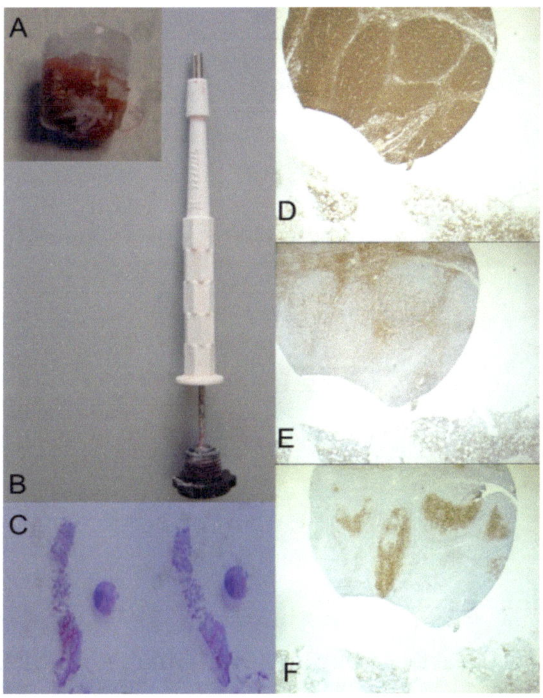

Figure 10.9. Quality control measures in immunohistochemistry (IHC).

Source: https://jcp.bmj.com/content/jclinpath/65/7/635/F1.large.jpg?width=800&height=600&carousel=1.

10.3. Applications of IHC in Diagnostics

Immunohistochemistry (IHC) revolutionized diagnostics, particularly pathology and oncology, as it allows for the detection and analysis of proteins in tissue sections. The specificity of IHC enables highly specific localization of antigens, thereby enhancing understanding of cell and tissue architecture. This technique has now become indispensable in various applications, such as the determination of tumor marker expression, which aids in cancer classification and the selection of therapeutic approaches. In breast cancer, for instance, determination of estrogen receptor (ER) and human epidermal growth factor receptor 2 (HER2) status by IHC plays an important role in determining the treatment regimen, such as the use of targeted drugs. Therefore, the application of IHC in diagnostic procedures not only increases the accuracy of tumor grading but also helps in the formation of targeted treatment based on individual cases. In infectious diseases, IHC has proved useful in pathogen diagnosis in tissue samples. It provides a way to visualize the presence of particular antigens associated with certain infectious pathogens, which can be priceless when standard methods like culture and serology are lacking. Through the assistance of specific antibodies, pathologists can directly detect viral, bacterial, and fungal infections from tissue sections, enabling timely and accurate diagnoses. For example, IHC may be employed to detect cytomegalovirus infection in organ biopsies, thereby facilitating appropriate treatment and management. Additionally, the ability of IHC to quantify the spatial distribution of the pathogens helps us understand the disease mechanisms and host responses, further enhancing the diagnostic value in infectious disease pathology. Furthermore, the advancement of IHC applications is also fueling innovation in precision medicine, particularly by combining with proteomics. Proteomics is interested in large-scale investigation into proteins that present the real-time dynamic status of molecular phenotypes in patients. By combining IHC results with proteomic data, clinicians can supply better stratification of patients, allowing them to customize treatment based on individual molecular profiles. In conditions such as bladder cancer, where heterogeneity is a clinically significant problem, biomarker identification by IHC can enable targeted therapies and improve patient outcomes. The potential for proteomics in being able to identify new therapeutic targets resonates with the evolving landscape of precision medicine. Hence, IHC is not just a diagnostic tool but also a foundation for the future development of individualized patient treatment, as described in current research on maximizing cancer therapies (Frantzi et al., 2017) and ongoing innovation in imaging technologies (Arzberger et al., 2020).

10.3.1. Role in Cancer Diagnosis and Classification

Immunohistochemistry (IHC) is a key component in the diagnosis and classification of cancer, supplementing the histopathological examination of tumors. IHC allows pathologists to view and verify the presence of certain proteins involved in malignancy through the application of specific antibodies that bind antigens in cancer cells. This process not only helps in cancer type identification but also helps in the determination of tumor origin, which is very important in those with atypical or indeterminate histology.

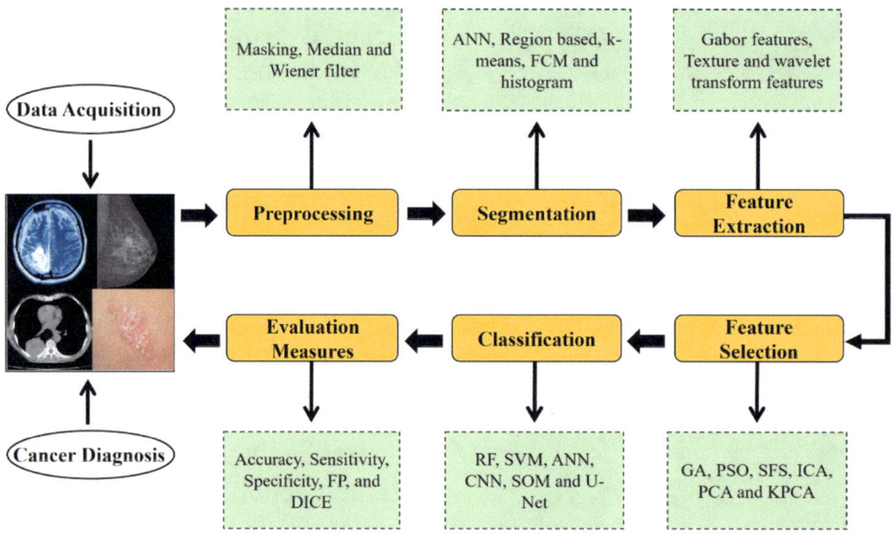

Figure 10.10. Role in cancer diagnosis and classification.

Source: https://www.mdpi.com/cancers/cancers-13-05546/article_deploy/html/images/cancers-13-05546-g001.png.

For instance, the application of IHC in pleural mesothelioma has been vital, where specific staining patterns can confirm a diagnosis that might otherwise prove elusive. In addition, IHC marker specificity improves classification accuracy to allow for more patient-specific treatment interventions based on distinctive tumor characteristics. Integration of IHC into clinical practice is important in facilitating personalized oncology practice. By characterizing the molecular profile of tumors, IHC assists oncologists in making informed decisions on treatment regimens. For example, research into protein expression, such as that of BAP1 and MTAP/CDKN2A, using IHC has been linked to increased pleural mesothelioma diagnosis levels, enabling medical practitioners to better predict patients' prognoses and adjust therapy to that effect (Lynch et al., 2024). Moreover, IHC may uncover predictive markers indicating sensitivity to some therapies, such as targeted drugs or immunotherapy. This approach not only gives a clearer understanding of tumor biology but also paves the way for novel treatment regimens that would be likely to increase patient survival and quality of life remarkably. Besides increasing the accuracy of diagnosis, IHC is also useful for ongoing classification of tumors with a better understanding of cancer biology. As scientists develop new evidence for the molecular etiology of cancer, IHC plays a critical role in updating classification systems based on newly discovered biomarkers. For instance, multimodal image analysis, including IHC techniques, has been integrated into whole-slide imaging (WSI) classification methods to significantly accelerate tumor recognition and classification (Lou et al., 2024). This innovative technique allows for additional inclusion of sources of data, in line with today's standards of precision medicine. As the science of diagnosing cancer continues to evolve, the application of IHC remains imperative, not only for accurate categorization, but also for guiding the evolution of subsequent studies and clinical approaches in oncology (Figure 10.10).

10.3.2. Use in Infectious Disease Identification

Immunohistochemistry (IHC) is an important tool in the diagnosis and detection of infectious diseases, particularly by allowing visualization of specific antigens in tissue sections. Through the use of labeled antibodies against antigens from pathogens, IHC permits the identification and localization of infectious agents within tissue specimens directly. It not only provides confirmation of diagnosis but also allows insight into the disease pathophysiology. IHC's antigen specificity enables it to distinguish among pathogens infecting the same tissue type and is of prime value in clinical settings, where rapid and accurate detection can have a crucial impact on treatment and outcomes. IHC, by application, has proven itself to be a useful tool, particularly in the diagnosis of new emerging infectious diseases when standard diagnostic methods often falter. Besides, the use of artificial intelligence (AI) and IHC has enhanced the diagnosis of infectious diseases to become more efficient and accurate. Recent advancements in AI, especially machine learning algorithms, make it easier to analyze complex tissue images produced by IHC. These algorithms can sift through large sets of data to find patterns and reveal faint changes missed by the naked eye. For instance, the utilization of AI with IHC could boost the precision in the detection of pathogens and antimicrobial resistance prediction and, therefore, guide effective therapeutic interventions. A future where AI's potential to automate processes in IHC is addressed is a bright future in infectious disease control, as it allows clinicians to make evidence-based decisions more rapidly than does current diagnostic methodology, thereby leading to better patient outcomes (Cesaro et al., 2025). Of equal interest is the focus on the difficulties and constraints inherent in utilizing IHC for the detection of infectious diseases. While IHC can be informative, issues such as the quality of existing antibodies, reproducibility of staining protocols, and the use of qualified operators to interpret results can, in theory, interfere with its use. Moreover, the emergence of new pathogens creates a demand for ongoing validation of antibodies and methods used in IHC. Combined, clinicians and researchers have addressed these challenges by exploring new biomarkers, as well as implementing novel technologies to enhance the sensitivity and specificity of assays. The integration of big data analytics, particularly those generated through AI methodology, can also benefit IHC by addressing the heterogeneity encountered with clinical specimens. Beating these pitfalls and enhancing practices will be crucial in ensuring the continued utility of IHCs as a valuable weapon in the war against infectious disease (Meslamani et al., 2024) (Figure 10.11).

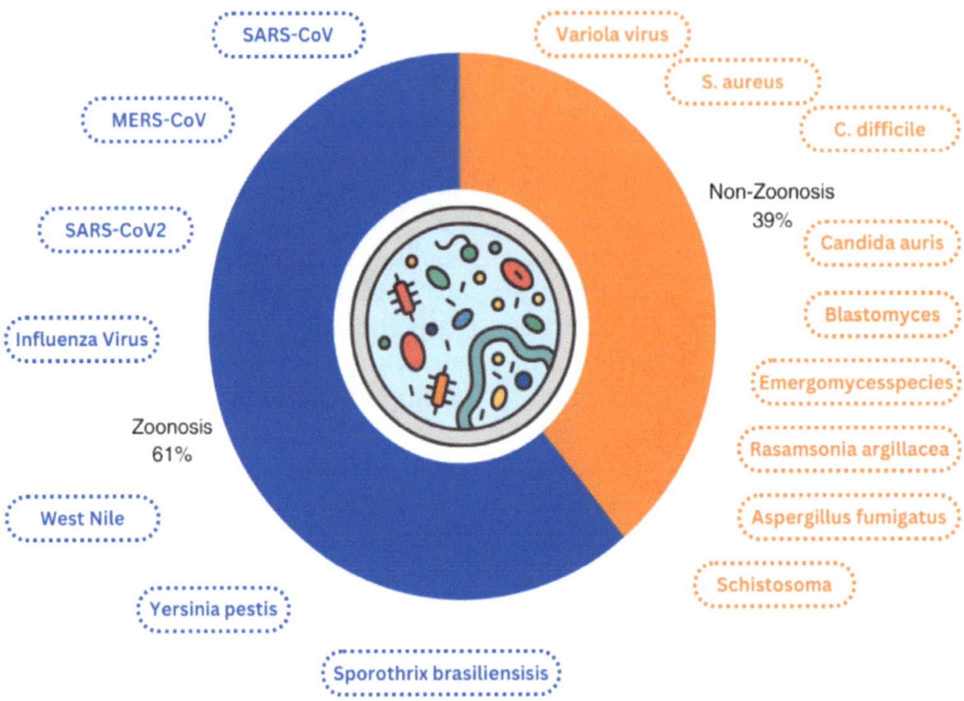

Figure 10.11. Use in infectious disease identification.

Source: https://www.mdpi.com/genes/genes-15-00908/article_deploy/html/images/genes-15-00908-g003.png.

10.3.3. Applications in Autoimmune Disease Research

Immunohistochemistry (IHC) has emerged as the core methodology in the study of autoimmune diseases over the past decades. Through histological analysis of tissue samples, IHC helps researchers identify specific antigens that are implicated in autoimmune processes. This role is particularly significant in elucidating the pathophysiology of such diseases as rheumatoid arthritis and systemic lupus erythematosus. By visualizing autoimmune-associated markers and inflammatory cells, researchers are able to gain insight into the disease process and underlying immunological mechanisms. For example, the expression of specific immune cells, as measured by IHC, can be used to distinguish active disease from remission, thereby guiding clinical management and patient stratification. The functional utility of IHC contributes to our understanding of the complexities of immune dysregulation underlying autoimmune diseases. Furthermore, IHC is a powerful tool for exploring disease markers and potential treatment targets in autoimmune research. Immune cell infiltrate comprehensive profiling, including T cells and macrophages, yields significant information for the identification of bioactive elements in affected tissues. Specifically, research on heparanase (HPSE) illustrates how IHC can characterize the roles of specific molecules involved in disease modulation. Increased HPSE expression in necro-inflammatory areas of fibrotic tissues suggests a role in immune-mediated liver damage, providing a target pathway for therapeutic targeting in autoimmune liver disease. All these observations reveal the function of IHC as complex, not only in the diagnosis of autoimmune diseases, but also in precluding interventions that specifically target singular molecular pathways of the immune system without inducing wider systemic effects, as reflected in investigations exploring proteomics and precision medicine (Frantzi et al., 2017).

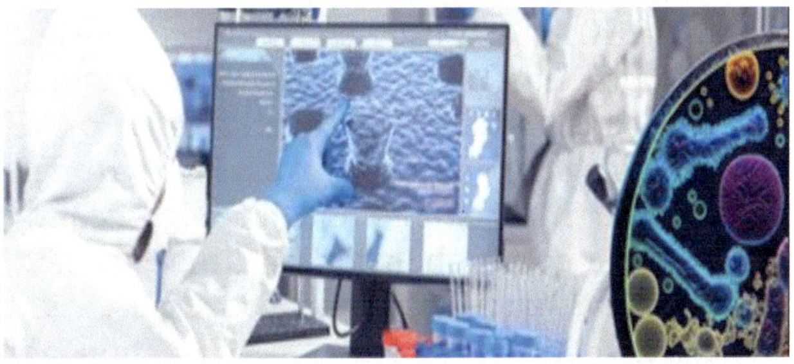

Figure 10.12. Applications in autoimmune disease research.

Source: https://external-content.duckduckgo.com/iu/?u=https%3A%2F%2Ftse3.mm.bing.net%2Fth%2Fid%2FOIP.2vAyLUhioKWsSppkbyg3_wHaD4%3Fpid%3DApi&f=1&ipt=882c5893d193c2999ef6d2f45444598f70e53dfa1f4fc5bd72a2b963f7f403d6.

Integrating IHC with emerging technologies is a promising means of further deciphering autoimmune diseases. For instance, multiplex IHC innovations enable the simultaneous identification of multiple markers from a single tissue section, revealing complex immunological maps that traditional methods may fail to detect. Such a broad-based strategy facilitates novel biomarker and therapeutic target discovery, thereby propelling personalized medicine initiatives. Such strategies may lead to more individualized patient treatments based on the individual's unique molecular signature of autoimmune disease. As established in studies of numerous pathologies, including cancers and inflammatory conditions, the transition towards more sophisticated, biomarker-driven treatment protocols is the future for research on autoimmune diseases employing IHC. Through continued exploration into these practices, researchers can increase diagnostic sensitivity and improve patient outcomes in the field of autoimmune disease (Crescenzi et al., 2017) (Figure 10.12).

10.4. IHC in Research

Immunohistochemistry (IHC) is crucial to scientific research as it enables scientists to see proteins in the cellular context. The technique relies on antigen-antibody interaction, with detectable visualization by a variety of detection means. The technique allows scientists to investigate the spatial localization and organization of proteins in tissue specimens. With the application of IHC, researchers have access to information on the molecular etiology of conditions like cancer and autoimmune illnesses, leading to an understanding of pathological processes. The advancement of IHC techniques, as noted, through monoclonal and polyclonal antibody combinations improves sensitivity and specificity, thus significantly contributing to experimental outcome consistency (Kohale et al., 2023). Thus, IHC is not only a diagnostic tool but also a fundamental research method that aims to identify cellular processes and interactions at the molecular level. The application of IHC is furthered by novel imaging technologies, such as three-dimensional (3D) X-ray histology. With laboratory facilities such as those at the University of Southampton, researchers can combine traditional IHC with advanced imaging techniques, significantly enhancing analysis of tissue structure and complex cellular interactions (Katsamenis et al., 2023). By pairing IHC with microfocus computed tomography (μCT), researchers can visualize whole-tissue sections in three dimensions, enabling them to have a better understanding of biological specimens. This union of methods not only increases the efficiency of data acquisition but also facilitates high-resolution spatial analysis of biomarker expression within tissue structure, thereby opening the doors for new knowledge in biomedical studies, with particular focus on the tumor microenvironment. Furthermore, the future of IHC in research is poised for great breakthroughs through the combination of automation and artificial intelligence.

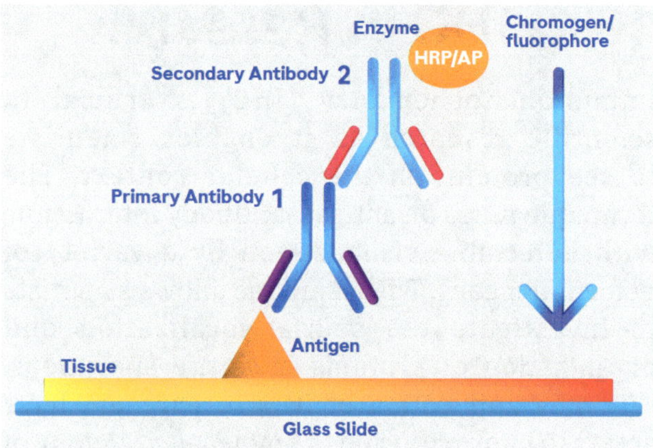

Figure 10.13. IHC in research.

Source: https://roche63-h.assetsadobe2.com/is/image/content/dam/diagnostics/us/en/products/i/immunohistochemistry-ihc/immunohistochemistry-graphic-no-bg-v5.png?scl=1&fmt=png-alpha.

Automated IHC platforms enhance reproducibility and throughput, i.e., large-scale analysis on numerous samples is possible. Additionally, machine learning algorithms can be used to quantify the intensity of staining and cellular context, enabling seamless data analysis and interpretation. The ongoing integration of IHC with next-generation sequencing technologies also holds the promise to transform research by facilitating simultaneous exploration of gene expression and protein localization in the same tissue context, an irreducible element of in-depth biomarker discovery and analysis (Kohale et al., 2023). Thus, the evolving landscape of IHC continues to extend its research applications, ultimately pushing the agenda for deciphering complex biological systems and diseases (Figure 10.13).

10.4.1. Utilization in Cellular and Molecular Biology Studies

The application of immunohistochemistry (IHC) to cellular and molecular biology has significantly enhanced our understanding of biological processes and disease conditions. By employing the use of specific antibodies for recognizing unique antigens within tissue sections, IHC allows researchers to visualize and identify proteins in their own native cellular context. This localization is critical in order to understand protein expression patterns and cellular interactions and has significantly aided in the comprehension of differentiation, proliferation, and apoptosis processes. As a critical imaging tool, IHC is fundamental not only to basic research but also to clinical diagnostics, particularly for identifying disease markers and therapeutic targets in conditions such as cancer and neurodegenerative diseases. The integration of IHC techniques into cellular and molecular biology enables a sensitive understanding of the molecular mechanisms of disease and health, highlighting the technique's critical position in furthering the biomedical sciences. Cellular response to biomaterials, as investigated by IHC, demonstrates the flexibility of the technique within cellular and molecular biology. For instance, studies have applied immunohistochemistry to investigate the foreign body reaction (FBR) elicited by injectable hydrogels designed for application in the central nervous system. The associated molecular interactions of the hydrogels with host cells are characterized by variability in stromal cell infiltration, inflammation, and resulting neural damage, which can be visualized through IHC approaches. This insight not only helps to elucidate the mechanism of FBRs but also provides help in the design of biomaterials that would be capable of enhancing therapeutic effects and safety. The finer points gathered from IHC research also direct towards the importance of decoding the host response at the molecular level, wherein it would give clues towards directions of progress in regenerative medicine and material sciences, as illustrated through the extensive work on cellular interaction with biomaterials (Ao et al., 2019).

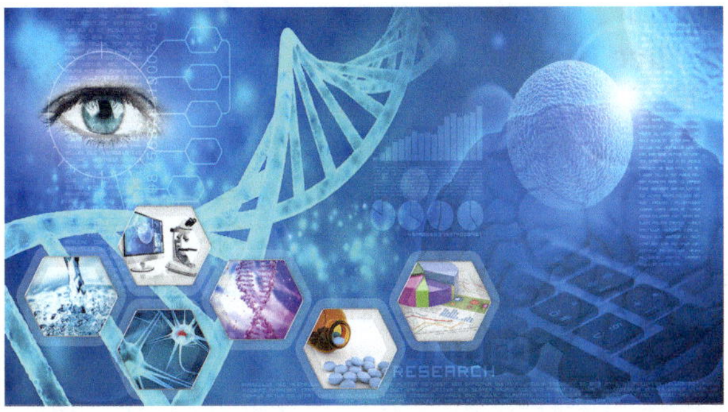

Figure 10.14. Utilization in cellular and molecular biology studies.

Source: https://cellmolbiol.org/public/journals/1/homepageImage_en_US.jpg.

Moreover, the identification of mutations in tumor suppressor genes, such as the p53 gene, underscores the role played by IHC in cancer biology. By applying the method, researchers have been able to associate specific mutations in the p53 gene with the development of adrenocortical carcinomas, which distinguish them from benign adenomas. IHC enables the detection of wild-type and mutant p53 proteins in tissue specimens with the capacity to identify their corresponding roles in tumorigenesis. It has been established that strong p53 immunoreactivity is strongly associated with mutations and malignant tumors, effectively equating protein presence with tumor behavior. This not only enhances the classification of neoplasms but also enhances prognosis estimations and treatments. The ability of IHC to expose such molecular interactions is a testament to its vital role in deciphering disease processes and designing targeted therapies, thus solidifying the techniques integral stature in modern-day biomolecular studies (Allolio et al., 1994) (Figure 10.14).

10.4.2. Role in Drug Development and Testing

The application of immunohistochemistry (IHC) in drug discovery and drug testing has grown increasingly important as researchers attempt to define specific biomolecular targets in tissues. IHC permits visualization of specific antigens in various cancer tissues and, in doing so, offers vital information regarding the tumor microenvironment and facilitates identification of possible drug targets. One of the most significant discoveries facilitated by IHC is the identification of overexpressed integrins, which are responsible for tumor growth and metastasis. By correlating IHC data with gene expression profiles in The Cancer Genome Atlas (TCGA), researchers can verify integrin targets for therapy. Thus, blocking these integrins with biologics or small molecules represents an exciting strategy for developing novel cancer therapies, ultimately streamlining the process from laboratory discovery to clinical therapy (Arun et al., 2018).

Also, IHC plays a critical role in predicting patient response to targeted therapy, particularly immuno-oncology. Use of IHC to quantify the expression of programmed death ligand 1 (PD-L1) on cancer cells has emerged as an emerging predictive biomarker for immune checkpoint inhibitor treatment. For example, in non-small-cell lung carcinoma (NSCLC), PD-L1 expression has been correlated with the response of PD-1/PD-L1 inhibitors. Proper interpretation and standardization of PD-L1 IHC testing allow for the stratification of patients in a way that only those who are expected to gain the most from the targeted treatments are given them. This integration of IHC in drug development allows for tailored delivery of treatment to maximize therapeutic response and patient outcome (Booton et al., 2016). The ongoing development of IHC technology has also enhanced its value in drug development by creating additional opportunities to identify new biomarkers and improving drug-testing processes with greater accuracy. Standardized IHC assays and new imaging modalities contribute to a better understanding of the intricate cellular processes involved in cancer. While scientists move forward with the preanalytical and analytical phases of IHC, the reproducibility and consistency of the results are improved, so that greater reproducibility of studies is guaranteed.

Furthermore, multidisciplinary collaborations that integrate IHC data with genomic and proteomic data are required for the entire biomarker identification. The common understandings of information obtained by IHC approaches not only enhance our understanding of disease pathology but also maximize drug development, resulting in more effective treatments that are specifically designed according to the specific needs of individual patients (Arun et al., 2018) (Figure 10.15).

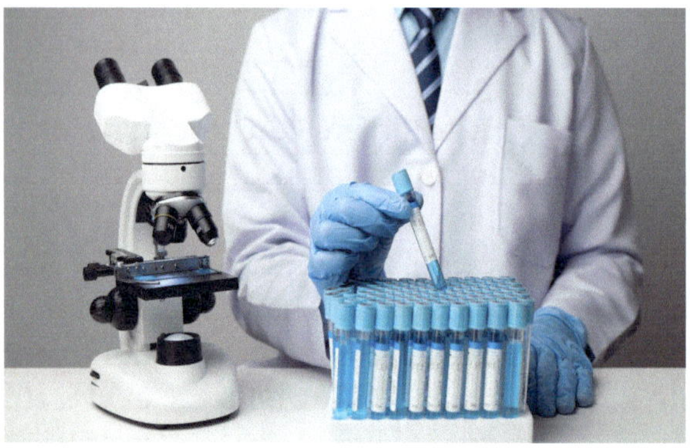

Figure 10.15. Role in drug development and testing.

Source: https://static.vecteezy.com/system/resources/previews/023/012/424/non_2x/close-up-view-of-scientist-analyzing-a-liquid-in-the-test-tubes-in-laboratory-free-photo.jpg.

10.4.3. Contribution to Understanding Disease Mechanisms

The application of immunohistochemistry (IHC) in the analysis of disease mechanisms has significantly expanded our understanding of pathologies, particularly in cancer studies. IHC enables the visualization of specific protein expressions in tissue samples and, therefore, gives a glimpse into the cellular and molecular pathways underlying disease formation. For instance, in osteosarcoma (OS), IHC analysis of MYC protein expression demonstrated its role in establishing an immunosuppressive tumor microenvironment. By co-associating the levels of MYC with the infiltration of tumor-associated macrophages and exclusion of T lymphocytes, researchers have demonstrated how oncogenic signaling affects immune evasion, thereby modifying treatment responses and clinical outcomes in canine and human patients (Makii et al., 2025). Thus, IHC is not only a diagnostic tool but also a key instrument to reveal the underlying mechanisms of disease. In addition to cancer, IHC has a pivotal function in research on the role of autophagy in disease mechanisms, particularly in neurodegenerative diseases. The ability to assess autophagy flux with IHC techniques allows cellular activities engaged in protein breakdown and recycling to be quantified. By using certain markers such as MAP1LC3 and SQSTM1, researchers can visualize autophagosomes and quantify the turnover of autophagosomes in tissue biopsies. This assists us in gaining vital information about how faulty autophagy contributes to cellular malfunction in neurodegenerative diseases like Alzheimer's and Parkinson's. The creation of inexpensive linear detection methods through chromogenic IHC also enhances the accessibility of such tests, reduces the disparity between clinics and research laboratories, and thus enhances our knowledge of disease mechanisms at a greater scale (Shojaei et al., 2025). Ultimately, the integration of IHC in disease mechanism research produces a superior understanding of pathology and therapy. By using IHC to examine molecular biomarkers, scientists can pinpoint pathways responsible for disease development and progression, enabling more specific treatment. The example of MYC in osteosarcoma demonstrates how IHC can expose tumor immunology insight, presenting options for increased effectiveness of immunotherapy (Makii et al., 2025). Besides, the measurement of autophagy processes provides us with rudimentary information on cellular responses to proteotoxic stress in various disorders (Shojaei et al., 2025). Being a multifactorial and highly potent tool, IHC not only enhances our insight into disease processes but also informs the development of new therapeutic options that are tailor-made to address such complex disorders effectively (Figure 10.16).

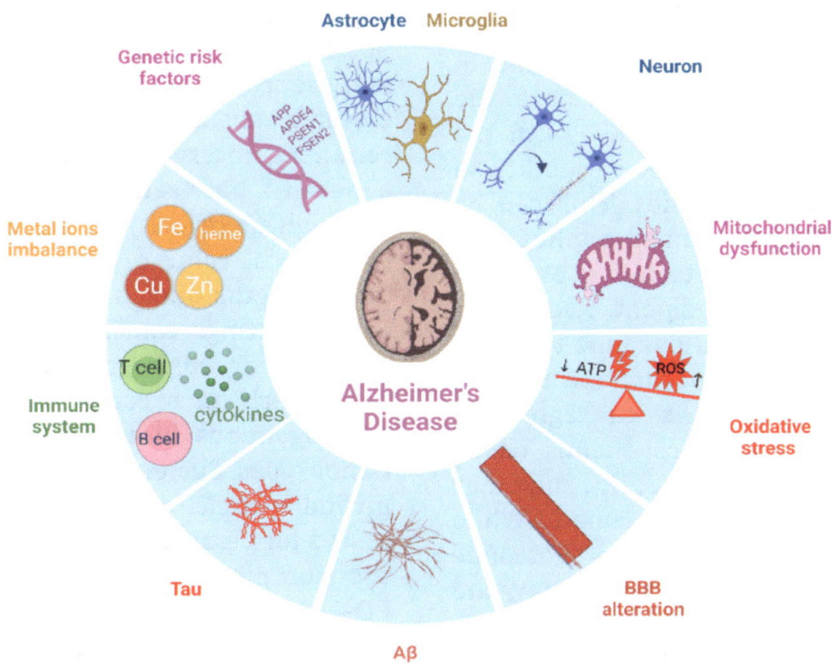

Figure 10.16. Contribution to understanding disease mechanisms.

Source: https://pub.mdpi-res.com/ijms/ijms-24-07258/article_deploy/html/images/ijms-24-07258-g001.png?1682386431.

10.5. Challenges and Limitations of IHC

Immunohistochemistry (IHC) is a powerful tool in modern pathology, providing extremely valuable information about disease processes and helping to make a diagnosis. However, it possesses several inherent limitations that can reduce its effectiveness and usefulness. One of them is variability resulting from variability in sample preparation, stain procedure, and interpretation between pathologists. These variations are capable of causing misdiagnosis or misdescription of tumor behavior and ultimately impacting patient management. Besides, the subjective component of visual assessments, especially when distinguishing between subtle differences in staining intensity or distribution, can lead to inconsistency in findings. Lack of standard protocols across laboratories exacerbates this, and thus, diagnostic laboratories have to engage in ongoing quality control exercises. Forming a consensus of best practices is thus crucial in avoiding these challenges and increasing the validity of IHC results. Another significant challenge of IHC is the built-in limitation of the specificity and sensitivity of the antibodies employed for the staining protocol. The selection of correct antibodies is critical, as their sensitivity may vary widely with regard to the target antigen, tissue type, and even the presence of cross-reacting antigens. These factors may lead to false positives or negatives, thereby concealing the true biological background of the sample being analyzed. Furthermore, the specificity of antibodies diminishes with the passage of time, with resultant variability in findings in longitudinal studies. This can be extremely frustrating in clinical applications where precise biomarker detection is essential for therapy-directed management. Redressing these limitations must be a dynamic research process to develop more specific and reliable antibodies and enhance the strategies for their validation within heterogeneous tissue microenvironments. The union of IHC and other molecular techniques is also problematic. While newer technologies in genomic and proteomic profiling have broadened tumor biology, the incorporation of these complex data types into IHC findings remains a challenge. IHC and molecular profiling union necessitates a multidisciplinary effort that does not always fit within the standard laboratory paradigm. In addition, the evolving landscape of precision medicine, in which treatment strategies are biomarker-specific, increases the burden on IHC to provide data that can be reliably interpreted alongside other diagnostic modalities. Being unable to overcome these integration challenges, the potential of IHC in the environment of precision medicine might be compromised. Therefore, the development of IHC methods will be essential in providing a response to contemporary oncology research and clinical practice requirements (Acquaviva et al., 2010; Fountzilas et al., 2020).

10.5.1. Specificity and Sensitivity Issues

In the context of immunohistochemistry (IHC), the two most important parameters influencing diagnostic outcome accuracy are specificity and sensitivity. Specificity refers to the ability of an assay to accurately state the absence of a target antigen, and sensitivity refers to its ability to detect true positive samples. High specificity is essential to minimize false positives, which could lead to misdiagnosis and inappropriate treatment regimens. Conversely, elevated sensitivity is required to identify cases requiring intervention effectively. Therefore, a best fit between these two parameters is the highest priority in optimally maximizing the clinical value of IHC assays. Investigating the strengths and limitations of IHC practice across settings can illuminate the challenges of achieving consistent diagnostic outcomes, particularly in a complex environment with heterogeneous biomarker expression across tumor types. Current studies have also indicated pivotal specificity and sensitivity issues in IHC assays for significant biomarkers. For instance, the complexities of several FDA-approved PD-L1 expression tests present variation in diagnostic performance. Failure to standardize several scoring systems across such tests has the tendency to cause confusion and inconsistent results. This assay performance variation can result in instances wherein disparate conclusions are derived by diverse labs regarding a patient's fit for immunotherapy, as has been demonstrated within the context of breast cancer diagnosis. This inconsistency eventually renders clinical decision-making more difficult and emphasizes the demand for specificity as well as sensitivity in the effective use of such diagnostic tools. It is critical that these standards are maintained by clinicians because they rely on proper information to guide therapeutic interventions, particularly in an era where precision medicine is becoming more integral to cancer care. Furthermore, future standardization tools for IHC assays might address issues of specificity and sensitivity. One recent example, like the application of NIST-calibrated microbeads to measure PD-L1, illustrates a novel method of measurement. Using predetermined concentration calibrators, laboratories can improve the reproducibility of results and track analytical sensitivity over time, thereby resolving variability inherent in many IHC protocols. While this tool does not squarely confront the interpretive challenges of pathologists in scoring IHC assays, it operates to fortify the foundations of specificity and sensitivity metrics. Yet, the achievement of universal implementation of such techniques will require synergism among clinical laboratories and research centers to ensure accurate biomarker identification within different settings. Through these advancements, ongoing optimization of IHC techniques continues to be pertinent in optimizing diagnostic accuracy in oncology (Martinez-Morilla et al., 2021; Aé-Besa et al., 2023) (Figure 10.17).

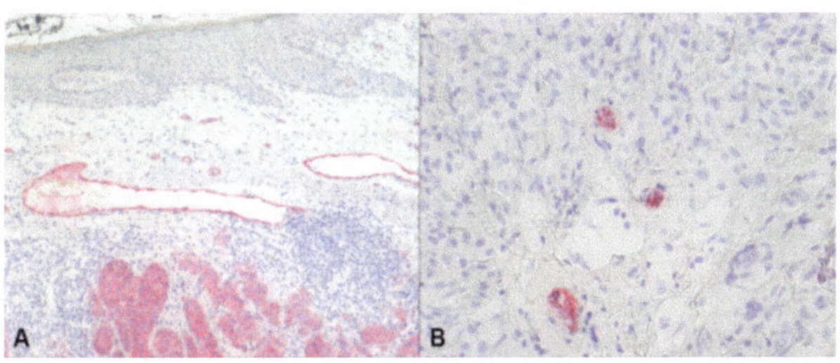

Figure 10.17. Specificity and sensitivity issues.

Source: https://www.jaad.org/cms/attachment/3ca2d94a-fa5a-4b55-85b1-4ebb96e151d4/gr1.jpg.

10.5.2. Variability in Results and Reproducibility

In the area of immunohistochemistry (IHC), protocol standardization remains a main issue considering the perceived heterogeneity of results obtained from various laboratories. Such heterogeneity may be due to variations in antigen retrieval methods, antibody titers, and detection systems applied. Various studies indicate that such variation not only affects the validity of IHC results but also negates reproducibility of results in a clinical context. Specifically, result interpretation among pathologists can be very different based on subjective judgment, hence cannot be made to provide strong diagnostic criteria. That variation highlights the need for stringent quality controls and standardized methods that can guarantee more reproducible outcomes when IHC use is involved. Continuous training and pathologists' proficiency testing may be employed to reduce variability and improve concordance in interpreting immunohistochemical stains. Moreover, the reproducibility of IHC results is also compromised by the intrinsic variability of biological samples. Notably, heterogeneity in tumor microenvironments, patient backgrounds, and treatment histories can affect availability and concentrations of target antigens and, indirectly, ensuing IHC results. In one study assessing lymphovascular space invasion (LVSI) in endometrial cancer, researchers tested interobserver concordance among pathologists reading IHC results for LVSI only. Interobserver concordance was found to be of high reproducibility with an intraclass correlation coefficient of 0.64 ($P < 0.001$) for LVSI assessment and 0.62 ($P < 0.001$) for LVSI grading, indicating that though differences exist, there are good protocols for consistent interpretation (Bartosch et al., 2019). Such observations point toward the necessity of robust methodologies to institute the reliability of IHC in clinical settings. Technological advancements are being used in important ways to address variability and reproducibility issues in IHC. Automated methodologies for processing and analyzing samples, such as fully automated membrane segmentation, enable a more objective assessment of stained cellular membranes that are difficult to visualize. Scientists can eliminate subjective errors typically associated with manual measurements by using precise algorithms that accurately segment cellular membranes and measure target proteins. In real applications, such computational systems have managed to show high accuracy in data across anatomical locations and thereby broadened the scope of IHC in cancer characterization and classification (Acquaviva et al., 2011). Such advances indicate a paradigm shift towards a quantitative, reproducible method in IHC, ultimately leading to improved outcomes in targeted therapy and precision medicine.

10.5.3. Limitations in Quantification and Interpretation

Immunohistochemistry (IHC), while a valuable tool in cellular and tissue research, poses significant limitations to quantifying and interpreting results. One of the overall concerns is the subjectivity of visual analysis because interpretation of the quality of the stain is primarily dependent upon the pathologist's experience and training. Variation in staining protocols, including antibody specificity and concentration, might generate non-reproducible results, and reproducibility issues between laboratories are a concern. Furthermore, as the discipline grew, the sheer volume of published studies has at times been allowed to outweigh rigorous methodological standards, leading to inconsistent treatment of the same data. The lack of consistency complicates the drawing of firm conclusions from immunohistochemical data and highlights the requirement of standardized protocols to enhance reliability and comparability of quantitative analysis (da Pinhal et al., 2010). Additionally, quantitative immunohistochemical staining is also plagued by technical issues inherent in the imaging and analysis method. For example, cellular membranes, critical in determining subcellular protein localization, can be weakly delineated within unstained areas, making accurate measurement of target proteins problematic. These problems require sophisticated image analysis; however, these are not universally established, and therefore, data analysis inconsistency ensues. An automated membrane segmentation technique, in its promise to enhance the accuracy of quantification, continues to be marred by inconsistency of membrane visibility across samples and staining conditions (Acquaviva et al., 2011). This mismatch between technological progress and standardization hinders the application of IHC in clinical settings, underscoring the need for methodological improvements and consensus on analytical methods. Beyond technical and interpretative concerns, biologically based limitations also complicate IHC quantification. Tumor heterogeneity, in which expression of the target protein may differ in disparate regions of a sample, is a cause of misinterpretation. This may be caused by differing microenvironmental conditions or point mutations within the tumor cells, and it is difficult to obtain a representative view of protein expression. Fixation time itself and antigen retrieval protocols may even influence the integrity of tissue samples, tending to lead to biased interpretation. Hence, a multidisciplinary approach that integrates general biological information with strict adherence to standardised procedures is essential for maximising the quantitative and interpretive validity of immunohistochemistry results (da Pinhal et al., 2010).

10.6. Future Directions in IHC

As the field of immunohistochemistry (IHC) advances, there are several exciting future directions that promise to reshape diagnostics and treatment in oncology. One key area of exploration is the integration of molecular techniques alongside traditional IHC methodologies. The dynamic evolution of lung cancer classification exemplifies this trend; in the past two decades, IHC has provided invaluable insights into tumor biology that extend beyond morphology alone. With the integration of IHC and a cutting-edge molecular armamentarium, pathologists can derive a clearer understanding of lung cancer subtypes and, consequently, inform personalized treatment protocols. Furthermore, the increasing complexity of cancer pathobiology necessitates a dimensional approach to analyze tumor behavior and thereby maximize patient outcomes through tailored treatments addressing the unique aspects of each subtype of cancer in a precise manner (Cangut et al., 2025). Another significant future direction is applying artificial intelligence (AI) to IHC result interpretation. AI technologies have the potential to transform histopathology, enabling pathologists to leverage their skills in image analysis and data interpretation better. Machine learning algorithms can examine large amounts of data in IHC images to identify patterns and anomalies undetectable by the human eye. As clinical workflows become more and more integrated with AI systems, they can also streamline diagnostic work and reduce the risk of human error. AI can also be employed to enable predictive models for pre-empting patient response to specific immunotherapies and therefore enacting more efficient treatments and more understanding of tumor behavior (Odeh et al., 2024). Lastly, the future of IHC shall witness the discovery of new biomarkers, thus further augmenting the diagnostic capability and enhancing therapeutic specificity. Research is already underway to identify novel IHC targets beyond conventional markers, particularly in immunotherapy. Such biomarkers directly reflecting changes in tumor microenvironment, immune cell infiltration, or even molecular changes will significantly increase the specificity of IHC in determining the treatment outcome. These advances place even greater emphasis on continued investment in basic and translational research to discover these new biomarkers. With our growing understanding of immune mechanisms within the tumor microenvironment, IHC will serve as the cornerstone for guiding clinical decisions and optimizing therapy outcomes in cancer-diagnosed patients (Cangut et al., 2025) (Figure 10.18).

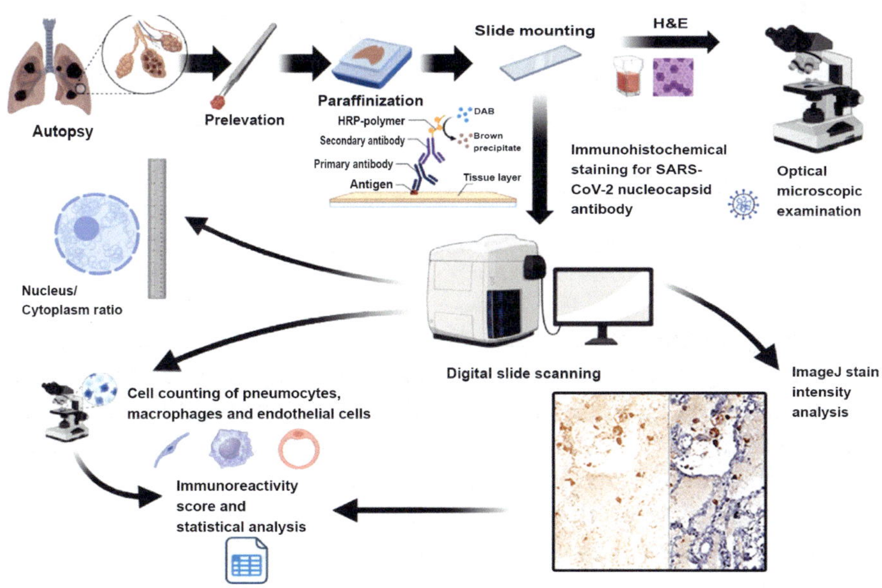

Figure 10.18. Future directions in IHC.

Source: https://pub.mdpi-res.com/diagnostics/diagnostics-14-00914/article_deploy/html/images/diagnostics-14-00914-g002.png?1714463848.

10.6.1. Advances in Technology and Methodology

Immunohistochemistry (IHC) has, to a great extent, been influenced by technological and methodological advances that have transformed both sensitivity and specificity of tissue analysis. Advances in imaging technologies have paved the way, and developments in digital pathology have facilitated high-resolution histology specimen scanning. A dramatic change has ushered in greater accuracy in biomarker identification, with resultant potential for greater diagnostic capability. In addition, the use of automated staining systems minimizes human error and maximizes reproducibility of experimental results. Rapid progress in multiplexing technologies, where multiple antigens are detected simultaneously on a single tissue section, is just one example of IHC technology development. Such capability not only enhances understanding of complex tissue environments but also opens wide opportunities for far-ranging studies in cancer biology, neurology, and other branches of medicine and biological sciences. Parallel with advances in molecular biology techniques, the methodological depth of IHC has been enriched considerably.

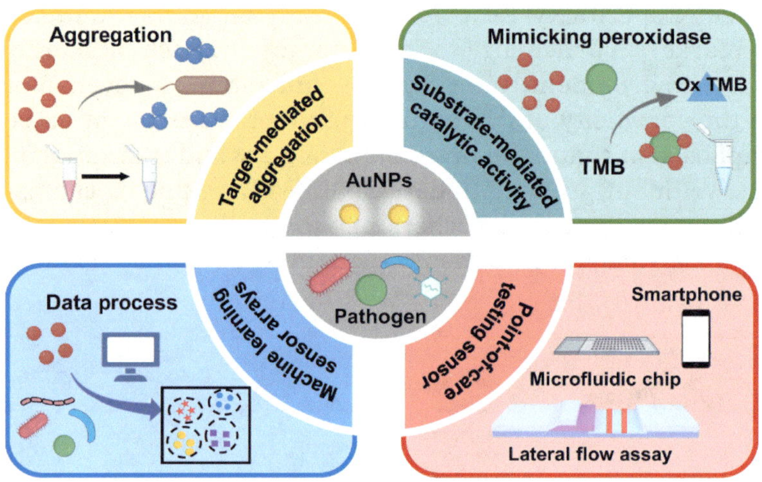

Figure 10.19. Advances in technology and methodology.

Source: https://www.mdpi.com/biosensors/biosensors-13-00029/article_deploy/html/images/biosensors-13-00029-g001.png.

The evolution of genetically engineered antibodies and nanobodies has introduced new possibilities for improved target specificity and reduced background staining. These sophisticated tools enable more precise protein localization mapping in the tissue with a direct influence on pathophysiological models of human diseases. Furthermore, applying quantitative analysis via image-processing software enables statistical confirmation of results, thereby enhancing the robustness of predominantly qualitative data. The combination of these methods not only enhances analysis but also allows researchers to conduct large-scale, data-driven studies, particularly in the field of personalized medicine. As demonstrated in technologies like neuroanatomical mapping, systematic approaches like tracers and viral vectors can generate a highly detailed comprehension of intricate biological systems (MacKenzie-Graham et al., 2009). Finally, the merging of physical and engineering sciences with health and life sciences highlights a collaborative atmosphere that enables much of IHC innovation. Studies in this interface have facilitated the design of new materials for enhanced tissue processing and imaging technologies that can facilitate accurate probing of molecular interactions in tissues. Utilization of techniques such as high-throughput screening and automated imaging boosts diagnostics and even accelerates knowledge of molecular mechanisms of disease. As mentioned, the incorporation of novel statistical techniques for data analysis can validate results and improve experimental designs. Therefore, continued investigation at the EPS-HLS interface highlights the pivotal role of multidisciplinary research in advancing immunohistochemistry toward more efficient therapeutic approaches (Smart et al., 2014) (Figure 10.19).

10.6.2. Integration with Other Diagnostic Techniques

The convergence of immunohistochemistry (IHC) with other diagnostic techniques is revolutionizing the field of pathological diagnostics, particularly in oncology. By marrying IHC with genetic analysis, for instance, pathologists can gain detailed insights into tumor biology. Molecular characterization, as outlined in Jones et al. (2018), allows for predictive testing and tumor subclassification, which are vital in personalized treatment protocols. This multidisciplinary approach enhances the accuracy of diagnosis and aids in clinical decision-making by correlating morphological data with genetic patterns. Through the integration of IHC and genomic analysis, clinicians can treat patients with targeted therapies, improving prognostication and cancer management. In addition, the combination of imaging techniques with IHC creates a synergy that benefits diagnostic oncology. Higher imaging modalities, such as PET scans and MRI, can provide histopathological results with spatial information, allowing enhanced comprehension of tumor heterogeneity and invasiveness. As evidenced in Berger et al. (2017), enhanced comprehension of the metabolic tumor profile, particularly low-grade gliomas, enhances patient stratification by genotype and expected response to therapy. Through the integration of these modalities, doctors can follow disease development and modify therapy, leading to more informed clinical decisions and, consequently, improved patient outcomes. Furthermore, the development of morphomolecular pathology, as described in Jones et al. (2018), indicates the necessity for an improved collaborative effort among pathology departments. Integration of IHC findings with genomic data is capable of initiating the identification of significant biomarkers and novel therapeutic targets. Bridge the gap between molecular diagnostics and classical cellular pathology by upskilling the workforce and re-evaluating pathology training programs. This holistic strategy not only maximizes the diagnostic pipeline but also positions pathology at the forefront of precision medicine, with the pathologist as the center of cancer care, as technology forges forward. Through encouraging collaboration among various diagnostic disciplines, the potential for improved patient care is endless.

10.6.3. Potential for Personalized Medicine Applications

The integration of immunohistochemistry (IHC) into personalized medicine applications represents a promising platform for enhancing patient care, particularly in oncology. By employing IHC techniques, clinicians can characterize individual protein expression patterns in tumor tissue, which remain a key factor in defining the biological character of a cancer. This information allows for the stratification of patients based on their unique molecular profiles and, therefore, personalizing therapeutic interventions to enhance treatment outcomes. Application of biomarker identification through IHC is essential because, besides guiding therapy decisions, it enhances the precision of treatment plans, such that patients are given tailored therapies that are aligned with the nature of their cancers. In this regard, studies have shown that the incorporation of proteomic data into IHC evaluation can reveal more insights about cancer dynamics and response to treatment, potentially shaping the future of personalized oncology medicine. Contributing to the utility from IHC, the application of proteomics reinforces the strength of personalized medicine in the management of cancer as well. Proteomics offers the ability to analyze protein dynamics that reflect real-time tumor biology status, as evidenced in the literature for use in various oncology conditions. More recent studies elucidate that employing a proteomics-informed approach to cancer treatment is beneficial in biomarker identification, patient stratification towards targeted intervention, and treatment outcome prediction (Frantzi et al., 2017). By integrating IHC results with advances in proteomics, clinicians can optimally use molecular data to inform clinical practice and optimize patient management and treatment efficacy overall. Being grounded in such integrated approaches, this not only maximizes therapeutic interventions but also renders viable treatment by addressing the intricacies of personalized patient care. Moreover, the landscape of clinical trials is also addressing precision medicine through the combination of new IHC techniques and biomarker evaluation. The shift to gene-targeted, histology-agnostic trials is the result of the demand for personalizing cancer treatment based on unique molecular profiles possible with the use of IHC techniques. By these developments, scientists demonstrate that matched therapies yield improved outcomes compared to the traditional, non-targeted therapies (Fountzilas et al., 2020). This paradigm will require the timely achievement of extensive tumor profiling to realize full benefits from individualized therapy approaches. Future clinical studies will focus on the integration of IHC with immunologically targeted therapy and other new agents to mitigate the complexity of cancer biology and improve patient prognoses. As technology continues to improve, accessing the potential of IHC combined with novel research will promote a robust framework for the utilization of personalized medicine (Figure 10.20).

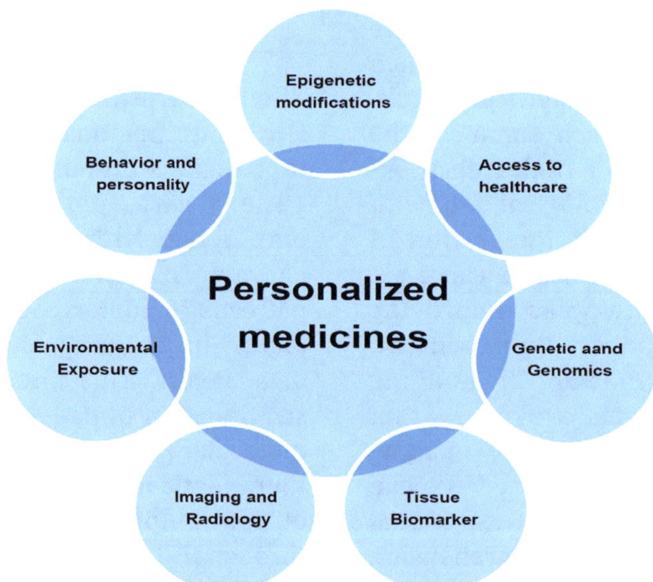

Figure 10.20. Potential for personalized medicine applications.

Source: https://edfuturetech.com/wp-content/uploads/2023/02/Personalized-Medicine.png.

SUMMARY

Lastly, immunohistochemistry (IHC) is a pillar of modern pathology and figures prominently in increasing diagnostic accuracy and guiding therapy in various types of cancer. Through the use of IHC techniques, it has been possible for physicians to identify specific biomarkers that are linked with the development of disease and response to therapy. As highlighted in recent studies, including investigations of serum AFP levels as prognostic indicators in hepatocellular carcinoma, IHC not only enables us to identify novel therapeutic targets, such as the FGF19 pathway, but also provides deeper insight into the molecular signatures of cancers. The positive correlation between high AFP levels and FGF19 IHC status points to the potential of the amalgamation of serological markers with IHC testing to more effectively guide patient care. Outside of hepatocellular carcinoma, the application of IHC is even broader in other cancers, including breast cancer. The breast cancer marker experience demonstrates the ability of IHC to provide essential information regarding tumor biology, guiding prognostic evaluation and treatment planning. As is evident from the report, which submits low percentages of ER and PR positivity in breast cancer patients, the role of IHC in characterizing tumor aggressiveness cannot be substituted. It not only determines the treatment modalities, such as endocrine therapy, but also points towards the need for certain treatment modalities for aggressive forms. The intricate relationship between IHC outcomes and clinical results proves the instrumental role that this technique assumes in optimizing cancer treatment. The future of IHC, ultimately, will rest with additional technical and methodological developments, which will allow for more precise cancer diagnosis and therapy personalization. While researchers strive to decipher the secrets of tumor biology, the integration of IHC into clinical routine will be a top priority. The potential of IHC to identify actionable biomarkers, as suggested by the findings on FGF19 in hepatocellular carcinoma and ER and PR levels in breast cancer, offers a huge promise in the prognoses of patients. With sustained research activity and clinical proof of principle, IHC can continue to advance personalized medicine strategies, ultimately revolutionizing paradigms in cancer therapy and resulting in improved survival rates in diverse populations.

Immunohistochemistry (IHC) is a significant tool in pathology that allows visualization of specific proteins in tissue sections. IHC employs antibodies that bind to target antigens, facilitating morphological examination of cells and tissues. The value of IHC lies in its application in the diagnosis of neoplastic disorders, including high-grade meningiomas. Recent studies demonstrate the feasibility of MTAP immunohistochemistry as a cost-effective alternative for the detection of CDKN2A/B loss, essential in grading meningiomas as WHO grade 3 tumors. Traditional testing methods, such as sequencing or FISH, although accurate, are problematic in terms of availability and cost. Thus, the research on IHC as a diagnosis tool not only makes the process easier but also enhances the diagnostic potential in the hands of clinicians in varied healthcare settings (Ozkizilkaya et al., 2024). Moreover, the versatility of IHC extends to image analysis, which is critical to reading staining results. As large-scale assessment often relies on integration of various imaging modalities, effective image registration is then imperative for effective co-localization analysis. Recent developments, such as the development of user-friendly software like the DS4H Image Alignment (DS4H-IA) plugin for ImageJ/Fiji, have simplified the process of registering more than a single image. This tool is particularly applicable in experimental setups for both immunofluorescence and immunohistochemistry. The DS4H-IA plugin is an accessible platform for scientists to use in order to make precise analyses without possessing advanced technical skills. Such tools significantly enhance the overall efficacy of IHC by addressing the common issue of image misalignment, thereby supporting its application in modern pathology (Piccinini et al., 2024). Overall, the application of immunohistochemistry to pathological testing not only presents a potential replacement for established diagnostic practices but also emphasizes the importance of technology innovation in imaging. The interrogation of MTAP as a surrogate marker with IHC presents a thrilling opportunity to further advance faster diagnostic testing in the instance of unruptured high-grade meningiomas. At the same time, programs like the DS4H-IA plugin represent a trend toward more affordable means of evaluating multi-modal images. Together, these developments are ready to enhance clinical outcomes through rapid, accurate diagnosis and the capacity to comprehend underlying biological processes better. Lastly, the convergence of IHC and image-processing technologies holds promise for enhancing diagnostic capabilities and enabling new areas of research in pathology and beyond (Ozkizilkaya et al., 2024; Piccinini et al., 2024).

A LOOK TO THE FUTURE:

FOREIGN BODY REACTION (FBR):

The foreign body reaction (FBR) is a fundamental biological process in which the body responds to the presence of a foreign object or material introduced into its tissues. Whether the object is a surgical implant, a fragment of a splinter, or a biomedical device, the host's immune system recognizes it as non-self and initiates a cascade of cellular and molecular events aimed at protecting the organism. This response is an evolved defensive strategy, but in clinical contexts it can limit the long-term success of medical implants and devices. At the onset of FBR, blood and interstitial proteins rapidly adsorb onto the surface of the implanted material almost immediately after implantation. This adsorbed protein layer serves as a signal that recruits immune cells to the site and sets the stage for subsequent inflammatory processes. Neutrophils — the body's first line of immune defense — arrive quickly, followed by monocytes that differentiate into macrophages, which persist at the material–tissue interface.

If the foreign material is too large for individual macrophages to engulf and clear through phagocytosis, these immune cells may fuse together to form multinucleated foreign-body giant cells (FBGCs). This fusion is a hallmark of FBR and reflects the chronic nature of the response, as the immune system attempts to degrade or isolate what it cannot remove. As the reaction progresses, continued macrophage and giant cell activity stimulates fibroblasts — cells responsible for forming connective tissue — to deposit collagen and other extracellular matrix components around the implant. Over weeks to months, this results in the formation of a dense, fibrous capsule that encases the foreign object. While this encapsulation isolates the material and protects surrounding tissues, it can also hinder the intended function of the implant. For example, fibrotic encapsulation can impede drug release from delivery systems or block electrical signals in neural interfaces.

Understanding FBR is especially important in biomedical engineering and regenerative medicine. The degree and nature of the reaction are influenced by myriad factors, including the material's chemical composition, surface properties, stiffness, and microstructure. Advances in biomaterials science aim to design surfaces and structures that mitigate adverse FBR by reducing protein adsorption or modulating cellular immune responses.

Despite decades of research, FBR remains a challenge for many implanted devices, often necessitating revision surgeries or device removal. However, ongoing studies into the molecular signals and cellular mechanisms driving FBR are opening pathways to improved biocompatibility and long-term implant success, underscoring the importance of this reaction in both basic biology and clinical practice.

REFERENCES

1. Di Cataldo, S., Ficarra, E., Acquaviva, A., & Macii, E. (2010b). Automated segmentation of tissue images for computerized IHC analysis. *Computer Methods and Programs in Biomedicine, 100*(1), 1–15. https://doi.org/10.1016/j.cmpb.2010.02.002Acquaviva, A., Di Cataldo, S., Ficarra, E., Macii, E., et al. (2011). Automated segmentation of cells with IHC membrane staining. https://core.ac.uk/download/pdf/11419237.pdf (accessed on 6th August 2025).
2. Al Meslamani, A. Z., Sobrino, I., de la Fuente, J. (2024). Machine learning in infectious diseases: Potential applications and limitations. *Annals of Medicine, 56*. https://www.semanticscholar.org/paper/07319e6b4ac52edcaccab070230b57b4f865d135 (accessed on 6th August 2025).
3. Allolio, B., Chrousos, G. P., Karl, M., Linehan, W. M., et al. (1994). P53 mutations in human adrenocortical neoplasms. https://core.ac.uk/download/12167816.pdf (accessed on 6th August 2025).
4. Ao, Y., Deming, T., Kim, J., O'Shea, T., et al. (2019). Foreign body responses in central nervous system mimic natural wound responses and alter biomaterial functions. https://core.ac.uk/download/323082685.pdf (accessed on 6th August 2025).
5. Arun, A. S., Lam, K. S., Tepper, C. G. (2018). Identification of integrin drug targets for 17 solid tumor types. https://core.ac.uk/download/323071824.pdf (accessed on 6th August 2025).
6. Arzberger, E., Bastos, P. M., Ferreira, J., Leal-Filipe, A., et al. (2020). Reflectance confocal microscopy for the diagnosis of skin infections and infestations. https://core.ac.uk/download/322493878.pdf (accessed on 6th August 2025).
7. Ayodele, S. D., Javid, F. A., Makanjuola, S. B. L., Obafunwa, J. O., et al. (2014). Breast cancer receptor status assessment and clinicopathological association in Nigerian women: A retrospective analysis. https://core.ac.uk/download/30729983.pdf (accessed on 6th August 2025).
8. Bartosch, C., Bosse, T., Genestie, C., Lax, S. F., et al. (2019). Reproducibility of lymphovascular space invasion (LVSI) assessment in endometrial cancer. https://core.ac.uk/download/322827724.pdf (accessed on 6th August 2025).
9. Benedetto, A., Biasibetti, E., Beltramo, C., Audino, V., Peletto, S., Bozzetta, E., Pezzolato, M. (2021). Regucalcin expression profiles in veal calf testis: Validation of histological and molecular tests to detect sex steroids illicit administration. *PeerJ, 9*. https://www.semanticscholar.org/paper/b0fafeb565f646ced99a15ba87e7b07312f70b3f (accessed on 6th August 2025).
10. Berger, M. S., Chang, S. M., Crane, J. C., Elkhaled, A., et al. (2017). Metabolic profiling of IDH mutation and malignant progression in infiltrating glioma. https://core.ac.uk/download/323074384.pdf (accessed on 6th August 2025).
11. Binch, A., Snuggs, J., Le Maitre, C. L. (2020). Immunohistochemical analysis of protein expression in formalin-fixed paraffin-embedded human intervertebral disc tissues. *JOR Spine, 3*. https://www.semanticscholar.org/paper/f51f9ab163e3bc68a3f21a5b8b0d05732f9f0122 (accessed on 6th August 2025).
12. Bommanavar, S. (2017). Historiography of immunology in oral pathology—a concise review. *Open Access Journal of Dental Sciences*. https://www.semanticscholar.org/paper/0be8b981173c3b9ed7fcee092dca05956f7c03c5 (accessed on 6th August 2025).

13. Booton, R., Cane, P., Cree, I. A., Gosney, J., et al. (2016). PD-L1 testing for lung cancer in the UK: Recognizing the challenges for implementation. https://core.ac.uk/download/77017413.pdf (accessed on 6th August 2025).

14. Cangut, B., Akinlusi, R., Mohseny, A., Ghesani, N., & Ghesani, M. (2025). Evolving paradigms in lung cancer: Latest trends in diagnosis, management, and radiopharmaceuticals. *Seminars in Nuclear Medicine*. https://www.semanticscholar.org/paper/118ac9b9119532b5dbad0f43828609bcd155c692 (accessed on 6th August 2025).

15. Cantarella, F., Mendoza Bertelli, A., Girotti, R., Marino, A. C., Brest, E., Dibarbora, D., Mahmoud, Y., et al. (2024). Clinical efficacy of a next-generation sequencing (NGS) and immunohistochemistry (IHC) panel in patients with advanced cancer in Argentina. *Journal of Clinical Oncology*. https://www.semanticscholar.org/paper/c95b7539a2e15bab5ceb04044492d4d90e4a263b (accessed on 6th August 2025).

16. Cao, Z., Li, J., Sun, L., Xu, Z., Ke, Y.-B., Shao, B., Guo, Y.-H., et al. (2022). GISTs with NTRK gene fusions: A clinicopathological, immunophenotypic, and molecular study. *Cancers, 15*. https://www.semanticscholar.org/paper/73c3c0025c3b09a48bc9f055e08eea6066a95344 (accessed on 6th August 2025).

17. Cesaro, A., Hoffman, S. C., Das, P., de la Fuente-Nunez, C. (2025). Challenges and applications of artificial intelligence in infectious diseases and antimicrobial resistance. *npj Antimicrobials and Resistance, 3*. https://www.semanticscholar.org/paper/d61855cd9af93c7328effdb491ada025ce57f8b9 (accessed on 6th August 2025).

18. Chen, Y., Zhang, H., Fan, Y., Yang, L., & Dong, Y.-B. (2024). Multiplex cyclic fluorescent immunohistochemistry. *Journal of Visualized Experiments: JoVE, 203*. https://www.semanticscholar.org/paper/c5e0cd710e0fd0b85fe4b7eb206fe09f5e68529d (accessed on 6th August 2025).

19. Clifford, C. (2017). A cross sectional analysis of the association between FGF19 tumor expression and serum AFP levels in advanced HCC patients. https://open.bu.edu/bitstream/2144/23745/5/Clifford_bu_0017N_12724.pdf (accessed on 6th August 2025).

20. Cohen, E. E. W., Farrow, A. D., Finn, S., Heitmann, J., et al. (2014). DNA repair biomarkers XPF and phospho-MAPKAP kinase 2 correlate with clinical outcome in advanced head and neck cancer. https://core.ac.uk/download/323064878.pdf (accessed on 6th August 2025).

21. Crescenzi, M., Floreani, A., Masola, V., & Onisto, M., et al. (2017). Heparanase and macrophage interplay in the onset of liver fibrosis. https://core.ac.uk/download/129592461.pdf (accessed on 6th August 2025).

22. da Silva Pinhal, M. A., de Matos, L. L., de Matos, M. G. L., & Trufelli, H., et al. (2010). Immunohistochemistry as an important tool in biomarkers detection and clinical practice. https://core.ac.uk/download/pdf/8385015.pdf (accessed on 6th August 2025).

23. Dinku, Y., & Dagnaw, G. G. (2024). Review of immunohistochemistry techniques: Applications, current status, and future perspectives. *Seminars in Diagnostic Pathology*. https://www.semanticscholar.org/paper/1b9787aa6ea6b91b0cf6a96766a16f474d4c404f (accessed on 6th August 2025).

24. Escalé-Besa, A., Yélamos, O., Vidal-Alaball, J., Fuster-Casanovas, A., Miró Catalina, Q., Börve, A., Ander-Egg Aguilar, R., et al. (2023). Exploring the potential of artificial intelligence in improving skin lesion diagnosis in primary care. *Scientific Reports, 13*. https://www.

semanticscholar.org/paper/bc5b4489fb694e7f703ea70e40de0ee0c4080404 (accessed on 6th August 2025).

25. Estep, J., Gong, Q., Hjelmeland, L. M., & Nguyen, H., et al. (2015). Localization of complement factor H gene expression and protein distribution in the mouse outer retina. https://core.ac.uk/download/323076013.pdf (accessed on 6th August 2025).

26. Fountzilas, E., Kurzrock, R., Nikanjam, M., & Tsimberidou, A. M. (2020). Review of precision cancer medicine: Evolution of the treatment paradigm. https://core.ac.uk/download/305124673.pdf (accessed on 6th August 2025).

27. Gallo, E., Ramieri, M., & Marino, M. (2022). Structural and functional thymic biomarkers are involved in the pathogenesis of thymic epithelial tumors: An overview. *Immuno*. https://www.semanticscholar.org/paper/77b014b945a7baa280609caf9bbd0e48469f77ce (accessed on 6th August 2025).

28. Gorris, M., Martynova, E., Sweep, M. W., van der Hoorn, I. A. E., Sultan, S., Claassens, M. J. D. E., van der Woude, L. L., et al. (2023). Multiplex immunohistochemical analysis of the spatial immune cell landscape of the tumor microenvironment. *Journal of Visualized Experiments: JoVE, 198*. https://www.semanticscholar.org/paper/442f84b6abfdcd0fae717546cd6cd85f7e065ece (accessed on 6th August 2025).

29. Jones, J. L., Lee, J. L., Moore, D. A., & Morris, R., et al. (2018). Time for change: A new training programme for morpho-molecular pathologists? https://core.ac.uk/download/132211774.pdf (accessed on 6th August 2025).

30. Katsamenis, O., Basford, P., Robinson, S. K., Boardman, R., Konstantinopoulou, E., Lackie, P., Page, A., et al. (2023). A high-throughput 3D X-ray histology facility for biomedical research and preclinical applications. *Wellcome Open Research, 8*. https://www.semanticscholar.org/paper/513e56b5eec97b8fac3ed6bde31f5ce462c2e91c (accessed on 6th August 2025).

31. Knudsen, B., Linden, M., Randolph, T., & Wang, J., et al. (2011). Statistical methods for tissue array images – algorithmic scoring and co-training. http://arxiv.org/abs/1102.0059 (accessed on 6th August 2025).

32. Kohale, M., Dhobale, A. V., Bankar, N. J., Noman, O., Hatgaonkar, K., & Mishra, V. H. (2023). Immunohistochemistry in pathology: A review. *Journal of Cellular Biotechnology, 9*, 131–138. https://www.semanticscholar.org/paper/370572f4a94c3243022134a5f07d752246650d8e (accessed on 6th August 2025).

33. Liu, X.-B., & Schumann, C. M. (2014). Optimization of electron microscopy for human brains with long-term fixation and fixed-frozen sections. https://core.ac.uk/download/323071028.pdf (accessed on 6th August 2025).

34. Lou, W., Li, G., Wan, X., & Li, H. (2024). Multi-modal denoising diffusion pre-training for whole-slide image classification. *Proceedings of the 32nd ACM International Conference on Multimedia*. https://www.semanticscholar.org/paper/5fbf1b442ad5fe1591e64920627f3ab356c96221 (accessed on 6th August 2025).

35. Lynch, G., Maskell, N. A., & Bibby, A. (2024). Recent advances in mesothelioma. *Current Pulmonology Reports*. https://www.semanticscholar.org/paper/61fc9ed56908673d6df3123418744c88de240f2b (accessed on 6th August 2025).

36. MacKenzie-Graham, A., Reiner, A., Vercelli, A., Visel, A., Jones, A., Hattox, A. M., Toga, A.

W., et al. (2009). A proposal for a coordinated effort for the determination of brainwide neuroanatomical connectivity in model organisms at a mesoscopic scale. https://core.ac.uk/download/4881776.pdf (accessed on 6th August 2025).

37. Makii, R., Ned, T., Underdown, M. J., Palmer, E., Wilky, B., & Regan, D. P. (2025). 582 A comparative approach to understanding the role of oncogenic MYC signaling in the metastatic osteosarcoma tumor immune microenvironment. *Journal of Clinical and Translational Science, 9*, 171. https://www.semanticscholar.org/paper/2d6121b86283d0394107611c36628763eee42d1a (accessed on 6th August 2025).

38. Martinez-Morilla, S., Moutafi, M., & Rimm, D. (2021). Standardization of PD-L1 immunohistochemistry. *Modern Pathology, 35*, 294–295. https://www.semanticscholar.org/paper/9d9b7ad2e5df06d88e27d5cec72a63f0962f3ef3 (accessed on 6th August 2025).

39. Nerlich, A., D'Ardenne, A. J., Unsworth, D. J., Macarak, E. J., Piérard, G. E., et al. (1992). Comparison of the solophenyl-red polarization method and the immunohistochemical analysis for collagen type III. https://core.ac.uk/download/12168261.pdf (accessed on 6th August 2025).

40. Odeh, A., Odeh, N., Mohammed, A. S. (2024). A comparative review of AI techniques for automated code generation in software development: Advancements, challenges, and future directions. *TEM Journal*. https://www.semanticscholar.org/paper/8281b1dcf71dac90a5c95a36f5c4b988ff1ec259 (accessed on 6th August 2025).

41. Ozkizilkaya, H. I., Vinocha, A., Dono, A., Ogunbona, O., Toruner, G. A., Aung, P. P., Kamiya Matsuoka, C., et al. (2024). MTAP and p16 IHC as markers for CDKN2A/B loss in meningiomas. *Cancers, 16*. https://www.semanticscholar.org/paper/d3a86b252ddaae3c6ed79a3e075573ad84d4c291 (accessed on 6th August 2025).

42. Piccinini, F., Tazzari, M., Tumedei, M., Stellato, M., Remondini, D., Giampieri, E., Martinelli, G., et al. (2024). Data science for health image alignment: A user-friendly open-source ImageJ/Fiji plugin for aligning multimodality/immunohistochemistry/immunofluorescence 2D microscopy images. *Sensors (Basel, Switzerland, 24)*. https://www.semanticscholar.org/paper/7249a96eb095f3f553924760308e495e19a6526d (accessed on 6th August 2025).

43. Seager, R., Ko, H., Pabla, S., Senosain, M., Van Roey, E., Gao, S., Strickland, K. C., et al. (2024). Abstract PO5-06-09: Metastatic triple negative breast cancer has distinct tumor immune landscape. *Cancer Research*. https://www.semanticscholar.org/paper/659cadbc355de6b6dbc329d360d9f05376156d7e (accessed on 6th August 2025).

44. Shojaei, S., Behrooz, A. B., Cordani, M., Aghaei, M., Azarpira, N., Klionsky, D., & Ghavami, S. (2025). A non-fluorescent immunohistochemistry method for measuring autophagy flux using MAP1LC3/LC3 and SQSTM1 as core markers. *FEBS Open Bio*. https://www.semanticscholar.org/paper/a3a0fd84ed0e30c62f7fa9fcf0db505fd8c468de (accessed on 6th August 2025).

45. Smart, S., van Raan, A. F. J., & Waltman, L. (2014). Exploring the relationship between the engineering and physical sciences and the health and life sciences by advanced bibliometric methods. https://core.ac.uk/download/388668614.pdf (accessed on 6th August 2025).

46. Watson, A. S., Le, C., Wertheimer, A. M., Escobedo, S., So, L., Siddegowda, B. B., Palting, J., et al. (2025). Precision detection of FGFR2b protein expression in solid tumors: A comprehensive assessment of staining parameters via automated immunohistochemistry. *Archives of Pathology & Laboratory Medicine*. https://www.semanticscholar.org/paper/07ec1df3b54e9a5e48c1f13e7f34436932c09abc (accessed on 6th August 2025).

47. Willies, B., Nalukurthi, A. R. K., Rayal, K. B. S., Ahamad, T., Roshinee, R., Gadi, P., Sarvani, R. V. D., et al. (2025). Immunohistochemistry and FISH in HER2-positive breast cancer: Diagnostic techniques and clinical implications. *International Journal of Current Research in Medical Sciences*. https://www.semanticscholar.org/paper/9456de4b5d274534bb9cfc061a58d72f6a533c18 (accessed on 6th August 2025).

48. Yeh, C.-C., Li, Y.-J., Liang, J.-S., & Liao, J.-B. (2024). Automated standardization of melanin bleaching procedures of heavily pigmented melanocytic lesions with low-concentration hydrogen peroxide on an automated platform. *Applied Immunohistochemistry & Molecular Morphology, 32*, 436–441. https://www.semanticscholar.org/paper/31f8b5e734bed65a69a955f7bfb2dfb3e4793dd7 (accessed on 6th August 2025).

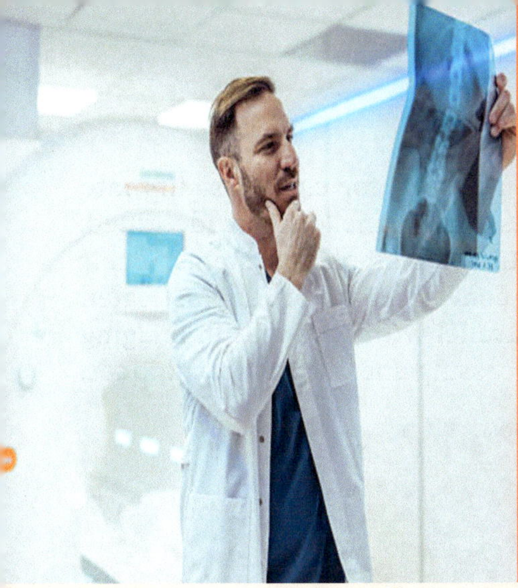

Chapter 11

ADVANCED IMAGING AND ANALYSIS TECHNIQUES

Contents

Introduction

Advanced imaging and analysis techniques have revolutionized the investigation of biological and medical occurrences. These new technologies provide powerful methods for visualizing complex structures and dynamic processes. By employing the synergy of cutting-edge imaging methods and analysis strategies, scientists are now able to dissect cellular interactions, trace molecular motion, and observe the functional response of biological systems in real time. These observations not only increase our understanding of intrinsic biological processes but also result in advances in medical diagnostics, thereby accelerating patient care and treatment protocols. **luorescence microscopy is at the forefront of these techniques**, allowing for **unprecedented** specificity and resolution in the study of biological specimens. Through the utilization of the inherent fluorescence characteristics, researchers can see intricate cellular morphology and observe their interactions in real-time (Abbe et al., 2012). Several advanced fluorescence techniques, including fluorescence recovery after photobleaching (FRAP) and Forster resonance energy transfer (FRET), are recognized as allowing for clear insights into cellular dynamics. These techniques enable minute variations in cells and organelles to be identified, giving them strong tools for investigating the multiscale character of biological systems. Their advancement with conventional imaging technologies lies in their convergence with sophisticated analysis technology to unlock complex biological information In parallel with advances in imaging techniques, there is an increasing need for sophisticated signal processing and analysis techniques.

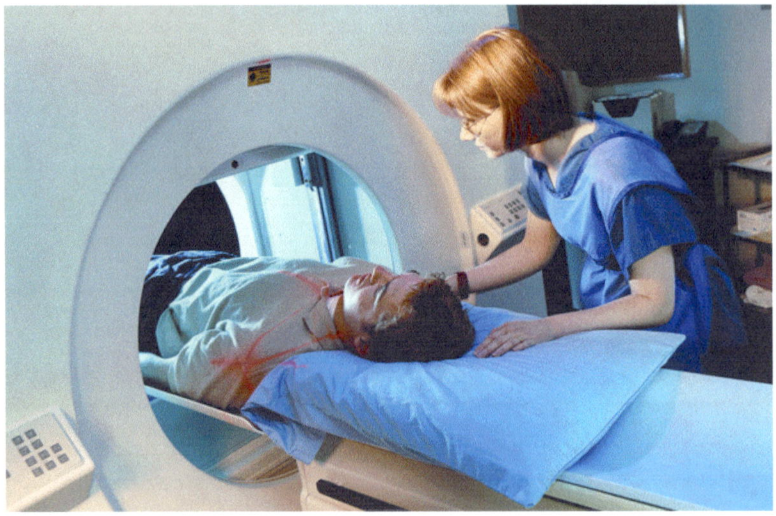

Figure 11.1. Advanced imaging and analysis techniques.

Source: https://cdn.expresshealthcare.in/wp-content/uploads/2017/05/27123918/201705ehm39.gif.

Biomedical data, which are often voluminous and complex in nature, require the application of sophisticated analysis systems to reap meaningful insights. (Cascio, D., & Raso, G., 2021) points towards the importance of machine learning techniques, more specifically deep learning, in bolstering the functionality of imaging analysis in medical applications. This transition towards computerized and intelligent processing of imaging data not only allows for efficient clinical diagnostics but also enables augmented precision in the detection and classification of disease. As scientists gain access to these powerful computational methods along with sophisticated imaging algorithms, the potential for revolutionary innovations both in research and in clinical practice is staggering, and thereby makes this multidisciplinary discipline relevant (Figure 11.1).

Definition of Advanced Imaging Techniques

Advanced imaging techniques refer to a variety of methods that significantly enhance the visualization and analysis of complex physical and biological systems. These techniques leverage advanced information and communications technologies to provide accurate insight that may not be achievable by traditional imaging means. Advanced techniques include, but are not limited to, medical imaging modalities such as magnetic resonance imaging (MRI), computed tomography (CT), and advanced optical imaging systems. In comparison with conventional imaging techniques, these advanced techniques not only capture images but also allow quantitative evaluation and recovery of significant parameters about the structures being imaged. Such capabilities enhance both the diagnostic accuracy and research potential in fields like medicine, material science, and environmental science. An exemplary advanced imaging technique is the application of DCE-MRI, which uses pharmacokinetic modeling for the quantification of relevant parameters. This specific technique provides information about contrast agent distribution kinetics in tissues, thus allowing for better characterization of tumors and other pathological conditions.. According to recent studies, the task of combining sophisticated software tools for image fitting and analysis plays an important role in optimizing the workflow of DCE-MRI. The tools can enable a detailed understanding of imaging data by abstracting fitting infrastructures and representation of results, and therefore, they are adaptable for heterogeneous imaging tasks and models. This versatility significantly enhances the capability of clinicians and researchers to perform analyses appropriate to specific needs within the medical imaging domain (Abdollahi et al., 2019). Moreover, advanced imaging techniques employ multidimensional imaging modalities that combine multiple imaging modalities to provide a more comprehensive understanding of the imaged objects. Such interaction results in higher sensitivity and specificity in analysis and diagnosis. For instance, the conjunction with other imaging technologies like CT or positron emission tomography (PET) and MRI facilitates the accumulation of complementary data to be established, which adds to general interpretation. As is explained in initiatives funded by organizations such as the Arts and Humanities Research Council (AHRC), the development of advanced imaging approaches is supported by systematic methodologies projecting technological assets onto artistic and research demands. It facilitates innovation in visual research and art by promoting the proper application of advanced imaging techniques to address the complexities of the day in various disciplines (Christie et al., 2007).

Importance in Various Fields

The development of imaging and analysis technologies is vitally significant across a broad range of applications, driving innovation and enhancing our understanding of complex systems. In materials science, for instance, advanced imaging technologies facilitate the determination of materials characteristics at resolutions previously unheard of, leads to a deeper comprehension of their structure-properties relations. This research capability is critical to the development and optimization of new materials and enables industries to develop stronger, more efficient products. With high-performance materials in greater demand, such advanced techniques become more and more vital in academic research and industry applications, emphasizing their importance in driving technological progress and solving materials design and use problems. In the area of biomedical applications, enhanced imaging techniques have revolutionized diagnostic practices, enabling non-invasive probing of biological systems. MRI and PET scan procedures are now medical imaging staples, enabling early disease identification and treatment. Integrating machine learning algorithms with imaging techniques further improves diagnostic accuracy and patient treatment by providing subtle insights into cellular reactions and organ function. This intersection of imaging science and advanced analysis provides individualized medicine approaches that fit singular patient needs, illustrating the dramatic impact of these techniques on medicine as a whole. The integration of experimental and computational approaches has also established new fronts in fields such as computational mechanics and materials science. The cooperative synergies that come from the combination of cutting-edge imaging technologies with predictive modeling capabilities provide a more extensive understanding of material behavior under varied conditions. The synergy is not only essential for validation and optimization of computation models but also propels innovation in next-generation technologies. According to the expanding literature, the role of experiments in multiscale models is increasingly emphasized, indicating computational approaches should serve as exploration tools instead of mere supportive elements in experimental science (Dingreville et al., 2015). Expanding innovations in these approaches ensure multidisciplinary approaches contribute their share in resolving complex science-associated problems.

11.1. Types of Advanced Imaging Techniques

The discipline of advanced imaging techniques encompasses a wide range of methods that significantly enhance the analysis of complex biomedical data. Conventional imaging modalities such as Magnetic Resonance Imaging (MRI) and Computed Tomography (CT) are widely used, providing high-resolution images of internal body structures. The addition of advanced signal processing methods is, however, essential in optimizing these images for greater clarity and improved diagnostic function. Recent studies underscore the importance of machine learning methods, particularly deep learning, which revolutionize medical image analysis. Such algorithms can automatically detect patterns and outliers in imaging data, leading to better clinical decision-making and novel applications in personalized medicine. Another groundbreaking field in advanced imaging is the evolution of three-dimensional (3D) histology techniques.

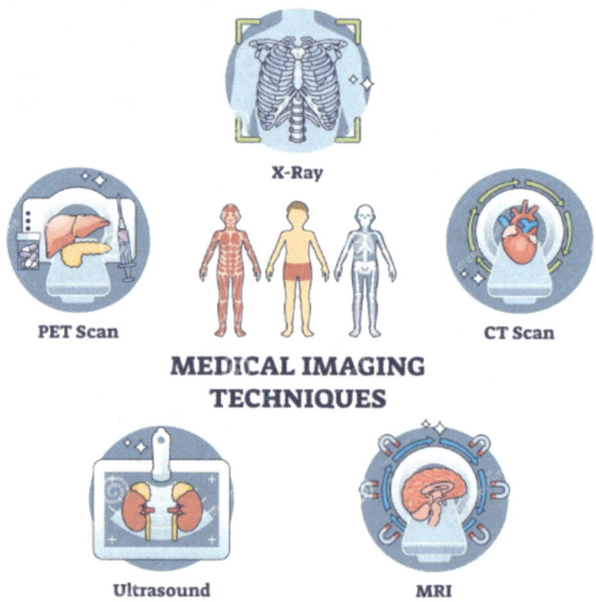

Figure 11.2. Types of advanced imaging techniques.

Source: https://thumbs.dreamstime.com/z/medical-imaging-techniques-body-diagnostics-outline-diagram-labeled-educational-scheme-types-bones-organs-inner-278873607.jpg.

Previously, histologic analysis was performed using two-dimensional tissue sections, which definitely limit the kind of disease that can be investigated. The advent of tissue clearing methods coupled with advanced fluorescence microscopy has transformed histopathology by enabling the visualization of biological tissues in 3D, providing pathologists with an unprecedented view of tissue architecture. This advancement allows for more accurate assessments of histological alterations, providing pathologists with unprecedented depth perception and spatial orientation in samples. Techniques that integrate classical hematoxylin and eosin (H&E) staining with computational reconstructions allow for similar insights of classical analyses but with enhanced depth perception and spatial orientation in samples (Cinci et al., 2023). Not only do these developments increase diagnostic accuracy, but they also elaborate on the potential clinical value of 3D histology in real-time use.

he rapid growth of imaging technologies also includes the development of functional imaging techniques, which quantify the body's physiological processes. The most significant functional imaging technology is Positron Emission Tomography (PET), which provides information about metabolic processes and gives insight into the biochemical determinants of disease and health. The method has been invaluable in the field of oncology, where it aids in cancer detection and monitoring of cancer growth and treatment response. In addition to anatomical imaging modalities like CT and MRI, PET-CT fusion imaging exploits the strengths of both techniques, offering combined diagnostic information. As image processing methods and machine learning continue to evolve, the overall effectiveness of functional imaging will improve, enabling earlier disease detection and tailored therapeutic approaches. In aggregate, the creation of such cutting-edge imaging techniques heralds a new era in medical diagnosis, which facilitates better patient outcomes and increased understanding of biological processes (Figure 11.2).

11.1.1. Magnetic Resonance Imaging (MRI)

Magnetic Resonance Imaging (MRI) has become a vital instrument in modern diagnostic imaging, particularly with the fact that it has the ability to provide high-quality anatomy information without ionizing radiation. The technique utilizes strong magnetic fields and radiofrequency pulses to generate high-resolution images of soft tissues, thereby making it very valuable in neurological, musculoskeletal, and oncological disease evaluation. One of the most important applications of MRI is in the evaluation of late cervical carcinoma, for which it has been shown to significantly enhance the detection of nodal involvement. Studies have also indicated that presurgical MRI assessment revealed pelvic nodal involvement in approximately 48.8% of the cases, a notably better detection compared to other imaging techniques. Despite its benefits, a note of caution is warranted: no imaging technique can entirely replace surgical evaluation, underscoring the need for a multidimensional approach in rigorous imaging practice (Diestro et al., 2013). In the realm of sophisticated MRI techniques, the study of non-enhancing peritumoral areas (NEPAs) has yielded beneficial avenues for distinguishing among brain tumor types. This hyperintense area surrounding tumors on T2-weighted and fluid-attenuated inversion recovery (FLAIR) images is indicative of heterogeneous pathological processes like vasogenic and infiltrative edema. Sophisticated analysis of NEPAs by MRI has been proven to be more accurate in the differentiation between high-grade gliomas from other malignancies like primary lymphomas and brain metastases. Consequently, the incorporation of innovative imaging methods, such as diffusion tensor imaging and dynamic contrast-enhanced perfusion imaging, has maximized the accuracy of MRI not just in tumor definition but also in prognosis and prediction of the response to treatment (Puppa et al., 2023). Continued advances in MRI technology represent a paradigmatic shift in the medical imaging terrain. Technological innovations such as functional MRI (fMRI) and MRI spectroscopy have broadened the applications of traditional MRI, allowing measurement of brain activity and metabolic function, respectively. These technologies offer superior insight into pathology at an integrated level, advancing treatment plans tailored to the individual and improving patient outcomes. Importantly, intermodal integration of structural and functional imaging modalities can yield synergistic interactions that improve overall diagnostic accuracy. While ongoing research still probes the ability of MRI in various clinical situations, the method continues to lead the way in advanced imaging and analysis techniques, highlighting its central place in contemporary medicine (Diestro et al., 2013) (Figure 11.3).

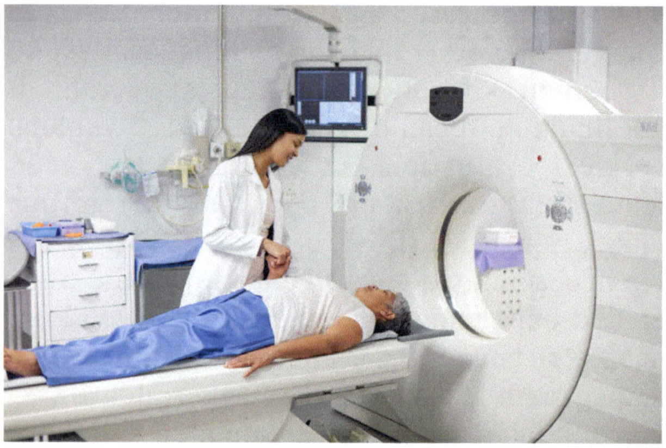

Figure 11.3. Magnetic resonance imaging (MRI).

Source: https://www.verywellhealth.com/thmb/0ju-aOTdy-UY9Gk4-nyW3FUaps0=/4203x2802/filters:fill(87E3EF,1)/it-ll-be-over-before-you-know-it-512702076-599cf073aad52b001104b457.jpg.

11.1.2. Computed Tomography (CT)

Computed Tomography (CT) has revolutionized medical imaging with the provision of excellent-quality cross-sectional images of the body. This advanced technique uses X-rays to generate highly accurate 3D models of internal structures, allowing medical professionals to make well-educated diagnoses and treatment choices. CT's lack of necessity for surgical intervention, coupled with its speed and accuracy, has made it an indispensable tool in emergency departments, cancer therapy, and surgical planning. With the ability to visualize soft tissues, organs, and even vascular structures, CT goes beyond traditional imaging modalities because it gives an overall assessment of pathological states. Also, the advances in technology have enhanced image quality and minimized exposure to radiation, further solidifying CT's role in modern medical diagnosis and treatment. CT's capacity to provide quantitative data ranks as one of the most beneficial contributions it makes to medical imaging. This is particularly pertinent in oncology, where precise measurement of volume and size of tumors is critical in monitoring response to treatment and disease progression. As an illustration, studies indicate that CT scans efficiently assess nodal involvement in cervical cancer and define results correlating imaging findings with pathological examination (Diestro et al., 2013). Although CT was beneficial for demonstrating pelvic nodal involvement in over 35% of cases, the statistics underscore the need for verification of imaging results through surgical evaluation to ensure accurate staging. In doing so, it is clear that not only is CT part of diagnostic procedures, but it is also critical when establishing treatment protocols based on quantitative data. Besides, the development of CT technology has also been used in non-clinical research, particularly in archaeology and material science. Its high-resolution imaging capability with sub-micron tomography can make precise examinations of material samples such as wood samples, providing important information on their structure and properties (Boone et al., 2009). This non-destructive method benefits both the interests of scholarly research and innovation in restoration and conservation treatments. Facilitating detailed examination without destroying the sample, CT shows greater insight into material structure and alterations, opening up interdisciplinary applications across a wide range of scientific disciplines. Therefore, CT's adaptability positions it as a central instrument for medical and materials research, encompassing the principles of advanced imaging and analytical techniques (Figure 11.4).

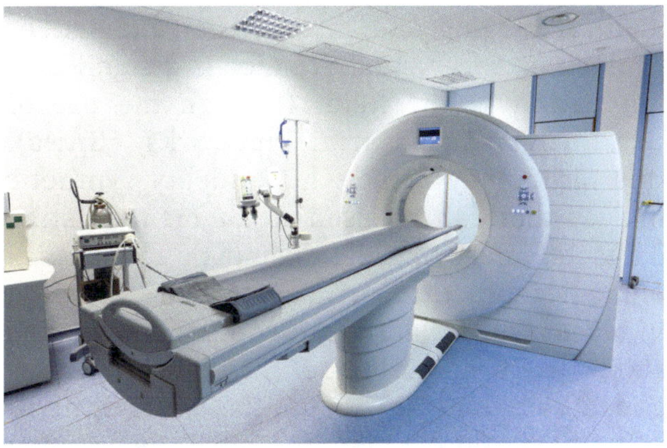

Figure 11.4. Computed tomography (CT).

Source: https://www.commonwealthradiologyassociates.com/wp-content/uploads/2016/06/shutterstock_204885118.jpg.

11.1.3. Positron Emission Tomography (PET)

Of the advanced imaging modalities, Positron Emission Tomography (PET) is a mainstay of diagnosis in many cancers. PET stands out for its ability to visualize metabolic processes in the body and thus provides data that other imaging modalities may not detect. With the assistance of radiotracers, most notably fluorodeoxyglucose (FDG), PET scans surface areas of increased cellular activity, which are characteristic of cancerous tumors. It is also critical for staging disease, evaluating the response to therapy, and detecting recurrence. To illustrate, in the treatment of prostate cancer, PET detection of oligometastatic disease affects decision making for treatment by allowing curative approaches rather than systemic therapy, which is potentially less specific to the patients' requirements. This highlights the extended role of PET imaging in the individualized treatment of oncology patients and guiding treatment plans, through the delivery of vital information to clinicians. PET imaging's application is not limited to oncology but can be used in various other clinical applications, such as in neurology and cardiology. In neurology, PET has played a pivotal role in diagnosing and distinguishing between diseases like Alzheimer's disease and epilepsy by monitoring changes in glucose metabolism within the brain. This feature is particularly crucial given the complexity of neurological disorders. where prompt and accurate diagnosis can affect therapeutic intervention. PET is applied in the assessment of myocardial perfusion and viability within cardiology to obtain heart disease-related information that can significantly improve therapeutic options. Furthermore, the recent introduction of innovations such as the integration of PET with magnetic resonance imaging (MRI) has served to further improve the imaging modality's capacity to provide improved anatomical information as well as functional data, in turn augmenting the diagnostic value and therapeutic planning in these diverse specialties. Despite its many advantages, the application of PET in clinical practice has its disadvantages. Accessibility is also a concern, as not all medical centers are equipped with the technology to carry out PET scans. PET imaging is also very costly and prevents the widespread utilization of PET imaging, particularly in underdeveloped countries. PET is also highly sensitive for detecting cancerous tumors but can yield false positives when metabolic activity is increased by infection or inflammation. These limitations highlight the importance of combining PET with other imaging modalities such as CT and MRI. This approach enhances overall diagnostic sensitivity With advancement in the field, ongoing exploration of novel radiotracers and their applications is predicted to further refine

PET's application in clinical practice, improving patient outcomes and diagnosis for an array of health conditions, as observed in recent studies in cancers such as bladder cancer and other neoplasms (Halpern et al., 2018; Bergh et al., 2019) (Figure 11.5).

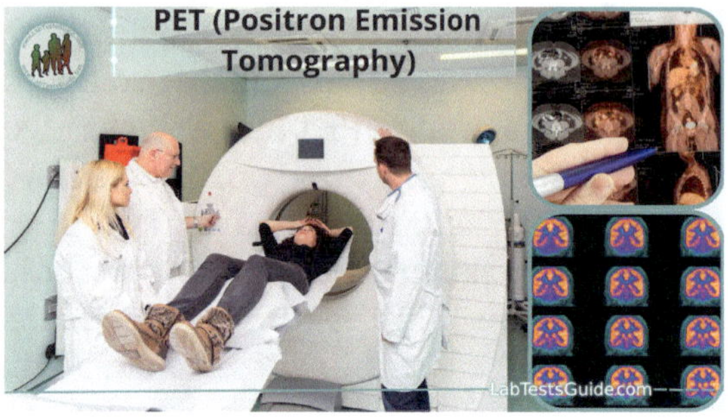

Figure 11.5. Positron emission tomography (PET).

Source: https://www.labtestsguide.com/wp-content/uploads/2023/03/PET-Positron-Emission-Tomography.webp.

11.2. Applications in Medical Diagnostics

The paradigm of medical diagnostics has been significantly reshaped by modern imaging and analysis technology, especially by the use of machine learning and artificial intelligence in radiology. Over the past decade, the adoption of deep learning algorithms has enabled rapid interpretation of complex medical images. Not only does this make it possible for improved screening and diagnosis of numerous medical conditions, but it also streamlines workflow in radiological departments. These devices are continuously trained on huge datasets, making them more accurate and reducing the scope for human error. Consequently, such innovations make the diagnosis of diseases such as cancer possible at an earlier stage, when early intervention can guarantee successful treatment. Tests have proven that diagnostic platforms based on AI can analyze imaging data with the same degree of accuracy as expert radiologists, demonstrating the widespread influence of such technologies on patient outcomes. Another exceptional use in medical diagnostics is the design of generative models, such as the Virtual Scanner, utilizing leading-edge generative AI to produce radiological scans. By addressing inherent limitations in medical imaging, data insufficiency, and patient protection, the Virtual Scanner is a significant innovation in the field. Through the use of Generative Adversarial Networks (GANs), this technology creates high-fidelity synthetic images that can be used to augment existing datasets, improving the diagnostic capabilities of medical practitioners. Furthermore, as noted in recent work, algorithmic robustness ensures stable performance under varying conditions and across imaging modalities. This shift to using high-end computation methods not only improves patient treatment but also improves radiological practice efficiency. The advantage of these technologies is vast, conjuring a future in which medical imaging becomes increasingly adaptive and holistic. Furthermore, the use of multiple imaging modalities, the so-called multimodal imaging techniques, is just one example of the power that advanced methods have to enhance the resolution of diagnosis. By combining information from different imaging modalities—MRI, CT scans, and PET scans, for example—the physicians can better know the patient's status. This general field assists in the more precise diagnosis and treatment planning, particularly for complex cases where one imaging modality may prove to be limiting. As the medical diagnostic imaging landscape is constantly evolving, combining advanced imaging modalities with innovative techniques like AI-based analytics will likely result in future treatment strategies. Ongoing development and validation of the methods reaffirm the promise of improved diagnostic outcomes, well-coupling technology with medicine for better patient management and care efficiency (Figure 11.6).

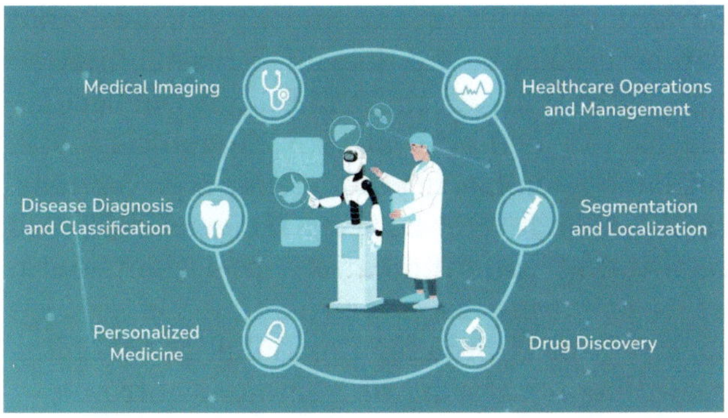

Figure 11.6. Applications in medical diagnostics.

Source: https://media.geeksforgeeks.org/wp-content/uploads/20240523171004/Applications-of-Deep-Learning-in-Healthcare.webp.

11.2.1. Early Detection of Diseases

Early detection of sickness is key to increasing treatment rates and patient survival rates. Advanced imaging and analysis techniques are key to the success of this objective, particularly in fields like medicine and agriculture. In agriculture, for instance, optical methods like RGB imaging and hyperspectral sensors enable early detection of plant diseases through precise diagnosis and quantification of disease.

These advancements encourage the transition to precision agriculture by providing the farmer with automated, objective, and repeatable detection systems that support the effective management of plant health. Providing non-destructive sensor-based methods has the potential not only to attain the highest possible yield but also to prolong the duration of plant production while avoiding the negative impact of pathogens. To this end, the convergence of imaging platforms from proximal to remote sensing enables comprehensive monitoring of plant health, highlighting the importance of early disease detection in agriculture. Early detection is also crucial in medicine, particularly through retinal imaging. The analysis of retinal fundus images, for instance, is a painless process that facilitates early diagnosis of ocular and vascular diseases. Such imaging provides significant information on patient health, typically identifying underlying disease states before they manifest as serious conditions. Employing advanced deep learning architectures to develop on such imaging enhances diagnostic data extraction embedded in the images, facilitating the detection of disease condition-associated abnormalities such as glaucoma and diabetes. This integration of medical image analysis and imaging techniques not only enhances diagnostic effectiveness but also enables timely interventions. By making it easier to assess retinal health, the likelihood of preventing irreversible outcomes is significantly increased, underscoring the importance of early detection in patient care (Motevali, 2023).

Moreover, the integration of machine learning and sophisticated imaging techniques transcends the limitations of traditional approaches, encouraging innovation in disease diagnosis. For example, the evolution of imaging paradigms, such as the advancement of 3D imaging techniques in brain MRI scan assessment, indicates a robust paradigm for the detection of attention disorders such as ADHD in children. This is a transdisciplinary approach that offers a broad-scale evaluation of various disease states through the implementation of advanced data analysis that generates actionable information using medical imaging. With continuing advances in technology, the application of sophisticated imaging will only grow, moving towards the development of automated systems to assist healthcare professionals with diagnoses. The innovations highlight the potential of early disease detection methods, reinforcing the conviction that continued innovation in imaging and processing is the way to go in improving healthcare outcomes and managing prevailing health challenges effectively (Figure 11.7).

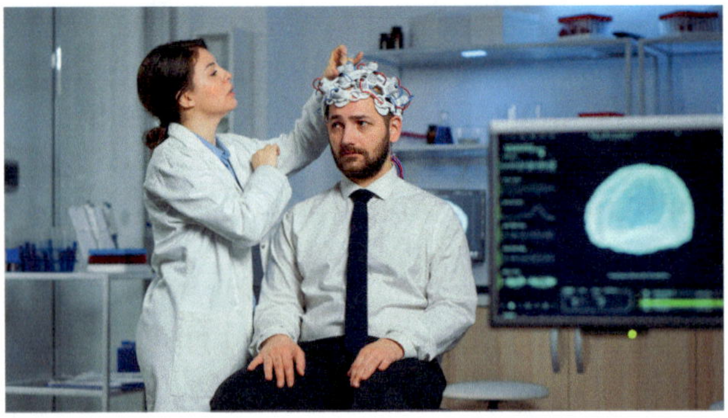

Figure 11.7. Early detection of diseases.

Source: https://zhl.org.in/blog/wp-content/uploads/2023/06/AI-and-EARLY-DISEASE-DETECTION.jpg.

11.2.2. Monitoring Treatment Effectiveness

The evaluation of treatment effect has become increasingly sophisticated with advances in imaging technologies that enable clinicians to monitor patient responses in real time. Quantitative ultrasound (QUS) parametric imaging is an excellent example in this regard, particularly in cancer. This imaging modality facilitates noninvasive assessment of tumor characteristics by monitoring alterations in tissue echogenicity over the course of treatment. In a study involving breast cancer patients, QUS demonstrated strong potential to predict treatment outcomes shortly after the initiation of chemotherapy. Specifically, QUS biomarkers, which assess spatial heterogeneities in the tumor tissue, were able to separate patient responses at 82 ± 0.7% to 89 ± 0.1% accuracies at different time points, indicating their strong potential as an effective tool in monitoring therapeutic efficacy (Ahmed et al., 2017). This early feedback on patient outcomes can lead to Beyond imaging technologies, the convergence of neurotechnologies is reshaping treatment efficacy monitoring, particularly in neurorehabilitation. Brain-computer interfaces (BCIs) are one such example of such convergence, enabling one to develop knowledge about a patient's cognitive and motor function that can be crucial in the tailoring of rehabilitation programs. With advances in BCIs, it will become feasible to combine human capabilities with technology, enhancing therapeutic interventions. In the near future, its uses are geared toward facilitating communication in patients with severe neurological impairment, while its long-term vision is broader functionality, including real-time monitoring of treatment outcome.

These technologies use behavioral and environmental data to provide clinicians with feedback on patient status, thereby aligning treatment modalities with individual needs (Kerick et al., 2012). By enabling adjustments by means of measurable parameters, BCIs are a novel approach to monitoring treatment effects. In addition, the integration of sophisticated analysis techniques with imaging modalities might more accurately assess treatment effectiveness. By applying sophisticated image processing algorithms and machine learning, clinicians can process complex datasets generated by heterogeneous imaging platforms. It is only through additional analysis that data can be optimized from treatment response within modalities, thereby understanding patient progress better. For instance, the utilization of QUS in combination with other imaging technologies could further explain the interaction between tumor characteristics and patient outcome. Such multi-dimensional diagnostics are able to uncover patterns not so clearly visible using traditional assessment methods by themselves, hence enabling the possibility of initiating early intervention once treatment is not effective. With these technologies evolving and merging, they also have the potential to revolutionize monitoring paradigms within clinics so that treatment to patients is both effective and individualized (Figure 11.8).

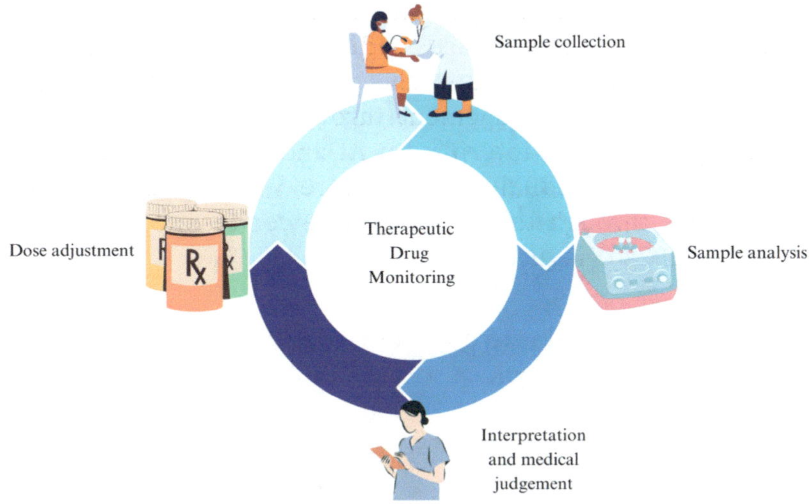

Figure 11.8. Monitoring treatment effectiveness.

Source: https://www.mdpi.com/pharmaceuticals/pharmaceuticals-17-00642/article_deploy/html/images/pharmaceuticals-17-00642-g001.png.

11.2.3. Personalized Medicine Approaches

Advances in imaging and analysis technology have ushered in a new phase of healthcare: personalized medicine. Individualization of medical treatment based on the specific attributes, needs, and preferences of patients is the aim of these methods. Using a patient's personal genetic information, lifestyle factors, and specific characteristics of the disease, physicians can develop very tailored treatment plans. This transition from a uniform approach to an individualized strategy allows physicians to predict outcomes to treatment and tailor treatments based on real-time patient data. The incorporation of new imaging modalities, such as MRI and CT scans, into oncologic evaluation provides a deeper understanding of tumor biology and disease progression, thereby facilitating more informed clinical decision-making. As science continues to advance, Bridging the gap between conventional and novel methods will open up new avenues for successful therapy." ssssss An important aspect of personalized medicine is the role of imaging technologies in maximizing the diagnostic process. Cutting-edge imaging modalities offer the capacity to visualize intricate biological processes in individuals, thereby enabling accurate disease characterization and prognosis. For instance, techniques such as multiparametric MRI can distinguish subtle differences in tumor phenotype, directing therapy and improving results. These imaging modalities produce dense datasets that, when put through sophisticated algorithms, make possible customized therapeutic approaches supported by robust empirical evidence. More importantly, the application of radiomics, a field that reaps tremendous data from medical scans, yields information on the tumor microenvironment that is reflective of structural and functional changes that are correlated with therapeutic response. The crossroads of data analytics and imaging thus places clinicians in a position to design interventions more in synchrony with individual patient profiles. Coupled with advanced imaging technologies, artificial intelligence (AI) increasingly plays a pivotal role in personalizing medicine, and that too through machine learning algorithms that sort through intricate datasets. By using supervised and unsupervised learning methods, researchers are developing prediction models with the capability to recognize the best treatment courses for patients in real-time. For instance, in breast cancer, AI can assess data from dynamic contrast-enhanced MRI to measure the likelihood of a pathological complete response to neoadjuvant chemotherapy. This predictive capability enhances not only clinical outcomes but also promotes patient engagement through individual patient data and feedback throughout the treatment process. The interplay of AI and personalized medicine is indicating a revolutionary shift towards more personalized healthcare, where patient empowerment and right treatment strategies converge through the support of newer technology, such as Mansoria et al. (2023) and Vocaturo et al. (2024) (Figure 11.9).

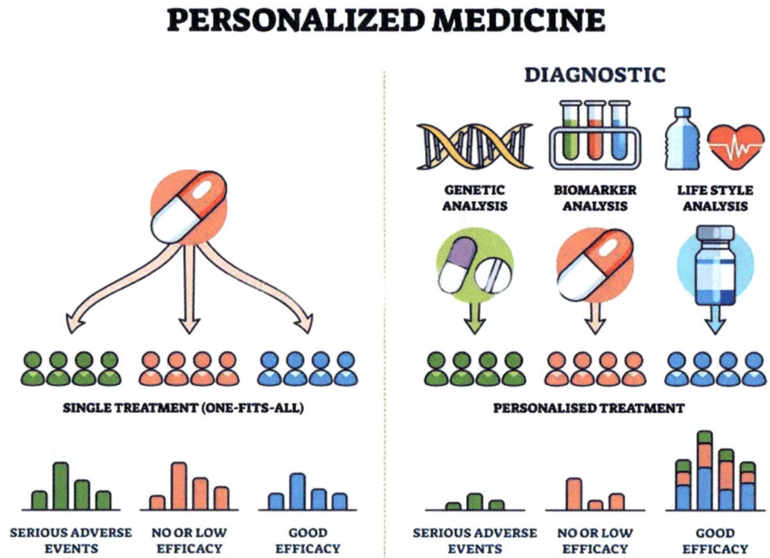

Figure 11.9. Personalized medicine approaches.

Source: https://thumbs.dreamstime.com/b/personalized-medicine-effective-individual-treatment-outline-diagram-labeled-educational-scheme-prescription-adjustment-280477671.jpg.

11.3. Imaging Techniques in Research

Imaging techniques in contemporary science find crucial application in medicine, biology, and materials science. The advances in imaging modalities, i.e., magnetic resonance imaging (MRI), computed tomography (CT), and scanning electron microscopy (SEM), allow scientists to image structures and processes at resolutions that were previously impossible. These capabilities not only enable us to gain a deeper understanding of complex systems but also spur advances in diagnostic methods and treatment protocols. Significantly, the use of machine learning algorithms in imaging techniques has transformed data analysis to enable researchers to process vast amounts of biomedical data generated. For instance, Cascio, D., & Raso, G. (2021) identify the significance of advanced analysis techniques in biomedical imaging with reference to the application of artificial intelligence in improving signal processing and classification of medical data. Additionally, advanced imaging techniques are not just confined to medical practice but are also at the core of nanotechnology. Techniques like STM allow scientists to visualize charge carrier distributions in silicon nanoscale devices at very high spatial resolution. Such capability is essential for fabricating nanoscale electronic devices that operate energy efficiently, exceeding the limits of conventional techniques. Through the application of sophisticated techniques such as the gap-modulation approach or dual-imaging technique, scientists can achieve precise information regarding nanoscale structures and thus facilitate breakthroughs in material science.

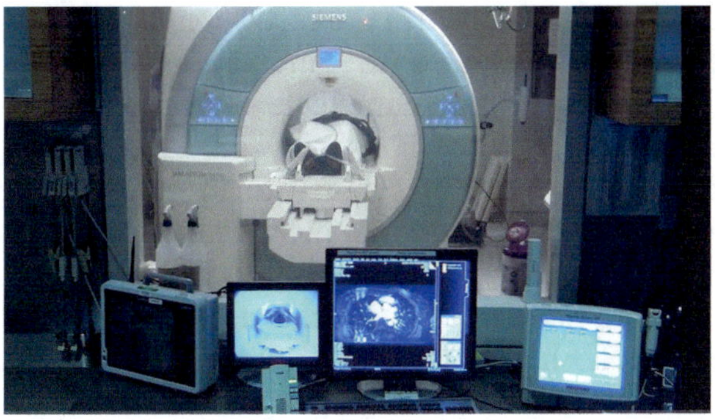

Figure 11.10. Imaging techniques in research.

Source: https://www.cedars-sinai.org/content/dam/cedars-sinai/depts-institutes/migrated-institutes/advanced-imaging-technologies-and-techniques.jpg.

The challenges and constraints provided by such sophisticated techniques against traditional imaging also have to be resolved. According to Bolotov et al. (2016), it is critical to comprehend such challenges in order to optimize the various applications of imaging. The innovation of machine learning and deep learning methodologies has revolutionized how data from images is treated and interpreted. These technologies enable patterns and anomalies to be identified within large data sets, increasing the diagnostic capability and research outcomes immensely. For example, machine learning algorithms can enable automatic classification of image data, doing away with processes that have always required extensive interpretation. This integration not only increases productivity but also increases the accuracy of analysis, as Cascio, D., & Raso, G. (2021) imply. In today's evolving world of research, there is little doubt that the combination of advanced imaging technology with computational methods will continue to transform our understanding of intricate phenomena, energizing scientific discovery and applications in practical life in numerous fields (Figure 11.10).

11.3.1. Biological Imaging in Cellular Studies

Biological imaging has become an essential tool in cellular studies, enabling observation of cellular activities in real time with unprecedented resolution. Two-photon microscopy and confocal imaging are some of the methods employed to observe dynamic cellular interactions and behavior within their natural habitat. This is particularly important when working with advanced tissues, where observing the spatial dynamics of diverse cell populations can yield valuable insights into physiological and pathological mechanisms. For example, technological progress in imaging enabled scientists to investigate the behavior of osteoclast precursors within bone marrow, monitoring their migratory patterns and interactions, which is important in bone remodelling and inflammation (Hasegawa et al., 2025). These sophisticated imaging modalities not only provide information about cellular dynamics but also enable scientists to conceptualize targeted therapies based on some observed cellular behavior in their studies. Advances in imaging methods have also significantly enhanced the study of developmental biology to the extent that a full understanding of embryonic development is now possible. Using fluorescent protein fusions, scientists can now see and track cell behavior and gene expression in three dimensions over time. High-resolution imaging allows researchers to see how individual cells talk to and cooperate with each other to form complex structures in organogenesis. Techniques like confocal and multi-photon time-lapse microscopy are changing how researchers examine developmental processes, from the fixed anatomical investigations to dynamic analysis of cell-cell communications (Aman et al., 2010). Not only do these new imaging techniques increase our understanding of fundamental biology, but they also have relevance for developmental disorders because they allow us to look into the underlying cellular abnormalities that may occur in early development.

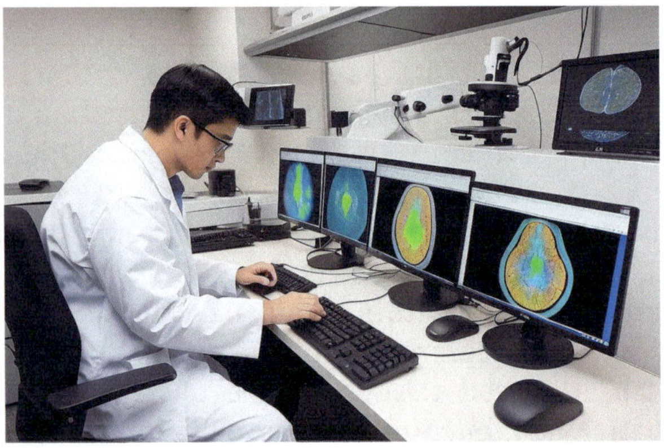

Figure 11.11. Biological imaging in cellular studies.

Source: https://img.freepik.com/premium-photo/students-using-advanced-imaging-techniques-detailed-cellular-studies_1108314-269177.jpg?w=900.

In parallel to these advances in imaging tools, the contribution of sound data analysis pipelines cannot be overstressed. The amount of information produced by such advanced imaging tools is so huge that custom computational software packages and analytical pipelines are required to interpret the captured data meaningfully. Advances in computational biology have introduced algorithms capable of processing multidimensional datasets to recover informative patterns and correlations that would otherwise be obscured. This integration of imaging and analysis is essential to grasping intricate biological processes, such as the dynamics of cellular signaling pathways or the effects of pharmacological manipulations on cellular behavior. By coupling advanced imaging technologies with robust data analysis, researchers can potentially enhance their capacity to draw conclusions from experimental data and increase their understanding of cellular processes in disease and health (Figure 11.11).

11.3.2. Material Science Applications

Material science is characterized by an intense reliance on advanced imaging and analysis techniques, which form the core of understanding the properties and the material's behavior at the atomic and nanoscale. Scanning probe microscopy (SPM) has emerged as a leading tool in this field of science to investigate the structural, electronic, and mechanical properties of a vast array of materials. New applications of SPM, particularly in characterizing oxide materials, have made possible breakthroughs in high-resolution imaging. For instance, research has demonstrated the potential of SPM to solve issues such as grain boundary transport in polycrystalline oxides. By employing advanced imaging technologies, researchers can manipulate and image ferroelectric domains, thereby advancing material manipulation and engineering capabilities in real-world materials applications (Bonnell et al., 2005). Apart from SPM, material science applications also depend on combining cutting-edge sensor technologies and analytical methods. Advances in sensor development, particularly CCD photometric array detectors and high-resolution imaging spectrometers, have led to new research projects aimed at studying materials under a wide range of conditions. These technologies offer a multi-faceted approach to material characterization that permits accurate measurement of composition and structure. For example, the combination of infrared spectroscopy and dual-polarization radar imaging has proven beneficial in investigating the nature of complex lunar surface materials. Such methods not only enhance our understanding of material structure but also provide potential ways of resource reconnaissance on other planets (Pieters, 2025). With increasing efforts of material scientists, the focus on the integration of heterogeneous sources of information from advanced imaging techniques also increases proportionally. Multimodal sensor data integration is the key to defining integral models that would thoroughly describe materials. Enhanced computing capability allows for the processing and fusion of data from diverse sources. This harmonization of data initiates pioneering uses in material science, where scientists are able to ask targeted questions regarding material properties and behavior. Moreover, the potential of using cutting-edge imaging techniques to study novel materials and nanostructures offers a platform for long-term breakthroughs, thereby broadening the scope of materials science and its applications in terrestrial and extraterrestrial settings (Pieters, 2025) (Figure 11.12).

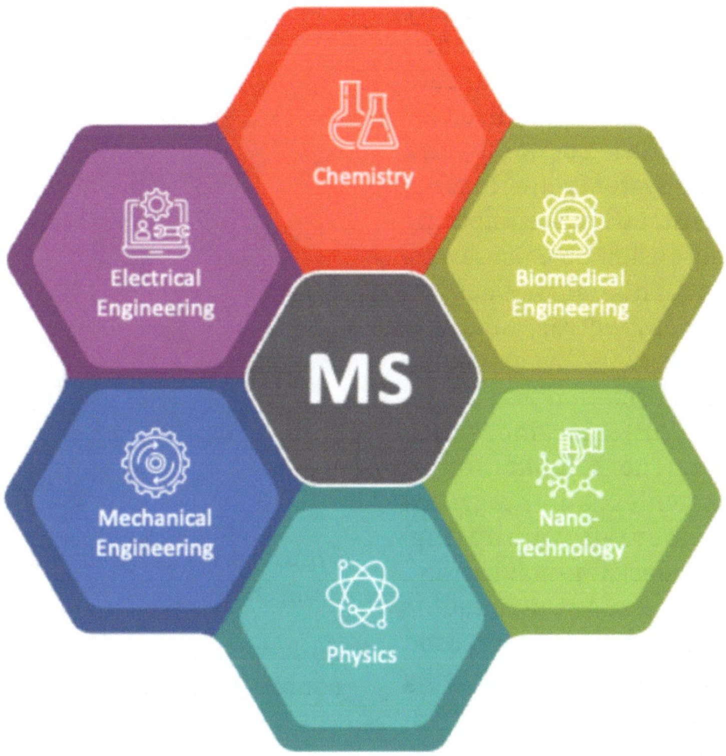

Figure 11.12. Material science applications.

Source: https://cdn.sketchbubble.com/pub/media/catalog/product/optimized1/0/5/0577acf8fadf939379beb8fa444339d81ded567de061db27bafadebda150c258/materials-science-mc-slide1.png.

11.3.3. Environmental Monitoring and Analysis

Good monitoring and analysis of the environment are essential to comprehend and deal with the impacts of human activities on nature. New technologies in imaging and analysis have revolutionized how environmental information is acquired and processed. For instance, high-resolution satellite imaging makes it possible for scientists to monitor land-use change, deforestation, and urbanization in near-real time. Such images can detect trends that can inform ecosystem management and conservation. Moreover, machine learning algorithms can enhance the efficiency of satellite data by facilitating predictive analytics, hence enabling proactive interventions that react to environmental degradation. These advances underscore technology's singular contribution toward encouraging a more advanced understanding of environmental dynamics, revealing hidden trends that otherwise would not be visible. Last but not least, the conjunction of artificial intelligence with environmental monitoring is a quantum leap. Modern environmental research benefits from AI's ability to act on data automatically and enhance interpretive precision. For instance, AI systems can analyze complex ecological data sets, identifying subtle variations in biodiversity and ecosystem health with economy and rapidity. In addition, the systems are capable of forecasting environmental trends, something that is integral to building sustainable processes. Progressive imaging technologies, such as multispectral and hyperspectral imaging, contribute to this mission also by capturing high-resolution spectral information that can be used to ascertain plant status, soil composition, and pollution gradients. The combination of these technologies provides an integrated approach to environmental monitoring, allowing more informed decision-making and policy implementation. As issues surrounding environmental sustainability gain increased attention, the use of sustainable imaging concepts cannot be overstated. Techniques that minimize environmental impact, such as the use of biodegradable contrast agents in imaging, are gaining popularity among researchers. These technologies address significant issues associated with pollutants commonly used in standard imaging techniques, as noted by Adadzi et al. (2024). Moreover, economic assessments highlight value for money in the form of goods, advanced imaging technologies for environmental observation that reveal a double benefit of augmented analytical capabilities and reduced ecological footprints. Institutions are increasingly considering ecologically friendly approaches in scientific investigation, as seen in initiatives such as the Advanced Diploma in Science with a focus on standards for sustainable learning outcomes, as witnessed in N/A (2010). This focus on sustainability in environmental monitoring not only encourages enhanced outcomes for ecosystems but also aids global efforts towards climate change reduction (Figure 11.13).

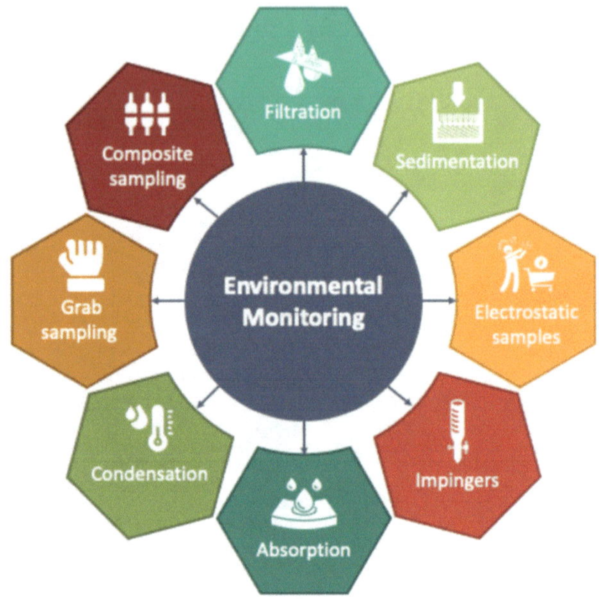

Figure 11.13. Environmental monitoring and analysis.

Source: https://www.ppsthane.com/wp-content/uploads/2022/11/image.png.

11.4. Data Analysis Methods

Advanced data analysis techniques are important in the area of imaging and analysis methods, especially in medicine. Modern approaches make use of the potential of high-level algorithms and computational processes to enhance the quality of images and provide meaningful interpretations of data. Machine learning, in particular, the application of deep learning, is among the prominent techniques where one can extract critical features from in-depth data. These technologies have enabled the development of innovative solutions that significantly improve diagnostic accuracy and clinical results. Importantly, the focus on high-resolution imaging and quantitative analysis has enhanced understanding of various conditions, underscoring the relationship between high-quality data and informed medical decisions (Sams, 2025). One major aspect of contemporary data analysis is the ability to handle vast amounts of diverse data types that are typically seen in biomedical research. Signal processing and classification methods play a crucial role in handling complexity. For instance, advanced modeling strategies allow researchers to retrieve information from intricate medical images through algorithms that are able to detect patterns and outliers. These methods not only make data interpretation easier but also yield predictive analysis that can potentially direct treatment avenues. Recent developments involve the application of integrating traditional machine learning methods with sophisticated statistical methodology. The resulting synergy offers a robust base that enables effective decision-making processes in clinical settings, subsequently enhancing the patient experience and outcomes (Cascio, D., & Raso, G.., 2021). Moreover, emphasis on applied, application-focused research in the field of data analysis cannot be overstressed. Through recent studies, as illustrated, the implementation of new methods plays a vital role in addressing specific issues in medical imaging diagnosis. Breaking down methods into signal processing, traditional machine learning, and deep learning categories, researchers may address complex medical puzzles systematically. Each category introduces unique strengths suited to particular imaging challenges, whether enhancing initial disease identification or characterizing conditions using advanced imaging data. Such all-encompassing characterization permits targeted improvement and facilitates multidisciplinary collaboration, ultimately stimulating innovation in diagnostic methods and medical imaging technology (Cascio, D., & Raso, G., 2021) (Figure 11.14).

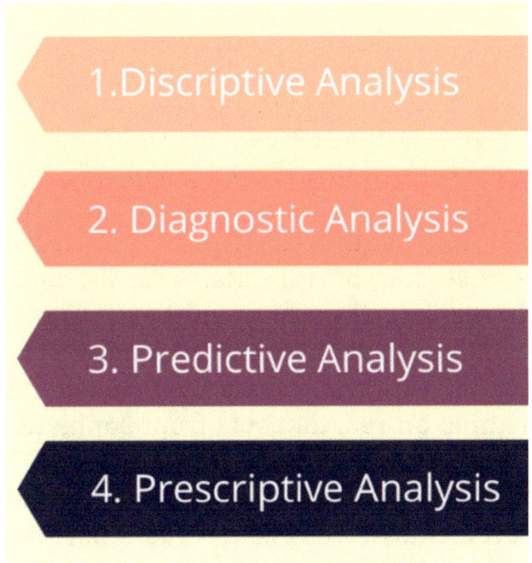
1.Discriptive Analysis
2. Diagnostic Analysis
3. Predictive Analysis
4. Prescriptive Analysis

Figure 11.14. Data analysis methods.

Source: https://cdn.hashnode.com/res/hashnode/image/upload/v1626704967564/YxbJMP5EY.png?auto=compress,format&format=webp.

11.4.1. Image Processing Algorithms

The quest for image processing algorithms has revolutionized the field of advanced imaging and analysis techniques, particularly in high-contrast imaging (HCI) systems. The algorithms have a significant impact on enhancing the performance of telescopes as well as HCI instruments designed for astronomical observations. By employing complex post-processing algorithms, researchers are able to significantly expand the detection limits of HCI instruments, thereby enabling the creation of science-ready images. Such advancements, in most instances, leverage unsupervised learning techniques to mimic the point spread function (PSF) and allow for the subtraction of residual starlight and speckle noise. This becomes significant while optimizing faint astronomical companion discovery rates, particularly in speckle-dominated regions, which are challenging to conventional imaging approaches and require new image processing strategies (Bleier et al., 2010). To further improve the performance of image processing algorithms, there has been a recent study that has advocated a move from unsupervised to supervised learning paradigms. This migration is more focused on the deployment of established machine learning models, such as random forests and neural networks, towards the post-processing of HCI data. With the building of these discriminative models, improved performance in distinguishing planetary signals from noise sources is facilitated. By using such algorithms on real datasets from sophisticated HCI instruments such as VLT/NACO and VLT/SPHERE, researchers have observed substantial improvements in true positive rates, particularly compared with traditional techniques such as ADI principal component analysis (ADI-PCA). Such a shift in methodology is required to enhance the detection capabilities of HCI instruments so that a more comprehensive understanding of astrophysical processes can be obtained (Bleier et al., 2010). The SPHERE Data Center is an essential gateway to improve scientific outcomes derived from HCI observations on the VLT. Through the provision of simplified reduction routines as well as user facilities, the Data Center improves the imaging process and significantly enhances the scientific return on data obtained. With a focus on providing freely accessible reduced datasets, the center is a treasure trove of information for researchers, contributing to a growing repository of processed imagery data. Established in 2017, the SPHERE Data Center has steadily enhanced its reduction processes, adapting its services based on the evolving needs of the astronomical community. With increasing experience of the hub in SPHERE data reduction and management, it is well positioned to cultivate improved reduction methods and more advanced data products and further advance the power of image processing algorithms for astronomical research (Figure 11.15).

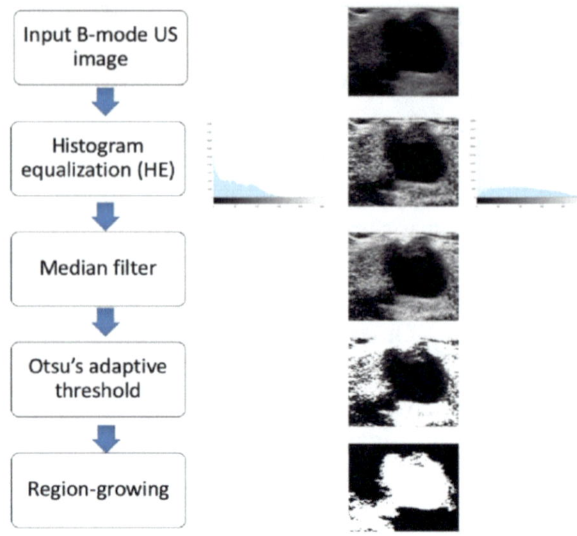

Figure 11.15. Image processing algorithms.

Source: https://www.researchgate.net/profile/Reham-Kaifi-4/publication/339628719/figure/fig3/AS:1063654703263744@1630606451909/Flowchart-of-image-processing-algorithm-From-top-to-bottom-the-following-steps-are.png.

11.4.2. Machine Learning in Image Analysis

The inclusion of machine learning (ML) in image analysis has transformed sectors across the globe, most notably in healthcare and diagnostics. Using sophisticated algorithms, specifically deep learning models, scientists can now glean valuable information from intricate visual data that was previously thought to be too complex for conventional analysis. Such algorithms are able to identify patterns in images, resulting in better diagnoses and treatment strategies. For instance, Convolutional Neural Networks (CNNs) have been applied very widely in urology image segmentation tasks to facilitate accurate volume measurements of the urinary bladder from medical images. This is an inspiring milestone toward quantitative examination, demonstrating that machine learning can enhance not only speed but also objectivity in medical assessment, particularly in fields where human error is a significant problem (Baradziej et al., 2024). Machine learning techniques are used much beyond urology and significantly impact hematology and oncology as well. The potential of classifying and predicting diseases through image analysis significantly improves diagnostic accuracy and enables timely interventions. Studies have indicated that ML models, including decision trees and support vector machines, are particularly suited to white blood cell classification in blood smear images and other clinical modalities, including MRIs and X-rays. These techniques not only enhance prediction effectiveness but also inform hematologists regarding potential diagnoses such as blood cancer or brain tumors. The growing use of advanced deep learning networks like Generative Adversarial Networks (GANs) and various iterations of CNNs indicates the ongoing quest to perfect image investigation protocols and works to respond to existing issues in data availability and model specificity (Asghar et al., 2023). With continuous developments in machine learning, its impact on image analysis is profound and extensive. The transition from conventional imaging practices to data-based techniques mirrors the increasing reliance on computational methods for accuracy and efficiency. However, obstacles remain, such as the need for massive datasets and the requirement for specialist training for researchers to employ such advanced techniques efficiently. Furthermore, incorporating data augmentation techniques can help overcome dataset limitations, enabling robust model training and validation. The ongoing convergence of sophisticated ML and deep learning approaches has the ability to bridge these impediments to deliver innovations to the practice and science of biomedical research. The machine learning history in image processing is one of gradual progress, with improvements potentially lying ahead for better healthcare diagnostics and beyond (Asghar et al., 2023) (Figure 11.16).

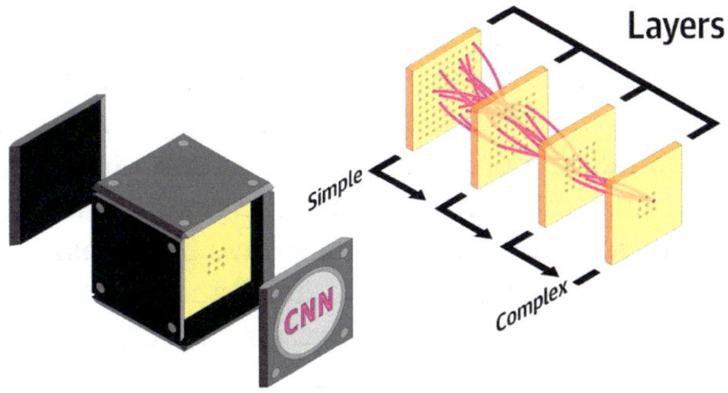

Figure 11.16. Machine learning in image analysis.

Source: https://i.ytimg.com/vi/VKnoyiNxflk/maxresdefault.jpg.

11.4.3. Statistical Methods for Data Interpretation

Statistical methods play an important role in interpreting data in advanced imaging and analysis protocols. By using highly effective statistical methods, researchers can learn important information from difficult imaging data, particularly in medical fields such as oncology. Advanced magnetic resonance imaging (MRI) techniques, for instance, including diffusion and perfusion imaging, produce extensive information on tumor activity and treatment response. Imaging data analysis is also complemented by the employment of statistical testing, such as unpaired t-tests and regression analyses. Through these methods, scientists can identify significant differences between patient groups and quantify significant variables that are related to clinical outcomes, as in research employing high-end imaging to predict glioma treatment response and tumor progression (Desideri, 2016). Furthermore, the addition of advanced statistical modeling adds more prognostic value to imaging in cancer treatment. Multivariate logistic regression allows the simultaneous examination of multiple predictors, providing a comprehensive understanding of the variables influencing patients. For example, values such as the Apparent Diffusion Coefficient (ADC) and relative Cerebral Blood Volume (rCBV) obtained through MRI can indicate tumor progression or a patient's response to chemoradiotherapy. Such predictors not only have a significant role to play in disease surveillance but even therapeutic decision-making. Interestingly, statistical methods also aid in the quantification of predictive performance of these models based on odds ratios and area under the curve (AUC) measures to further enhance the prediction of treatment efficacy (Desideri, 2016). In breast cancer, advanced statistical methods have been instrumental in enhancing the imaging data interpretative value. Intra-tumor heterogeneity analysis by voxel-wise analysis is one such example of the nuances of quantifying DCE-MRI metrics that combine traditional features neglected by methods based on simple design. Logistic and Cox regression models support pathologic complete response (pCR) and recurrence-free survival (RFS) evaluation, equating imaging features to clinical outcomes. Results indicate that voxel-wise features possess much greater predictability capacity compared to conventional methods, as evidenced by superior AUC and C-statistic values. This demonstrates how sophisticated statistical methods can enable scientists to reap usable information from imaging data and thus enable improved treatment planning and patient management in locally advanced breast cancer (Figure 11.17).

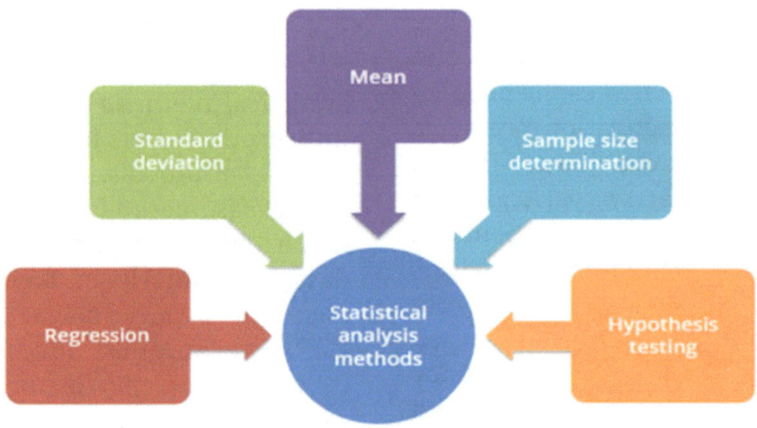

Figure 11.17. Statistical methods for data interpretation.

Source: https://lh5.googleusercontent.com/proxy/fauLgg6kCIBrV9HXOOOYaW6OmBroyPcpl2gf-CIxn17OXXhibfk6ZY_im9GxIYTkJkn7FDWC0TkDeh_Tw-ZIRZZydPwk0KgQgvDjTHzwPg3dj-irHklcTQ.

11.5. Challenges in Advanced Imaging

Advanced imaging has, certainly, brought with it revolutionary innovations, but also has enormous challenges. The entry point for new technologies, like volumetric laser endomicroscopy (VLE), presents a paramount clinical challenge: ensuring uniform user competency and understanding of the modalities of the imaging. Since VLE procedures demand highly advanced training, healthcare practitioners usually must ascend daunting learning curves that predispose patients to heterogeneity in diagnostic precision. The employment of technologies that produce high volumes of data only complicates the interpretative process. As imaging techniques become more advanced, professionals are not just expected to gain technical competence but also acquire the analytical skill to blend hard interpretation. Such reasons verify the need for comprehensive education systems capable of empowering professionals with expertise in advanced imaging techniques as well as improving patient outcomes. Another significant challenge in advanced imaging is managing the enormous volumes of data generated by imaging tests. For instance, information obtained through VLE imaging provides millimeter-sized detail of ailments such as Barrett's esophagus (BE), and research has indicated that VLE led to a 700% increase in neoplasia detection compared to standard processes. Though the information it provides is useful, manipulating and analyzing the same is daunting for practitioners and prevents timely decision-making. The challenge of integrating VLE outcomes into existing clinical work processes is also an obstacle, as physicians may need to struggle to integrate results into treatment programs. Thus, advanced imaging technologies do not only have to look towards enhancing diagnostic capability but also towards reducing data management solutions. These will be crucial to overcome in order to achieve maximum benefits of advanced imaging in clinical practice. Also, the financial implications of implementing advanced imaging techniques are formidable barriers that can prevent their global use. The initial costs of acquiring advanced imaging equipment and setting up operating units can be colossal, especially for smaller hospitals. Also, payment plans lag behind technological advancements, and thus, organizations investing in advanced modalities are not certain of reimbursement. As the VLE registry portrays, while improving diagnostic yield and patient care, the economic climate of these innovations remains precarious. To realize the full promise of advanced imaging, it is important to advocate for policy measures that promote fair reimbursement for diagnostic modalities that significantly improve clinical outcomes. Balancing advanced imaging costs with its wide benefits is key to stimulating a climate of innovation and greater patient care (Figure 11.18).

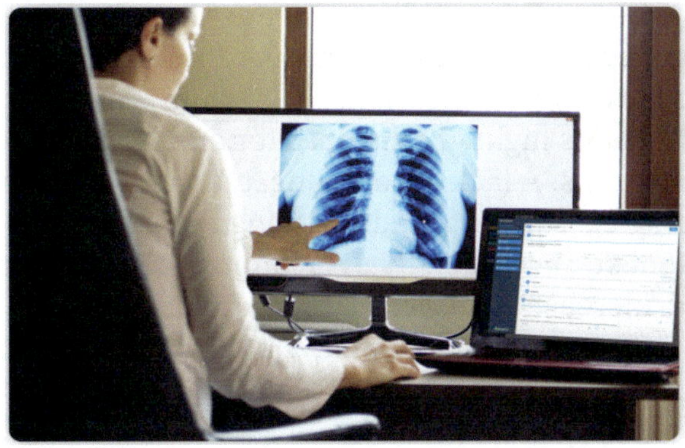

Figure 11.18. Challenges in advanced imaging.

Source: https://www.abbadox.com/hubfs/Radiology%20Workflows%20image-Feb-09-2023-10-35-02-0459-AM.png.

11.5.1. Technical Limitations and Artifacts

In the case of advanced imaging techniques, understanding of the technical restrictions is highly crucial for optimal application. All modern techniques, such as electron tomography, are susceptible to many artifacts that can conceal the image interpretation of complex structures. For instance, standard reconstruction algorithms like weighted back projection will show favored artifacts when limited projections are employed, which results in a distortion of the actual morphology of the specimen. The sparsity-exploiting algorithms that emerge through the prism of compressed sensing do promise some in this regard, and yet the practicals still need to be all-encompassing in theoretical exploration so as not to be among the pitfalls to the fidelity of the reconstructed images. Numerical calculations indicate that structural feature complexity impacts the number of projections needed for high-quality reconstructions, as seen in the sensitive balance between resolution and dose in imaging applications (Hovden et al., 2018). Artifacts also yield state-of-the-art imaging due to limitations in measurement tools, particularly biophotonics. The interaction of biological processes and photons presents unique challenges for accurate diagnostics. For instance, the National Institute of Standards and Technology has realized the necessity of improved measurement devices to further develop biophotonic applications, especially in cell and tissue diagnostics. The findings from several workshops highlight the need for an efficient measurement system that addresses these technological limitations. A lack of sophisticated measurement equipment can be responsible for the distortion of biological samples, underscoring the critically significant interface between imaging technology and diagnostic accuracy. By overcoming these limitations, scientists can foster innovation in biophotonics and increase the overall reliability of imaging techniques applied in life sciences (Brownstein et al., 2007). In addition, analysis of sample optimization parameters is required to decrease artifacts and improve reconstructed image quality. In electron tomography, to cite an instance, application of techniques such as l_1-norm and total-variation minimization has placed in the limelight the susceptibility of sparsity-based reconstructions to artifact deformations, particularly in the case of using limited tilt angles. As illustrated by studies, a limited tilt angle can significantly affect reconstructed images, underscoring the need to optimize reconstruction algorithms and acquisition parameters, such as projection direction and beam dose distribution. The assumption that splitting beam doses across more projections produces improved images is falsified when adequate data are collected, confirming the importance of a considered strategy to imaging conditions. Therefore, resolving the technical constraints and artifacts present in sophisticated imaging methodologies is critical in achieving deeper insights into complex materials and biological systems (Hovden et al., 2018) (Figure 11.19).

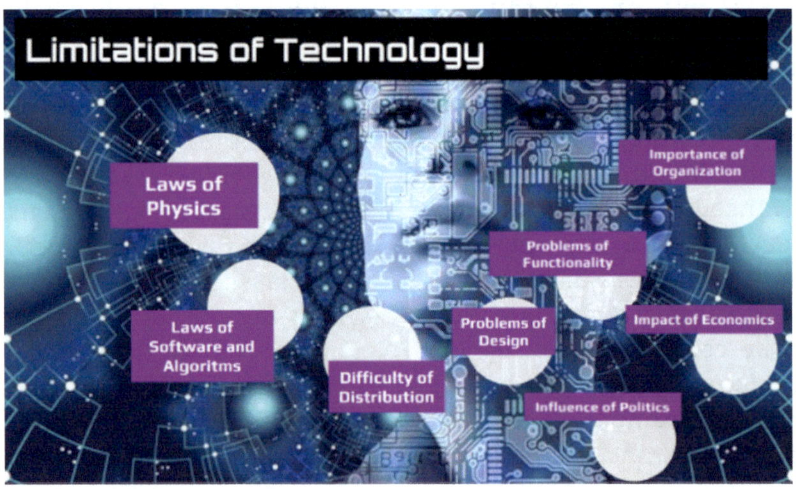

Figure 11.19. Technical limitations and artifacts.

Source: https://0701.static.prezi.com/preview/v2/yqjont xs64cilc v7pknl ycdtzx6jc3sachvcdoaizecfr3dnitcq_3_0.png.

11.5.2. Ethical Considerations in Imaging

The dramatic evolution of imaging technology has posed significant ethical challenges that must be addressed with caution. As technology advances, issues regarding the social implications of brain imaging and analysis become relevant with increasing urgency. The first is privacy and consent, whereby imaging studies reveal results that can open up private information that may be better left unknown. Researchers, when they conduct research, have an obligation to inform participants about the potential risks involved in giving their neural data. Participants may not clearly understand the implications when researchers fail to provide appropriate information, which can compromise autonomy and the right to decide what happens to one's information. As mandated in current guidelines, the ethical control of imaging techniques calls for openness and respect for individual rights for the purpose of building up trust among the research community and the general public (N/A, 2010). Beyond issues of privacy, the ethical aspects of imaging extend to the accuracy and interpretation of data. The outcomes of misinterpretation can be very dire, not only for research results but also for individuals' lives. For instance, outcomes of research from imaging studies may affect clinical practice or social perception of mental well-being and cognitive function, and result in stigmatization or unnecessary concern. Scientists, therefore, need to assume ethical responsibility for the publication and release of imaging results without deceiving individuals by sensationalizing results or making conclusions that are unwarranted. Scientific integrity demands that scientists issue an even account of their results based on the limitations of imaging techniques. By adhering to these ethical guidelines, scientists can avoid misrepresentation that may arise from oversimplifying complex data for the public (Mitchener-Nissen et al., 2014). Furthermore, the intersection of neuroscience and ethics calls on us to act proactively towards the future implications of imaging technologies. As we ponder progress in brain modulation and imaging techniques, issues around the potential for misuse come up. For example, neurotechnology to verify lying through imaging poses severe challenges to due process and human rights. In forensic contexts, the integrity of the justice system can be jeopardized by overreliance on imaging data. Ethical standards need to meet these challenges, forcing scientists to consider the broader social impact of their research. It is important to weigh the pursuit of scientific knowledge against moral responsibilities; therefore, cross-disciplinary discussions among policymakers, ethicists, and neuroscientists are required in order to make sense of complexities brought about by advanced imaging technologies (N/A, 2010; Mitchener-Nissen et al., 2014) (Figure 11.20).

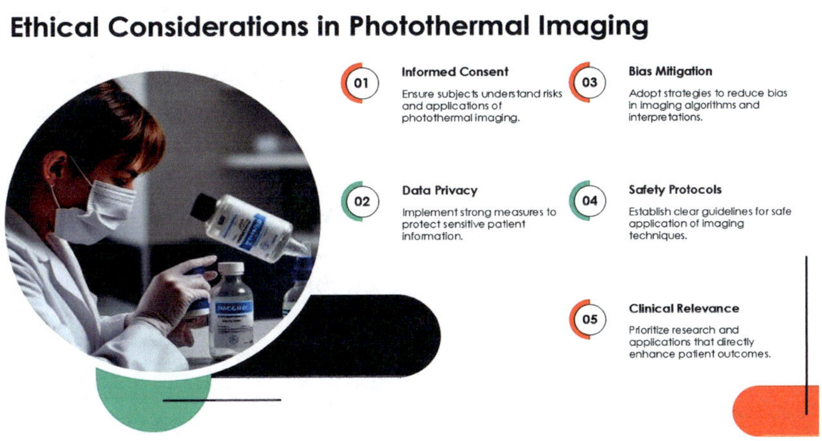

Figure 11.20. Ethical considerations in imaging.

Source: https://www.slideteam.net/media/catalog/product/cache/1280x720/e/t/ethical_considerations_in_photothermal_imaging_ppt_example_st_ai_ss_slide01.jpg.

11.5.3. Cost and Accessibility Issues

The synergy of advanced imaging techniques, particularly mobile thermal imaging, has significantly enhanced our ability to scan materials in real time. The cost and accessibility of such technologies, however, are still significant issues. An example of such advancement is the use of inexpensive mobile thermal cameras, which can be used to supplement standard smartphones, thereby making more advanced imaging capabilities more accessible (Anind et al., 2018). While this innovation brings down the price of traditional high-end thermal cameras, there remain constraints to their broader usage. Many individuals and organizations must grapple with the expense of training staff on how to utilize these devices optimally, which can limit their use in real-world applications to field settings. Therefore, lowering costs and increasing training programs are pivotal in facilitating these advanced imaging techniques to reach their full potential in a wide variety of industries. Besides, access to advanced imaging modalities is not just a matter of economic factors; it also largely depends on social factors. Almost 50 million individuals in the United States suffer from disabilities that can be enhanced using better imaging techniques (Arnoldussen et al., 2017). These individuals often lack access to advanced technologies that can greatly improve their lifestyle. While rehabilitation technologies play a critical role in supporting persons with disabilities, the mismatch between investment in resources and accessibility is a concern. The investments made in clinical and engineering resources, in most instances, have not been commensurate, which has caused disparities in respect of access. Addressing these disparities requires an integrative approach that goes beyond investment to a just technology development method, whereby solutions are designed to address diverse needs. Finally, the technological development of rehabilitation through programs like the Rehabilitation Engineering Research Centers indicates that there is an initiative towards resolving these factors of cost and access. These centers aim to form an interdisciplinary team that creates a connection between engineering and the individual with the disability's unique needs (Arnoldussen et al., 2017). By bringing in user perspectives and focusing on information technology, such projects have the potential to democratize advanced imaging solutions. But there is a growing need to ensure that innovations are not just theoretical but practical, usable applications. Future research activities need to be focused on developing cost-efficient solutions that consider the user experience and ensure integration of state-of-the-art imaging technology into people's lives with varying abilities, eventually redefining the accessibility horizon of advanced imaging.

11.6. Future Trends in Imaging Technology

The landscape of imaging technology is changing rapidly, driven by advances in computational capabilities and algorithmic complexity. Perhaps the most important trend is the embedding of artificial intelligence (AI) and machine learning (ML) into imaging systems. These technologies advance image processing performance, permitting higher precision and speed in many uses, from medical diagnosis to agricultural surveillance. For instance, images can today be processed by algorithms in real-time and enable instant decision and automated response in crisis situations. With increasingly smarter imaging systems, single-image analysis is not only enhanced but also enables correlation of data from diverse sources to provide end-to-end insights. This convergence of imaging technology and AI is leading the way to sophisticated analytics that are capable of predicting trends, optimizing outcomes, and streamlining processes across a multitude of industries, illustrating the depth to which technology is transforming our ability to visualize and decipher data. Another trend in imaging technology worth mentioning is the increasing importance of remote sensing and aerial imagery. This synergy of technology is transforming industries like agriculture and environmental observation to a great extent, where timely received data can bring a significant change. One such example is the use of high-resolution sensors on drones that capture high-resolution aerial shots, which, when run through advanced imaging methods, can yield valuable insights regarding crop health and soil health. Additionally, data gathered by satellites and UAVs can be processed using machine vision technologies to identify issues such as pest infestations or water shortages. Not only is the automation of data analysis more accurate in agricultural pursuits, but it also encourages sustainability in that it optimizes the use of resources. As scientists continue to make new discoveries in this area, the possibility of enhancing environmental monitoring and farm efficiency through enhanced imaging capability becomes increasingly evident, signaling a new era of data-driven decision-making. The future of imaging is also envisioned to encompass breakthroughs in real-time visualization and 3D imaging techniques, which have the potential to transform many areas of endeavor. Holography and volumetric imaging technologies enable a more complete understanding of complex shapes, which is invaluable in medicine and engineering. For example, the ability to visualize anatomical structures, as in 3D, assists surgeons during preoperative planning, leading to enhanced surgical success. Furthermore, during the engineering design process, 3D imaging supports prototype verification and the identification of failure opportunities before actual failure. The continuous development of such approaches, further amplified by increasing computing capabilities, will make real-time and interactive imaging ubiquitous, enabling specialists to interact with information in natural and convenient ways. As the techniques advance, they will stand to enhance not only the rate of analysis but also comprehension itself in millions of fields, thereby revolutionizing practices reliant on correct visualization and effective examination of complex systems (Figure 11.21).

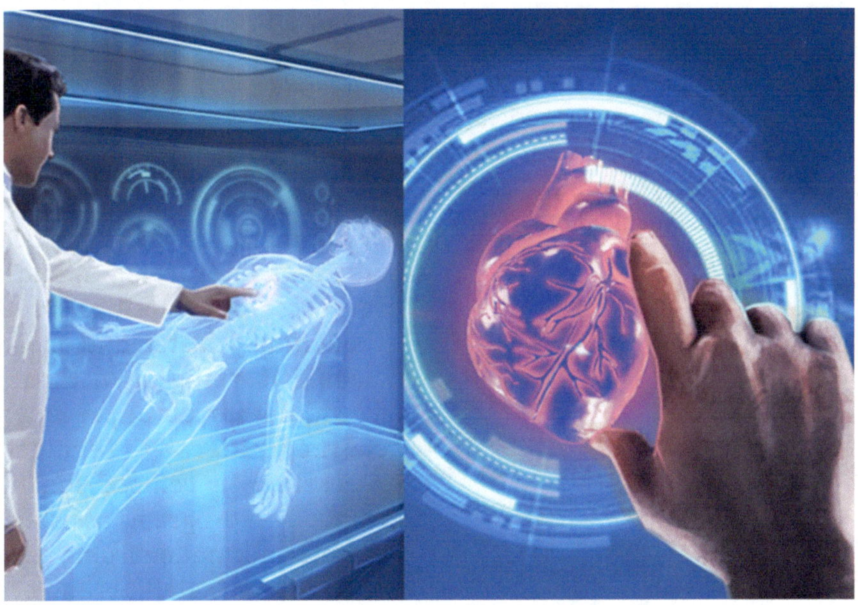

Figure 11.21. Future trends in imaging technology.

Source: https://www.appstudio.ca/blog/wp-content/uploads/2020/08/Major-AI-Trends-Revolutionizing-Healthcare-in-The-Future.jpg.

11.6.1. Innovations in Imaging Hardware

New technology in imaging devices has completely changed the conditions for medical diagnosis and treatment, promoting higher accuracy of analysis. The application of three-dimensional imaging systems has made it possible for practitioners to assess complicated anatomical structures with unprecedented accuracy. The innovation is particularly helpful in fields like reconstructive surgery, where sophisticated planning is essential for good outcomes. For example, in rhinoplasty in facial cleft patients, 3D imaging offers a bottom-up approach to surgical planning in the sense that the surgeon reconstructs the underlying bone structures first, prior to addressing soft tissue. Such improvements not only improve the process of preoperative evaluation but also the surgical execution process, such that there are more predictable and favorable clinical outcomes. The integration of novel imaging technology and thoughtful planning in a harmonious manner underscores the pivotal role of imaging hardware innovations in contemporary surgical interventions (Codazzi et al., 2019). Beyond improvements in visualization, recent developments in medical imaging hardware have addressed computational limitations that could constrain the capabilities of new imaging technologies. Several ultrasound, X-ray, and MRI imaging methods have been enhanced by technology advancements spurred by architectural developments, allowing more advanced algorithms to be processed more efficiently to create better images. The availability of MIRAQLE, a medical image reconstruction benchmarking toolkit, reflects the thrust toward democratizing access to high-end imaging technology. MIRAQLE tries to encourage hardware designers toward more accessible and cost-effective solutions by supplying detailed background information and parallel implementations for a wide variety of imaging tasks. In return, there is an increase in the adoption rate of these technologies by a larger number of healthcare facilities, thus reducing the disparities in diagnostic capabilities among different institutions and enhancing patient care across various settings (II et al., 2025). Lastly, the convergence of high-end imaging technology with innovative hardware thinking is driving tailored solutions in medical imaging. Effective co-design methods that consider both hardware capability as well as software algorithms can yield huge efficiency and image-quality gains. The Sonic Millip3De project, for instance, illustrates the extreme power efficiency gains possible when hardware is carefully designed for 3D ultrasound imaging. These advances not only reduce the cost of operation but also facilitate greater processing speed, allowing for real-time imaging required for a variety of clinical applications. As researchers continue to improve these technologies and expand their fields of application, the potential of more advanced imaging devices to enable breakthrough innovations in medical diagnosis and treatment becomes increasingly clear, rendering their vital contribution to modern medicine ever more evident (II et al., 2025).

11.6.2. Integration of Artificial Intelligence

The integration of artificial intelligence (AI) into advanced imaging and analytical techniques has made data interpretation and decision-making processes for practitioners and researchers exponentially faster and more accurate. With machine learning algorithms, AI can analyze large datasets at unprecedented speed and accuracy, thereby revolutionizing image processing. In remote sensing, for example, computer AI programs assist in the derivation of valuable information from very complicated data obtained from satellites and other sensors. This feature is particularly important in applications such as land-use and environmental monitoring, where timely and accurate data interpretation is required to support effective management and planning. These advanced imaging techniques, when combined with AI, improve the quality of the outcome as well as mechanize processes for ensuring effective resource utilization in scientific and practical applications. Moreover, the combination of AI with imaging showcases numerous advantages because it solves issues associated with data overloads, popularly referred to as the data glut problem. In the context of Earth Observing System (Eos) applications, the proposed Information Sciences Experiment System (ISES) highlights the potential of AI in revolutionizing data management and analysis processes. The ISES aims at maximizing capability in order to address real-time needs for data, benefiting researchers by giving them instruments that facilitate the timely processing and interpretation of massive amounts of data. By embedding AI within existing frameworks, scientists will be able to implement state-of-the-art image processing and data management capabilities to mitigate data saturation. Not only does this improve decision-making as more information is available, but it also sets the door ajar for innovative and effective practices in fields like environmental science and urban development. In addition to improving analytical abilities, the combination of AI with imaging technologies also fosters the development of new solutions for novel issues. For instance, the Civil Space Technology Initiative (CSTI) has taken a leading role in examining AI's application in space technology through the establishment of inclusive programs that have been developed with the aim of improving imaging systems. CSTI supports the introduction of AI-based techniques appropriate to enhance imaging systems utilized in planetary research and Earth observation. Through continuous research on the underlying technologies and methodologies, CSTI embodies the visionary character required to meet increasing requirements for precision and accuracy in data acquisition and interpretation. This forward-thinking method not only contributes to the scientific body of knowledge of varied phenomena but also encourages interdisciplinary collaboration, bolstering further the potential of AI for advanced imaging and analysis techniques.

11.6.3. Potential For Real-Time Imaging

Real-time imaging technology has changed the face of medicine, particularly in the field of interventional procedures. It has enabled precise, patient-specific planning that improves surgical outcomes and safety. Integration of real-time imaging with computer-assisted surgery (CAS) has facilitated easier navigation of complex anatomy by surgeons. As Haidegger et al. (2017) show, the history of advanced imaging techniques formed the groundwork for real-time navigation of surgical trajectories, integrating visual feedback with steps of the procedure. This simultaneous coordination among imaging and surgical action not only makes the procedure performed more accurate but also enhances the potential for minimally invasive procedures. By providing enhanced visualization, real-time imaging thus facilitates less patient trauma and shorter recovery times, and is evidence of its vital role in modern surgical practice. The capability of real-time imaging, however, extends beyond the short-term context of surgery; it has potential for application in all areas of medicine, most certainly emergency and critical care. In emergency and critical care environments, visualizing microcirculation in real-time could be extraordinarily important. According to Najarian (2012), advanced imaging technologies are capable of offering earlier detection of conditions and injuries that affect microcirculation. This can be employed to guide the implementation of real-time intervention strategies. Real-time monitoring of microvascular dynamics not only aids in diagnosis but can also enhance therapeutic endpoints for resuscitation. By digitizing microvascular extraction and quantitative analysis, these imaging systems provide physicians with immediate insights that can improve patient outcomes in emergent situations, demonstrating the real-time imaging methodologies' multidisciplinary utility. Real-time imaging combined with automated algorithms is a breakthrough marvel that enhances the reliability and effectiveness of medical assessments. These algorithms allow for stabilization of imaging data and segmentation of vascular networks, thereby allowing for extensive analysis with little intervention. As detailed in Najarian (2012), the automated system allows for accurate segmentation of microvascular networks and identification of blood flow changes, thereby providing decision-enabling insights without inconsistencies arising from manual interventions. The capacity to calculate functional capillary density (FCD) values in real-time provides a significant diagnostic tool with a productive capability to differentiate between pathology and health. By minimizing computation time and maximizing diagnostic accuracy, these computerized imaging techniques are well placed to strongly promote clinical decision-making and intervention planning, demonstrating the revolutionary potential of real-time imaging in medicine.

SUMMARY

The combination of innovative imaging and analytical techniques has the power to revolutionize several fields, but especially in the health sector. As demonstrated by several studies, the use of advanced imaging technologies in healthcare institutions can significantly enhance patient outcomes and organizational efficiency. A particular research study that critically analyzed the internal and external hospital environments of Malaysian hospitals, resulting in the effective implementation of medical imaging systems such as PACS and RIS/HIS. This highlights an important connection between organizational design and the deployment of technology, representing a critical frontier for research and practice in the future. The evidence suggests that something more than pure technological potential influences the manner in which such tools are applied to overcome intricate health problems, highlighting the need for comprehensive planning in healthcare technology implementation (Nor et al., 2010). Furthermore, highly sophisticated imaging techniques—when coupled with personalized treatment, i.e., exercise protocols—can improve patient quality of life significantly, especially in advanced disease such as end-stage breast cancer. There is evidence to suggest that inclusion of mechanical loading through exercise not only inhibits the growth of tumors but also improves bone density in patients with osteolytic lesions. The implications of this dual-pronged approach highlight the importance of cross-disciplinary approaches combining imaging and intervention methodologies. Such advanced techniques are not just diagnostic but have the potential to be part of integral therapeutic steps to treat both biological and physiological sides of patient treatment. The potential to attain greater treatment efficacy and patient quality of life is a classic illustration of the transformative power of synergistic merging of advanced imaging with focused treatment modalities (Chee et al., 2018). Lastly, image and analysis methodology development acts as a stepping stone for emerging healthcare and other medical advancements. The ongoing innovation of these technologies holds great potential to enhance diagnostic precision, treatment efficacy, and health care management. However, it is crucial to note that successful integration not only requires attention to technology but also a solid comprehension of the organizational, social, and environmental determinants of implementation. Future studies should focus on examining these interlinks more deeply, drawing on current research to inform best practice. By facilitating collaboration among heterogeneous healthcare providers and promoting evidence-based care, the full potential of innovative imaging technologies can be realized, thereby improving outcomes at both clinical and systemic levels (Nor et al., 2010; Chee et al., 2018).

Modern imaging and analysis methods have greatly transformed the understanding of many medical diseases, especially ischemic stroke. Emerging technology provides continuous monitoring of cerebral blood flow, making it critical to monitor changes over time and not necessarily strict time-based therapeutic windows. This paradigm shift enables timely intervention tailored to the patient's presentation, as demonstrated by the successful deployment of imaging protocols that warn clinicians of ischemia progression. Furthermore, knowledge of collateral circulation enhances the prediction of clinical outcomes because continuous imaging studies can minutely describe perfusion dynamics and the efficacy of endovascular treatments. As these technologies advance, they have the potential to simplify reperfusion therapies by identifying optimal methods for modulating brain reperfusion with minimal risk of adverse outcomes, underscoring the clinical value of newer imaging in optimizing stroke treatment (Ip et al., 2014). In orthopedic studies, sophisticated imaging techniques, such as laser scanning confocal microscopy (LSCM), have provided important insights into joint degeneration, particularly osteoarthritis (OA). With the ability of three-dimensional visualization of wear particles from cartilage, LSCM makes possible the whole-characterization analyses of mechanical properties and surface morphology under wear conditions. It has opened new avenues for systematic quantification of wear debris, promoting understanding of the wear process. Dramatic correlations between surface textures on wear particles and degrees of wear conditions have been constructed, leading to the identification of critical surface descriptors reflecting underlying disease processes. The innovative use of field and feature parameters as outlined in ISO/FDIS 25178-2 illustrates the promise of image-based measurements for informing clinical treatment and intervention in joint diseases (Aigner et al., 2012). Lastly, deployment of high-tech imaging and analysis technology into clinical medicine is a quantum advance in patient care delivery in most medical specialties. Visualization and quantification of physiological alterations offer an unprecedented level of comprehension that can guide treatment protocols and improve patient outcomes. Through continued research, constant refinement of these imaging modalities will undoubtedly deliver even more insightful predictive models and treatment algorithms. Clinical practice and evidence from data still need to be balanced, as inter-disciplinary cooperation has the potential to develop imaging technologies further while ensuring that results in effective manners are brought into clinical application. Further research in advanced imaging and analysis, hence, allows clinicians to adopt more personal and efficient treatments, further enhancing the general efficacy of modern medicine (Aigner et al., 2012; Ip et al., 2014).

A LOOK TO THE FUTURE:

PROSTATE CANCER:

Prostate cancer is one of the most common cancers affecting men worldwide — a malignant growth that begins in the prostate, a small gland of the male reproductive system located just below the bladder and surrounding the urethra. The prostate's primary role is to produce seminal fluid, and although it is small in size, cancer arising in this gland carries profound implications for health and quality of life as men age. The disease usually develops slowly; in many cases, it remains confined to the prostate for years without causing noticeable symptoms. Because of this, early stages of prostate cancer are often detected through screening tests such as the prostate-specific antigen (PSA) blood test or digital rectal examination (DRE), rather than symptoms alone. When identified early, localized prostate cancer often has a favorable prognosis and a variety of treatment options.

The risk of developing prostate cancer increases with age, particularly after the age of 50, making age one of the most significant risk factors. Family history — especially having a father or brother diagnosed with the disease — also raises risk, and certain racial groups, such as Black men, tend to have higher rates and poorer outcomes compared with others. Genetic factors, including inherited mutations in genes like BRCA1 and BRCA2, can further influence susceptibility.

Early stages of prostate cancer may cause no symptoms at all. When symptoms do appear, they often relate to urinary function and can include frequent urination, especially at night, difficulty starting or stopping urination, weak urine flow, or even blood in the urine or semen. As the disease advances and potentially spreads (metastasizes) beyond the prostate, symptoms such as pelvic or bone pain, fatigue, and unexplained weight loss may emerge. Diagnosis typically involves a combination of screening tests, imaging, and biopsy to confirm the presence and aggressiveness of cancer cells. Once diagnosed, treatment pathways vary widely based on stage, patient age, overall health, and personal preferences. Active surveillance may be appropriate for slow-growing tumors, while more aggressive cases may be treated with surgery, radiation therapy, hormone therapy to block testosterone (which often fuels

prostate cancer growth), chemotherapy, or newer approaches such as immunotherapy and targeted agents. Public health efforts emphasize awareness and early detection, particularly as global cases are projected to rise in coming decades due to aging populations. This makes education about risk factors and routine screening vital components in reducing advanced-stage diagnoses and improving long-term outcomes for affected men.

REFERENCES

1. shikawa-Ankerhold, H. C., Ankerhold, R., & Drummen, G. P. C. (2012). Advanced Fluorescence Microscopy Techniques—FRAP, FLIP, FLAP, FRET and FLIM. *Molecules, 17*(4), 4047–4132. https://doi.org/10.3390/molecules17044047Abdollahi, A., Debus, C., Floca, R., & Ingrisch, M., et al. (2019). MITK-ModelFit: A generic open-source framework for model fits and their exploration in medical imaging—Design, implementation and application on the example of DCE-MRI. http://arxiv.org/abs/1807.07353 (accessed on 6th August 2025).
2. Adadzi, J., Anderson II, J., & Azi, C. I., et al. (2024). Transformative advancements in diagnostic imaging: Reducing risks, enhancing accuracy, and promoting sustainability. https://core.ac.uk/download/621451782.pdf (accessed on 6th August 2025).
3. Adornato, C., Assolito, C., Ayllon, E. M., Cordelli, E., Di Feola, F., Guarrasi, V., Iannello, G., et al. (2024). Virtual scanner: Leveraging resilient generative AI for radiological imaging in the era of medical digital twins. https://core.ac.uk/download/643638812.pdf (accessed on 6th August 2025).
4. Ahmed, A., Guimond, A., & Sadeghi-Naini, A., et al. (2017). Chemotherapy-response monitoring of breast cancer patients using quantitative ultrasound-based intra-tumour heterogeneities. https://core.ac.uk/download/286714031.pdf (accessed on 6th August 2025).
5. Aigner, T., Ballantine, G., Blunt, L., Buckland-Wright, J., Chan, E., & Chiffre, L., et al. (2012). A new approach to numerical characterisation of wear particle surfaces in three-dimensions for wear study. https://core.ac.uk/download/30732623.pdf (accessed on 6th August 2025).
6. Albert, D., Beuzit, J.-L., Boccaletti, A., & Chauvin, G., et al. (2017). The SPHERE data center: A reference for high contrast imaging processing. https://core.ac.uk/download/484031117.pdf (accessed on 6th August 2025).
7. Aman, A., Bianco, A., & Czirok, A., et al. (2010). Advanced optical imaging in living embryos. https://core.ac.uk/download/4886369.pdf (accessed on 6th August 2025).
8. Anind, C. W. D., Cho, Y., Hendriks, A., Holone, H., & Jaderberg, M., et al. (2018). Deep thermal imaging: Proximate material type recognition in the wild through deep learning of spatial surface temperature patterns. https://core.ac.uk/download/154747826.pdf (accessed on 6th August 2025).
9. Arnoldussen, A., Hansen, A., & Hansen, A., et al. (2017). How a diverse research ecosystem has generated new rehabilitation technologies: Review of NIDILRR's Rehabilitation Engineering Research Centers. https://core.ac.uk/download/213086708.pdf (accessed on 6th August 2025).
10. Asghar, R., Kumar, S., & Shaukat, A. (2023). A review on classification of white blood cells using machine learning models. http://arxiv.org/abs/2308.06296 (accessed on 6th August 2025).
11. Baradziej, D., Chodyka, M., & Mosorov, V. (2024). Bladder volume estimation based on USG images. https://core.ac.uk/download/622110694.pdf (accessed on 6th August 2025).
12. Bergh, R. van den, Borgmann, H., Briganti, A., & Futterer, J., et al. (2019). Imaging modalities in synchronous oligometastatic prostate cancer. https://core.ac.uk/download/210534351.pdf (accessed on 6th August 2025).

13. Berzin, T., Cash, B., Chang, K., DeMeester, S., et al. (2019). Volumetric laser endomicroscopy and its application to Barrett's esophagus: Results from a 1,000 patient registry. https://core.ac.uk/download/286362760.pdf (accessed on 6th August 2025).

14. Bleier, L., Wittig, I., Brandt, U., & Dröse, S., et al. (2010). Measuring mitochondria-derived reactive oxygen species in cell culture: Challenges and limitations. https://core.ac.uk/download/pdf/82333005.pdf (accessed on 6th August 2025).

15. Bonnell, D. A., Kalinin, S. V., & Shao, R. (2005). Local phenomena in oxides by advanced scanning probe microscopy. https://core.ac.uk/download/76363009.pdf (accessed on 6th August 2025).

16. Boone, M., Stevens, M., Van Acker, J., & Van den Bulcke, J., et al. (2009). X-ray tomography as a tool for detailed anatomical analysis. https://core.ac.uk/download/55837758.pdf (accessed on 6th August 2025).

17. Brownstein, M., Dowell, M. L., Gaigalas, A. K., & Hoffman, R., et al. (2007). Biophotonic tools in cell and tissue diagnostics. https://core.ac.uk/download/323070689.pdf (accessed on 6th August 2025).

18. Cascio, D., & Raso, G. (2021). Special issue on signal processing and machine learning for biomedical data. https://core.ac.uk/download/427519287.pdf (accessed on 6th August 2025).

19. Chee, R., Clay, T., Feeney, K. T., & Galvao, T., et al. (2018). Mechanical suppression of osteolytic bone metastases in advanced breast cancer patients: A randomised controlled study protocol. https://core.ac.uk/download/213607862.pdf (accessed on 6th August 2025).

20. Christie, P., Pringle, M., & Shepherd, R. (2007). The hunt for submarines in classical art: Mappings between scientific invention and artistic interpretation. https://core.ac.uk/download/9427963.pdf (accessed on 6th August 2025).

21. Cinci, L., Costantini, I., Franceschini, A., Laurino, A., Mazzamuto, G., Montalbano, A., Nesi, G., et al. (2023). A guide to perform 3D histology of biological tissues with fluorescence microscopy. https://core.ac.uk/download/576923411.pdf (accessed on 6th August 2025).

22. Codazzi, T., Han, S., Hierl, T., Inanli, A., Koc, M., Ogino, T., Ong, H., et al. (2019). New technologies in rhinoplasty: A comprehensive workflow for computer-assisted planning and execution. https://core.ac.uk/download/323232725.pdf (accessed on 6th August 2025).

23. Cohen, E., Davatzikos, C., Hsieh, M.-K., & Hylton, N., et al. (2019). Prediction of treatment response to neoadjuvant chemotherapy for breast cancer via early changes in tumor heterogeneity captured by DCE-MRI registration. https://core.ac.uk/download/323063042.pdf (accessed on 6th August 2025).

24. Debackere, K., Monard, E., Raspoet, D., & Ratinckx, K., et al. (2025). Technologie en innovatie in Vlaanderen: Prioriteiten. https://core.ac.uk/download/pdf/6468460.pdf (accessed on 6th August 2025).

25. Della Puppa, A., Bianchi, A., Gadda, D., Carlesi, E., Scola, E., Fainardi, E., Busto, G., et al. (2023). Conventional and advanced magnetic resonance imaging assessment of non-enhancing peritumoral area in brain tumor. https://core.ac.uk/download/610293895.pdf (accessed on 6th August 2025).

26. Desideri, I. (2016). Role of advanced MR techniques in predicting response to chemoradiotherapy in glioblastomas. https://core.ac.uk/download/79621994.pdf (accessed on 6th August 2025).

27. Devi, M. K. A. (2021). Plant disease identification using the unmanned aerial vehicle images. https://core.ac.uk/download/621412633.pdf (accessed on 6th August 2025).

28. Diestro, M. D., González-Benítez, C., Hernández, A., & Salas, R., et al. (2013). Nodal involvement evaluation in advanced cervical cancer: A single institutional experience. https://repositorio.uam.es/bitstream/10486/664927/1/nodal_gonzalez_EJGO_2013.pdf (accessed on 6th August 2025).

29. Dingreville, R., Karnesky, R. A., Puel, G., & Schmitt, B., et al. (2015). Review of the synergies between computational modeling and experimental characterization of materials across length scales. http://arxiv.org/abs/1509.03892 (accessed on 6th August 2025).

30. Haidegger, T., Nagy, D. Á., & Rudas, I. (2017). Surgical data science, an emerging field of medicine. https://core.ac.uk/download/148786989.pdf (accessed on 6th August 2025).

31. Halpern, E. J., Kim, S., Salmanoglu, E., & Thakur, M., et al. (2018). A glance at imaging bladder cancer. https://core.ac.uk/download/227055407.pdf (accessed on 6th August 2025).

32. Hasegawa, T., Ishii, M., & Kikuta, J. (2025). Imaging the bone-immune cell interaction in bone destruction. https://core.ac.uk/download/592758910.pdf (accessed on 6th August 2025).

33. Hovden, R., Jiang, Y., Muller, D. A., & Padgett, J., et al. (2018). Sampling limits for electron tomography with sparsity-exploiting reconstructions. http://arxiv.org/abs/1904.02614 (accessed on 6th August 2025).

34. Ip, H. L., & Liebeskind, D. S. (2014). The future of ischemic stroke: Flow from prehospital neuroprotection to definitive reperfusion. https://core.ac.uk/download/323076634.pdf (accessed on 6th August 2025).

35. Kerick, S. E., Lance, B. J., McDowell, K., & Oie, K., et al. (2012). Brain computer interface technologies in the coming decades. http://arxiv.org/abs/1211.0886 (accessed on 6th August 2025).

36. Mansoria, P., Singh, S. B., & Hada, S. S. (2023). Urine analysis in Ayurveda and modern medicine: Exploring convergence and divergence. https://core.ac.uk/download/617189589.pdf (accessed on 6th August 2025).

37. Mitchener-Nissen, T., & Rusconi, E. (2014). The role of expectations, hype and ethics in neuroimaging and neuromodulation futures. https://core.ac.uk/download/228177242.pdf (accessed on 6th August 2025).

38. Mohd Nor, R. (2010). The organizational implications of medical imaging in the context of Malaysian hospitals. https://core.ac.uk/download/1588563.pdf (accessed on 6th August 2025).

39. Motevali, S. (2023). Towards non-vascular fundus image analysis and disease detection. https://core.ac.uk/download/579994448.pdf (accessed on 6th August 2025).

40. N/A. (2010). Criteria for the diploma qualifications in science at advanced level: Principal learning. https://core.ac.uk/download/4151080.pdf (accessed on 6th August 2025).

41. Nagel, M. (2019). Computational contributions to the automation of agriculture. https://core.ac.uk/download/213463714.pdf (accessed on 6th August 2025).

42. Najarian, K. (2012). An automated method for analysis of microcirculation videos for accurate assessment of tissue perfusion. https://core.ac.uk/download/51287059.pdf (accessed on 6th August 2025).

43. Pieters, C. M. (2025). The quickest, lowest-cost lunar resource assessment program: Integrated high-tech Earth-based astronomy. https://core.ac.uk/download/pdf/10447868.pdf (accessed on 6th August 2025).

44. Sampson II, R. (2025). Architectural support for medical imaging. http://deepblue.lib.umich.edu/bitstream/2027.42/137105/1/rsamp_1.pdf (accessed on 6th August 2025).

45. Sams, C. F. (2025). Multidimensional processing and visual rendering of complex 3D biomedical images. https://core.ac.uk/download/pdf/141519205.pdf (accessed on 6th August 2025).

46. Vocaturro, M. F. (2024). MR-radiomic-based pathological response prediction to neoadjuvant chemotherapy in breast cancer. https://core.ac.uk/download/613214233.pdf (accessed on 6th August 2025).

47. Welch, A., Platt, B., Billings, L., Borchelt, D., Brankack, J., Drzezga, A., Dubois, B., et al. (2012). FDG-PET imaging, EEG and sleep phenotypes as translational biomarkers for research in Alzheimer's disease. https://core.ac.uk/download/370450.pdf (accessed on 6th August 2025).

48. Wilson, R. G. (2025). Applications of ISES for vegetation and land use. https://core.ac.uk/download/pdf/42822563.pdf (accessed on 6th August 2025).

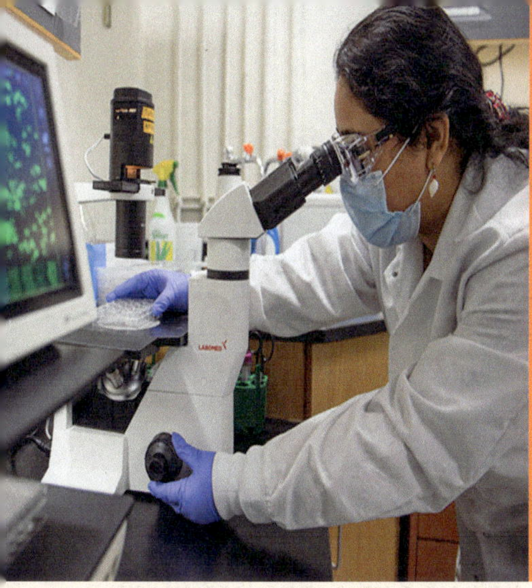

Chapter 12

IN SITU HYBRIDIZATION AND MOLECULAR MORPHOLOGY

Contents

Introduction

The discipline of molecular biology has greatly evolved ever since the invention of new techniques, among which is the *in situ* hybridization (ISH). ISH has made it possible for investigators to visualize a sequence of nucleic acid within their natural cellular or tissue environment, bridging what was otherwise a gap between morphological information and molecular information. Using fluorescent probes, ISH enables the identification of gene-expression localization, thereby allowing researchers to dissect complex biological processes at a resolution that would otherwise be unattainable. This is crucial in the task of unraveling gene function, cellular architecture, and genetic-morphological interaction, ultimately giving us a better understanding of , developmental biology, and disease mechanisms. *In situ* hybridizations versatility is exemplified by its applications in different model organisms that lead to evolutionary conservation and divergence insights. For example, the comparative band mapping approach was able to effectively illustrate the conservation of subchromosomal regions among species, like humans and primates, reflecting evolutionary synteny persistence over millions of years (Jauch et al., 1991). Such studies illustrate the breadth of information accessible via ISH, ranging from determining chromosomal morphology to characterizing single-gene expression patterns. As ISH becomes more commonly used in research, the integration of findings from taxa enhances not merely our understanding of single species but also illustrates the general principles underlying molecular morphology and genetic regulatory networks. However, while *in situ* hybridization is informative, the techniques employed must continue to innovate with novel problems in functional genomics.

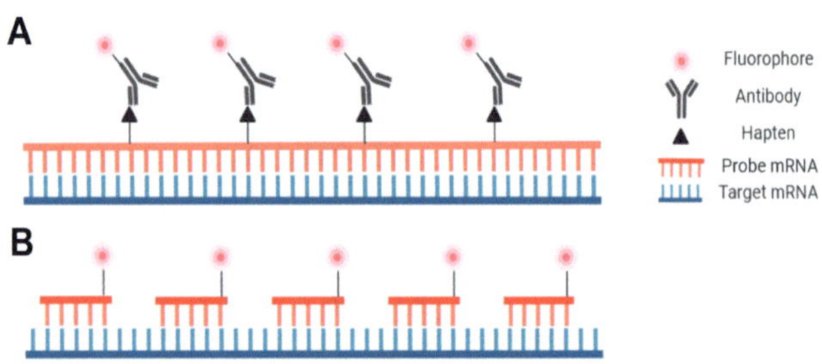

Figure 12.1. *In situ* hybridization and molecular morphology.

Source: https://media.springernature.com/lw785/springer-static/image/chp:10.1007%2F978-0-387-89626-7_12/MediaObjects/978-0-387-89626-7_12_Fig2_HTML.gif.

Novel techniques have branched into employing RNA interference (RNAi) techniques in conjunction with ISH to explore gene function during development. Research has indicated that while advancements have been achieved, RNAi-induced morphological changes in chick embryos are subtle and often undetectable (Torrens et al., 2013). This limitation underscores perhaps the most significant characteristic of contemporary molecular biology: the necessity for robust experimental systems that can reproducibly link gene expression silencing and unmistakable phenotypic effects. To this end, as the technology of ISH and ancillary methods improves, they will necessitate robust standards for determining how molecular changes correspond to morphologically discernible change, further establishing the science of molecular morphology (Figure 12.1).

Definition of *In Situ* Hybridization

In situ hybridization (ISH) is a cost-effective technique applied in molecular biology to detect specific nucleic acid sequences in fixed tissues or cells. ISH helps researchers study the spatial relationships between genes and mRNA in their native cellular context, acquiring insights into gene expression patterns and genome organization. Using labeled probes that hybridize to complementary nucleic acid targets, ISH allows for the localization of genetic material at the microscopic level. The resolution and specificity provided by *in situ* hybridization render it a valuable tool for the examination of many biological processes and abnormalities, especially in developmental biology, cancer biology, and genetics. This method not only confirms the presence of specific genes but also their expression dynamics, contributing a lot to the realm of molecular morphology of living creatures. One of the major advancements in the field of ISH is the development of fluorescence *in situ* hybridization (FISH), which uses fluorescent probes for improved visualization. FISH is particularly beneficial in the identification of chromosome disorders and studies on the structure of the genome. For example, the application of chromosome bar codes produced by FISH allows for the recognition of chromosomes with precision and the detection of inter- and intra-chromosomal rearrangements. This molecular cytogenetic technique is an important tool in clinical diagnostics and research, as it enables rapid and precise identification of chromosomal changes. FISH and ISH, in this case, not only complement our understanding of genetic arrangement but also aid in the diagnostic processes of various chromosomal disorders, as indicative of their primary functions in contemporary molecular morphology studies (Müller, S., & Wienberg, J., 2006). Extending the usefulness of ISH, studies using the method have been able to provide valuable insights into the realm of chromatin in many organisms, such as the tomato plant. Using FISH with different DNA probes, scientists can visualize repetitive sequences and assess chromosomal structures such as heterochromatin, euchromatin, and nucleolar organizer regions. These studies demonstrate fundamental correlations among types of chromatin and genetic activity. Principal classes of chromatin and their specific distribution have been determined in an attempt to make clear the tomato plant's and other species' genome organization. With further understanding of chromatin dynamics via ISH, scientists are able to investigate the effects of such structural characteristics on gene expression and overall organismal development (Chang et al., 2008). ISH is therefore a core method in molecular morphology studies, integrating genetic data with structural data (Figure 12.2).

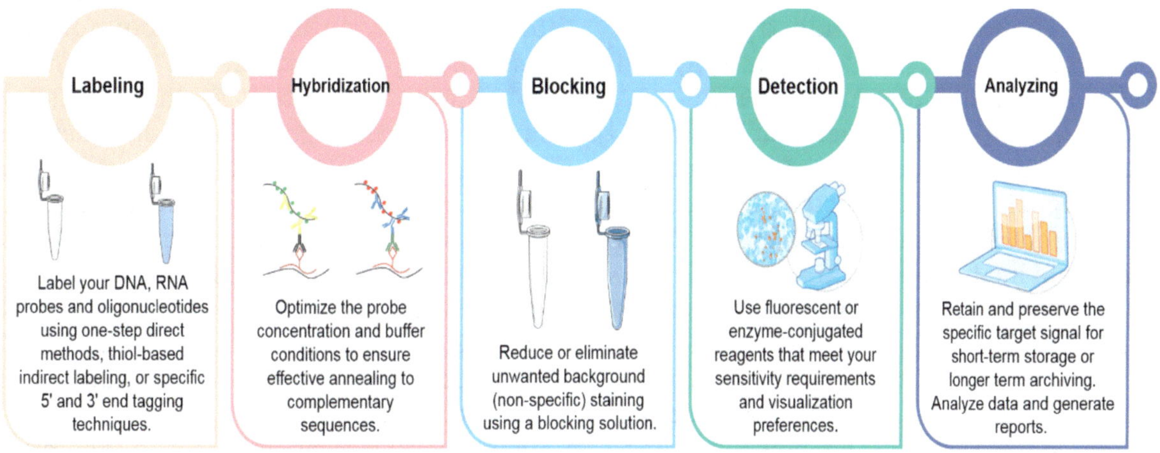

Figure 12.2. *In situ* hybridization.

Source: https://www.histobiolab.com/upload/image/20190516/In-Situ-Hybridization-1_7404396.png.

Importance of Molecular Morphology

The significance of molecular form extends deeply into the realm of biological science, particularly within the contextual environment of *in situ* hybridization. This technique enables one to observe specific nucleic acid sequences in the cellular environment and, hence, to understand gene expression patterns in their natural spatial context. Through molecular morphological analysis, researchers can correlate functional activity with cellular structural properties, thereby enabling the determination of pathological states and developmental processes. For instance, changes in cellular structure morphology can indicate changes in gene expression that are predictive of disease. These data are precious for the further explanation of complex biological processes and could lead to novel therapeutic strategies or diagnostic procedures aimed at specific morphological changes that are part of disease development. In addition to the medical application, molecular morphology is of central relevance in material science and bioengineering. The invention of conductive polymers is an example of the relationship between molecular structure and purpose, where the nanoscale characteristics of the polymers are key to their functionality. The present work highlights the unique attributes of nanostructured conductive polymers, such as increased surface area and enhanced charge transport capabilities, which are a result of their engineered molecular morphology. These properties not only render them desirable for energy conversion and storage applications, but also for sensors and biomedical devices. Knowing how molecular morphology affects these properties enables design criteria to make informed decisions that can result in high-performance device innovation, highlighting the multifaceted significance of molecular morphology in developing technology and industry. Besides, molecular morphology is needed for the physical interactions within biological systems, such as the role of the extracellular matrix (ECM). Experiments have demonstrated the importance of ECM composition and structure in vascular homeostasis; alterations of these morphological properties will likely trigger dramatic biological reactions. For example, studies on basal chordate *Botryllus schlosseri* show that even subtle changes in the collagen fibers of the ECM can cause a concerted vascular structure regression via apoptosis and cell extrusion. This finding introduces the role of molecular morphology in dictating cellular response and tissue integrity and its contribution to modifying physiological processes. Hence, the correlation between molecular morphology and biological functionality also substantiates the requirement of this concept in fundamental research as well as in applied sciences to finally contribute to an all-encompassing understanding of living systems.

12.1. Historical Background

The historical development of *in situ* hybridization (ISH) and its subsequent expansion into molecular morphology are rooted in the emergence of powerful molecular probes for analyzing genetic data in tissues. Initially characterized in the late 1960s and early 1970s, ISH provided the ability to detect individual nucleic acid sequences within fixed tissue samples. This radical method resulted from the realization of a necessity to visualize gene expression patterns within cellular structure. Early applications were primarily interested in the detection of viral RNA and ribosomal RNA gene mapping and were the basis for further refinement. Over the decades, improvements in probe design, signal amplification, and imaging technology have greatly expanded the scope of ISH, making it an invaluable tool not only for basic biological research but also for clinical and cancer diagnostics. As the technique has improved, *in situ* hybridization has increasingly become integrated with other molecular techniques to make it more specific and valuable. For instance, the development of fluorescent *in situ* hybridization (FISH) in the late 1980s transformed gene mapping and chromosomal analysis by enabling one to visualize defined DNA sequences on the background of intact chromosomes. In clinical use, FISH has been fairly successful in the detection of chromosomal abnormalities in various cancers, including cancers of blood and bone marrow (hematological malignancies) and solid tumors. FISH research, including comparative genomic hybridization (CGH), has provided critical information on genetic imbalances in various cancers. Combining CGH with FISH has enabled more comprehensive studies of chromosomal alterations, confirming the place of *in situ* hybridization techniques in modern genetics and oncology research (Bakar et al., 2004). Recent technologies have further developed *in situ* hybridization methods, resulting in higher levels of automation and better throughput in clinical laboratories. Automated brightfield double *in situ* hybridization (BDISH) applications, for instance, rationalize the process of target examination, like HER2 gene expression in breast cancer tissues, and provide substantial upgrades over conventional manual FISH procedures. This transition not only enhances efficiency but also facilitates better and reproducible analysis of gene alterations in cancer prognosis and treatment. Manufacturing BDISH has made evident the merit of merging molecular techniques with histopathologic evaluation, obtaining data impossible to collect previously. These advances are part of a wider trend towards the implementation of molecular morphology as a disease mechanism paradigm, establishing a necessary interface between molecular biology and clinical practice (Murillo et al., 2008) (Figure 12.3).

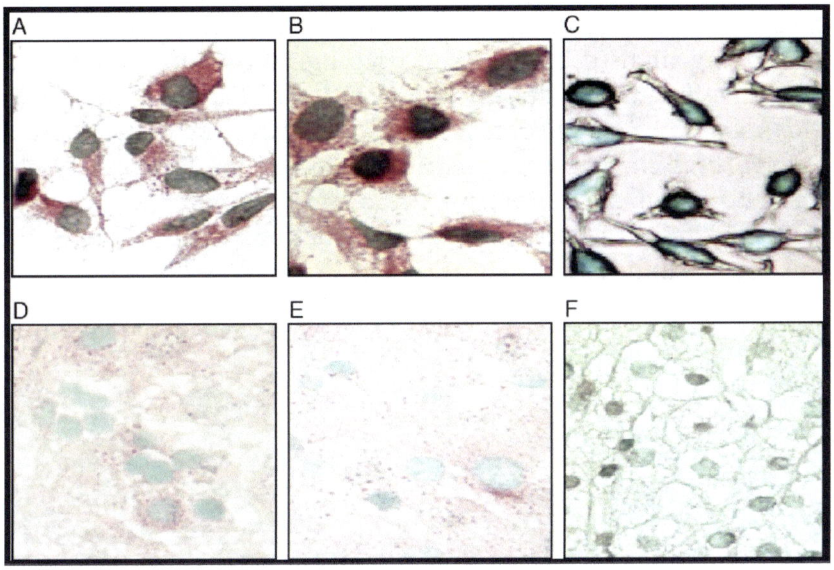

Figure 12.3. The historical background of *in situ* hybridization (ISH).

Source: https://www.researchgate.net/profile/Kathie-Anne-Walters/publication/7205586/figure/fig1/AS:280791817965568@1443957394195/n-situ-hybridization-ISH-staining-of-HCV-RNAs-in-control-cell-lines-panels-A-through.png.

12.1.1. Development of In Situ Hybridization Techniques

The development of *in situ* hybridization techniques has transformed molecular morphology by allowing researchers to visibly observe patterns of gene expression within the framework of cell structure. Initially optimized for model organism research, the techniques have proven extremely versatile, being applied to a variety of biological questions. The initial techniques primarily used radioactive probes, which, while sensitive, raised significant safety and practical issues. The emergence of non-radioactive detection techniques, such as fluorescent probes, was a great milestone. These fluorescence *in situ* hybridization (FISH) techniques went beyond safer lab practices, allowing the localization of multiple gene expressions simultaneously and thereby providing great insight into developmental processes. This evolution represents the transition from gene discovery to analysis of their functions in complex biological systems. The application of in situ hybridization techniques across various model organisms has yielded valuable insights into developmental biology. In the chick embryo, research has shown that it is difficult to quantitatively silence gene expression, particularly with RNAi. Recent studies in the field indicate that tools like microinjection of double-stranded RNA (dsRNA) and small interfering RNA (siRNA) into chick embryos turn out to be ineffective at creating the evident and clear null-like mutant phenotypes required for functional analyses. Interestingly, fgf8 gene expression has been discovered to be resistant to these silencing methods, casting questions on its effectiveness and applicability in different model systems. These findings emphasize the need for improved tools and techniques to reproducibly regulate gene expression in developmental studies, an essential area for future exploration (Torrens et al., 2013). Other than chick embryos, application of *in situ* hybridization techniques has been essential in the study of the genetic organization of non-chordate deuterostomes such as the purple sea urchin. It was only in recent times that the initial attempts at placing gene loci on chromosomes were successful, and a significant breakthrough for sea urchin genetics was realized. By employing high-resolution karyotyping and fluorescence *in situ* hybridization methods, researchers have begun to identify the positions of developmentally important genes such as brachyury, foxA, and foxB on chromosomes. Specifically, the genes were found on different *Strongylocentrotus purpuratus* chromosomes, which indicated the complexity of gene architecture in the organism. The successful application of these methods not only enables individual gene mapping but promises to extend research into the interactions of genes as well as developmental problems in marine species (Eno, 2009) (Figure 12.4).

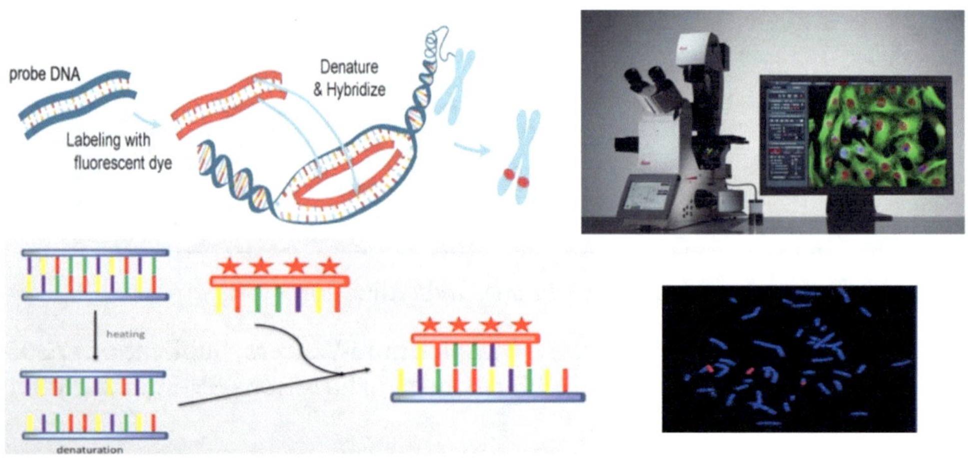

Figure 12.4. Development of *in situ* hybridization techniques.

Source: https://i.ytimg.com/vi/MdY95VxrTUw/maxresdefault.jpg.

12.1.2. Key Milestones in Molecular Morphology

Morphological milestones of significance come on the heels of the principal advances in understanding cell structure and function at the molecular level. Early findings on microscopic anatomy laid the groundwork for current approaches, enabling researchers to "see" cellular contexts for greater insights into biological processes. Mid-20th-century electron microscopy transformed the science with its unprecedented resolution and ability to probe subcellular structures. This innovation introduced the integration of molecular biology and morphological studies, yielding new methods such as in situ hybridization (ISH), which allows the specific localization of nucleic acid sequences within fixed tissue or cells. The development of ISH techniques has yielded foundational information about gene expression patterns and cellular morphology, making it a critical tool for demystifying molecular morphology complexities and making its contribution to histopathology significant. Moreover, the availability of hybridization techniques has significantly influenced molecular pathology, a critical field where molecular morphology is a necessary contribution. As recorded in academic works, molecular pathology converts molecular biology methods into traditional pathology to provide information on the ethical and biological aspects of disease states (Maanoja, 2024). The marriage has been core in cancer diagnostics and therapeutic approaches so that specific biomarkers that inform prognosis and treatment can be identified. Techniques such as fluorescent *in situ* hybridization (FISH) are representative of this integration, enhancing visualization capability for chromosomal abnormalities in relation to cancer. These advances complement not just the applicability of proper morphological assessment but also indicate trends towards precision medicine. Taken together, these developments represent further improvements in techniques that shed greater light on the molecular bases across diverse biological contexts. Finally, the interdisciplinary approach of integrating molecular biology and morphological techniques recommends further advancements in clinical practice as well as research. Integration of nano-bioelectronics is a new boundary in this area with promise to revolutionize biomolecular sensing and imaging technologies. As there is development in silicon nanowires and graphene technologies, they bring solutions that integrate the biological system with advanced molecular imaging techniques (Kim et al., 2024). This convergence will allow greater interaction within biological ecosystems, paving the way for innovations in biomedical therapy and environmental applications. With growing molecular morphology, these innovations will unlock doors for new comprehension of cellular processes, ultimately affecting such fields as drug discovery, ecosystem management, and crop production. Overall, the future of molecular morphology holds breakthrough applications integrating theoretical research with problem-solving functions in complex biological systems.

12.1.3. Evolution of Research Methods in Biology

The history of research methods in biology has been marked by major advances that have radically reshaped our understanding of biological form and function. The antiquated methods, being more centered on histological approaches, have since been replaced with more sophisticated molecular methods, hence enhancing our ability to venture into the complexity of cell structure and gene expression. Among these developments, *in situ* hybridization was a milestone technique by which scientists were able to visualize and localize the presence of particular RNA molecules within fixed tissues. Not only did this technological innovation enable spatial investigation of gene expression, but it also enabled investigation of developmental processes across various taxa. Therefore, the incorporation of *in situ* hybridization within molecular morphology attests to a growing trend towards conjoining molecular techniques with classical morphological endeavors to create an integrated perspective on organismal biology. Over the past few years, molecular morphology has emerged as more significant since scientists endeavored to learn about the relations between structure and function at the molecular level. The creation of novel imaging techniques, including the application of fluorescent markers, has revolutionized the capability of recording real-time visualization of biological processes. An example is the use of genetically encoded fluorescence that enabled researchers to follow cellular events dynamically and provide information regarding cellular structure and tissue organization previously unavailable. In addition, the application of *in situ* hybridization in most model organisms, including insects and vertebrates, indicates its versatility and uses in diverse biological systems. This shift towards molecular methodologies is a paradigm shift of significant proportions in biology that emphasizes the necessity to integrate morphological examination with molecular techniques to study the intricate interactions defining biological processes. These research advances are very well demonstrated in recent research that has made basic biological truths using new applications. Vertebral segmentation research, for instance, has been greatly advanced by the new techniques since researchers have applied *in situ* hybridization and cell lineage marking to explain developmental processes. Specifically, vertebral skeleton resegmentation studies in different taxa have concluded that the trait is an ancestral one shared by jawed vertebrates, as indicated by current evidence in skates (Criswell et al., 2020). Moreover, the identification of tandemly-repeated DNAs, namely those coding in *Drosophila melanogaster*, confirms satellite RNAs' central role in the biology of an organism, highlighting their role in male fertility and chromatin structure (Allshire et al., 2019). These instances affirm the significant influence of altering research methods in biology, with them making it easier to comprehend complex biological processes and interdisciplinary coordination towards knowledge attainment (Figure 12.5).

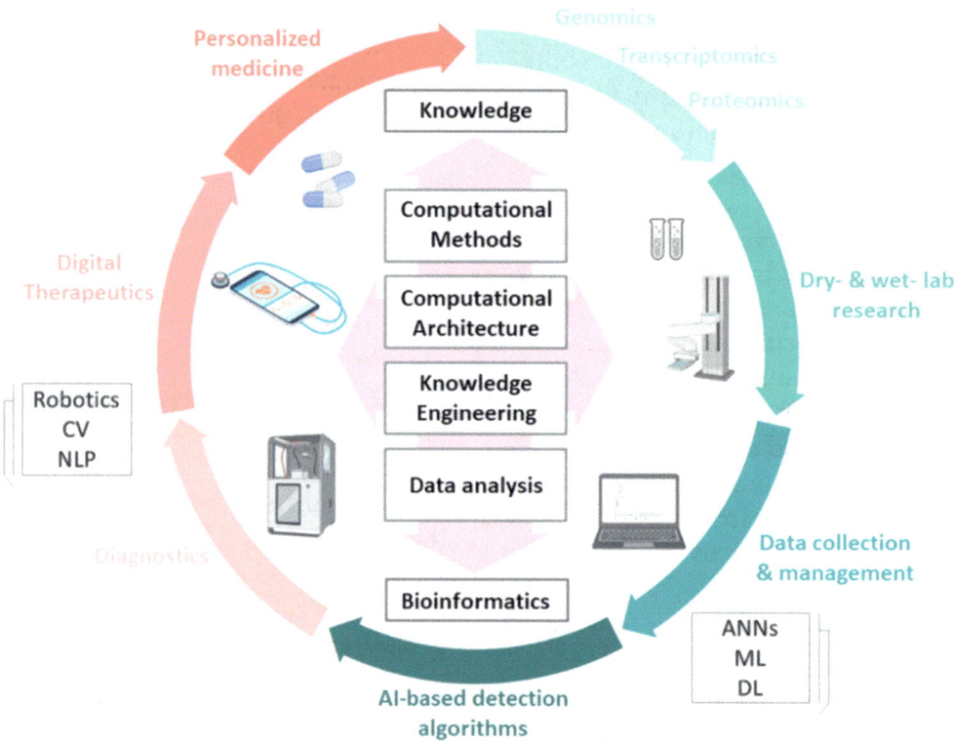

Figure 12.5. Evolution of research methods in biology.

Source: https://www.researchgate.net/publication/366422158/figure/fig2/AS:11431281318938887@1742574999539/Illustration-depicting-the-involvement-of-AI-based-tools-in-the-different-levels-of.tif.

12.2. Principles of In Situ Hybridization

In situ hybridization (ISH) is an important technique in molecular morphology, by which researchers can observe specific nucleic acid sequences in fixed tissue or cells. It is founded on the principle that complementary nucleic acid strands will hybridize to and bind to each other under specific conditions and create localized patches of hybridization that may be visualized using various labeling methods, such as fluorescence or isotopic labeling. The precision of ISH provides the ability to identify gene expression patterns and RNA and DNA locations in various stages of cellular and developmental advancement. This aspect is particularly critical in measurements of spatial dynamics of gene expression, greatly uncovering the tissue structure and cellular function. With the use of ISH, scientists are able to clarify molecular marker-phenotypic trait relationships, thus contributing to developmental biology and human genetics. ISH's flexibility opens doors for potential applications within a wide range of biological studies, such as developmental biology, cancer biology, and genetic disease. Applications such as chromosomal *in situ* suppression (CISS) hybridization are exemplary of this flexibility. CISS facilitates the selective staining of chromosomes, as emphasized in research that examines aberrations in cultured human cells. For example, differential staining of the euchromatic areas of the Y chromosome and the examination of translocations, e.g., in XX-males, emphasizes the powerful potential of ISH in diagnosing chromosomal abnormalities. Besides, the sensitivity of CISS hybridization also offers the ability to identify minimal chromosomal changes, which are imperative in cancer investigations and prenatal diagnosis, where identification of minimal genomic changes can inform prognostic approaches and therapeutic strategies. With this multidimensional ability, ISH fuels its position as a core technique in contemporary genetic research. In addition to its superior sensitivity and specificity, ISH is increasingly being paired with live-cell imaging to gain insights into nucleic acid motion within living tissue. Current fluorescent labeling methods, required to visualize RNA and plasmid DNA, complement ISH by providing real-time feedback on cell processes. The integration of these techniques radicalizes the ability to trace mRNA localization and translation in situ, thus enabling a more dynamic study of gene expression previously not possible. The concurrent employment of ISH with innovative imaging techniques not only contributes to a better understanding of cellular dynamics but also underscores the need for scientists to be abreast of the most recent labeling techniques. As outlined in recent critiques, the correct selection of the fluorescent labeling technique is critical to maximizing experiment results, thereby guiding scientists on how to advance exploring the complexity of molecular and cellular interactions (Rombouts et al., 2016) (Figure 12.6).

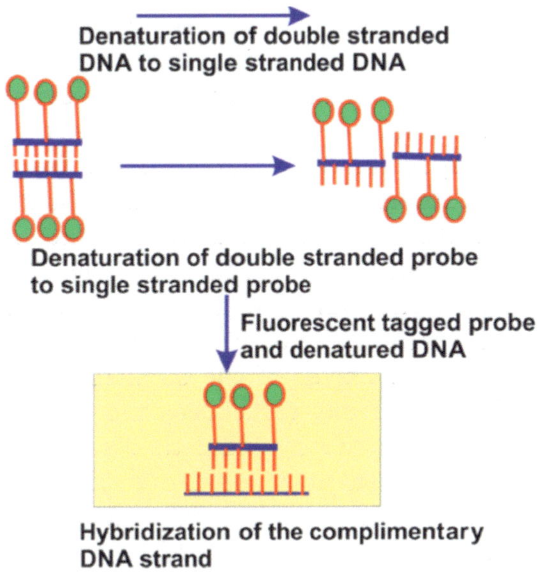

Figure 12.6. Principles of *in situ* hybridization.

Source: https://media.springernature.com/lw685/springer-static/image/chp%3A10.1007%2F978-981-10-8252-8_21/MediaObjects/456657_1_En_21_Fig1_HTML.png.

12.2.1. Mechanism of Hybridization

Hybridization is a major aspect of the in situ hybridization component and molecular morphology. Hybridization refers to the process whereby the complementary nucleic acid strands interact and form a double helix, a basic function that enables accurate targeting and visualization of specific RNA or DNA sequences within biological samples. This approach is much facilitated by the advances in molecular probes, which are designed to bind target sequences with high specificity. The success of hybridization is influenced by several biochemical parameters, including temperature, salt concentration, and probe concentration, each of which is crucial for controlling the stability of the resulting nucleic acid complexes. Determining the best conditions for hybridization is critically essential, since slight changes in them may lead to nonspecific interaction or failure to generate adequate signal intensity, further complicating the interpretation of morphological data from such research. The increasing scope of molecular morphology makes an understanding of hybridization mechanisms' nuances extremely relevant for understanding developmental processes in a broad spectrum of organisms. For instance, current studies have established that the unique vertebral segmentation architecture and somite development can be traced using hybridization methods. The four-limbed tetrapods exhibited resegmentation where a recombination between the adjacent halves of the somites occurs to produce different vertebrae; the process is evaluated by the hybridization studies that allow scientists to trace the tissue lineage. Specifically, recent findings regarding the skate (Leucoraja erinacea) have revealed a conserved hybridization mechanism that contributes to our existing understanding of vertebrate evolution and implies that hybridization processes are not necessarily tetrapod-specific but are, in fact, ancestral features of jawed vertebrates (Criswell et al., 2020). The effects of hybridization cut across biological systems and include both plants and animals. Plant molecular-genetic dynamics of hybridization can reveal the mechanisms underlying morphological diversity, such as the homeotic floral structure transformations. Deviations from normal floral organ patterns can be explained by hybridization of gene-expression patterns, as demonstrated in research on *Lacandonia schismatica*. The ability of some B- and C-function genes to interact in hybridization experiments gives us a useful insight into how small changes in molecules can lead to dramatic morphological changes in natural populations. The richness and flexibility of hybridization mechanisms, thus, not only tell us more about molecular morphology but also give us a glimpse into the mechanisms of diversity evolution (Ambrose et al., 2010).

12.2.2. Types of Probes Used

The use of various types of probes is at the heart of *in situ* hybridization (ISH) because they facilitate accurate localization of specific nucleic acid sequences in cells or tissue sections. Probes are categorized according to their biological origin, label type, and size. Riboprobes, for instance, are made from RNA polymerase transcription, allowing synthesis of labeled RNA that is capable of recognizing complementary target sequences. Alternatively, DNA probes are generated from polymerase chain reaction (PCR) techniques, which are highly specific and flexible. The choice among such probes often depends on the nature of the target sequences and the degree of sensitivity required in the assay. Consequently, the appropriate probe type is crucial in getting reproducible results when performing ISH experiments, as supported by various studies examining various probes under various biological contexts. Probe labeling is also an important factor in ISH that impacts detection sensitivity and visualization. Probes are labeled with either fluorescent dyes or enzymes for catalyzing color reactions, allowing researchers to easily visually identify hybridization events. Fluorescent probes enable researchers to leverage sophisticated imaging techniques, such as confocal microscopy, which produces images of labeled cells at very high resolution. In contrast, enzyme probe labeling provides a less complicated observation technique through colorimetric reactions that form visible precipitates. Whether one type of labeling is preferable to another is a point that can be a decisive factor in the ease with which results are interpretable, and whether background noise or non-specific binding can pose problems may mean difficulties. Hence, both probe type and labeling are essential to successful ISH and must be planned out carefully in an experiment.

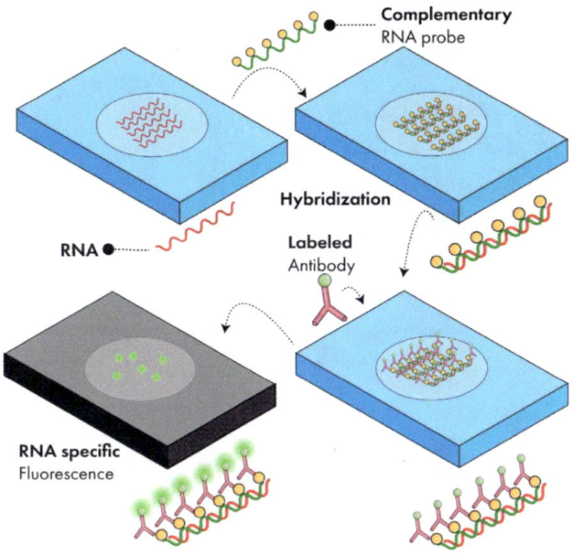

Figure 12.7. Types of probes used.

Source: https://www.histobiolab.com/upload/image/5-what-are-the-different-types-of-ish.jpg.

The specificity and sensitivity of *in situ* hybridization tests are significantly enhanced with the addition of techniques such as competitive hybridization and the use of altered probes. Competitive hybridization is the method of adding an excess of unlabeled probes to make the non-specific binding sites unavailable, thereby enhancing the overall signal-to-noise ratio. Moreover, modified probes, such as locked nucleic acid (LNA) or peptide nucleic acid (PNA), offer higher binding stability, allowing even the detection of challenging targets in the context of high genetic complexity. Such new methods have been demonstrated to improve the resolution of ISH to investigate patterns of gene expression with better accuracy. Typically, studies on various molecular targets have demonstrated the effectiveness of such techniques, wherein scientists documented drastic elevation of hybridization signals and specific localization of gene expression, illustrating the sophistication of ISH techniques in contemporary molecular biology research (Figure 12.7).

12.2.3. Detection Methods

Under molecular morphology, detection methods are a valuable resource for elucidating structural and functional relationships among the components of biological samples. Central to this is in situ hybridization (ISH), a technique that combines nucleic acid hybridization with microscopic visualization to localize specific DNA or RNA sequences within their cellular context. FISH is a type of ISH, and it employs fluorescent probes to locate genetic material and allow researchers to visualize chromosomal aberrations and genetic rearrangements. FISH is particularly valuable in comparative genomics as it permits the quantification of evolutionary conservation among species. For example, FISH has been utilized to unveil chromosomal rearrangements within primates, illuminating the phylogenetic affiliations marking our evolutionary clade, thereby underscoring the greater relevance of detection technologies in deciphering biological evolution and diversity (Baldini et al., 1994). Another effective detection method in in situ hybridization is genomic in situ hybridization (GISH), which elucidates genome content and hybridization events. This technique has been pivotal in the study of interspecific hybrids, including those between the *Begonia* species. By the marking of genomic DNA fragments and their utilization as probes, GISH allows discrimination among chromosomal contributions from various ancestral species present within hybrid organisms. The mapping of genome presence and composition in hybrids like the *Elatior-begonias* allows researchers to assess genomic integrity in addition to demystifying the complexities surrounding hybridization processes. Consequently, GISH can enable more in-depth exploration of genomic interaction and can inform breeding tactics in horticulture and agriculture, noting the importance of comprehensive detection methodologies in genomic research and applied research (Laak et al., 2010). Further, the development of dual-color FISH and other multiplexed detection methods further enhanced the capacity to analyze genomic structures in situ.

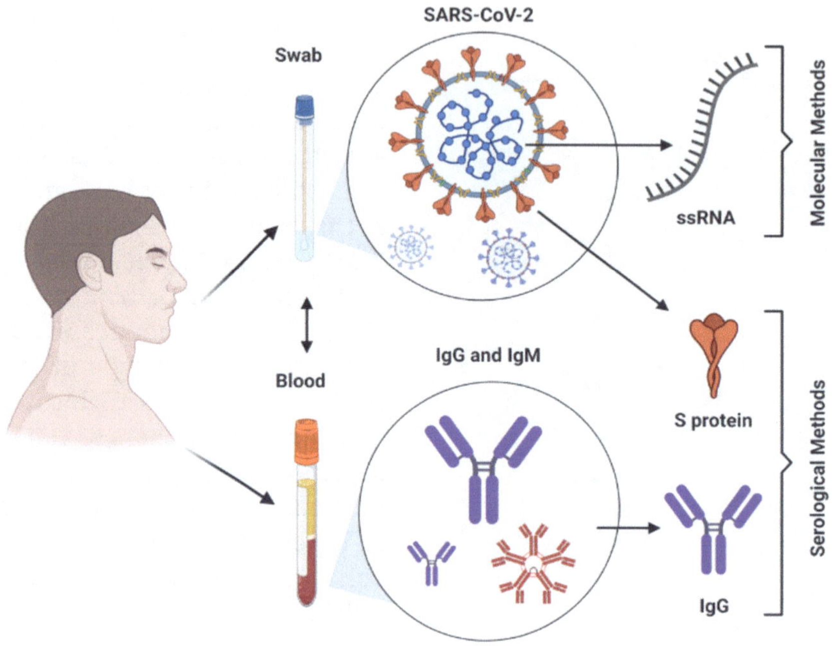

Figure 12.8. Detection methods.

Source: https://external-content.duckduckgo.com/iu/?u=https%3A%2F%2Fdfzljdn9uc3pi.cloudfront.net%2F2020%2F10180%2F1%2Ffig-1-2x.jpg&f=1&nofb=1&ipt=828078be48776e6399e509960a5aed0780b88f10021b8f346e1965825e3e241c.

These advanced techniques allow researchers to study a vast number of genetic locations in a single sample simultaneously, which allows for closer comparisons and functional characterization. The coupling of fluorescence tagging with high-resolution microscopy provides an upgraded technique for probing chromosomal dynamics in the course of cell division and differentiation processes. By employing these more advanced detection tools, scientists are able to decipher the complexities of gene expression and regulation at specific stages of development and report valuable information on cellular function and disease. To this end, ongoing advancements in detection tools further advance the molecular morphology area, offering potent tools to reveal the subtle interactions that underlie the life sciences (Figure 12.8).

12.3. Applications in Developmental Biology

The applications of *in situ* hybridization in developmental biology are profound, as the technique enables imaging of gene-expression patterns within intact tissue architecture. This spatial information is crucial for understanding the complex events of development because temporally and spatially controlled gene expression dictates cellular behavior. For instance, zebrafish models have been used in research demonstrating the ways calcium regulation is disrupted and can impact the integrity of myofibrils in cardiac development. The findings from these experiments reveal the relationship between gene expression and cellular structural transformation, justifying the pivotal role of *in situ* hybridization in unraveling the molecular mechanisms of development (Chen et al., 2017). By equating gene expression to morphological change, scientists can examine the extremely intricate interplay of signaling pathways and gene networks responsible for embryonic development and tissue regeneration. *In situ* hybridization is also an effective technique for investigating genetic variation involved in specific diseases, particularly in model systems like the zebrafish. The genetic manipulation of the relevant pathways allows researchers to have closely similar models to human conditions, such as type 2 diabetes. The tcf7l2 mutant zebrafish line is a case in point for such application, as it learns about the impact of TCF7L2 variants on insulin secretion and pancreatic development (Argenton et al., 2017). With the aid of *in situ* hybridization, researchers can investigate how mutations in genes influence gene expression in different cell types and developmental phases. Not only does it explain the mechanism behind the disease, but it also provides a platform for assessing the efficacy of potential treatments in reversing or mitigating developmental defects resulting from metabolic conditions. In addition, the integration of *in situ* hybridization with other molecular morphological techniques offers new opportunities for the investigation of developmental biology. By applying advanced imaging methods, such as confocal microscopy, it is now possible to generate detailed three-dimensional representations of gene expression during the development of tissues. Multimodal analysis can increase our understanding of the manner in which cells interact and coordinate their behavior within a dynamic environment. With the capture of cell context in gene expression, researchers can identify sites for intervention of disease-associated with developmental origins. An example is how revelations from investigating the dysregulation of genes that manage myofibril stability are translated into innovation in cardiac well-being, still reflecting the central role of *in situ* hybridization and molecular morphology in developmental biology (Chen et al., 2017). With these integrative approaches, nuances of disease and development are addressed more optimally, resulting in prevention and treatment innovations (Figure 12.9).

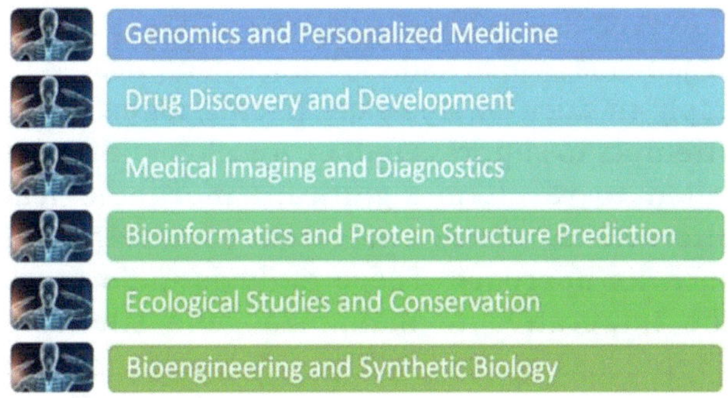

Figure 12.9. Applications in developmental biology.

Source: https://www.easybiologyclass.com/wp-content/uploads/2023/09/applications-of-ai-in-biology.jpg.

12.3.1. Gene Expression Analysis

Gene expression analysis is pivotal to understanding the complex regulatory mechanisms that govern morphological transformation in development. ISH is a powerful means of visualizing spatial and temporal gene expression patterns in tissue settings. Most importantly, it allows one to envision how modifications in gene expression correlate with specific morphological features. For instance, during the investigation of gene functions involved in organ development, ISH reveals the site-specific locations of transcriptional activity, thereby elucidating the potential pathways through which genes influence cellular behavior and tissue structure. By combining ISH with the latest imaging technologies, researchers are able to link gene expression profiles more closely to morphological consequences, thereby facilitating an increased understanding of developmental biology complexity. RNA interference (RNAi) application in gene expression studies further advances the understanding of molecular mechanisms governing morphology, as exemplified by recent studies. Whereas traditional ISH techniques show gene expression patterns, RNAi can silence the target genes, allowing functional analysis of their activities. However, RNAi efficiency can vary across model organisms, which makes it more complicated to apply. In chick embryo experiments, for example, attempts to suppress fgf8 expression with RNAi failed to result in significant morphological alterations, which indicated constraints of such an approach. These findings underscore the imperative to maximize gene silencing approaches, as contradictory data may obscure our understanding of gene function relative to quantifiable phenotypic effects, thereby affecting the overarching goal of correlating gene expression with morphological development (Torrens et al., 2013). In addition, the relationship between morphological development and gene expression can be characterized by evolutionary pressures, as seen through various adaptations across species. For instance, the ABC model conserved floral organ identity illustrates how gene function reorganization can generate far-reaching morphological diversifications. In illustrating this to be true, the unusual floral architecture of *Lacandonia schismatica* in comparison to *Arabidopsis thaliana* illustrates how minor genetic variations are capable of yielding radical alterations in morphology. The reality that interactions among B-function genes are conserved within these species illustrates how small genetic variations are capable of producing widespread phenotypic diversities. Thus, the analysis of gene expression not only promotes morphological development but also sheds light on the evolutionary forces that determine biodiversity (Ambrose et al., 2010). This integrated approach, integrating conclusions gathered by means of ISH, RNAi, and comparative genomics, is required to decode the intricate interactions that determine gene expression and morphological traits (Figure 12.10).

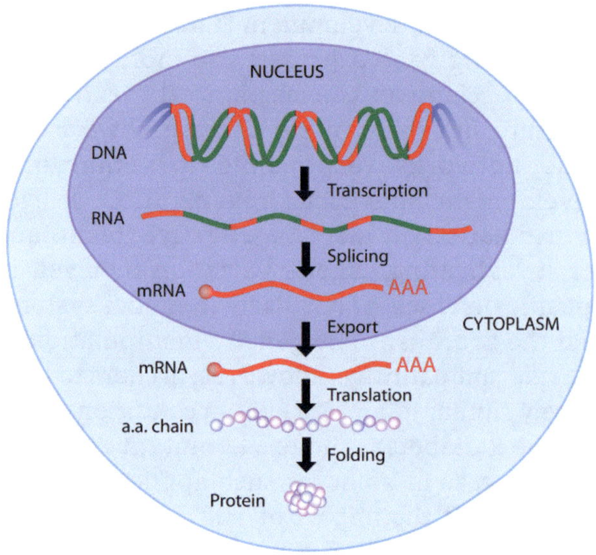

Figure 12.10. Gene expression analysis.

Source: https://m3.healio.com/~/media/af4f5577ac97c532df467711c1837aae.jpg.

12.3.2. Visualization of Cellular Structures

Visualization of cellular organelles is an important aspect of molecular morphology that provides insight into the intricate dynamics of cellular processes and the localization of specific molecules. Immunohistochemistry and *in situ* hybridization can be utilized to carry out direct mapping of proteins and nucleic acids in the cellular architecture, respectively. These methods enable researchers to define the position of molecular components, which is crucial for understanding physiological and pathological mechanisms. For instance, the differential intracellular localization of the A-SUCL protein encoded by SUCLA2 in neurons, as revealed by immunoreactivity experiments, illustrates the necessity of site-specific measurements in defining the functional role of proteins in a cellular context. These findings provide a framework for correlating molecular biology with clinical presentation with genetic mutations, illustrating the role of visualization techniques in comprehending pathologies (Kowluru et al., 2013). Live-cell imaging over the past few decades has greatly enhanced our ability to study cellular morphology in real time and the possibility of visualizing dynamic processes that were previously difficult to see.

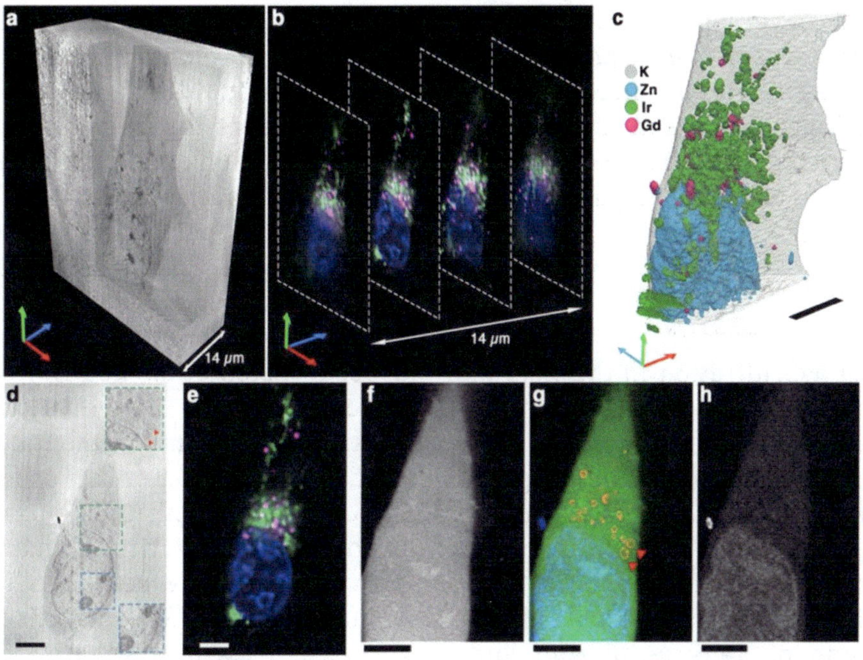

Figure 12.11. Visualization of cellular structures.

Source: https://www.researchgate.net/publication/392063568/figure/fig2/AS:11431281458350986@1748089118851/Three-dimensional-visualization-of-the-cellular-structures-with-the-proposed.jpg.

The application of fluorescent tagging of nucleic acids and other cellular constituents makes it possible for scientists to track the movement and interaction of molecules in their natural settings. Fluorescent techniques, particularly those developed for the labeling of mRNA, are found to be valuable tools for a wide variety of scientific investigations ranging from cellular development to cancer studies. By adopting appropriate fluorescent approaches, researchers are able to make informed choices that optimize their experimental outcomes towards furthering our knowledge about molecular interactions in living organisms. The use of these new imaging techniques, complemented by the classical techniques, such as *in situ* hybridization, makes the area of molecular morphology richer because it provides a multi-dimensional perspective of cellular dynamics (Rombouts et al., 2016). In disease contexts, visualization of cellular architecture is critical in the context of gaining insight into abnormal cellular processes that might lead to pathological conditions. For example, research into the role of SUCLA2s in neuronal cells has provided critical information regarding their involvement in mitochondrial disorders. By demarcating the specific expression of A-SUCL-protein in neurons and corresponding absence in glial cells, the research not only explains the functional importance of SUCLA2 but also highlights the importance of selective targeting of molecules for mechanism studies of diseases. In addition, combining such analyses with *in situ* hybridization techniques offers an integrated insight into cellular morphology during health and disease. Such a convergence of visualisation methods drives our capacity to document and describe cellular life's complexity, necessary for research advancement as well as the build-up of therapeutically targeted therapies (Kowluru et al., 2013; Rombouts et al., 2016) (Figure 12.11).

12.3.3. Role in Understanding Developmental Processes

The role of *in situ* hybridization in the field of investigating developmental processes cannot be overstated, particularly in determining the spatial and temporal regulation of gene expression during various stages of organism development. Through *in situ* hybridization, researchers can visualize the specific RNA sequences within fixed tissue, which aids in the comprehension of gene regulation and functional gene functions in developmental processes. For instance, signaling protein-coding gene expression patterns reveal how these components regulate interactions between various cell populations during development. The ability to recognize the domains of expression of these genes emphasizes the complexity of developmental processes as cells interact and specialize based on molecular instructions. As highlighted by studies of neural circuits, proper expression of guidance cues is paramount for cellular guidance and connectivity in developing tissues, mirroring the profound impact of *in situ* hybridization on developmental biology. In addition, implications of cytoplasmic signaling adaptors such as members of the Cas family offer insights into the molecular mechanisms of axon guidance and fasciculation within the peripheral nervous system. Understanding the roles of these signaling molecules is significant in understanding how axons establish connections during development. Phosphorylation status of these adaptors in various cellular contexts indicates that they are controlled by extracellular signals. By synthesizing data from molecular morphology and *in situ* hybridization, researchers can outline how certain gene expression and molecular interactions give rise to certain developmental consequences, such as the formation of functional neural circuits. Thus, the cross-talk between cellular responses and gene expression profiles significantly enhances the understanding of developmental processes, supporting the pivotal contribution of *in situ* hybridization techniques towards our enrichment of understanding complex biological systems, particularly in neurodevelopmental aspects (Estep et al., 2018). Apart from neural development, it is worth considering the contribution of environmental factors towards guiding developmental processes through molecular mechanisms. As an example, subtle exposure to antibiotics in aquatic environments provokes immune reactions involving NF-κB signaling pathway activation, an adaptive response to extrinsic stressors of developmental integrity. This necessitates critical questions to understand the mechanisms through which environmental contaminants disrupt the developmental pathways of aquatic animals. Visualization of pathway activation via in situ hybridization enables scientists to link environmental exposures to specific gene-expression changes. These are the types of information that have to be created to put the broader implications of environmental health into developmental biology. By associating molecular response to environmental stimuli and familiarizing ourselves with the direction of developmental progression, *in situ* hybridization is a valuable tool in understanding how organisms change or respond to dynamic environments and continues to deepen our understanding of the complicated layers of developmental biology (Chen et al., 2020).

12.4. Applications in Disease Research

Advanced methods, such as in situ hybridization (ISH), have greatly influenced disease research by making it possible to locate gene expression with excellent accuracy within tissues. The technique makes it possible for researchers to see the spatial and temporal RNA molecule pattern, offering information on developmental mechanisms and disease processes. For instance, in T2D, the use of ISH methods in identifying the Tcf7l2 variant has furnished critical information regarding the disruption of insulin secretion. The demonstration of morphological alterations in tcf7l2 zebrafish mutants in pancreatic islet development has shown the capability of ISH in ascertaining the intrinsic genetic basis of disease pathology. Such findings enhance our understanding of multicomponent diseases, continuing to guide therapeutic intervention and genetic engineering according to an individual patient's profile, ultimately leading to better management and outcomes of disease. Another well-established application of *in situ* hybridization to the study of disease involves defining the molecular heterogeneity of disease tissue. By mapping expression patterns of genes, researchers are capable of establishing how such patterns correspond to disease phenotypes. For instance, in coffee, the environmentally pressure-controlled genetic variation is a metaphor for describing the genetic basis of disease susceptibility. As in the molecular genetic diversity study of *Coffea arabica* populations of Ethiopia, similar approaches can be a powerful basis for assessing genetic variation and resistance to disease. Blending ISH with genomic approaches can uncover molecular markers impacting agronomic traits, just as disease-inducing genetic markers can be discovered in human populations. Overall, taking advantage of the capability of ISH in disease research emphasizes the importance of genetic diversity in informing conservation and treatment. In addition to the direct examination of gene expression, *in situ* hybridization can be applied to investigate functional consequences in the disease process. Identification of vascular changes within Tcf7l2 mutant zebrafish, represented by impaired islet-related capillary development, illustrates the interaction between gene expression and physiological responses to pathology. The combined evaluation provides researchers with aid in relating genetic change to systemic expression of pathology. Similarly, in the case of natural *Coffea arabica*, its genetic loss due to environmental threats points to the need for conservation measures to enhance agricultural resistance to plant diseases. Whenever methods such as ISH are applied alongside molecular biology techniques, they promote an integrative understanding of disease mechanisms, ultimately facilitating the integration of specific interventions that can reduce disease effects across various biological systems.

12.4.1. Cancer Research and Diagnostics

Cancer diagnostic science has undergone a significant transformation with the advent of molecular techniques, particularly *in situ* hybridization (ISH). ISH is now an indispensable tool for the identification of specific nucleic acid sequences within tissue to precisely localize the genetic abnormalities unique to various cancers. By hybridizing labeled probes to homologous DNA or RNA in tissue sections, ISH enables visualization of chromosomal alterations that are often pivotal to cancerogenesis. These alterations, including amplifications or deletions of specific oncogenes and tumor suppressors, provide valuable information on the disease's molecular basis, which guides treatment modalities and prognostic evaluation. Therefore, *in situ* hybridization not only enhances the understanding of cancer biology but also serves as a vital tool within the pathology laboratory, becoming a vital component of contemporary cancer diagnosis. The integration of molecular morphology with cancer research has greatly enhanced our understanding of tumor biology. This is achieved by looking at the cancer cells' molecular structure using advanced imaging techniques along with traditional histopathology. For instance, studies on components of the extracellular matrix (ECM), such as collagen, have revealed that alterations in the structure of collagen can influence tumor development and metastasis (Goldbloom-Helzner et al., 2019). With methods like collagen-targeting peptides, researchers can study the therapeutic potential of such ECM structures in cancer treatments. Molecular morphology of the tumor microenvironment plays a significant role in planning individualized therapeutic plans and patient prognosis evaluation. The molecular morphology approaches thus promote cancer in a more subtle aspect by promoting innovative diagnostic approaches and treatments. In addition, the role played by gene mutations in leukemia highlights the need for robust diagnostic methods in cancer research. Chromosome alterations have been identified as key predictors in leukemia prediction and diagnosis, as well as for monitoring minimal residual disease in follow-up studies of patients (Tyybäkinoja, 2009). Conventional cytogenetic analysis, although powerful, is often inadequate in resolution to permit extensive genome analysis. With the advent of high-throughput technologies such as array comparative genomic hybridization (array-CGH) and SNP microarrays, scientists have gained unprecedented insights into the genetic landscape of leukemias and have identified new oncogene candidates and tumor suppressors that may inform future therapy. These innovations underscore the imperative for ongoing development in cancer diagnosis, as clarity regarding the genomic background of diverse malignancies continues to play a central role in maximizing patient outcomes and developing more successful treatment strategies (Figure 12.12).

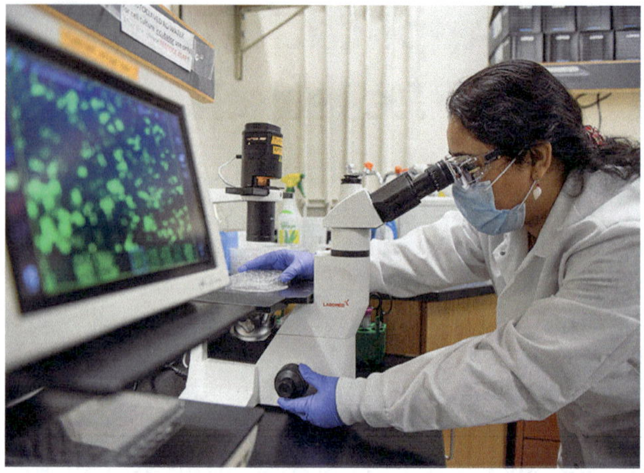

Figure 12.12. Cancer research and diagnostics.

Source: https://www.purdue.edu/uns/images/2021/cancer-data-scienceLO.jpg.

12.4.2. Infectious Disease Studies

Infectious disease investigation has expanded significantly with advances in molecular techniques, particularly *in situ* hybridization and molecular morphology. These methods enable researchers to visualize and examine the spatial arrangement of pathogens at tissue and cellular levels and provide insights into the multifaceted dynamics of host-pathogen interactions. With the help of *in situ* hybridization, scientists can detect specific nucleic acid sequences in tissues and consequently detect viral components such as those that are part of post-transplant lymphoproliferative disorders (PTLD). This disease, commonly associated with Epstein – Barr Virus (EBV) in immunocompromised patients, underscores the fine balance between the presence of the virus and the immune response of the host, as discussed in recent research on the mechanisms related to PTLD (Nalesnik et al., 1994). Other than tracking viral infections, the employment of molecular morphology is applied to detect other causative agents of infections, still enhancing our understanding of their pathophysiology. For instance, the rise of *Arcobacter* species as emerging foodborne pathogens has portrayed the demand for more effective detection methods in infectious disease research. Poultry having been identified as a significant reservoir, occurrence of *Arcobacter* among retail meats indicates the demand for accurate isolation procedures in order to ensure food safety (Bhandari, 2006). Multiplex PCR and sequencing not only aid in the determination of species identification but also give information regarding the genetic diversity of such organisms in foodstuffs. With continued studies revealing the complexities of such pathogens, the integration of molecular tools becomes essential in formulating effective public health measures.

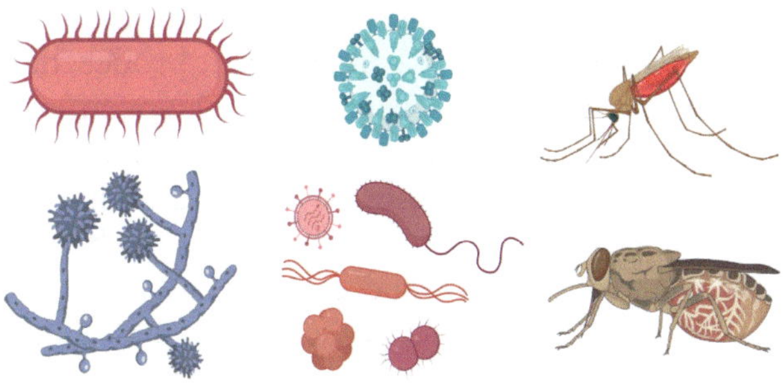

Figure 12.13. Infectious disease studies.

Source: https://microbenotes.com/wp-content/uploads/2024/04/Infectious-Diseases.jpeg.

The interaction between molecular morphology and *in situ* hybridization and infectious disease investigation has far-reaching significance for public health and for epidemiologic research. Pathogen action, particularly in the context of host defense suppression, is illuminating as to mechanisms of infection and disease development. The basis on which specific immunosuppressive regimens allow for opportunistic infection, for example, is concrete proof that informs organ transplant clinical practice (Nalesnik et al., 1994). Moreover, the integration of these molecular tools in the routine monitoring of pathogens like *Arcobacter* promotes proactive steps to reduce the risks that come with foodborne illness (Bhandari, 2006). As the scientific community continues to develop such technologies, thorough research into infectious diseases will help guide targeted prevention, diagnosis, and treatment strategies in the increasingly complex global health landscape (Figure 12.13).

12.4.3. Genetic Disorders and Anomalies

To understand genetic disorders and anomalies is the clue to molecular morphology because the disorders all too frequently illuminate intricate biological processes. Genetic anomalies, most commonly resulting from chromosomal aberrations, are expressed in many different forms, normally impairing cell function and the organism's well-being. Chromosomal deletions, for instance, such as those occurring in chronic lymphocytic leukemia (CLL), are accountable for generating high disease variability among patients. Studies employing techniques like fluorescence *in situ* hybridization (FISH) have indicated that nearly 51.7% of CLL patients present with chromosomal abnormalities, of which deletion of 13q14 is relatively prevalent. Not only do these findings highlight the importance of accurate genetic testing in prognostic evaluation, but they also emphasize the importance of targeted treatment interventions that account for variability in the genetic presentation, ultimately dictating patient treatment and outcomes (Chauffaille et al., 2006). In another example, dysmorphias such as cleidocranial dysplasia (CCD) illustrate the tremendous impact of specific genetic mutations on anatomical development. CCD most commonly results from mutations in the RUNX2 gene, which is crucial for osteoblast differentiation and craniofacial development. Remarkably, about 70% of CCD cases arise through RUNX2 mutation, providing a clue to its primary role in skeletal development. The presence of supernumerary teeth and normal craniofacial malformations, commonly determined through molecular morphological examination, also advocates for the necessity of identifying genetic impacts on body defects. The application of advanced techniques, such as comparative genomic hybridization, has also further established genotype-phenotype correlations among CCD patients and illustrated the complex interaction among genes and morphologic features, thereby enhancing our understanding of this infrequent disorder (Greene, 2017). Genetic disease implications extend to such fields as therapeutic intervention strategies and individualized medicine. The technique of *in situ* hybridization and genetic profiling enables the identification of specific mutations and chromosomal aberrations that potentially can direct therapy in one's own genetic profile. As an example, in the field of oncology, the detection of chromosomal abnormalities in CLL can dictate the course of therapy, with possible prognostic advantage to the patient. In addition, advances in molecular morphology have also revolutionized the study of diseases like CCD, which has made it possible to conduct extensive studies of structural dysmorphias as well as genetic influences. The confluence of genetic study and morphological analysis, thus, provides a firm basis for further diagnosis, treatment, and understanding of genetic disorders, pushing forward significant progress in medical science and patient care practice (Chauffaille et al., 2006; Greene, 2017).

12.5. Advantages of In Situ Hybridization

In situ hybridization (ISH) is blessed with several strengths that make it extremely useful in molecular morphology. Perhaps the strongest of these is the possibility of providing spatial localization of nucleic acids within the biological framework of intact tissues. Unlike other traditional approaches that may provide gross overviews of gene expression, ISH allows one to see the precise cellular and tissue distributions of specific RNA or DNA targets. This spatial resolution is important for understanding gene function in developmental pathology and biology because it indicates how gene-expression changes are linked to morphological changes. Unique patterns of expressions identified can be used to acquire information about cellular behavior, differentiation, and disease progression, which gives a lot of value to ISH in molecular research. ISH is also very versatile for probing all kinds of targets. This approach accommodates a wide range of nucleic acid types, such as mRNA and non-coding RNA, both required for complete gene expression analysis. Its application may also be adapted to species and sample diversity, from plant tissues to human biopsies. Development of novel labeling approaches, like fluorescent probes, has also enhanced the sensitivity and specificity of ISH to detect low-abundance transcripts that would go undetected using alternative strategies. This versatility creates broad research prospects, from ecological research that examines transcriptional reactions in plants like *Coffea arabica* to clinical research into human health genetic variation, as in the case of the background for ISH uses within these areas (Aga, 2005; Müller, S., & Wienberg, J., 2006). ISH is also crucial in the investigation of chromosomal arrangement and genome structure. Scientists can see chromosomal structure and detect genomic abnormalities that cause various diseases, such as cancer, using fluorescence *in situ* hybridization (FISH). This application is particularly crucial in cytogenetics, as it enables detection of known oncogenic chromosomal translocations, duplications, and deletions. For example, the use of chromosomal bar codes in FISH provides an exact method of mapping intra- and inter-chromosomal rearrangements, improving the accuracy of diagnosis and treatment strategies. The combination of ISH with other analytical methods for molecular analysis improves its analytical capability and provides a complete approach to understanding molecular mechanisms and their implications in health and disease. Such varied applications underscore the prime role of ISH in accelerating research as well as clinical work in molecular morphology (Figure 12.14).

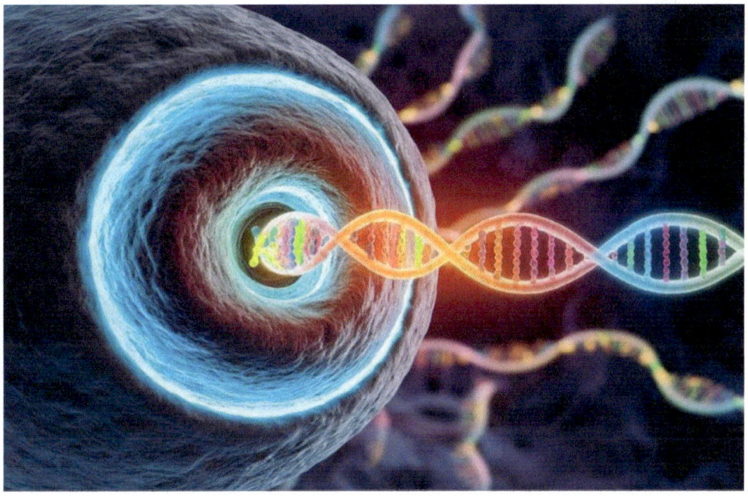

Figure 12.14. Advantages of *in situ* hybridization.

Source: https://notesforbiology.com/wp-content/uploads/2024/07/Fluorescent-In-Situ-Hybridization_11zon-1024x683.jpg.

12.5.1. Spatial Resolution of Gene Expression

With the exploration of the spatial resolution of gene expression, the technique employed becomes crucial to establishing findings presented on molecular morphology. A prominent method adopted to visualize targeted nucleic acid sequences in cellular structure is *in situ* hybridization (ISH). ISH equips scientists with the power to target gene expression within the complex tissue environments of organisms, significantly expanding our understanding of developmental processes and states of disease. High-resolution imaging technologies, when combined with ISH, have revolutionized the spatial resolution at which gene expression can be observed. By enabling accurate charting of gene activity in these incredibly complex biological contexts, ISH is an absolute requirement to establish detailed molecular maps that characterize cellular heterogeneity within multicellular organisms. Advances in technologies such as Fluorescent In Situ Sequencing of Barcoded Individual Neuronal Connections (FISSEQ-BOINC) have significantly enhanced our ability to understand the spatial component of gene expression. The method leverages the traditional *in situ* hybridization techniques but introduces a scalable framework to chart sophisticated neural networks with rich molecular definitions. With fluorescent *in situ* nucleic acid sequencing, FISSEQ-BOINC provides a method that reveals differential cellular interactions without compromising high spatial resolution. These approaches not only expand our knowledge of gene expression patterns in fixed tissue but also enable comparative analysis of molecular information across various developmental stages, potentially revealing the delicate interrelationship between gene expression and morphological transformation during organismal development (Boyden et al., 2014). In a practical application of these techniques, researchers localized clusters of histone genes in *Drosophila melanogaster* nuclei with very high spatial resolution by means of ISH techniques. With a 4.8-kb biotinylated probe favorable for high-resolution, three-dimensional fluorescence microscopy, investigators observed dynamic locus organization of homologous loci for genes throughout different phases of developmental cycles. Above all, these experiments revealed that homologous clusters, though divergent in earlier stages, exhibit strong colocalization at a specific stage of zygotic transcription. This extreme nuclear repositioning demonstrates that gene expression is not a fixed state but an active process dependent on cellular context and timing. These findings highlight the importance of spatial resolution to molecular comprehension of gene expression and emphasize the potential of revolutionary breakthroughs in molecular morphology (Agard et al., 1993) (Figure 12.15).

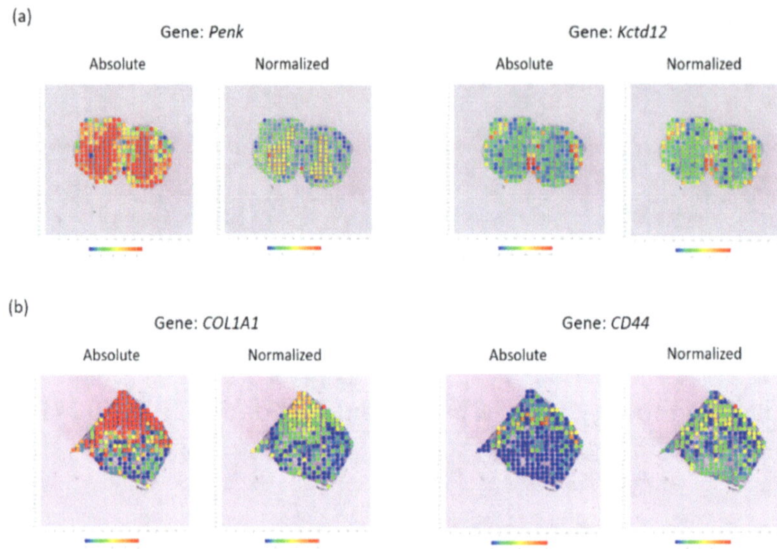

Figure 12.15. Spatial resolution of gene expression.

Source: https://www.researchgate.net/publication/369187197/figure/fig3/AS:11431281126408642@1678711641279/Examples-of-visual-examination-of-gene-expressions-on-STAr-Spatial-expression-pattern.ppm.

12.5.2. Preservation of Tissue Architecture

Preservation of tissue architecture is of first priority in the study of molecular morphology, especially with methods such as *in situ* hybridization. Conventional techniques tend to destroy the structural integrity of tissues and, therefore, lead to false interpretation of spatial contacts between cells and their molecular structures. Recent advances circumvented these flaws by introducing innovative chemical and physical methods that ensure optimal preservation of phenotypic information. For instance, high-resolution imaging techniques are now capable of taking detailed data for gene expression at single-cell resolution without disrupting three-dimensional tissue architecture. This methodological shift substantially enhances our understanding of complex metazoan systems and enables us to visualize and dissect cellular interrelations with unprecedented detail, which is crucial for accurate descriptions of molecular morphology across multiple biological contexts (Deisseroth et al., 2018). Utilization of tissue clearing techniques has revolutionized the preservation of tissue architecture, such that it is possible to achieve whole-organ imaging without sacrificing critical anatomical information. Methods such as the passive clarity technique (PACT) allow for the optical clearing of whole organs and bodies, thereby allowing visualization of intact cellular structures without destruction and their connectivity. These approaches enhance compatibility with various imaging modalities like immunohistochemistry and RNA single-molecule fluorescence *in situ* hybridization (FISH). Utilizing such sophisticated methodologies, scientists can create in-depth 3D anatomical maps that uncover the structure-function relationships of various organ systems. This ability is notably important for detecting pathological alterations in tissues, allowing for better-informed explanations of disease processes while having a complex understanding of tissue structure (Cai et al., 2014). Ultimately, the maintenance of tissue structure is an important consideration in furthering our understanding of molecular morphology and its implications in biomedical research. The union of high-resolution imaging and tissue clearing techniques not only facilitates the observation of fine cellular interactions but also opens doors to phenomenal advances in deciphering intricate biological systems. By revisiting the traditional methods of tissue examination, researchers can now construct vast phenotypic maps that yield information on normal and pathological states. This innovation in technique highlights the importance of maintaining structural integrity in the analysis of molecular interactions, and future prospects for exploration in cell biology, neuroscience, and other fields lie ahead. As we continue to develop these techniques, the landscape of potential advances in understanding cellular dynamics and disease processes will expand, with new and exciting possibilities (Cai et al., 2014; Deisseroth et al., 2018) (Figure 12.16).

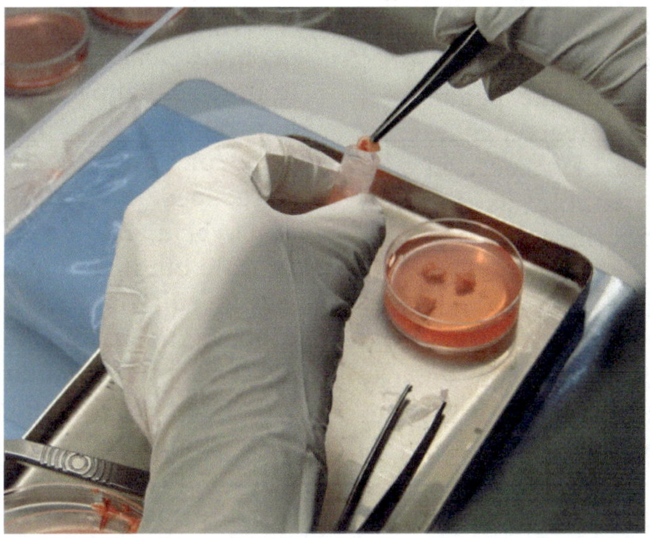

Figure 12.16. Preservation of tissue architecture.

Source: https://external-content.duckduckgo.com/iu/?u=https%3A%2F%2Flookformedical.com%2Fimg%2Fe%2Fed%2FPetefszekszvet-cskok_fagyaszt_oldatba_helyezse.jpg&f=1&nofb=1&ipt=dcfc174b0eedf121d0949bb548cd2124dd92bba450cd0a4956801cb28f96bfec.

12.5.3. Versatility Across Different Organisms

The ability to apply molecular techniques to a wide range of organisms underlines the utility and versatility of *in situ* hybridization in the biological sciences. It has emerged as a valuable tool for the visualization of gene expression and cellular distribution, providing information on developmental processes and functional dynamics. Even though long linked to animal models, advances in technology have now made the *in situ* hybridization field possible in plant studies using new methods such as the Expansion Microscopy in Plant Protoplast Systems (ExPOSE). This method enhances our understanding of plant biology since it facilitates high-resolution imaging of biomolecules, a critical need for studying complex interactions in plant cells. By demonstrating its utility in other organisms, ExOSE highlights the expansiveness of *in situ* hybridization techniques outside of classic organisms and thereby enhances our appreciation for molecular morphology across the biological spectrum (Cox et al., 2025). Beyond their application in plant systems, *in situ* hybridization techniques have also been extremely useful in the study of multicellular animal systems, evoking intricate patterns of gene expression and cell behavior. The new advances in hydrogel-tissue chemistry have allowed researchers to acquire high-resolution datasets from whole organisms, merging single-cell gene expression and three-dimensional spatial structure. This technique provides a revolutionary new perspective on metazoan biology, where syntheses of structural and functional information enable us to gain insights into cellular networks and their roles in physiology. Notably, this method has provided informative analyses of vertebrate neuronal activities, which inform the fundamental principles that govern cognition and sensory processing. Accordingly, the versatility of *in situ* hybridization not only adds depth to animal and plant biology but also fosters a multidisciplinary approach that gives crossovers between fields of investigation (Deisseroth et al., 2018). As researchers refine and expand in situ hybridization techniques, the potential for use across diverse organisms is poised to increase substantially. New technology and adaptations, such as improvements in imaging resolution and accessibility, can be made to a wide variety of biological systems, ranging from unicellular life to intricate metazoans. The capacity to visualize interactions and expressions at previously unimaginable levels of resolution enables a better comprehension of the underlying principles that drive life processes. Moreover, these breakthroughs enable cross-pollination of ideas between scientific disciplines, catalyzing innovation in experimental design and theory. Lastly, the ubiquity of *in situ* hybridization and its applications to diverse organisms attest to an ever-growing interconnectivity of biological principles, setting the stage for research that is less encumbered by traditional boundaries in the life sciences.

12.6. Limitations and Challenges

Limitations and challenges of in situ hybridization (ISH) techniques have far-reaching implications for the practice of molecular morphology. The most glaring limitation is the inherent challenge of biological specimens, resulting in non-uniform labeling and interpretation. Because ISH relies on the specificity of hybridization between nucleic acid probes and target sequences, variations in sample preparation and hybridization conditions can result in non-specific binding or poor signal detection. Such issues can obscure the true morphological topography at the cellular level and hinder correlating molecular data with anatomical characteristics. Isolation of single mRNA or DNA sequences may also overlook broader cellular patterns and interactions that might provide more informative data on organism development and functional complexity. The other flaw of ISH is its reproducibility and scalability, particularly for large biological samples or complex tissues such as whole-brain connectomes. Although techniques such as Fluorescent In-Situ Sequencing of Barcoded Individual Neuronal Connections (FISSEQ-BOINC) have been suggested to enhance mapping resolutions, they may not necessarily suppress the issues surrounding high-throughput analysis (Boyden et al., 2014). The need for accurate probe design, optimal hybridization parameters, and optimal imaging technology can create substantial bottlenecks in detailed molecular map construction. As researchers try to extend these methodologies, they are faced with the challenge of optimizing probe specificity and multiplexing capability, which effectively limits the amount of molecular information achievable from such advanced imaging methods. Finally, the association of *in situ* hybridization with other imaging technologies presents additional challenges that could undermine the overall precision and worth of molecular morphology studies. While imaging and image analysis technologies have improved, trade-offs persist among sample size, resolution, and throughput. For instance, higher resolution imaging could supply more detailed morphological data, but often at the expense of investigation of larger sample sizes (Abbas-Zadeh et al., 2014). This condition puts into question the representativeness of findings to the entire biological system under investigation. Transcending these challenges, researchers will be forced to come up with ways of integrating various imaging systems and correlating diverse data sets, hence gaining a holistic perception of the intricate interface between molecular structure and cell morphology.

12.6.1. Technical Difficulties in Probe Design

The design of probes for *in situ* hybridization (ISH) is fraught with technical difficulties that can significantly influence the accuracy and utility of molecular morphology studies. Probes must be optimized to demonstrate specificity for their target nucleic acid sequences, a task complicated by the presence of homologous sequences in the genome. Such cross-reactivity can result in non-specific binding and inaccurate conclusions. In addition, optimal probe length and incorporation of modifications, such as fluorescent dyes, can contribute to the complexities. Balancing specificity and sensitivity is paramount to obtain consistent results in tissue localization research. Technologies such as synthetic nucleic acids and dual-labeled probes are being pursued to circumvent these issues, but the leeway for error remains an issue in the diverse biological contexts in which ISH is applied, particularly within complex tissue architectures where the spatial context of molecules can influence interpretation. Second, one of the most persistent problems in probe design is probe affinity and thermal stability for binding under hybridization conditions. Ionic strength and temperature, for instance, can have large effects on hybridization rate and the probe-target complex stability. Such unfavorable conditions may lead to premature probe dissociation or, conversely, augment non-specific binding. Thus, researchers have the challenging task of laboriously optimizing all facets of the hybridization assay, a labor-intensive process. Inclusion of sophisticated signal amplification techniques, such as tyramide signal amplification, in the scenario adds an additional level of complexity to probe design, requiring demanding calibration of concentration and reaction time to perform optimally. These technical difficulties highlight the necessity for continued innovation in probe design strategies, which are required to maximize the precision of ISH in molecular morphology studies (Boyden et al., 2014). Novel strategies in probe design are beginning to overcome these technical difficulties and promise more robust and informative *in situ* hybridization assays. For instance, the development of fluorescence-based techniques, such as Fluorescent In-Situ Sequencing of Barcoded Individual Neuronal Connections (FISSEQ-BOINC), is a significant direction towards more complex methodologies with multi-aspect probe designs that are capable of sensing complex tissue environments. The methods rely on the premise of integrating molecular and morphological data to pave the way for a more sophisticated comprehension of cellular interactions and structure. But the technical demand and complexity involved in those methods being integrated into existing paradigms of *in situ* hybridization pose ongoing challenges with regard to usability and feasibility for the population of researchers. The development of probe design, particularly with these new techniques in mind, continues to redefine the landscape of the field of molecular morphology research (Boyden et al., 2014) (Figure 12.17).

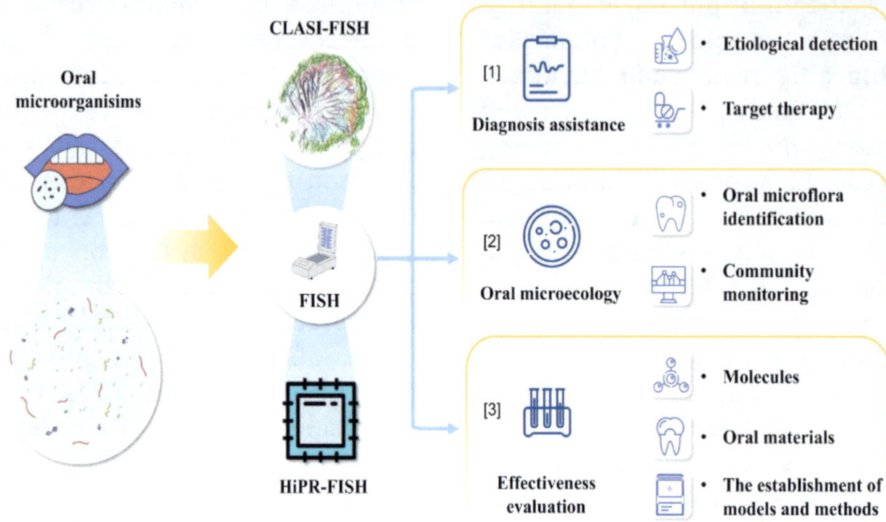

Figure 12.17. Technical difficulties in probe design.

Source: https://pub.mdpi-res.com/pathogens/pathogens-11-01450/article_deploy/html/images/pathogens-11-01450-ag.png?1669883827.

12.6.2. Interpretation of Results

The interpretation of results in the context of *in situ* hybridization and molecular morphology is an important factor in understanding chromosomal evolution and phylogenetic interrelation among species. With techniques such as fluorescence *in situ* hybridization (FISH), researchers can analyze chromosomal conservation and rearrangements across primate lineages. For instance, research on hybridization patterns observed in the long arm of human chromosome 2 differs when compared to those of great apes and Old World monkey chromosomes. The recognition of inversions in the pericentric region among the great apes highlights the chromosomal changes that have accompanied primate evolution. These observations not only unveil the shared genetic architecture among species but also provide valuable information about evolutionary dynamics driving primate genomes in contemporary times (Baldini et al., 1994). Apart from data analysis on chromosomal changes, data interpretation is crucial in uncovering the molecular-genetic process responsible for morphological variation in plant species. The ABC floral organ identity model depicts how *in situ* hybridization can reveal complex expression patterns of significant functional genes. While normal in flowering plants, Lacandonia schismatica possesses a unique floral structure due to an altered expression of B- and C-function genes. This homeotic alteration, where stamens occur in the center of flowers surrounded by carpels, emphasizes the significance of molecular alterations during morphogenesis. By linking gene expression patterns to morphological phenotypes, researchers can enhance our understanding of how single genetic changes can lead to fundamental alterations in floral anatomy across taxa (Ambrose et al., 2010). Ultimately, the interpretation of data that result from the employment of *in situ* hybridization studies is at the heart of integrating molecular biology with evolutionary morphology. The ability to visualize and analyze spatial patterns of gene expression not only teaches us about organismal development but also highlights the evolutionary influences that shape these events. Through comparative analysis across species, researchers can identify conserved genetic elements and ascertain their functions in producing phenotypic variation. These are not only helping us better comprehend the evolutionary past of life organisms but also enabling us to construct a scheme by which predictions can be made regarding how genetic variations can be manifested in future morphological changes, thus complementing the significance of *in situ* hybridization in contemporary biological sciences.

12.6.3. Limitations in Sensitivity and Specificity

In the instance of *in situ* hybridization (ISH) methods, sensitivity and specificity constraints are a serious obstacle that can hamper the reliability of molecular morphology assessments. Sensitivity is the power of techniques to detect the presence of a target nucleic acid sequence, while specificity is the power to distinguish between similar sequences. Sensitivity is needed when detecting low-abundance targets in highly complex biological specimens, but its achievement can lead to false positives if specificity is compromised. For instance, in certain applications using peptide nucleic acid (PNA) probes, through the achievement of theoretical sensitivities of 100% and specificities of 100%, there exist practical challenges with biofilms. Direct detection is complicated by autofluorescence from support materials, making precise quantification challenging and underscoring the delicate balance between maximizing sensitivity and ensuring the required specificity in hybridization assays (Almeida et al., 2008). Furthermore, the complexity of distinguishing closely related sequences tends to exacerbate limitations in specificity when using *in situ* hybridization. For example, comparative genomic *in situ* hybridization (CGH) provides valuable data on differences in genetic material between control and test genomes. However, estimation of relative copy numbers using fluorescent ratios has an intrinsic potential for misinterpretation, especially in cases of segmental duplications or genetic rearrangements. Such kinds of chromosomal aberrations can provide misleading fluorescence intensities that make it difficult to establish a correct state of a genome. Therefore, while CGH holds promise for the assessment of genomic imbalances, its drawback in specificity and, consequently, sensitivity necessitates rigorous methodological improvement to ensure accurate data interpretation in the area of molecular morphology (Cremer et al., 1993). Furthermore, the correction of these limitations demands the use of more sophisticated methods and approaches. Recent advances, e.g., better sonication protocols to be applied in biofilm disruption, have boosted the sensitivity of the hybridization signal by minimizing autofluorescence background noise from support material. Continued refinement of probe design also has the potential for further boosting specificity by minimizing cross-reactivity with non-target sequences. Coupled with other modalities, such as confocal microscopy or better image analysis software, such advances are designed to boost both sensitivity and specificity of ISH applications. Lastly, an overall understanding of the natural limitations is needed by researchers to design good experiments and interpret the resulting data properly. Greater knowledge about sensitivity and specificity problems aids in providing good insights into molecular morphology, which is of more significance for application in diagnostic pathology and genetic studies (Cremer et al., 1993; Almeida et al., 2008).

SUMMARY

In summarizing the discussion of *in situ* hybridization and molecular morphology, it is essential to highlight the profound implications these techniques have for the comprehension of genetic architecture and evolutionary biology. Genomic *in situ* hybridization (GISH) has deciphered the complexity of hybrid genomes, particularly in genera such as the Elatior-begonias, which represent complex interspecific hybridization systems. The results of such studies reveal the diversity of chromosome numbers and the extent of ploidy levels found in hybrids, all of which feed into a better understanding of plant genetics. This not only promotes breeding for the *Begonia* genus but also provides entry into better agricultural techniques with the help of the development of genetic potential. As the figure shows, GISH arises as an important tool for labeling genomic constitutions and making researchers aware of novel approaches to explaining hybrid vigor and adaptability (Laak et al., 2010). Beyond botany, the application of such molecular tools extends to broader biological contexts, including vertebrate evolution. Research in Acipenseriformes, particularly on paddlefishes and sturgeons, illustrates the intricate role of whole genome duplications in creating evolutionary lines. The findings related to the rediploidization events in paddlefish genomes are of prime significance to comprehend how genomic features are retained or altered over evolutionary timescales. By cytogenetic mapping and exploring the paralog gene clusters, researchers can document the evolutionary history of these creatures, and past and recent polyploidy events are of significant relevance in this situation. Such thorough analyses not only enhance our understanding of the individual species but also contribute to the broader narrative of vertebrate evolution, showing us the dynamic power of genetic diversity (Amemiya et al., 2017). Finally, the intersection of *in situ* hybridization and molecular morphology has transformed the biological sciences and inspired many practical and theoretical innovations. Such methods allow scientists to investigate genomic complexities with hitherto unprecedented precision, facilitating the untangling of evolutionary connections and mechanisms of species adaptation. The ramifications of this research extend far beyond academic interest, providing the foundations for applied genetics to agriculture, conservation, and maintenance of biodiversity. As molecular techniques continue to evolve, they promise to uncover further layers of complexity in genomes, enabling a further understanding of life's intricate brocade. Ultimately, the continuous exploration of *in situ* hybridization and molecular morphology will remain critical to unravel the mysteries of genetic inheritance and evolutionary history.

It has increased significantly since the discovery of *in situ* hybridization techniques. The method allows the localization of specific nucleic acid sequences in tissue sections with the provision of information on gene expression patterns in situ. The application of *in situ* hybridization in the study of vascular development, such as during early postnatal retina, has suggested the role of vascular endothelial growth factor A (VEGF-A) during angiogenesis. As demonstrated, cellular response through VEGF-A is regulated by various mechanisms, where tip cells are affected by directed migration by temporal gradients, while stalk cells demonstrate proliferative responses to concentration levels of VEGF-A. This cell behavior demarcation highlights how variations in spatial distributions of signaling molecules are able to bring about complex morphogenetic events in developing tissues (Abramsson et al., 2003). Another significant feature highlighted by *in situ* hybridization is the development of neural crest cells. Earlier work has documented significant regulatory roles of hindbrain neural tube cells that can respond to changing developmental contexts. In particular, after the removal of sections of the dorsal hindbrain surgically, neural crest cells exhibit robust migratory behavior and altered patterns of gene expression. In contrast, misdirecting them through experimental manipulations has different effects upon gene expression, such as upregulation of Hoxa-3 in response to specific migratory stimuli. These findings emphasize the plasticity of neural crest progenitors to adjust developmental processes in response to environmental perturbations, making them crucial in the overall context of vertebrate development (Bronner-Fraser et al., 1997). Furthermore, an integration of *in situ* hybridization and molecular morphological analysis elucidates the complex interconnection between tissue structure and gene expression. The dynamic cellular behaviors of endothelial and neural crest cells in response to signaling molecules are paradigmatic of the regulatory complexity of developmental networks. Understanding such processes not only contributes to further elucidating elementary biological principles but also lays the groundwork for the creation of future therapeutic interventions for abnormal development and disease. These findings related to VEGF-A's role in angiogenesis and neural crest cell responsiveness bring to the fore the function of molecular signaling in tissue structure. This knowledge goes further to advance the area of developmental biology and to understand tissue organization and function better (Bronner-Fraser et al., 1997; Abramsson et al., 2003).

A LOOK TO THE FUTURE:

MOLECULAR GENETICS:

Molecular genetics stands at the forefront of modern biological science, uniting traditional concepts of heredity with the tools and insights of molecular biology. At its core, this discipline explores the structure, function, and regulation of genetic material — particularly DNA and RNA — at the molecular level. By examining how genes are encoded, expressed, and altered, molecular genetics provides a conceptual bridge between the microscopic architecture of biological molecules and the macroscopic outcomes seen in organisms, populations, and ecosystems. The inception of molecular genetics in the mid-20th century marked a watershed moment in scientific thought. With the identification of DNA as the hereditary material and the elucidation of its double-helical structure, researchers gained a new vantage point from which to interrogate the mechanisms of life itself. Far from being an abstract theoretical endeavor, molecular genetics quickly became transformative, influencing fields as diverse as medicine, agriculture, forensics, and biotechnology. Its methodologies — ranging from polymerase chain reaction (PCR) and DNA sequencing to gene editing and genomic mapping — have revolutionized our ability to isolate, alter, and understand genes.

This field is fundamentally interdisciplinary, drawing upon classical genetics, biochemistry, cellular biology, and computational science. By doing so, molecular genetics addresses fundamental questions about how living organisms inherit traits, how genes are regulated, and how genetic variation arises and persists within populations. For example, the concept of the *central dogma* — that genetic information flows from DNA to RNA to protein — remains a guiding principle, shaping how scientists understand gene expression and cellular function. Yet beyond this basic framework, researchers now investigate complex regulatory systems, epigenetic modifications, and interactions between genes and the environment.

The practical applications of molecular genetics are profound. In medicine, insights into the molecular basis of disease have enabled the development of genetic diagnostics, targeted therapies, and personalized medicine. In agriculture, molecular markers and genome editing accelerate crop improvement, increasing yields and resilience. In environmental sciences, genetic tools help track biodiversity and understand evolutionary processes. Collectively, these advancements underscore both the scientific significance and societal impact of the field.

This book is designed to introduce readers to the foundational concepts, historical developments, and cutting-edge techniques of molecular genetics. It aims to cultivate scientific literacy and inspire further inquiry into this dynamic and ever-evolving domain of life sciences.

REFERENCES

1. Downie, H. F., Adu, M. O., Schmidt, S., Otten, W., Dupuy, L. X., White, P. J., & Valentine, T. A. (2014b). Challenges and opportunities for quantifying roots and rhizosphere interactions through imaging and image analysis. *Plant Cell & Environment*, *38*(7), 1213–1232. https://doi.org/10.1111/pce.12448Abramsson, A., Alitalo, K., Betsholtz, C., Fruttiger, et al. (2003). VEGF guides angiogenic sprouting utilizing endothelial tip cell filopodia. https://core.ac.uk/download/1685251.pdf (accessed on 6th August 2025).
2. Abu Bakar, S. (2004). Application of comparative genomic hybridization and fluorescent *in situ* hybridization techniques on human glioma cell lines treated with bis[S-methyl-A-N-(2-furylmethylketone) dithiocarbazato] cadmium (II). https://core.ac.uk/download/42993475.pdf (accessed on 6th August 2025).
3. Aga, E. (2005). Molecular genetic diversity study of forest coffee tree (*Coffea arabica* L.) populations in Ethiopia: Implications for conservation and breeding. https://core.ac.uk/download/11694916.pdf (accessed on 6th August 2025).
4. Agard, D. A., Dernburg, A. F., Hiraoka, Y., Parmelee, et al. (1993). The onset of homologous chromosome pairing during *Drosophila melanogaster* embryogenesis. https://core.ac.uk/download/323081477.pdf (accessed on 6th August 2025).
5. Allshire, Brown, Cai, Chen, Demarco, Dernburg, Ding, et al. (2019). RNA from a simple-tandem repeat is required for sperm maturation and male fertility in *Drosophila melanogaster*. https://core.ac.uk/download/286362222.pdf (accessed on 6th August 2025).
6. Almeida, C., Azevedo, N. F., Keevil, C. W., Vieira, et al. (2008). A fluorescence *in situ* hybridization method using a peptide nucleic acid probe for the detection of *Salmonella* spp. in biofilms. https://core.ac.uk/download/55618254.pdf (accessed on 6th August 2025).
7. Ambrose, B. A., de la Torre-Bárcena, E., Englund, M., Engström, et al. (2010). B-function expression in the flower center underlies the homeotic phenotype of *Lacandonia schismatica* (Triuridaceae). https://core.ac.uk/download/4887783.pdf (accessed on 6th August 2025).
8. Amemiya, C. T., Flajšhans, M., Gela, D., Havelka, et al. (2017). Molecular cytogenetic differentiation of paralogs of *Hox* paralogs in duplicated and re-diploidized genome of the North American paddlefish (*Polyodon spathula*). https://core.ac.uk/download/323063824.pdf (accessed on 6th August 2025).
9. Argenton, F., Ek, O. F. D., Facchinello, N., Grisan, et al. (2017). *Tcf7l2* plays pleiotropic roles in the control of glucose homeostasis, pancreas morphology, vascularization and regeneration. https://core.ac.uk/download/84923362.pdf (accessed on 6th August 2025).
10. Baldini, A., Jauch, A., Dutrillaux, B., Horsthemke, B., Lengauer, C., & others. (1994). The origin of human chromosome 2 analyzed by comparative chromosome mapping with a DNA microlibrary. https://core.ac.uk/download/12170141.pdf (accessed on 6th August 2025).
11. Bhandari, S. (2006). Prevalence and diversity of *Arcobacter* spp. in poultry meat in New Zealand: A thesis presented in partial fulfillment of the requirements for the degree of Master of Science in Veterinary Microbiology and Public Health at Massey University, Palmerston North, New Zealand. https://core.ac.uk/download/157568849.pdf (accessed on 6th August 2025).

12. Boyden, E. S., Church, G. M., Daugharthy, E. R., Kalhor, et al. (2014). Rosetta brains: A strategy for molecularly-annotated connectomics. http://arxiv.org/abs/1404.5103 (accessed on 6th August 2025).
13. Bronner-Fraser, M., Krull, C. E., Ruffins, S., Saldivar, et al. (1997). Dorsal hindbrain ablation results in rerouting of neural crest migration and changes in gene expression, but normal hyoid development. https://core.ac.uk/download/4893372.pdf (accessed on 6th August 2025).
14. Bueno i Torrens, D., & Hernández Hernández, V. (2013). RNA interference is ineffective as a routine method for gene silencing in chick embryos as monitored by *fgf8* silencing. http://hdl.handle.net/2445/43814 (accessed on 6th August 2025).
15. Cai, L., Chen, C.-K., Deverman, B. E., Gradinaru, et al. (2014). Single-cell phenotyping within transparent intact tissue through whole-body clearing. https://core.ac.uk/download/33111836.pdf (accessed on 6th August 2025).
16. Chang, S. B., Datema, E., Jacobsen, E., Jong, et al. (2008). FISH mapping and molecular organization of the major repetitive sequences of tomato. https://core.ac.uk/download/pdf/29258318.pdf (accessed on 6th August 2025).
17. Chauffaille, M. L. L. F., Figueiredo, V. L. P., Franco, L. F., Kimura, et al. (2006). Leucemia linfocítica crônica: Anormalidades cromossômicas e a sua relação com o estágio clínico CD38 e o ZAP-70. https://core.ac.uk/download/37706307.pdf (accessed on 6th August 2025).
18. Chen, J.-N., Geisler, R., Huang, J., Langenbacher, et al. (2017). The Calcineurin-FoxO-MuRF1 signaling pathway regulates myofibril integrity in cardiomyocytes. https://core.ac.uk/download/323066728.pdf (accessed on 6th August 2025).
19. Chen, Q., Fang, M., Greer, J., Hu, et al. (2020). Evidence linking exposure of fish primary macrophages to antibiotics activates the NF-kB pathway. https://core.ac.uk/download/305123972.pdf (accessed on 6th August 2025).
20. Cox, K., Czymmek, K., Huss, D., Klebanovych, et al. (2025). ExPOSE: A comprehensive toolkit to perform expansion microscopy in plant protoplast systems. https://core.ac.uk/download/649473272.pdf (accessed on 6th August 2025).
21. Cremer, T., Daumer, C., Jauch, A., Lichter, et al. (1990). Chromosomal *in situ* suppression hybridization of human gonosomes and autosomes and its use in clinical cytogenetics. https://core.ac.uk/download/12170028.pdf (accessed on 6th August 2025).
22. Cremer, T., Döhner, H., Joos, S., Kovacs, et al. (1993). Detection of complete and partial chromosome gains and losses by comparative genomic *in situ* hybridization. https://core.ac.uk/download/12170033.pdf (accessed on 6th August 2025).
23. Criswell, K. E., & Gillis, J. A. (2020). Resegmentation is an ancestral feature of the gnathostome vertebral skeleton. https://core.ac.uk/download/305121129.pdf (accessed on 6th August 2025).
24. David, C. N., Engel, J., Holstein, T. W., Kurz, et al. (1991). Mini-collagens in *Hydra* nematocytes. https://core.ac.uk/download/12164244.pdf (accessed on 6th August 2025).
25. Deisseroth, K., Gradinaru, V., Overton, K., Treweek, et al. (2018). Hydrogel-tissue chemistry: Principles and applications. https://core.ac.uk/download/211377600.pdf (accessed on 6th August 2025).

26. Ding, Y., Peng, L., Shi, Y., Yu, et al. (2015). Nanostructured conductive polymers for advanced energy storage. https://core.ac.uk/download/211336648.pdf (accessed on 6th August 2025).

27. Eno, C. C. (2009). Karyotyping and localization of genes on the chromosomes of the sea urchins, *Strongylocentrotus drobachiensis* and *Strongylocentrotus purpuratus*. https://core.ac.uk/download/215515698.pdf (accessed on 6th August 2025).

28. Estep, J. A., Riccomagno, M. M., Rosette, K. A., Rutlin, et al. (2018). Cas adaptor proteins coordinate sensory axon fasciculation. https://core.ac.uk/download/323067842.pdf (accessed on 6th August 2025).

29. Frisk, A.-L., Kreutzer, R., Lemarchand, T., Lezmi, et al. (2023). European Society of Toxicologic Pathology (Pathology 2.0 Molecular Pathology Special Interest Group): Review of *in situ* hybridization techniques for drug research and development. https://www.zora.uzh.ch/id/eprint/236094/1/monne_rodriguez_et_al_2023_european_society_of_toxicologic_pathology_pathology_2_0_molecular_pathology_special_interest__1_.pdf (accessed on 6th August 2025).

30. Goldbloom-Helzner, L., Hao, D., & Wang, A. (2019). Developing regenerative treatments for developmental defects, injuries, and diseases using extracellular matrix collagen-targeting peptides. https://core.ac.uk/download/323068929.pdf (accessed on 6th August 2025).

31. Greene, S. L. (2017). Evaluating the genotype phenotype correlations in cleidocranial dysplasia. https://core.ac.uk/download/640970031.pdf (accessed on 6th August 2025).

32. Jauch, A., Dutrillaux, B., Horsthemke, B., Lengauer, C., Pinkel, D., et al. (1991). Comparative chromosome band mapping in primates by *in situ* suppression hybridization of band specific DNA microlibraries. https://core.ac.uk/download/12170097.pdf (accessed on 6th August 2025).

33. Kim, S., Li, P., & Tian, B. (2024). Beyond 25 years of biomedical innovation in nano-bioelectronics. https://core.ac.uk/download/613853123.pdf (accessed on 6th August 2025).

34. Kowluru, A., Minelli, A., Navarro-Sastre, A., Rotig, A., Vozza, A., Gerencser, A. A., Yu, A. C., et al. (2013). Exclusive neuronal expression of *SUCLA2* in the human brain. https://core.ac.uk/download/18405730.pdf (accessed on 6th August 2025).

35. Laak, W. A., Marasek Ciolakowska, A. R., Ramanna, M. S., Tuyl, et al. (2010). Genome composition of 'Elatior'-*begonia* hybrids analyzed by genomic *in situ* hybridisation. https://core.ac.uk/download/pdf/29238194.pdf (accessed on 6th August 2025).

36. Maanoja, A. (2024). Molekyylipatologiset menetelmät: Tarkastelua onkologian näkökulmasta. https://core.ac.uk/download/638718587.pdf (accessed on 6th August 2025).

37. Müller, S., & Wienberg, J. (2006). Multicolor chromosome bar codes. https://core.ac.uk/download/16432836.pdf (accessed on 6th August 2025).

38. Murillo, A. E., Hauss-Wegrzyniak, B., Walk, E., Gaire, F., Penault-Llorca, F., Nitta, H., Pettay, J., et al. (2008). Development of automated brightfield double *in situ* hybridization (BDISH) application for *HER2* gene and chromosome 17 centromere (CEN 17) for breast carcinomas and an assay performance comparison to manual dual color *HER2* fluorescence *in situ* hybridization (FISH). https://core.ac.uk/download/pdf/81832682.pdf (accessed on 6th August 2025).

39. Nalesnik, M. A., & Starzl, T. E. (1994). Epstein-Barr virus, infectious mononucleosis, and posttransplant lymphoproliferative disorders. https://core.ac.uk/download/12205238.pdf (accessed on 6th August 2025).

40. Rombouts, K., Braeckmans, K., & Remaut, K. (2016). Fluorescent labeling of plasmid DNA and mRNA: Gains and losses of current labeling strategies. https://core.ac.uk/download/55851519.pdf (accessed on 6th August 2025).

41. Tyybäkinoja, A. (2009). Genomic microarrays in chromosomal analysis of leukemia. https://core.ac.uk/download/14916055.pdf (accessed on 6th August 2025).

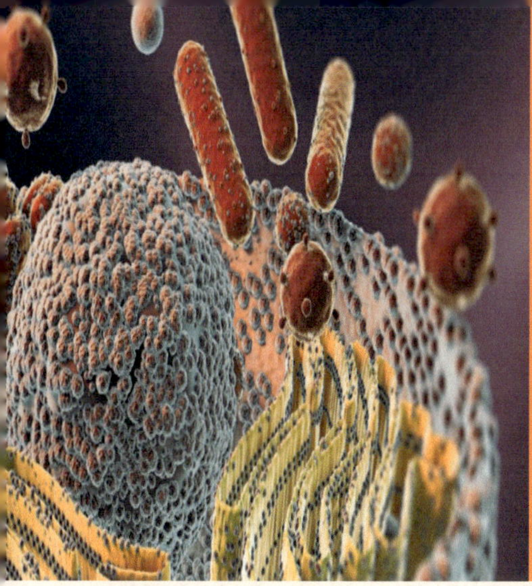

Chapter 13

MORPHOMETRIC ANALYSIS AND QUANTIFICATION

Contents

Introduction

Morphometric analysis is a key tool in biological research, enabling quantitative description of biological structure and form. Morphometric analysis involves the measurement of spatial parameters, which can provide valuable information on developmental biology, ecology, and physiology. With the addition of statistical and geometrical tools, morphometric analysis facilitates the understanding of variability among and within species, hence enabling evolutionary biology and conservation research. Among the main values of morphometric analysis is the reliance on landmarks as well as semi-landmarks in order to capture shape. Techniques such as geometric morphometrics allow researchers to capture these nuances in a way that is more than conventional morphometry, leading to systematic and objective form and function analyses in organisms. The application of morphometric techniques extends beyond ecological and evolutionary research and finds notable relevance in medical research. For example, morphometric analysis is very valuable in assessing pathological changes that occur as a result of disease states. A good case in point is use of morphometric parameters to assess heart damage in patients with cancer who receive chemotherapy with doxorubicin. As experimental findings elicit, quantifications of the nuclear index and cross-sectional area of myocytes provide quantifiable data that emphasize the drug's cardiotoxicity. Specifically, quantitative comparisons of morphometrics between treated and controls enlighten us on how doxorubicin impacts not only cardiomyocyte morphology but also myocardial capillary density, justifying the method's contribution toward a deeper understanding of drug-induced cardiomyopathy and endorsing the need for careful analysis in pharmacological science (Feijen et al., 1988). Besides, the development of technologies such as microcomputed tomography (μCT) has revolutionized morphometric analysis by providing three-dimensional visualization of biological structures.

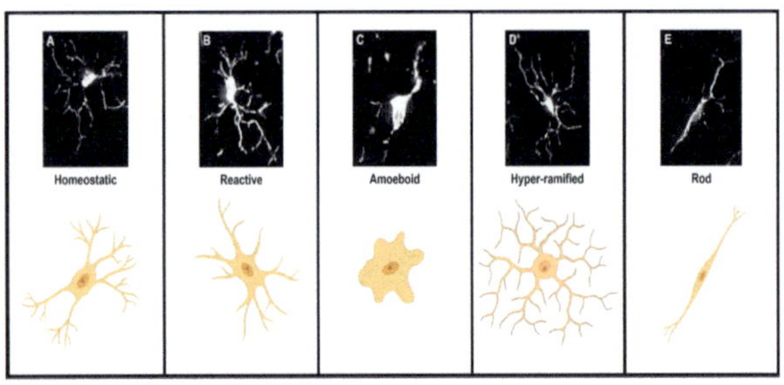

Figure 13.1. Morphometric analysis and quantification.

Source: https://www.frontiersin.org/files/Articles/1211188/fninf-17-1211188-HTML/image_m/fninf-17-1211188-g001.jpg.

While histomorphometry, being a conventional approach, is precise, it has limitations such as being destructive and time-consuming. The integration of μCT in morphometric studies has been effective in evaluating parameters such as bone-implant contact and bone area in dental implants. Comparisons with histomorphometry indicate that although μCT has its drawbacks, it is a quicker and less invasive procedure with a good correlation with the traditional histological technique. This advancement in morphometric devices is the hallmark of ongoing progress in quantification methods, and this reinforces the objective measurement of biological shapes and broadens their applications to all medical and biological sciences (Coelho et al., 2013) (Figure 13.1).

Definition of Morphometric Analysis

Morphometric analysis is a quantitative technique to study and describe the form and structure of biological phenomena, in this case, organisms. The study examines morphological details and, based on research, discusses the variations resulting from evolutionary processes, environmental factors, and functional adaptations. Using geometric morphometric approaches, researchers can study the overall shape of the biological phenomenon; with these approaches, variation in form can be investigated using landmark-based or outline-based methods. The ability to represent complicated biological shapes in a mathematically valid manner enhances the precision of analyses, it is a critical instrument in ecological, anthropological, and evolutionary biology. Morphometric analysis thus enables understanding of evolutionary relationships and can potentially identify species' special adaptations to their environments. One of the principal aspects of morphometric analysis is that it relies upon geometric concepts in order to quantify shape differences, which is required for interspecific comparisons. This is very advantageous in analyzing anatomical variation within a wide variety of organisms, such as fossils and contemporary species, using techniques such as sliding semi-landmarks to outline shape without the inelasticity of traditional landmark-based methods. The application of software packages, such as Edgewarp and Morpho, facilitates accurate analyses demonstrating the biological variability within morphospaces. Although both software packages yield similar outcomes in biological interpretation, their usage efficiencies differ significantly, demonstrating the importance of selecting the right tools for analyzing intricate biological data (Botton-Divet et al., 2015). Lastly, such procedures allow researchers to fill gaps in morphological variation and add to the ongoing debate surrounding the evolution and classification of species. In addition to its intrinsic role in evolutionary biology, morphometric analysis assists in addressing problems of application for researchers. Conventional techniques are extremely hard to master and involve lots of training to determine anatomical markers precisely, rendering them inaccessible to most researchers. The advent of new algorithms that circumvent conventional landmark marking has made it possible, allowing morphometric research to be undertaken by the masses (Boyer et al., 2011). Not only does it make analysis of larger data sets faster, but it also encourages interdisciplinary collaboration among morphologists and researchers in genomics, allowing us to better understand evolutionary trends. With narrowing disparities between phenomics and genomics, morphometric analysis is still critical in accounting for the continuity of the biological forms that link the wide variety of life, stressing its significance in contemporary scientific inquiry.

Historical Background and Development

The morphometric analysis has its roots in the early work in biometrics and quantifying the forms of biology. Pioneering researchers like Karl Pearson and Francis Galton established the foundation for statistical analysis of biological shapes with the use of early geometric and statistical methods. These initial works developed into an even more sophisticated system with the advent of geometric morphometrics, which allows the global analysis of biological shape from landmark and outline information. Digital imaging methods additionally revolutionized this discipline, allowing precise data capture and display. Over time, morphometric analysis advanced not only in scientific research but also in practical applications, influencing fields such as anthropology, paleontology, and evolutionary biology. Morphometric analysis revealed a narrow link between shape variation and evolutionary change, demonstrating that morphology serves as a significant marker of biological processes. With improved innovations in software tools and approaches, as morphometric analysis became mature, efficiency and precision in data interpretation improved. The use of sliding semi-landmarks in morphometric analysis was a significant improvement. The landmarks allow the acquisition of detailed shapes while allowing scientists to deal with datasets that have few or sparsely occurring anatomical landmarks. Comparing software packages, such as Edgewarp and Morpho, is one illustration of a commitment to improving operational efficiency in morphometric analysis. Interestingly, research has determined that Morpho handily surpasses Edgewarp in terms of delivering faster computational outcomes while retaining descriptive integrity of biological variability. Such developments not only simplify the analysis process but also increase our range of inquiry in the field of morphometric studies, enhancing our knowledge of morphological variation and the evolutionary pathways upon which it is based (Botton-Divet et al., 2015). The successful application of morphometric analysis also became intrinsically tied to the evolution of neuroimaging techniques, particularly when working with complex biological systems, e.g., the human brain. Today's research emphasizes the potential of multimodal neuroimaging, in which structural and functional imaging, volumetric and morphometric analyses, and other methods are combined to investigate the consequences of traumatic brain injury (TBI). This cross-disciplinary approach illuminates how advanced imaging modalities have the potential to further our knowledge of structural pathology and brain connectivity. By combining concurrent morphometric analysis, biomarkers of outcome in TBI can be established and, ultimately, greater insight into the neurobiological processes involved. These developments mark a sea change in morphometric research, where interdisciplinary collaboration brings with it new methods and greater insight into human anatomy (Aylward et al., 2012) (Figure 13.2).

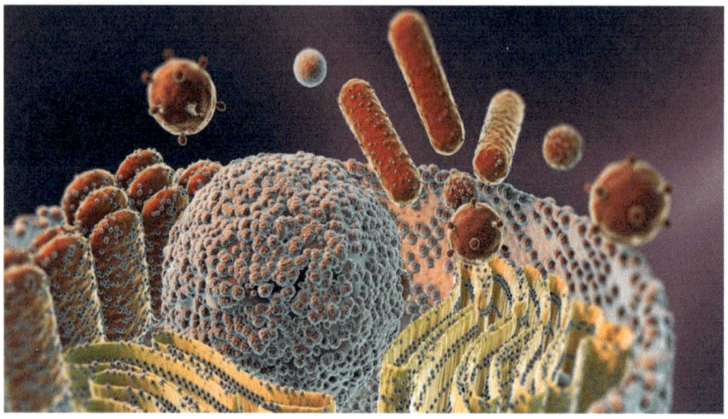

Figure 13.2. Historical background and development.

Source: https://bitesizebio.com/wp-content/uploads/2007/11/BSB-History-of-cell-bio-featured.jpg.

Importance in Various Scientific Fields

The relevance of morphometric analysis pervades numerous scientific disciplines, but notably so in biomedical science, where it aids the acquisition of insight into the structure and function of cells. Quantifying the morphology, such analysis assists in distinguishing between various cell types and conditions when exposed to stimulations. This has been observed particularly in studies investigating the effects of inhaled drugs, where macrophage morphology alterations are both adaptative and detrimental. As an illustration, research has demonstrated the ability of high-content image analysis to differentiate between the foamy macrophage phenotypes of some drugs, such as amiodarone and staurosporine, enabling improved decision-making during the development of new drugs. These developments are noteworthy in that they inform researchers on potential therapeutic impacts and safety profiles of emerging drugs, eventually determining clinical practices and patient treatment (Hoffman et al., 2020). The application of morphometric principles is also highly influential in genetics and developmental biology. By quantifying changes in morphological characteristics, researchers can identify genotype-phenotype correlations that illuminate mechanisms of numerous genetic disorders. For example, in Pompe disease, researchers applied morphometric techniques to evaluate muscle and heart pathology and parameters of functional performance in experimental animal models. In this particular study, the efficacy of TFEB gene therapy on symptom mitigation was quantified by assessing cellular morphology and muscle integrity post-treatment. Such morphometric analysis not only provides insights into the pathogenesis of disease but also highlights the potential of accurate genetic therapies. Also, the possibility of monitoring structural evolution over time aids in developing more appropriate therapeutic solutions tailored to the specific needs of individual patients (Alvino et al., 2017). Besides, ecological and environmental sciences appreciate the application of morphometric analysis, especially in biodiversity assessment and habitat analysis. Through the measurement of morphological aspects of organisms within their habitats, scientists can draw conclusions about indicators of health and ecological processes. For example, a difference in body size, form, or population structure of specific species may reflect variation in environmental aspects, such as climate change or loss of habitats. These morphometric analyses not only enhance understanding of species responses to environmental stress but also inform conservation planning. Biodiversity still continues to face threats from human activities, and the use of morphometric analysis in ecological studies provides the necessary information informing policies applied to conserve ecosystems and maintain biodiversity.

Hence, its application is fundamental not only for building scientific knowledge but also in an effort to address current environmental problems on our planet.

13.1. Types of Morphometric Techniques

Morphometric procedures are diverse and encompass many methodologies utilized in examining shape, size, and structural variation in biological organisms. Classic morphometrics is one of the dominant forms, employing linear dimensions and angles to specify the geometry of samples. It is mostly straightforward, making use of simple statistical models for the analysis of the connection between measurements. Its limitation is that it does not work well in documenting complicated shape variations. On the other hand, geometric morphometrics has been more significant due to its ability to quantify differences in shape in terms of landmark configurations. It employs landmarks that correspond to biologically meaningful points on the specimens' surfaces, thereby enabling high-resolution shape comparisons between populations or species. With researchers advancing with these advanced techniques, morphometric variability is better known to offer increased insights into ecological and evolutionary processes.

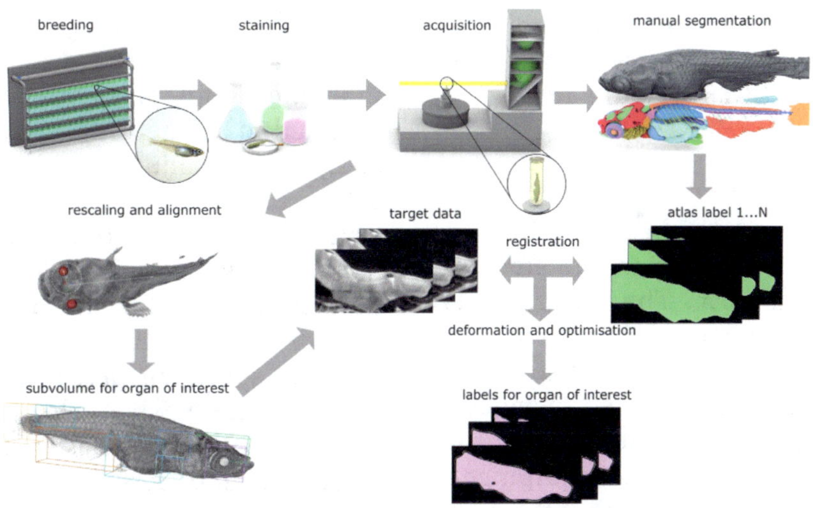

Figure 13.3. Types of Morphometric Techniques.

Source: https://www.nature.com/articles/s41598-018-34848-z/figures/1.

In geometric morphometrics, a key aspect is data collection accuracy. Researchers often measure the error of landmark configuration datasets, which affects statistical analysis results considerably. One study emphasized how differences in data acquisition, including specimen presentation variations and differences in imaging instruments, can contribute to more than 30% of the total variation that can be seen among datasets. This indicates the importance of stringent methodologies that minimize error at the collection stage. Measurement error evaluation not only informs on the reliability of the morphometric analysis but also maintains the integrity of the conclusions drawn from these studies. These cautions, taken into consideration, help standardize procedure across research studies as well as enhance the application of morphometric methods in evolutionary and ecological studies (Adams et al., 2020). Additionally, dedicated morphometric techniques have evolved to address specific biological questions. For instance, synchrotron radiation-based computed tomography is utilized for assessing three-dimensional structures in cortical bone, which suggests extremely minute information of vascular networks and osteocyte lacunae with respect to bone condition. Such techniques offer information about alterations with age and microstructural features of bone, which are valuable for studies of conditions like osteoporosis. Through the use of advanced imaging technology, scientists can combine morphometric evaluation with physiological information to achieve an enhanced perception of skeletal variation at different life stages. With the improvement of morphometric protocols, the implementation of novel imaging and analysis techniques is likely to expand the scope of biological investigation and enable the investigation of more complex morphological events (Goring et al., 2018) (Figure 13.3).

13.1.1. Traditional Morphometrics

Traditional morphometrics has long been a standard method of analysis in the field of biological shape and form. The technique is generally the measurement of lengths, angles, and proportions from samples of biology. Scientists can determine means, variances, and differences between populations with the utilization of calipers or similar equipment, hence a comparative framework through which to analyze differences in morphologies. Despite its antiquity, traditional morphometrics has been severely faulted for relying on a limited number of measurements that could be inefficient in capturing shape complexity. Consequently, its application could overlook possibly complex and important differences to evolutionary adaptation. In order to improve the interpretive ability of this technique, researchers must use caution in the measures picked so that they are suitable for questions posed in evolutionary biology and systematics. As scientific knowledge has developed, the limitations of traditional morphometrics have brought into question new approaches, such as geometric morphometrics. This new paradigm utilizes a more quantitative mathematical system to describe shape change with landmarks in shapes. Through the use of coordinate data, scientists are able to provide a comprehensive description of shape and obtain richer interpretations of morphological diversity. For instance, plant morphology research has been significantly improved through the integration of 3D geometric representation and conventional methods, thereby ensuring enrichment of floral structure research. Recent research has shown that the application of geometric morphometrics yields more comprehensive inquiries into ecological and evolutionary processes, and, by doing so, enhances resolution in quantitative analyses of variation among taxa (Johnson et al., 2010). This change in approach stresses the necessity that methodologies need to be realigned to maximize the fidelity of morphometric analysis. In conjunction with methodological advances, the detection of measurement error in morphometric analysis is becoming increasingly important. Traditional analyses neither account for the potential differences due to data capture methods nor consider variable specimen presentations and imaging hardware. Research emphasizes the significance that measurement error has on statistical inference and categorizing conclusions. To illustrate, milestone coordinate-based research into mammalian teeth has revealed that data acquisition errors can account for over 30% of overall variability between sets (Adams D C et al., 2020). This finding underscores the need for standardized protocol in the taking of morphometric measurements so that resulting analyses are representative of true biological variation and not a product of measurement error. By eliminating these sources of bias, scientists can make their findings more robust, thereby advancing morphometric analysis and contributing to a greater understanding of biological diversity.

13.1.2. Geometric Morphometrics

In biological science, geometric morphometrics is a useful analytical method for measuring and interpreting variation in shape among organisms. Geometric morphometrics is landmark-based and is designed to capture subtle details of biological form, allowing researchers to quantify morphological variation among and within species and populations. Geometric morphometrics is distinct from traditional morphometrics, which prefers linear measurements. It employs coordinate positions of landmarks. These landmarks, chosen for their specific anatomical relevance, provide a robust scaffold to which statistical analysis can be applied, enabling shape change to be visualized in an array of multidimensional spaces. Through this methodological precision, researchers can examine complex biological forms, thereby facilitating more refined interpretations of evolutionary relationships and functional adaptations. Although it has its advantages, using geometric morphometrics is not without its limitations, particularly in terms of measurement precision and potential for error. Recent research has determined that how data is collected can introduce significant variance to results, in some cases up to 30% of total variation between datasets (Adams et al., 2020). This highlights the need for proper standardization in data collection procedures, including specimen presentation and digitization protocols. Variation between different observers or imaging conditions can lead to conflicting classifications and undermine the reliability of conclusions drawn. Accordingly, in performing morphometric analyses, researchers must remain conscious of such likely sources of error and take active measures to minimize them to enhance the fidelity of results. In addition, the use of geometric morphometrics is not only restricted to taxonomy and evolutionary biology. For instance, its use in elucidating craniofacial characteristics of genetic disorders, such as 22q11.2 deletion syndrome, offers crucial insights into underlying developmental mechanisms of dysmorphology (Aggarwal et al., 2015). Utilizing advanced landmarking techniques and three-dimensional imaging, not only can facial morphology between affected patients be contrasted, but also comparisons can be drawn between facial dysmorphology and other disorders, such as schizophrenia. This similarity in facial dysmorphology provides new insight into the complex interplay between genetics and phenotype, once again reinforcing the relevance of geometric morphometrics in clinical practice. Having these applications in view, it is essential that scientists leverage geometric morphometrics, both its methodological constraints and potential for advancing our understanding of biological shapes (Figure 13.4).

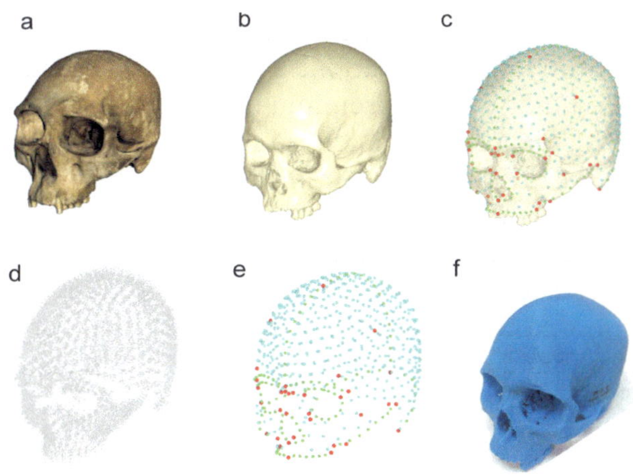

Figure 13.4. Geometric morphometrics.

Source: https://www.researchgate.net/publication/335056957/figure/fig1/AS:11431281222193082@1707128414847/A-typical-workflow-in-virtual-morphology-for-geometric-morphometric-research-in-digital.jpg.

13.1.3. Landmark-Based Morphometrics

Landmark-Based Morphometrics is a landmark advance in the morphometric analysis and measurement science, from linear measurement to a sophisticated geometric model. This technique employs fixed points, or landmarks, on biological material to measure their size and shape precisely. By superimposing these landmarks with Procrustes, researchers can remove scale, rotation, and translation effects and concentrate analysis purely on shape differences. The importance of landmark-based morphometrics has been clearly demonstrated in studies of domestic animal populations, where differences in cranial morphology can be used to characterize breeds and evolutionary trajectories. Remarkably, the geometric morphometrics approach has been demonstrated to provide higher discrimination and greater classification accuracy between groups, as indicated from comparative studies of several horse skulls that reveal hidden morphological differences not always highlighted by standard methods (Bentez-Molano et al., 2020). The core methodology of Landmark-Based Morphometrics has evolved substantially, from the simple linear analyses of earlier work to the sophisticated multivariate techniques of the present day. This is evident in numerous studies where shape quantification has played a pivotal role in understanding ecological and evolutionary processes. For instance, in studying cranial morphology among populations, scientists are able to quantify phenotypic adaptations in relation to environmental pressures. The higher accuracy of this method allows for analysis that can capture subtle morphological differences that can be lost to more traditional linear measurements. Furthermore, the blend of digital imaging and automatic landmark recognition has made the step of data collection easier, allowing for large sample sizes with less human error. This methodological advantage positions landmark-based morphometrics at the pinnacle of tools employed in contemporary biological research (Adams et al., 2018). Considering its utility, the applications of Landmark-Based Morphometrics bring it to transdisciplinary fields of study that place a premium on accurate morphological examination. For instance, in paleobiology, fossils can be examined in order to infer phylogenetic relations among extinct groups based on cranial morphology. Similarly, in forensic science, this technique can help identify species and support individual identification in court. The broad applicability of this approach indicates its significance in enriching our understanding with respect to biodiversity, evolutionary past, and species identification. As research continues to improve, the creation of landmark-based approaches will continue to yield more information on morphological structure across taxa, solidifying its position as a foundational approach within the broader field of morphometric analysis and quantification (Bentez-Molano et al., 2020) (Figure 13.5).

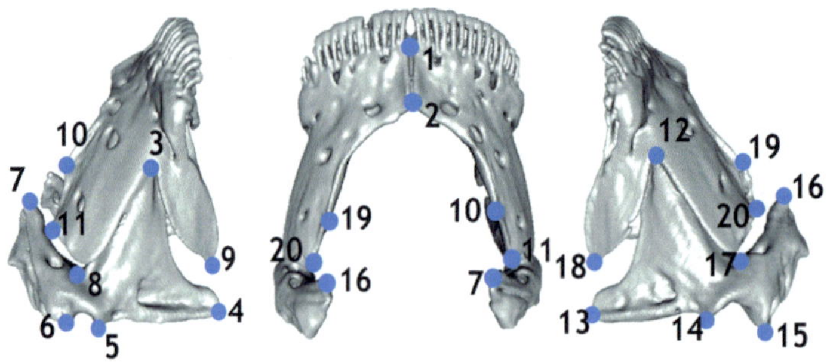

Figure 13.5. Landmark-based morphometrics.

Source: https://www.researchgate.net/publication/359402687/figure/fig1/AS:1160536741945350@1653704929386/Landmarks-used-for-morphometrics-analysis-Each-landmark-represents-a-functionally.png.

13.2. Data Collection Methods

The value of morphometric analysis and quantification lies in the reliability of the methods for gathering the data. These can be as uncomplicated as hand measurements using more involved digital approaches, such as geometric morphometrics and three-dimensional (3D) imaging. Hand measuring employs calipers and rulers, which are well known and simple, but are open to human interpretation and potential human error. On the other hand, advanced imaging techniques utilize computer programs to obtain accurate information from samples, making results more accurate and reproducible. Accuracy in data collection is of maximal significance because any degree of inaccuracy may lead to incorrect conclusions and interpretations. Thus, the use of innovative methods in morphometric investigations considerably enhances the quality and reliability of the obtained data, giving a crucial basis for analysis. Furthermore, technology has changed the processes by which data are gathered in morphometric studies. For instance, the use of machine learning algorithms is a transformative development in the discipline, enabling the efficient and accurate processing of vast morphometric datasets. A good example is the QuantiMus software, which enables quantification of muscle morphology with high precision. With advanced machine learning algorithms, QuantiMus can measure cross-sectional areas of myofibers and other morphological characteristics, thereby providing previously unattainable results using conventional techniques. This software demonstrates how simplifying the data collection process mitigates observer bias and increases reproducibility, an essential for scientific research. Developments such as these signal the beginning of a new era in morphometrics, with more objective and consistent data-collection procedures, ultimately leading to a more robust field. At the same time, the classic gathering of morphometric data still has relevance where technology is unaffordable or inappropriate. Traditional methods can be used as a foundation on which new technologies can be created. For instance, systematic observation and careful measurements carried out on bone artifacts can yield highly useful qualitative information on morphology, just like in the case of stone tool use in chimpanzees, as provided in palaeoanthropology research. These works highlight the importance of damage pattern recognition and differentiation among different usage types as the foundation for an enhanced understanding of prehistoric and modern organisms' adaptive strategies. The union of manual and automatic methods thus becomes an intertwined data accumulation strategy that not only enhances precision but also preserves the interpretive knowledge gleaned from well-gathered empirical information, becoming a cornerstone of morphometric analysis and quantification.

13.2.1. Measurement Techniques

Morphometric analysis relies heavily on precise measurement techniques that enable the reproducible quantification of biological structures. Modern medical imaging technologies, such as multidimensional visualization instruments, enable the creation of voluminous amounts of data that require sophisticated computational tools for evaluation. For instance, Krenz et al. (2010) developed an automatic algorithm for morphometric analysis that integrates cutting-edge image processing libraries to segment three-dimensional structures and form hierarchical structures. This not only enhances the speed at which the data is processed but also eradicates operator bias, thus providing accurate and reliable measurements obtained. Through the employment of robust techniques, scientists can draw meaningful inferences about the structural and functional characteristics of various biological systems and thereby contribute to enhanced knowledge about their physiology and pathology. Following advancements in imaging technology, machine learning algorithms have emerged as effective agents for maximizing measurement techniques in morphometric analysis. Machine learning algorithms can enable fast measurement of morphological attributes, as exemplified by software such as QuantiMus. QuantiMus, according to Ayer et al. (2019), enables precise measurement of myofiber cross-sectional area (CSA) and quantification of other traits more accurately than traditional manual evaluations. The ability of the software to analyze entire muscle sections irrespective of sampling ensures greater rigor and reproducibility when estimating muscle regeneration and pathology.

These new measurement techniques are necessary for distinguishing minute morphological differences that may signal underlying pathological change and thereby enhance our interpretative capacity in biological research. The combination of these sophisticated measurement techniques with morphometric analysis is necessary for advancing the understanding of complex biological systems. The application of automated image analysis combined with machine learning gives rise to a synergistic effect that not only accelerates morphometric assessments but also enhances their precision. As epitomized by the approaches presented in Krenz et al. (2010) and Ayer et al. (2019), automating the process of measurement not only facilitates research in morphology but also provides means for conducting large-scale studies across different fields. By doing so, therefore, the application of advanced measurement techniques not only improves the level of accuracy in morphometric analysis but also provides a window for paradigm-changing discoveries in health, disease, and developmental biology, a testament to the immense power of technology in scientific research (Figure 13.6).

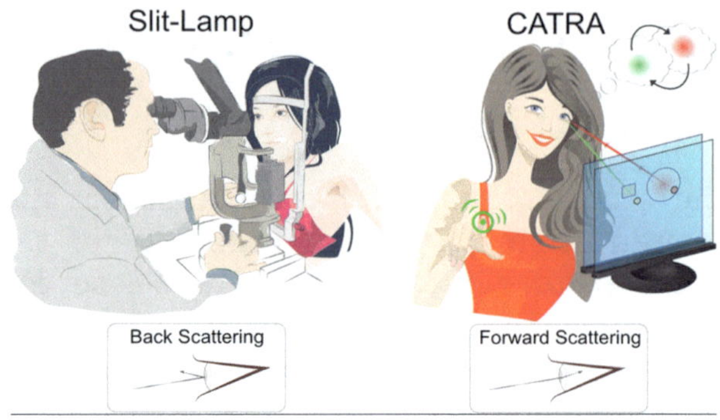

Figure 13.6. Measurement techniques.

Source: https://www.researchgate.net/profile/Vitor-Pamplona/publication/338582759/figure/fig17/AS:847288721211401@1579020781414/Can-one-create-a-device-that-makes-people-aware-of-their-early-cataract-condition-Using.ppm.

13.2.2. Imaging Technologies

The development of advanced imaging technologies has significantly influenced morphometric analysis and quantification by enabling scientists to obtain detailed information on structural parameters in biological systems. Advanced magnetic resonance imaging (MRI) and computed tomography (CT) technologies can generate multidimensional datasets that accurately describe anatomical traits. This precision is essential to identify minute morphological changes, particularly in disease development or anatomical variability research. By utilizing a combination of these technologies, morphometric analysis algorithms are designed to automate the process and enhance accuracy. As noted by Krenz et al. (2010), such algorithms facilitate three-dimensional segmentation and vessel diameter optimization, which is the key to comprehending the biomechanics of vascular structures and therefore demonstrating their invaluable contribution to the research methodologies of today. Furthermore, the use of imaging technology transcends visualization to enable a profound quantification of morphological characteristics. At research centers and hospitals, like the Medical Imaging Laboratory, Hospital General Universitario Gregorio Marañón, there has been emphasis on bringing imaging breakthroughs into clinically useful applications. The creation of software tools that can quantify multimodal brain images is a notable step in this direction. With their ability to process morphometric and functional data, these tools not only illuminate complex biological systems but also enable translational studies aimed at addressing real-world clinical issues. As described in Déndez et al. (2009), the ability to analyze multidimensional data on high-end imaging platforms is a critical advance for cognitive neuroscience and other fields of medicine.

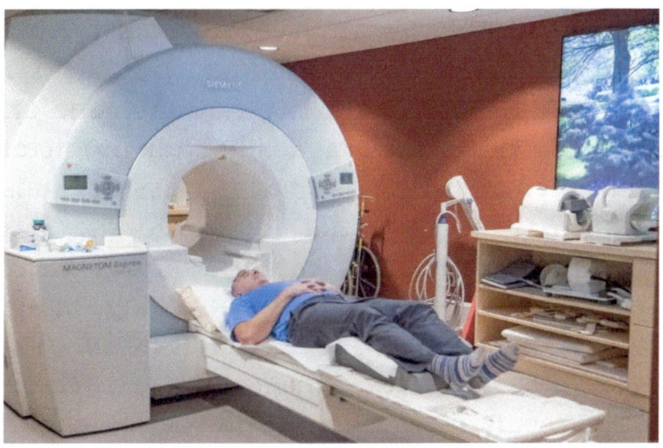

Figure 13.7. Imaging technologies.

Source: https://camiscare.ca/wp-content/uploads/2018/10/DSC01623_1-e1557173112825.jpg.

The creation of imaging tools for use in morphometric analysis also poses challenges and possibilities in data management. The sheer volume of data generated needs to be retained and processed well to facilitate useful inferences from results. Advanced computational techniques, including models of machine learning, are increasingly being employed to manage the richness of data. Furthermore, computerization of morphometric analysis, as explained in Krenz et al. (2010), minimizes human error and time required for data evaluation, enabling researchers to focus on acquiring biological conclusions rather than lengthy measurements. With accelerating progress in the field, the integration of powerful imaging modalities and advanced computational capabilities not only enhances the accuracy of morphometric measurements but also provides new directions toward cutting-edge applications in precision medicine, thereby reinforcing the value of imaging technologies in current research (Figure 13.7).

13.2.3. Software Tools for Data Acquisition

The advent of advanced data acquisition software has revolutionized morphometric analysis, with more precise and effective measurements and quantifications of biological form than previously possible. Software packages such as QuantiMus show how machine learning algorithms are applied to enhance muscle morphology evaluation. This software not only facilitates quantification of myofiber cross-sectional area (CSA) but also provides efficient analysis of central nucleation, a valuable measure of muscle regeneration. By automating what has been a labor-intensive task, QuantiMus increases the speed and accuracy of data retrieval and therefore enhances the reproducibility of research results. Such software development enables researchers to scrutinize muscle pathologies more rigorously, gaining a greater insight into the underlying biology and permitting the production of targeted therapeutic interventions (Ayer et al., 2019). In addition to muscle analysis, data acquisition software is also required to study complex vascular networks. Recent advances have introduced algorithms permitting automated morphometric examination of three-dimensional datasets from advanced imaging techniques. These algorithms effectively segment, image, and quantify the intricate tree-like structures of vascular trees, revealing important information regarding their biomechanical characteristics.

By incorporating computational libraries for image processing, these programs not only streamline the analytical process but also eliminate operator bias, a common source of error in manual measurement techniques. For instance, computer-aided techniques for pulmonary vascular morphology analysis enable researchers to perform meaningful comparisons between health and disease, significantly easing the research study of lung diseases (Krenz et al., 2010). The far-reaching effects of these packages extend beyond data collection only; they mark a revolution in morphometric research methods. Studies made possible through cutting-edge data acquisition devices improve the reproducibility of outcomes, which is especially important in the case of preclinical research and drug development. Rapid analyses, such as those offered by QuantiMus or automated vascular morphology, make it possible to conduct large studies that can detect subtle morphological alterations with high statistical power. By. Increasing the quantity and quality of information collected, these software packages allow investigators to address complex biological problems more effectively and, as a result, push the frontiers of human understanding in such fields as muscle physiology and vascular biology (Krenz et al., 2010; Ayer et al., 2019).

13.3. Statistical Approaches in Morphometric Analysis

The application of statistical techniques in morphometric analysis is crucial to appropriately measure and interpret biological shape and form. Central among such techniques is geometric morphometrics, a statistical framework for analyzing differences in shape using landmark coordinates. Such a technique has come quite a long way in being applied for fine analyses in evolutionary biology, ecology, and taxonomy. Nevertheless, the accuracy of geometric morphometric analyses is dependent on methodological dependability and precision of data collection methods. Every time measurement error is uncontrolled, analyses resulting from it can be deceptive. A study that contrasted error in 2D landmark coordinate data illustrates this point well, showing that data-collection error can account for over 30% of total variation within datasets and highlighting the fundamental need for rigorous standardization in morphometric studies (Adams et al., 2020). Furthermore, multiple sources of measurement error will have a profound impact on the statistical outcomes of morphometric analysis. For instance, discrepancies can arise from specimen presentation, imaging devices, and interobserver or intraobserver variability. When evaluating these factors in landmark datasets, it becomes apparent that no two measurements are identical, which can drastically alter predicted group memberships in species classifications. As such, it is essential for researchers to implement consistent methodologies when digitizing landmarks and capturing image data to minimize potential biases. The research indicates that neglecting such errors would result in substantial misclassification, underscoring the importance of methodological rigor in morphometric analysis (Adams et al., 2020). In addition to measurement error control, statistical procedures used in morphometric analysis must also be deliberately selected to answer specific study queries. For instance, linear discriminant analysis is extensively applied in the classification of species from landmark data, but the prevalence of measurement error can affect its efficiency. As scientists proceed to analyze diverse morphological features, knowledge of the limitations and potential biases of different statistical tests is important. With the use of robust statistical models and the testing of errors in a strict manner, not only are the validity of the morphometric studies enhanced, but science as a whole advances since the findings make meaningful contributions to our knowledge of biological variance and evolutionary processes (Figure 13.8).

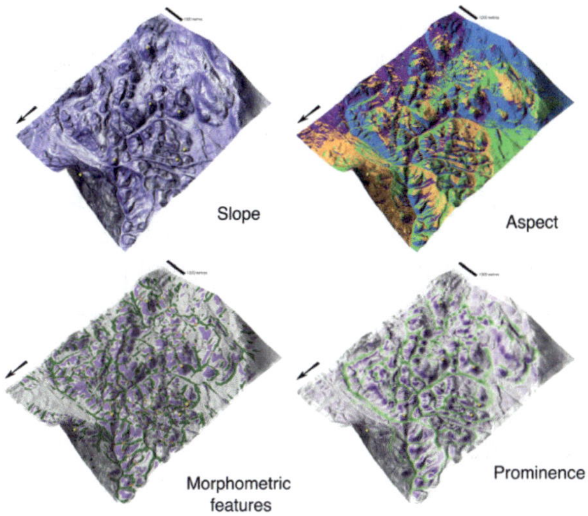

Figure 13.8. Statistical approaches in morphometric analysis.

Source: https://www.researchgate.net/profile/Silvia-Polla/publication/322735016/figure/fig3/AS:1136441694388228@1647960222964/Morphometric-analyses-of-the-topography-of-accessibility.ppm.

13.3.1. Descriptive Statistics

In the field of morphometric quantification and analysis, descriptive statistics are crucial in aggregating intricate multidimensional datasets acquired via cutting-edge imaging technologies. By aggregating data into insightful values, i.e., means, medians, standard deviations, and ranges, scientists are able to draw meaningful conclusions about the structural properties of biological samples. The early statistical examination allows patterns and irregularities in the dataset to be identified, giving an initial basis for the knowledge of phenotypic differences. As an example, the application of descriptive statistics to volumetric analysis allows one to identify structural abnormalities in different conditions, for example, traumatic brain injury (TBI). In this context, descriptive statistics-driven measures may provide insight into the exploration of structural changes involved in clinical outcomes, ultimately contributing to enhanced prognostication and therapy (Aylward et al., 2012). Descriptive statistics not only ease the interpretation of data but also facilitate an initial evaluation of morphometric measures. By generating summary statistics for different morphological parameters, such as vessel diameter or pulmonary surface area in vascular research, scientists can determine required standards and baseline characteristics. Quantification is significant, particularly in research depending on advanced imaging modalities, where huge volumes of data will overwhelm the analytical process. Techniques described in current methodologies, such as computer-based algorithms to conduct morphometric analysis, are significantly facilitated by a sound descriptive statistical basis. By establishing consistent measures prior to conducting multivariate statistical analyses, researchers can ensure adequate representation of the dataset's key traits, thereby increasing the reliability of findings (Krenz et al., 2010). Furthermore, the inclusion of descriptive statistics in morphometric analysis provides a broader study of correlations among the structural components and the functional outcomes. For instance, contrasting morphological profiles between conditions can reveal significant associations that give insights into biological behavior. In the case of TBI patients, examining the relationship between structural variables from neuroimaging and cognitive performance captures the research value of this statistical technique. Employing descriptive statistics to interpret such relationships enables researchers to uncover biomarkers that are predictors of clinical outcomes. In the context of shifting approaches, descriptive statistics are important not only to summarize the data but also to establish a template for future studies with an eye towards expanding the predictive power of morphometric analyses (Aylward et al., 2012).

13.3.2. Multivariate Analysis

Multivariate analysis is a critical tool in morphometric analysis and quantification, and it allows researchers to investigate intricate relationships in data involving more than one variable. The technique is most useful in the evaluation of biological forms because it can examine multiple morphological characteristics simultaneously. By applying techniques such as principal component analysis (PCA) and canonical variate analysis (CVA), scientists can reduce dimensionality without losing important information about variance among specimens. Through these analyses, scientists can identify patterns that could be hidden in univariate methods and thereby develop a better understanding of the evolutionary and functional relevance of morphological variation. The integration of multivariate statistics is vital in advancing the field, facilitating a deeper interpretation of the relationships between different morphological features and their ecological contexts. The implementation of advanced imaging techniques alongside multivariate analysis has significantly enhanced the accuracy of morphometric studies. For instance, 3D geometry obtained from micro-computed tomography scanning reveals the intricate details of biological structures that would be challenging to quantify using traditional methods. This innovation dovetails with multivariate statistical techniques, which can analyze the resulting geometric data effectively. Researchers investigating traumatic brain injury (TBI) outcomes have increasingly combined volumetric/morphometric analysis with advanced neuroimaging methods. Emerging studies indicate that integrating these approaches has substantial potential to identify biomarkers that predict clinical outcomes, thereby illuminating the mechanisms of TBI. This exemplifies how the synergistic application of morphometrics and multivariate analysis can lead to significant advancements in biomedical research, particularly in prognostication. Moreover, the application of multivariate analysis extends beyond medical research into various biological disciplines, such as evolutionary biology and plant systematics. The quantification of shape variation in angiosperm flowers, for instance, benefits from multivariate techniques that can handle the complexities of three-dimensional forms. By embracing geometric morphometric approaches, scientists are able to quantify floral diversity, throwing light on evolutionary adaptation and pollination strategies. Mentioned by recent research, the marriage of multivariate analysis with advanced imaging technologies enables robust visualization and elucidation of morphological information and therefore catalyzes a better understanding of biological diversification. This not only increases the analytical capabilities within the field but also emphasizes the dynamic interplay between form and function across diverse biological systems, reinforcing the importance of integrating multivariate analysis into standard morphometric practices.

13.3.3. Hypothesis Testing

Hypothesis testing is a key approach that helps in validating results from morphometric analysis. In such an approach, scientists are enabled to reach conclusions based on statistical evidence rather than intuition and speculation. This work on biological shape quantification allows scientists to determine whether the observed differences in morphological features among species were statistically significant. Using methods like linear discriminant analysis, researchers are able to determine the degree to which shape differences help differentiate classes in a dataset. Measurement error implications, as indicated by Adams et al. (2020), demonstrate that errors can account for large differences in outcomes, thereby underscoring the importance of hypothesis testing as a sound framework for accurate data interpretation. By testing specific hypotheses related to morphometric variations, scientists can enhance the fidelity of their analyses and bolster the credibility of their findings within broader biological contexts. The design of a robust hypothesis testing framework is essential for making sound inferences from morphometric datasets. This includes the selection of appropriate statistical tests to evaluate the null hypotheses against alternative hypotheses that postulate specific morphological traits. For instance, in addressing the species differentiation within the morphometric method, the tendency isto construct null hypotheses. These null hypotheses could claim that there is no meaningful difference in shape characteristics between the species under study. This relies on how well these tests control for intervening variables, such as specimen presentation and imaging equipment, as recommended by Adams et al. (2020). Failure to adequately control these factors may result in inappropriate conclusions about species classification. Therefore, the addition of hypothesis testing to the approach for morphometric analysis not only makes shape variation analytical work more orderly but also highlights the need for methodological rigor in biology.

Beyond its utility in checking the validity of experimental results, hypothesis testing enhances the effective communication of scientific findings within the morphometric analysis community. By providing a quantitative assessment of morphological differences, researchers can present their results in a manner that is both transparent and reproducible. In addition, as the literature on morphometric analysis grows, the application of hypothesis testing becomes increasingly important for comparing varying methods and results across studies. For example, in scaffold design for tissue engineering, as illustrated by the mechanical properties and degradation rates, can be statistically tested to affirm their viability for specific applications. Thus, incorporation of hypothesis testing in morphometric analysis not only forms the foundation for scientific research but also sets the stage for potential development in the field of biological shape science as well as practical applications in tissue engineering, thus proving the intrinsic worth of proper statistical approaches (Figure 13.9).

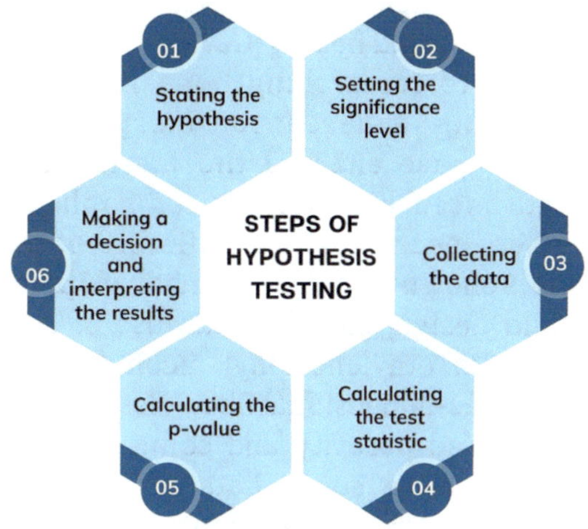

Figure 13.9. Hypothesis testing.

Source: https://miro.medium.com/v2/resize:fit:1200/0*ZoXKfS4jVaGPGCsQ.jpg.

13.4. Applications in Biological Research

The use of morphometric analysis in biological research has proven very helpful in describing many physiological processes, especially in relation to bone disease and health. Research published in recent years, for example, has shown the influence of age on bone porosity by the use of advanced imaging technologies such as synchrotron radiation-based computed tomography. Using this method, scientists can actually quantify the vascular canals and osteocyte lacunae distribution in mouse cortical bone. Results show dramatic age-related changes, with young and old specimens exhibiting striking differences in vascular density and structural integrity, most remarkably at important skeletal junctures. These findings further our understanding of the microarchitectural changes of aging and their impact on bone strength and fracture healing, and point towards therapeutic targets for degenerative disease conditions like osteoporosis. This emphasizes the importance of morphometric methods as primary instruments in biological research on skeletal disease and health (Goring et al., 2018). In addition to researching bone remodeling accompanying senescence, morphometric approaches have enabled the fabrication of highly advanced biomaterials for application in tissue engineering. The significance of these methods is shown by more recent developments in scaffold design, including the use of starch blended with ethylene-vinyl alcohol. By the design of three-dimensional fiber-mesh scaffolds with controlled porosity and connectivity, the researchers have succeeded in replicating the natural extracellular matrix. Scanning electron microscopy and microcomputed tomography provide detailed insight into scaffold morphology and are instrumental in highlighting key features such as pore size and interconnectivity. Such studies have proven the biocompatibility and structural integrity of scaffolds produced, rendering them as first-choice candidates for application in regenerative medicine. Quantification of these characteristics appropriately is essential for the purposes of advancing tissue engineering research (Athanasiou et al., 2014). Besides structural testing, the influence of morphometric analysis also encompasses functional testing in biological systems. The degradation behavior of the newly developed 3D scaffolds demonstrates the dynamic interactions between the biological and material environments. Enzymatic biodegradation of the scaffolds by alpha-amylase has been thoroughly studied, which shows a progressive increase in porosity and interconnectivity with continuous aging. Such biocompatibility is also supported by *in vitro* cell studies, which show an encouraging cellular response. The biological behavior of scaffolds is aligned with their morphometric attributes, which subsequently enables closer tailoring of their design to realize the maximum achievable effectiveness in tissue engineering. While thereby, such a methodology enhances our knowledge with respect to material characteristics, it also aids in unearthing the significance of morphometric measurement in making effective biology research methodologies (Athanasiou et al., 2014 Goring et al., 2018) (Figure 13.10).

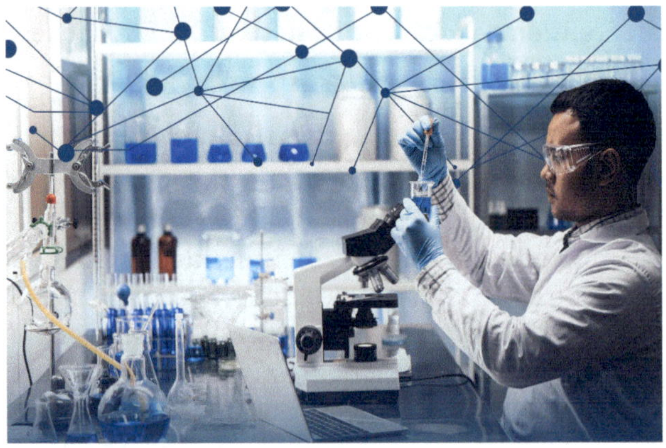

Figure 13.10. Applications in biological r.

Source: https://www.ucc.ie/en/media/research/abcrf/UCCFutures_Pharmaceuticals_MobileBanner_1024x640px_AW__5.jpg.

13.4.1. Evolutionary Biology

Evolutionary biology forms the core of explanation for the complexity of life forms through the application of morphometric analysis and quantification. Evolutionary biology entails the study of shape, size, and structural variation among living organisms, which can be quantified and analyzed to establish phylogenetic patterns and evolutionary directions. Morphometric techniques, geometric and traditional, allow scientists to convert the intricacy of biological structures into numeric information, and consequently engage in comparison both between species and lineages. By using such techniques, scientists are able to show how evolutionary pressures affect anatomical structures, and thus comprehend adaptation and speciation processes. Such examinations also allow one to study functional relationships and ecological interactions, which are critical to comprehending dynamic biodiversity patterns. In current research, novel uses of technologies have pushed morphometric analysis forward, increasing our knowledge of evolutionary biology significantly. For instance, new high-throughput imaging and sophisticated statistical models have revolutionized the capture and analysis of morphological data. By the use of geometric morphometrics, major advancements have been made in studying brittle anatomical structures, including vertebrate skeletons and insect wings. This technique not only enhances data collection accuracy but can also allow for visualization of shape and size variation that might be associated with environmental factors. Greater analytical capabilities have brought new insights to evolutionary processes by showing correlations between morphological features and their associated adaptive value, thereby adding richness to the theoretical underpinnings of evolutionary biology. Furthermore, interdisciplinary studies have begun to integrate morphometric analyses with genomic research and have progressed our understanding of evolutionary paths between species. Studies have proven the genetic basis of phenotypic variability, which has allowed an overall assessment of evolution that takes into account both form and function. For instance, comparing the olfactory receptors of mice, chimpanzees, and humans has revealed how slight genetic differences create morphological differences that can be accounted for with fractal analysis and mathematical morphology. Such research shows how the union of genomic data and morphometric tools enhances our potential to interpret the complexities of evolutionary history and dynamics of biodiversity, ascertaining the value of quantitative estimates in evolutionary biology (Goswami et al., 2011; Arroyo et al., 2015) (Figure 13.11).

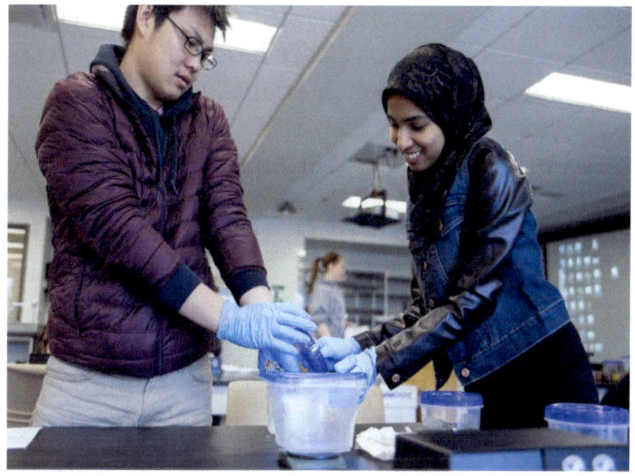

Figure 13.11. Evolutionary biology.

Source: https://semo.edu/colleges-departments/stem/biological-and-environmental-sciences/_images/2014-biology-lab-mp-0306-025-980x654.jpg.

13.4.2. Ecology and Environmental Studies

Research on morphometric analysis in environmental science and ecology is crucial because it provides valuable information on how organisms adapt to different environments. Biological differences can be measured and visualized using morphometric techniques, which may be a reflection of environmental pressure-evoked evolutionary processes. For instance, research on the body size of species might reveal adaptations in specific habitats, available resources, and threat by predators. In ecological studies, morphometric information also contributes to monitoring biodiversity and assessing the impact of habitat degradation. With the use of advanced analytical tools, ecologists can gain an integrated understanding of species interaction within their habitats, which sheds more light on ecological dynamics and serves to identify conservation measures for the maintenance of biodiversity. Moreover, the integration of technical development within morphometric analysis significantly reinforces ecological investigation. The application of geographic information systems (GIS) in this field facilitates the intricate modeling of species distribution and spatial analysis of anatomical features among populations. Numerous methods, for instance, automatic morphometric GIS classification, have been demonstrated to systematically investigate patterns of wear on tools used by chimpanzees in the wild, thus creating a new avenue for comparative studies with early human artefacts (Arroyo et al., 2015). Such between-species analyses are not only essential to determining behavioral evolution but also emphasize the role of technological proficiency in the persistence of species. By correlating morphometric variables directly with ecological outcomes, researchers can develop predictive models that better inform conservation efforts. Measurement error in morphometric analysis remains an important issue within the discipline as well. Recent studies demonstrate that many aspects, such as interobserver variability and imaging protocols, have the potential to bring tremendous variation in data quality and resulting statistical outcomes (Adams et al., 2020). It is important for researchers to recognize the implications of such kind of errors when they try to draw strong conclusions about ecological relationships and evolutionary trends. Because mistakes sometimes account for over 30% of variation in morphometric information, it is critically necessary to standardize procedures of data collection in an effort to enhance the dependability of results. By applying precise measurement protocols and consistent methodologies in research, ecologists can provide strong empirical evidence supporting substantial ecological interpretation as well as conservation actions, which ultimately support a sustainable future for rich ecosystems.

13.4.3. Medical and Clinical Applications

Morphometric analysis is a crucial part of medical and clinical applications, particularly in medical imaging. As imaging modalities have evolved, so has the need for competent analysis tools, particularly for assessing complex structures in the human body. Such tools are vital in distinguishing between normal and pathological conditions, thereby increasing diagnosis accuracy and the effectiveness of treatment protocols. For instance, research groups such as the Medical Imaging Laboratory at Hospital General Universitario Gregorio Marañón have developed advanced methods focused on the application of medical imaging. These works emphasize the importance of developing image analysis tools that allow the quantification of multimodal brain images and thus directly address clinical issues facing specialists (Déndez et al., 2009). The increase in multidimensional data sets that are produced by modern medical imaging scanners necessitates fast and reliable mechanistic studies. Computerized morphometric analysis has emerged as a solution to speed up the process, minimizing human bias and measurement errors. The development of an automated algorithm for three-dimensional segmentation of vascular structures and quantification is one such breakthrough area. These innovations enable scientists to observe biological systems more intensively in terms of structural and functional properties, particularly in the context of pulmonary vascular morphology. For example, the algorithm employs specialized processing libraries to estimate vessel diameters automatically, obtaining repeated measurements that are essential for analyzing variation in vascular properties across disease states (Krenz et al., 2010). Moreover, the application of these advanced analysis techniques to medical practice has the potential to improve outcomes for patients. By providing clinicians with more advanced tools for analysis, morphometric analysis enables health professionals with vital information necessary for the early detection of disease and monitoring of treatment efficacy. Utilization of morphometric software in clinical procedures can yield considerable benefits in chronic disease management, where the monitoring of exact anatomical changes is crucial. As witnessed by the efforts of research projects crossing basic science and clinical practices, such as those mentioned in funding research from various health ministries, continuous improvement in morphometric techniques is expected to continue providing more valuable applications in medical diagnosis and therapy interventions (Déndez et al., 2009) (Figure 13.12).

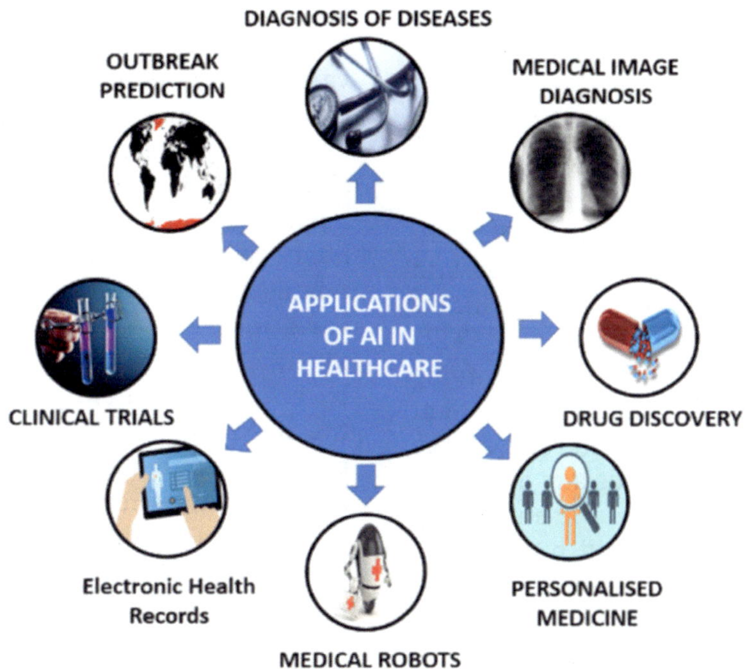

Figure 13.12. Medical and clinical applications.

Source: https://www.researchgate.net/publication/355954943/figure/fig3/AS:1094702044577792@1638008714362/A-representation-of-various-applications-of-AI-in-healthcare.png.

13.5. Challenges in Morphometric Analysis

The intricacy of morphometric analysis is hand in hand with several outstanding challenges that researchers need to overcome in order to get correct and enlightening results. One of the main challenges is the heterogeneity of biological systems affecting the validity and reproducibility of morphometric data. This heterogeneity can be caused by a broad host of variables, including genetic differences, environmental determinants, and methodological variations across studies. Moreover, phenotypically equivalent structures are difficult to distinguish, necessitating sophisticated imaging modalities and evaluations that may not be available to everyone. The complexity involved in accurate quantification of measurements such as cellular morphology, size, and vacuolar type introduces complexity, particularly when investigating reactions against various compounds. The work of researchers on foamy macrophages underscores the need for high-content image analysis to identify subtle morphological changes induced by drug exposure, highlighting the difficulty of obtaining consistent results across different contexts (Hoffman et al., 2020). Another challenge with morphometric analysis lies in gathering data from diverse imaging modalities and from a variety of data types. Sophisticated techniques such as structural and functional magnetic resonance imaging (MRI), diffusion tensor imaging (DTI), and volumetric analysis have to work together to provide a precise description of morphological alterations. Discrepancies in data alignment and interpretation, however, could be excellent obstacles and lead to inconclusive results or misinterpretations. The unification of multimodal neuroimaging techniques and morphometric analysis is particularly significant in fields such as traumatic brain injury (TBI) research, wherein the focus is on identifying biomarkers that will enable forecasting of patient outcomes. As mentioned in current reviews, the integration of statistical methods and advanced image processing is essential in enhancing morphometric analysis in this field, but requires rigorous standardization and verification for addressing the challenges involved (Aylward et al., 2012). Moreover, the interpretative nature of morphometric data further complicates the process of analysis. Researchers must struggle with defining clinically relevant thresholds and parameters that capture suitable biological significance, which proves to be subjective. For instance, while some morphometric changes are linked to pathological conditions, the judgment about what is an abnormal phenotype could vary depending on context. Such subjectivity can work against the reproducibility of results between studies or clinical settings. Additionally, application of statistical methods to discern patterns in morphometric data demands a strong understanding of multivariate analysis to reduce threats of overfitting or misidentification. Overcoming these interpretative difficulties is essential to optimizing the reliability of morphometric measurements and allowing further advances in the ways these analyses can inform therapy and clinical outcomes.

13.5.1. Variability in Biological Samples

Biological sample variation significantly affects the outcome of morphometric analysis, and a thorough knowledge of its causes and effects is needed. Accuracy in measurements, particularly in geometric morphometrics, is influenced by various parameters like specimen presentation, imaging techniques, and observer systematic error. Consideration of such variables becomes significant as data capture errors can lead to misinterpretation of the morphological features, hence twisting statistical findings. For instance, Adams et al. (2020) emphasize the case that variations in landmark precision are most pronounced when data are being digitized by two independent people, which indicates the need for standardization throughout the entire morphometric process. By recognizing and accounting for such sources of variability, scientists can make their analyses more reliable to ensure that the described variations truly indicate real biological differences and not artifacts of measurement. Furthermore, the biological stability of morphometric features often relies on their stability routinely, particularly for complex objects such as tumors. In studies such as those discussed by Jamshidi et al. (2017), stability concerning semi-automated segmentation of biological tissues demonstrates that many morphometric features indeed have high stability, but it remains the case that the quality of feature extraction is paramount. The experiments reveal that over 90% of the tested features were consistent well, but features like normalized dynamic range (NDR) indicated redundancy problems. This heterogeneity requires rigorous inspection of feature quality because redundant measurements can mask underlying biological signals. Thus, researchers are motivated to test and optimize their analytic processes for reliable and interpretable results, again illustrating the need for controlling variability in biological samples. Lastly, the nuances of variability also find their way into the preparation and analysis of samples on other platforms or in other studies. Differences may arise from minor variations in specimen handling, including fixation procedures, imaging parameters, and the software used for analysis. Such differences may create huge classification issues, particularly in morphometric studies that critically rely upon accurate shape descriptors to distinguish species or conditions. Addressing these challenges requires integrated procedures that bring data collection processes into alignment within different research settings. In addition, as noted in Adams et al. (2020), high error contribution to total variation in datasets requires strict controls in preventing potential biases. By creating consistency and dependability in the morphometric analysis process, researchers can achieve stronger conclusions regarding biological variability and eventually further the field's knowledge of function and shape within living organisms (Figure 13.13).

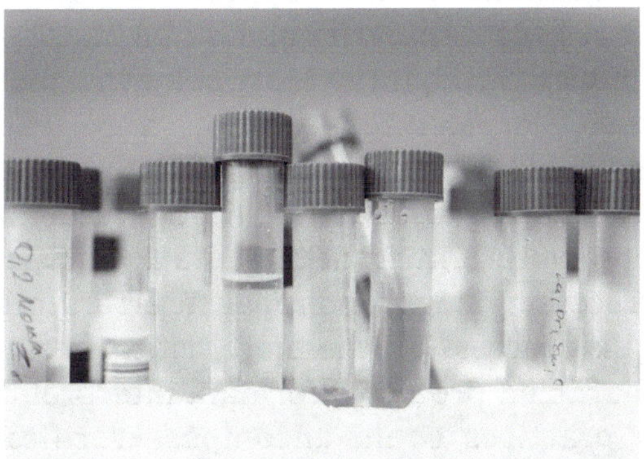

Figure 13.13. Variability in biological samples.

Source: https://area9lyceum.com/laboratorymedicine/wp-content/uploads/2020/05/samples-in-test-tubes-3735699.jpg.

13.5.2. Limitations of Measurement Techniques

Measurement techniques used in morphometric analysis, though imperative to measure biological structures, are not without limitations that can influence the accuracy and validity of findings. Traditional techniques such as histology have lengthy turnaround times as well as sample destruction, which can limit reproducibility as well as comparative studies. The inherent variability in processing and sectioning tissues may reduce the accuracy of measurements, particularly in heterogeneous tissues with "patchy" distribution of disease conditions. This inconsistency necessitates other techniques that can yield greater fidelity measurement, as seen in the creation of advanced software like QuantiMus. Through application of machine learning algorithms to the measurement of properties such as myofiber cross-sectional area, QuantiMus avoids some inherent disadvantages of manual measurement, which add analysis beyond that which can be achieved by more traditional methods in isolation, and ultimately improves rigor in the assessment of muscle pathology (Ayer et al., 2019). One significant limitation arises when comparing measurement strategies, for instance, when comparing microcomputed tomography (μCT) and histology. While histology has remained a gold standard for anatomical structure assessment for decades, it is limited by its destructive nature and reliance on two-dimensional interpretation. Compared to this, μCT offers three dimensions and faster processing, hence enabling more detailed analyses of bone integration to dental implants. However, despite the advantages of μCT, the latter still awaits being fully validated for histomorphometric parameters. Studies have revealed differences in measurements derived from these two approaches, where μCT may yield results different from histological assessments in some instances. The recognition and realization of these differences are of fundamental importance in the appropriate interpretation of morphometric data, particularly in studies carried out on complex biological interactions and materials (Coelho et al., 2013). Moreover, the incorporation of new techniques into morphometric analysis threatens the reproducibility of findings across studies and laboratories. Different measurement techniques may have their own bias and limitations, leading to differences when conclusions are being compared or transferred from one situation to another. For instance, the ease of use and scope for customization available in a tool like QuantiMus are of great advantage, yet they also have to be subjected to critical examination so that variability is not imposed by user-defined parameters. Appreciation of the inherent restrictions of each measurement technique is essential for researchers who aim to deliver solid conclusions from morphometric data. By encouraging an appreciation of these limitations, the scientific community will be better able to deal with the complexity of quantification in biological research and provide results that will have a useful place within our understanding of morphology and pathological process (Ayer et al., 2019).

13.5.3. Data Interpretation Issues

In morphometric analysis and quantification, data interpretation is a genuine limitation on the validity of conclusions drawn from high-dimensional datasets. Such problems are usually also further exacerbated by the natural complexity of multidimensional datasets routinely encountered in scientific research. For instance, the dynamic raster surface presentations of geographically and socio-economically oriented data, while appealing visually, have a tendency to mask the essential information required for proper decision-making. Some key limitations of the method include poor information presentation and difficulties establishing spatial and temporal continuity, both of which are essential for valid analysis. The research work offered by scholars suggests that the visualization methods, including representing surfaces as morphometric features, can overcome these limitations, thus improving the interpretability of complex data sets and enabling more improved analytical results (Dykes, J. & Rana, S., 2002). A second pressing issue in the interpretation of data in morphometric studies involves the handling of voluminous datasets generated with the help of advancements in imaging technology. Such datasets, typically abundant in numerous variables, need sophisticated analysis tools and effective methodologies to interpret with utmost accuracy. Automated algorithms in morphometric analysis have demonstrated significant potential to address these gaps by enabling high-speed analysis and integrating image processing libraries to perform data segmentation accurately. Such technological advancements allow for the measurement of complex anatomical structures, such as vascular trees, and minimize user bias and operator variation. Furthermore, continuous validation with established methods subjects the effectiveness of advances to greater scrutiny, suggesting that automatic data interpretation is crucial for resolving the inherent challenges of conventional manual approaches (Krenz et al., 2010). Data integrity should be maintained all the way through the morphometric analysis process, as misinterpretation may lead to wrong conclusions that can influence research outcomes and subsequent utilization. Inability to give proper attention at the data acquisition or preprocessing stage can propagate errors into the analysis process. It is therefore critical to employ standardized protocols for data interpretation. Such practices could encompass verification techniques evidenced to cross-check findings and identify potential inconsistencies early in the analysis. Secondly, the vital examination of metrics produced, combined with the enhancement in visualization techniques, holds the promise to provide better insight into the relations in data. By solving these problems in data interpretation, the validity of results can be improved by researchers, which consequently contributes to a more robust body of knowledge in morphometric analysis (Dykes, J. & Rana, S., 2002) (Figure 13.14).

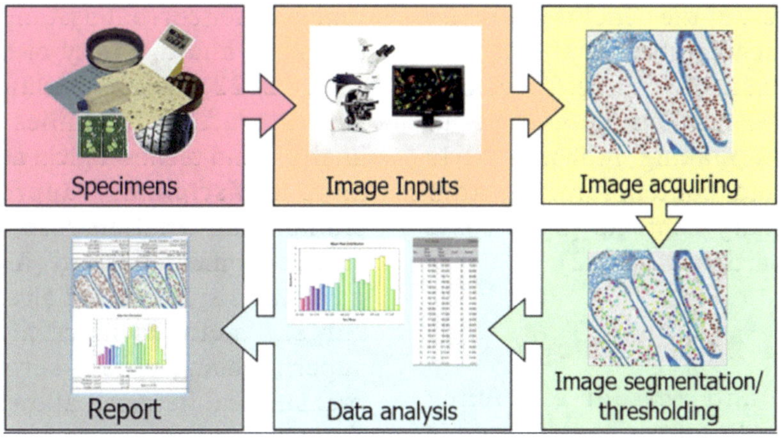

Figure 13.14. Data interpretation issues.

Source: https://media.springernature.com/lw685/springer-static/image/chp%3A10.1007%2F978-3-031-36850-9_2/MediaObjects/541053_1_En_2_Fig1_HTML.png.

13.6. Future Directions in Morphometric Research

With advances in morphometric science, the integration of novel imaging technologies is leading the charge of future research directions within the field. The integration of structural and functional neuroimaging modalities, such as MRI and DTI, has opened up new lines of inquiry into the elucidation of complex biological structure. Specifically, the examination of ways in which these imaging modalities may be integrated with volumetric and morphometric measures enables one to identify nuanced differences between biological systems. This multimodal approach not only enhances the accuracy of morphometric measurements but also allows for the identification of new biomarkers that are predictive of a particular physiological or pathological status. In this respect, embracing multimodal imaging is poised to revolutionize morphometric studies and expand its relevance across different scientific fields. As part of the evolving technological landscape, the use of machine learning and artificial intelligence in morphometric assessment holds tremendous promise. These computational methods can handle large sets of data with great speed, revealing subtle patterns not found by traditional analytical techniques. By using algorithms trained on morphometric data, scientists can improve data interpretation and enhance predictive modeling across contexts ranging from anthropology to medicine. Additionally, using such technologies can improve real-time interactivity and dynamic visualization of morphometric attributes, enhancing the applied utility of research findings. Consequently, the future of morphometric research lies in such developments, because they offer greater understanding and knowledge of the dynamics of form and structure in biology. Finally, the solution to problems with visualizing dynamic raster surfaces remains an important subject for future morphometric research. Conventional models are not always able to present comprehensive, interactive data, which limits the possibilities for effective data provision. But recent developments attempting to re-describe surfaces in terms of morphometric structures hugely improve this aspect of research. Graphic lag and spatial generalization are methods that offer novel ways of representing complex datasets, hence facilitating interpretative potential. By improving visualization methods and tools, researchers are able to increase stakeholder involvement, such as policymakers and the general public, so that morphometric scholarship may penetrate more deeply into societal discourse. Therefore, making graphical presentations more powerful will be essential in making morphometric research relevant and contemporary within various interdisciplinary contexts (Dykes, J. & Rana, S., 2002; Aylward et al., 2012).

13.6.1. Advances in Technology

Higher-precision and higher-efficiency technology in morphometric analysis has greatly advanced in the field. High-resolution imaging methods, like high-resolution micro-computed tomography (μCT), enable capturing the anatomical structure in greater detail than ever. Not only does it facilitate visualization of the intricate morphology within the cranial perspective, but it also makes it possible to extract finer landmark data required for more robust shape analysis. Such imaging of high resolution is critical for surgical planning and assessment, particularly in congenital correction like craniosynostosis. As reported in recent studies, the confluence of automated surgical planning based on these imaging modalities demonstrates the technology's capacity to overcome variability in surgical prognosis among surgeons, thereby improving surgical outcomes through personalized preoperative planning (Mato et al., 2021). In addition to imaging innovation, the adoption of geometric morphometrics as part of the morphometric analysis toolkit is a reflection of the underlying paradigm shift involved in seeing anatomical variations. With this methodology, computational techniques are employed to measure shape change and clarify discrete clusters of anatomical information that cannot be resolved using traditional classification. For instance, new research on human mandibular shape variation highlights how genetic and environmental factors interact to control craniofacial growth. With 3D scanning coupled with morphometric analysis, researchers have determined new shape clusters that counter current assumptions regarding the evolution and diversity of humans (Sivakumar et al., 2023). These findings are reflective of the interactive dynamics of morphological analysis and technological advances and require an interdisciplinary approach in explaining craniofacial variation. Also, newer technologies such as augmented reality (AR) and intraoperative navigation systems are already revolutionizing surgery methods in craniofacial surgery. By superimposing virtual surgical plans onto the real surgical field, AR allows surgeons to guide their instruments with phenomenal precision, enhancing the precision of osteotomy and remodeling phases in craniosynostosis surgery. Meanwhile, intraoperative optical tracking-based navigation offers real-time feedback, aligning remodeled bone fragments to preoperative targets, thus ensuring compliance with patient-specific surgical plans. These technological innovations not only make the surgical process easier but also reduce complications and improve overall patient outcomes. Incorporating such advanced equipment in clinical settings is a testament to how much technology has impacted morphometric analysis, leading the way in developing our understanding of surgical anatomical considerations in craniofacial procedures (Mato et al., 2021).

13.6.2. Integration with Genomic Data

The integration of genomic data into morphometric analysis is a milestone towards the attainment of biological diversity and evolutionary processes. By the use of precise genomic data, researchers can unveil the genetic factors underlying morphological variation experienced in populations. The analysis method is one that moves beyond the traditional morphometrics, where form and shape were primarily analyzed without regard for the genetic factors. For instance, improvements in imaging technology and genetic sequencing enable full datasets that are able to correlate physical characteristics with identified genetic markers. The value of such an integration emerges in craniofacial structure studies, where knowing the genetic factors can reveal patterns and differences that are insusceptible to traditional groupings. These findings not only augment our understanding of human evolution but also provide a foundation for a better understanding of functional anatomy across contexts, thereby focusing on the intricate interaction between morphology and genetics in shaping organismal diversity (Sivakumar et al., 2023). Furthermore, the application of genomic data in morphometric analysis assists in establishing adaptive traits in various environments. By integrating genetic markers linked to specific phenotypic expressions, researchers can investigate how particular morphological traits confer survival advantages in specific ecological niches. This integration also intersects with the field of bioinformatics, where complex datasets integrate environmental conditions and genetics to further model adaptive evolution. For instance, the knowledge of divergence in male and female mandible shape can reveal more general patterns related to sexual selection and ecological adaptation. This type of analysis allows researchers to challenge dominant paradigms as well as inform conservation strategies aimed at safeguarding new phenotypic variation, which may harbor critical genetic diversity. Therefore, the effective integration of morphometric investigations within broader ecological contexts serves to emphasize the need for multidisciplinary approaches to the interpretation of adaptation (Berg et al., 2020). The uses of the integration of genomic data with morphometric analysis extend into clinical and applied science, particularly in personalized medicine and evolutionary biology. With growing understanding of the genetic basis of phenotypic variation, there is huge potential for new diagnostics and interventions tailored to specific genetic profiles. This convergence not only enables better prediction of health outcomes but also enhances our capacity to design treatment plans for morphological and genetic characteristics. Moreover, the study of the relationship between genetic variation and phenotypic characteristics provides new avenues of research in evolutionary biology, where this knowledge can explain speciation processes and flexibility over time. By relating morphometric analysis with genetic data, researchers can further validate the significance of conservation of genetic diversity among species, which is crucial in ecological resilience and adaptation in the course of global change (Sivakumar et al., 2023) (Figure 13.15).

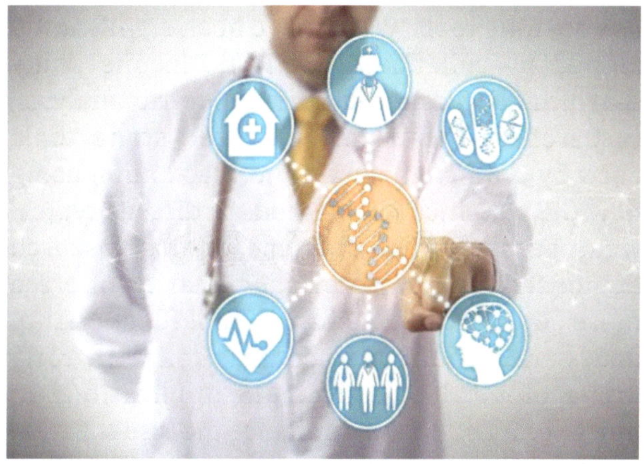

Figure 13.15. Integration with genomic data.

Source: https://thumbs.dreamstime.com/b/unrecognizable-male-clinician-integrating-genomic-data-clinical-workflow-healthcare-concept-pharmacogenomics-118645604.jpg.

13.6.3. Interdisciplinary Approaches

Inter-disciplinary investigation is central to advancing morphometric analysis and quantification, encouraging inter-disciplinary exchange in progressing across disciplines. By integrating biological, geological, and computational approaches, researchers are in a better position to extract more complex insight into the variability of shape and functional morphology. For example, the application of geographic information systems (GIS) for spatial analysis enhances the understanding of how morphological traits are distributed at the population level and how they respond to environmental pressures. This progressive methodology is able to evaluate the evolutionary significance of form and structure in a highly integrated fashion. Because such collaborations expand not only the datasets but also the creation of new instruments and frameworks required to investigate complex biological processes, the differing methodological outlooks affect stronger interpretations when working with ancient artifacts or modern specimens. Interdisciplinary approaches are shown in studies of chimpanzee use of stone tools, which have been significantly helped by collaborative efforts. In one study that utilized advanced morphometric analysis, researchers thoroughly analyzed stone tools used by wild chimpanzees to crack nuts, using new GIS classification methods to discern typical wear patterns. The outcome of this research demonstrates how interdisciplinarity offers a more sophisticated picture of tool functionality and, hence, the ease of comparison with early archaeological evidence. GIS applications in morphometric analysis enhance the visualization and interpretation of morphological differences, both in the present and in the past. In effect, these cross-disciplinary researches create a shared pool of knowledge that enriches anthropology and archaeology by connecting evolutionary biology and material culture to reveal the intricate interactions between species and their tools (Arroyo et al., 2015). Cross-disciplinary applications are also relevant in fisheries science, particularly with stock identification methods. The Stock Identification Methods Working Group (SIMWG) is yet another instance of interdisciplinary collaboration towards improving the understanding of fish population structure and dynamics. Employing a range of analytical tools, from genetics to morphometrics to tagging methods, SIMWG produces valuable information to aid management decision-making on resources. The integration of multiple methodologies enables improved estimation of stock boundaries, which underpins fisheries management success. Additionally, interdisciplinarity in discussions among researchers ensures that the issues brought about by climate-induced changes in stock compositions are properly tackled. Ultimately, the collaborative skills outlined in such collaborations ensure an optimization of the rigor in morphometric research, and thus a more substantial understanding of ecological and evolutionary dynamics in aquatic systems (Berg et al., 2020) (Figure 13.16).

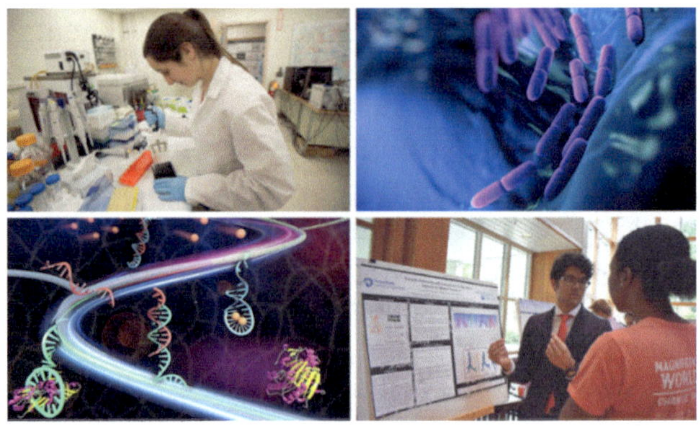

Figure 13.16. Interdisciplinary approaches.

Source: https://www.bme.psu.edu/assets/images/news/2018/BME-interdisciplinary-collage.png.

SUMMARY

In conclusion, the application of morphometric analysis and quantification plays a crucial role in explaining how biological structures evolve and their functions. By employing techniques such as scanning electron microscopy (SEM) and microcomputed tomography (μCT), researchers can delineate and quantify key parameters, including porosity, interconnectivity, and pore size, in biomaterials. The outcomes of experiments performed on scaffolds, such as those obtained from a blend of starch and ethylene-vinyl alcohol, tell us a great deal about their mechanical performance and degradation behavior, both of which are essential for their application in tissue engineering. Notably, scaffold synthesis of highly elastic and rapidly degrading materials under physiological conditions underscores the importance of morphometric approaches in advancing biomaterials for regenerative medicine (Athanasiou et al., 2014). Secondly, the integration of morphometric analysis with advanced imaging modalities provides insights into the complexities of structural change within various biological systems, notably in traumatic brain injury (TBI) research. Recent studies suggest the importance of multimodal neuroimaging methods like MRI, fMRI, and DTI in studying the interaction between morphometric changes and their functional implications. Connectome-level quantification enables researchers to set up novel biomarkers for better prediction of TBI outcome. Such developments attest to the evolving climate of neuroimaging and emphasize the call for an interdisciplinary framework that pairs morphometric analysis with cutting-edge imaging technology to respond to overarching questions about brain health and trauma (Aylward et al., 2012). Finally, uses of morphometric analysis are sweeping past basic science and influencing clinical practice and treatment intervention. As researchers delineate the structural correlations with functional outcomes, the search for precision medicine in fields such as tissue engineering and neurology becomes increasingly feasible. The identification of unique morphometric parameters as biomarkers not only clarifies disease mechanisms but also unlocks the potential for targeted therapies. In conclusion, the future of morphometric quantification and analysis is promising, with potential to fill knowledge gaps and pave the way towards innovations in biomaterials and neurological well-being. Continued exploration of these techniques will be paramount as we transition to continue refining our approaches towards solving complex biological challenges and improving patient outcomes in a number of disciplines.

Considering the intricacies of cerebral anatomy in neonates gives us the preliminary picture of the developing brain in early life and emphasizes the significance of morphometric inspection and quantification. Formulating cerebral anatomy is difficult and necessitates sophisticated methodologies that employ sophisticated imaging modalities. Image analysis algorithm development enables automatic vessel tree extraction and modeling of the cerebral vessels, including vessel tracking from strategically seeded locations and generation of fully representative vascular reconstructions. These techniques are central to vasculature development investigation because they can uncover vital transitions in the neonatal stage and provide better insight into cerebral structure growth patterns, effectively enabling pediatric neurodevelopmental studies (Xue, 2008). Further advancing neonatal cortex research, segmentation techniques developed with respect to the unique characteristics of the neonatal brain are paramount. Traditional adult-based algorithms will mislabel gray and white matter in neonates due to varying tissue characteristics, such as mixed pixel type mislabeling. A novel expectation-maximization method has been introduced to address this issue and improve cortical segmentation by eliminating partial volume mislabeling. After segmentation, the implicit evolution method of reconstructing the cortex results in a closer representation of its true form.

This precise approach not only enhances morphometric analysis but also enables more reliable quantification of cortical properties to better analyze developmental patterns in the neonatal brain (Xue, 2008). Aside from imaging technology improvements, understanding of morphometric alteration in geologic environments—e.g., long-runout landslides—confirms the varied application of quantification tools. Experiments in Valles Marineris have revealed distinctive morphological features and transport mechanisms of such landslides, for which geological mapping and analysis have provided comprehensive insight into the transport process. Scientific exploration has revealed that the morphology of landslides is characterized by a two-zone model with a varying degree of mobility with reference to mass and transport distances. Besides, the presence of hydrated silicates in these marginal regions of the landslide indicates a relationship between mobility and mineral composition, wherein the quantification methods are able to shed light on complex relationships in the geological ground. These analyses point to the cross-disciplinary relevance of morphometric analysis, ranging from neuroimaging to geology, indicating its fundamental role in driving scientific knowledge as well as applied fields.

A LOOK TO THE FUTURE:

MEDICAL IMAGING LABORATORY:

The field of medical imaging has revolutionized modern healthcare by enabling clinicians and researchers to see inside the human body with unprecedented clarity and precision. A Medical Imaging Laboratory is at the heart of this transformative discipline: a specialized environment where advanced imaging technologies, computational methods, and scientific inquiry converge to improve diagnostic accuracy, guide therapeutic decisions, and drive innovation in medicine and biomedical research. Medical imaging itself refers to the use of various physical principles to visualize internal anatomy and physiological processes for clinical analysis and the assessment of disease and injury. Medical imaging laboratories serve multiple purposes across academic, clinical, and research settings. In educational institutions, such laboratories provide students and trainees with hands-on experience in acquiring, processing, and interpreting images produced by modalities such as X-ray radiography, computed tomography (CT), magnetic resonance imaging (MRI), ultrasound, and nuclear imaging techniques. By facilitating practical understanding of imaging physics, instrument operation, and image visualization tools, these labs play a crucial role in preparing future radiologic technologists, biomedical engineers, and clinicians.

Beyond education, medical imaging laboratories are central to cutting-edge research and innovation. They integrate technologies from engineering, computer science, and artificial intelligence to develop new imaging methods and enhance existing ones. For example, research in image processing and analysis focuses on improving segmentation, registration, and quantitative interpretation of complex datasets, enabling automated detection of abnormalities and supporting decision-making in clinical contexts. Some labs also pursue interdisciplinary projects that combine imaging with bioinformatics and machine learning to extract meaningful biomarkers and predictive models from large volumes of imaging data. These laboratories contribute not only to diagnostic imaging but also to the advancement of personalized medicine. By enabling earlier detection of disease, more accurate characterization of pathological conditions, and better monitoring of treatment response, imaging research is directly linked to improved patient outcomes. The integration of artificial intelligence and computational analysis into imaging workflows further enhances efficiency and precision, reducing the time needed for interpretation and expanding the potential for real-time clinical applications.

Importantly, the Medical Imaging Laboratory is a hub of collaboration, bringing together clinicians, scientists, and technologists who share a common goal: to expand the boundaries of what can be seen and understood within the living human body. By fostering innovation and translating scientific discoveries into clinical practice, these laboratories continue to shape the future of healthcare and biomedical research.

REFERENCES

1. Macleod, N., Hall, M. J. R., & Wardhana, A. H. (2018). Towards the automated identification of Chrysomya blow flies from wing images. *Medical and Veterinary Entomology*, *32*(3), 323–333. https://doi.org/10.1111/mve.12302Adams, D. C., Arnqvist, G., Cardini, A., Chapman, R. E., Fox, N. S., Patterson, B. D., Rohlf, F. J., et al. (2020). Are geometric morphometric analyses replicable? Evaluating landmark measurement error and its impact on extant and fossil *Microtus* classification. http://core.ac.uk/download/323063854.pdf (accessed on 6th August 2025).
2. Aggarwal, Allanson, Antshel, Armando, Bassett, Bayer, et al. (2015). Craniofacial dysmorphology in 22q11.2 deletion syndrome by 3D laser surface imaging and geometric morphometrics: Illuminating the developmental relationship to risk for psychosis. http://core.ac.uk/download/42358302.pdf (accessed on 6th August 2025).
3. Aldave, A. J., Azimov, R., Boere, P. M., Chung, et al. (2020). Phenotypic and functional characterization of corneal endothelial cells during *in vitro* expansion. http://core.ac.uk/download/323311032.pdf (accessed on 6th August 2025).
4. Alvino, F. G., Auricchio, A., Ballabio, A., Carrella, et al. (2017). AAV-mediated transcription factor EB (TFEB) gene delivery ameliorates muscle pathology and function in the murine model of Pompe disease. http://core.ac.uk/download/132157116.pdf (accessed on 6th August 2025).
5. Arroyo, A., Benito-Calvo, A., Carvalho, S., de la Torre, et al. (2015). First GIS analysis of modern stone tools used by wild chimpanzees (*Pan troglodytes verus*) in Bossou, Guinea, West Africa. http://core.ac.uk/download/187434286.pdf (accessed on 6th August 2025).
6. Athanasiou, Azevedo, Bobyn, Chen, Chung, Cordell, et al. (2014). Elastic biodegradable starch/ethylene-co-vinyl alcohol fibre-mesh scaffolds for tissue engineering applications. http://core.ac.uk/download/30698010.pdf (accessed on 6th August 2025).
7. Ayer, R. E., Ellefsen, K. L., Giebel, J. J., Kastenschmidt, et al. (2019). QuantiMus: A machine learning-based approach for high precision analysis of skeletal muscle morphology. http://core.ac.uk/download/323310928.pdf (accessed on 6th August 2025).
8. Aylward, S. R., Gerig, G., Hovda, D. A., Irimia, et al. (2012). Neuroimaging of structural pathology and connectomics in traumatic brain injury: Toward personalized outcome prediction. http://core.ac.uk/download/323078685.pdf (accessed on 6th August 2025).
9. Bentez-Molano, J., Crosby-Granados, R., Parés Casanova, P.-M., Salamanca-Carreño, et al. (2020). A comparison of traditional and geometric morphometric techniques for the study of basicranial morphology in horses: A case study of the Araucanian horse from Colombia. http://core.ac.uk/download/286577454.pdf (accessed on 6th August 2025).
10. Berg, F., Cadrin, S., Gras, M., Hidalgo, M., et al. (2020). Stock Identification Methods Working Group (SIMWG). http://core.ac.uk/download/481437789.pdf (accessed on 6th August 2025).
11. Botton-Divet, L., Cornette, R., Fabre, A.-C., Herrel, et al. (2015). Tools for quantitative form description: An evaluation of different software packages for semi-landmark analysis. http://core.ac.uk/download/55846768.pdf (accessed on 6th August 2025).
12. Boyer, D., St. Clair, E., Daubechies, I., Funkhouser, et al. (2011). Algorithms to automatically quantify the geometric similarity of anatomical surfaces. http://arxiv.org/abs/1110.3649 (accessed on 6th August 2025).

13. Coelho, P. G., Jimbo, R., Vandeweghe, S., Vanhove, et al. (2013). Utilizing micro-computed tomography to evaluate bone structure surrounding dental implants: A comparison with histomorphometry. http://core.ac.uk/download/55848647.pdf (accessed on 6th August 2025).

14. Desco Menéndez, M., García Barreno, P., Pascau González Garzón, J., Reig, et al. (2009). Research at the medical imaging laboratory, CIBERSAM CB07/09/0031. http://core.ac.uk/download/30044588.pdf (accessed on 6th August 2025).

15. Dykes, J. & Rana, S. (2002). Techniques for augmenting the visualisation of dynamic raster surfaces. http://core.ac.uk/download/1668902.pdf (accessed on 6th August 2025).

16. Ehlmann, B. L., Watkins, J. A., Yin, A. (2020). Spatiotemporal evolution, mineralogical composition, and transport mechanisms of long-runout landslides in Valles Marineris, Mars. http://core.ac.uk/download/323312328.pdf (accessed on 6th August 2025).

17. Feijen, J., Mross, K., Pinedo, H. M., Poort, et al. (1988). Morphometric study of myocardial changes during doxorubicin-induced cardiomyopathy in mice. http://core.ac.uk/download/pdf/11473806.pdf (accessed on 6th August 2025).

18. García Mato, D. (2021). Optimization of craniosynostosis surgery: Virtual planning, intraoperative 3D photography and surgical navigation. http://core.ac.uk/download/541360700.pdf (accessed on 6th August 2025).

19. Goring, A., Pitsillides, A. A., Javaheri, B., Clarkin, C. E., Gomez-Nicola, D., Hesse, E., Razi, H., et al. (2018). Regional diversity in the murine cortical vascular network is revealed by synchrotron X-ray tomography and is amplified with age. http://core.ac.uk/download/161124277.pdf (accessed on 6th August 2025).

20. Goswami, A., Dayasagar, B. S., Choudhury, P. P., Guha, R., Chakraborty, S., Hassan, S. S. (2011). Understanding genomic evolution of olfactory receptors through fractal and mathematical morphology. http://core.ac.uk/download/pdf/289843.pdf (accessed on 6th August 2025).

21. Hoffman, E., Hutter, V., Murnane, D. (2020). Investigating the suitability of high content image analysis as a tool to assess the reversibility of foamy alveolar macrophage phenotypes *in vitro*. http://core.ac.uk/download/288394148.pdf (accessed on 6th August 2025).

22. Jamshidi, N., Kim, J. H., Kuo, M. D., Lee, et al. (2017). Quality of radiomic features in glioblastoma multiforme: Impact of semi-automated tumor segmentation software. http://core.ac.uk/download/323079133.pdf (accessed on 6th August 2025).

23. Johnson, S. D., Linder, H. P., Ponce de León, M. S., Van der Niet, et al. (2010). Three-dimensional geometric morphometrics for studying floral shape variation. http://www.zora.uzh.ch/42648/4/Niet_Trends_Plant_Science_2010_V.pdf (accessed on 6th August 2025).

24. Krenz, G. S., Molthen, R., Shingrani, R. (2010). Automation process for morphometric analysis of volumetric CT data from pulmonary vasculature in rats. http://core.ac.uk/download/213079048.pdf (accessed on 6th August 2025).

25. Sakthiya Sivakumar, S., Vennila, G., Sathish Kumar, L., Deenadayalan, A. (2023). A comprehensive morphometric analysis of mandibular variations: Unveiling novel insights through advanced techniques. http://core.ac.uk/download/603896768.pdf (accessed on 6th August 2025).

26. Xue, H. (2008). Computerized analysis of magnetic resonance images to study cerebral anatomy in developing neonates. http://core.ac.uk/download/295780.pdf (accessed on 6th August 2025).

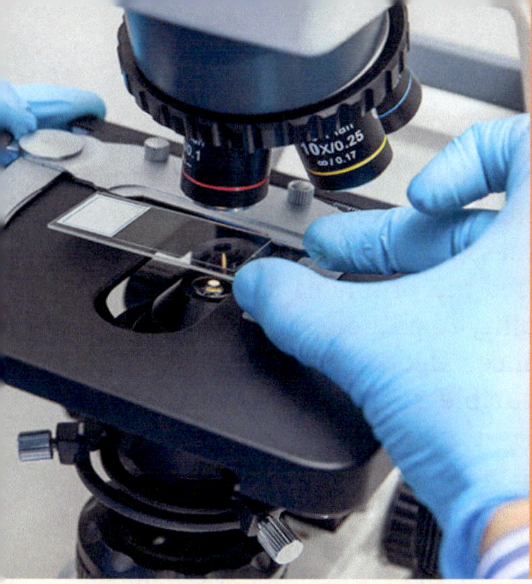

Chapter 14

PATHOLOGICAL TISSUE MORPHOLOGY

Contents

Introduction

Pathological tissue morphology is the basic foundation for investigating the complexities of tissue diseases. It involves the investigation of cellular structure alterations, Pathological tissue morphology refers to the investigation of cellular structure alterations, which may signal the presence of disease processes like cancer. This area of research is of utmost significance not just for diagnostic reasoning but also for the direction of therapeutic processes. With advancing imaging techniques in medicine and computational algorithms, the analysis of tissue morphology becomes increasingly accurate and dependable, which eventually translates to enhanced diagnostic accuracy and therapeutic outcomes. Advances in imaging and segmentation technology have revolutionized the realm of pathological tissue morphology. Automated methods have been fashioned, which allow for detailed analysis of immunohistochemical images presenting various challenges, including tissue complexity and staining heterogeneity. Segmentation of nuclear membranes in cancerous tissue, for instance, is essential to establish protein activities concerning cellular function and abnormalities within malignancies. Research has established the superiority of fully automated morphology-based approaches compared to standard methods such as semi-automated active contours, which, though beneficial, do not possess precision and efficacy.

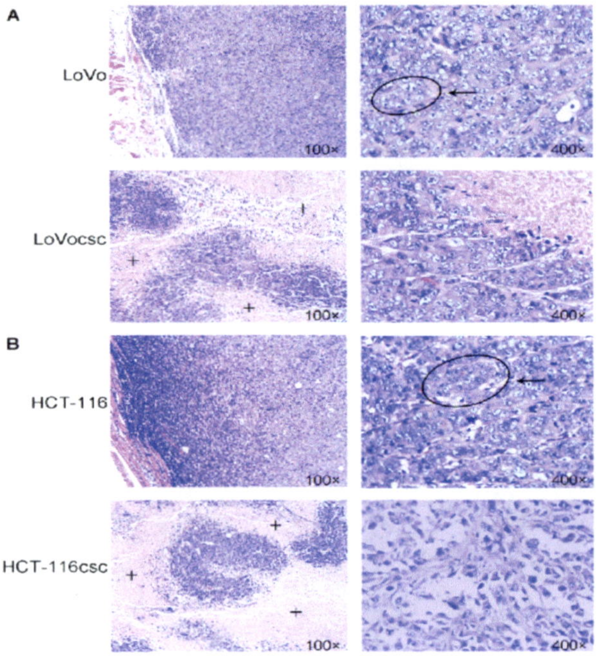

Figure 14.1. Pathological tissue morphology.

Source: https://www.researchgate.net/publication/325427278/figure/fig4/AS:631678951247926@1527615406732/Pathological-morphology-of-tumor-tissues-was-investigated-via-H-E-staining-of-A-LoVo.png.

By promoting innovation in image analysis, scientists have a higher likelihood of exploring tissue characteristics with more fidelity, paving the way for improved diagnostics as well as personalized therapeutic interventions (Acquaviva et al., 2010). The interplay between technology and biological analysis indicates the need to develop accurate and efficient segmentation methods in pathological tissue morphology. enhance the identification of cancerous areas and the impact of the adjacent stroma. This transition from manual to computerized techniques not only allows for quantitative assessments of tissue specimens but also bypasses the problems caused by the inherent variability of pathological samples. By employing advanced algorithms, researchers can achieve reproducible segmentation outcomes, enabling more in-depth exploration of specific cellular processes and molecular expression. Lastly, these innovations are also responsible for promoting the understanding of multifactorial genetic pathologies and developing personalized therapeutic treatments, underpinning the place of automated approaches in pathological tissue morphology in the future (Acquaviva et al., 2010) (Figure 14.1).

Definition of Pathological Tissue Morphology

pathological tissue morphology requires a consideration of the structural and functional alterations. Pathological tissue morphology is interested in how tissues deviate from normal anatomy in a way that reflects the related pathology of various health sicknesses. Notably, these alterations may vary significantly based on the specific disease process, to inform clinical diagnosis and treatment. in malignant cancer tissues, morphological changes include **cellular atypia, increased mitotic activity, and the presence of necrosis**, all of which are used to distinguish malignant from benign tumors.. Similarly, investigations of tissues associated with metabolic disorders reveal irregular cellular architecture and abnormal extracellular matrix deposition, demonstrating the far-reaching impact of these pathologies on tissue structure and function. The use of enhanced imaging modalities has significantly enhanced our understanding of pathological tissue morphology. X-ray Micro-Tomography (XMT) allow researchers to observe internal structures with high resolution and identify specific micro-level changes that evolve in pathological tissues. For example, studies on femoral heads have utilized XMT to differentiate between healthy and disease states, with results showing changes in bone mineral density and microcallus formations that signify damage and repair mechanisms (Ahmed et al., 2011). Furthermore, the imaging techniques enable the establishment of the relationship between pathological changes and clinical outcome, which serves as useful information in the context of the mechanical properties and structural integrity of diseased tissues. Thus, the deployment of novel imaging techniques is crucial for better defining tissue morphology in disease. Moreover, the role of genetic and molecular determinants in the development of pathological tissue morphology is further appreciated. Cell responses to disease are regulated by specific genes and pathways for control, hence altering tissue structure and function. For example, in *Caenorhabditis* elegans models, forkhead transcription factor DAF-16 has been implicated in longevity determination and stress response ssssss(Buckley et al., 2010). By studying how these molecular processes affect morphology, scientists can more accurately describe the relationships between genetics, pathology, and structure. In summary, a sound understanding of pathological tissue morphology is crucial in formulating specific therapies and developing diagnostic techniques, hence improving patient care in various areas of medicine.

Importance in Medical Diagnosis

The role of pathological morphology of tissue in clinical diagnosis is pivotal, since it is the basis of detection and categorization of diseases at the cellular level. Through thorough examination of tissue specimens, pathologists can identify abnormal cellular characteristics that suggest various pathological conditions, such as neoplasia or inflammation. This microscopic examination not only aids in initial diagnosis but also guides decisions on treatment and prognosis. The convergence of the latest technologies, such as digital histopathology and machine learning, has further augmented the diagnostic potential of tissue morphology. With increasing ease of access to digital histopathological images, there is a continuous need to employ advanced analytical tools to analyze these images successfully, thereby enhancing diagnostic accuracy and reducing human error. This ongoing innovation in diagnostic technology underscores the paramount position of pathological tissue morphology in contemporary medicine. The advent of molecular pathology has revolutionized the discipline of diagnostics by bringing together the old histology and genetic testing in a manner that reconciles their values. The relationship between morphological assessment and molecular characterization has intensified in scale, particularly in the field of oncology. For instance, the application of next-generation sequencing technology allows extensive genomic characterizations of tumors to facilitate personalized treatment plans that address the genetic causes of an individual's cancer. But the integration is not without challenges since the majority of the healthcare centers continue to have a lack of integration between molecular testing and cellular pathology departments. Closing the knowledge and skills gap among workers will be crucial in establishing a morphemolecular pathology specialty with both cellular morphology and genomic knowledge. This will enhance the applicability of cellular pathology in patient management and enhance a more integrated approach to precision medicine in cancer therapy (Jones et al., 2018). The increasing occurrence of digital pathology and the accompanying increase in the use of machine learning are among the main trends towards improved diagnostic precision. Digital pictures of histopathological samples are submitted to advanced computational analysis that can detect subtle morphological changes, typically beyond human sight. Difficulties still dominate, however, including the complexities associated with image interpretation and the risk of algorithmic bias. Researchers address these problems by creating machine learning algorithms that are capable of effectively analyzing digital pathological images and taking into account variability in image quality and staining. The potential of machine learning to enhance traditional diagnostic practices makes it important to maintain pace with technological advancements in pathology. With these methods evolving, they are going to further cement the role of pathological tissue morphology in medical diagnostics as well as redefine the future of clinical pathology (Ishikawa, S., & Komura, D., 2017) (Figure 14.2).

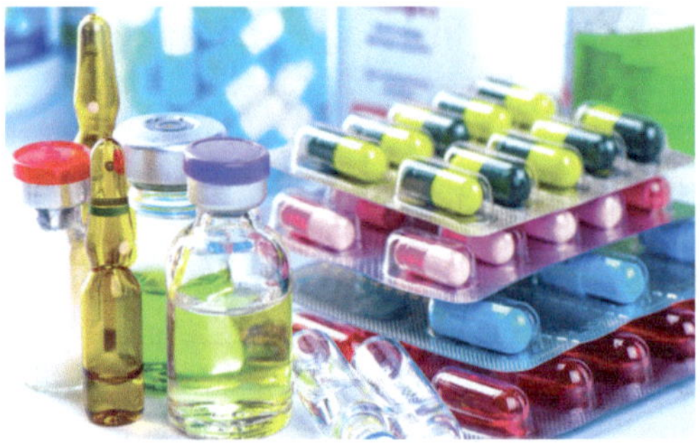

Figure 14.2. Importance in medical diagnosis.

Source: https://infinitabiotech.com/wp-content/uploads/2021/05/Importance-Of-Enzymes-In-Medicine.jpg.

14.1. Historical Background

The pathological tissue morphology's clinical history has been a significant story of medical science, reflecting the evolution in disease mechanisms and technology. Pathology initially was greatly reliant upon gross inspection of specimens, with limited techniques for detailed study of tissue structure. This rudimentary method was gradually altered as the microscope was introduced in the 17th century, enabling more study of cellular structures. By the 19th century, histological staining techniques further refined, distinguishing normal from diseased tissue, leading to the thorough classification of diseases. Such early achievement paved the way for the official recognition of cellular pathology as a medical branch that uses morphological study in conjunction with clinical medicine, paving the path towards subsequent higher-level concepts of disease in subsequent generations. With the progression of the 20th century, the interfacing of pathological tissue morphology with emerging molecular and genetic insights profoundly changed the discipline. The realization that cancer was not merely a structural derangement but a genetically heterogeneous disease spurred the trend toward increasing integration in pathology. The trend toward molecular typing of specimens introduced the age of precision medicine, where treatment could be individualized based on genetic profiles. These developments have required the integration of genomic data with morphological observations increasingly, fostering a new paradigm known as morphomolecular pathology. This conceptual shift accentuates the importance of interdisciplinary training and teamwork since the practitioners in the field must now deal with cellular structures and molecular mechanisms to effectively diagnose and manage complex diseases such as cancer, and thus consolidate the application of cellular pathology in contemporary medicine (Jones et al., 2018). Also, ongoing programs identify gaps in the current knowledge and training that are required to maximize the potential of an integrated pathology service that spans both morphological and molecular areas. For instance, the way in which the CM-Path program in the UK has emphasized the need for upskilling the existing workforce to cover the gap between the genomic laboratory and the cellular pathology department. This identification of training deficit is important, with the future of pathology increasingly involving itself with genomic advancement. Such integration is also underscored by initiatives like the 100,000 Genome Project, which facilitates the application of whole-genome sequencing into routine practice. It is vital that education models evolve to combat these challenges and provide a workforce trained in the application of morphomolecular techniques to ensure that pathologists remain an integral part not only of cancer diagnosis but also of research and discovery in medical science (Masic et al., 2012).

14.1.1. Early Studies in Histopathology

The field of histopathology has evolved significantly since its inception, driven primarily by the need to understand disease at the cellular level. The initial research provided a foundation for systematic processing of tissues bearing pathologies of different kinds, with the major focus being microscopic examination for the diagnosis of disease. Pathbreaking workers in the discipline employed rudimentary techniques to stain and prepare tissue specimens so that cellular architecture and disease alterations could be seen. Such an underpinning was essential, as it not only made tumor detection possible but also provided a foundation for discussion on the cellular basis of disease processes. Such early work emphasized the use of strict methodological paradigms, which would be built upon by later studies, demonstrating just how instrumental the use of advanced staining techniques and microscopy were in the advancement of histopathological analysis. Ongoing innovation within this field continues to reveal the complex relationships with the tissue on which many disease states are based. As histopathology developed, technological improvements were essential to upgrading diagnostic insight. The introduction of digital pathology and computerized image analysis has expanded the range of methodologies at the disposal of pathologists, and this allows for more nuanced interpretations of tissue morphology. The technology allows for the characterization of tumors and their microenvironments with greater accuracy, which is essential for the understanding of tumor behavior and patient prognosis. The classical qualitative tests were usually lacking in detecting the intricate interactions between the tumor and the surrounding tissues; however, with automated techniques, researchers can now quantify such interactions. Early studies demonstrated the lack of adequacy of mere visual observations, with an obligatory shift towards more extensive analytical processes. This advancement is consistent with the contemporary push toward multi-disciplinary approaches to patient care and also symbolizes the discipline's allegiance to the advancement of diagnostic accuracy and therapeutic interventions through technology integration.

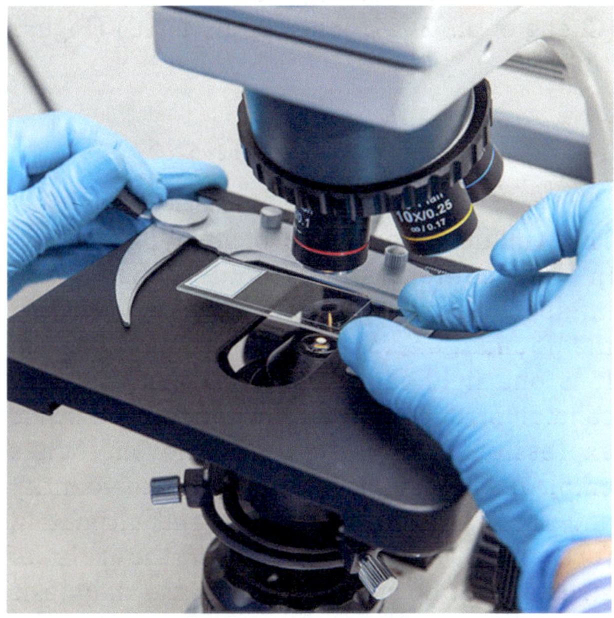

Figure 14.3. Early studies in histopathology.

Source: https://mlecl.com/wp-content/uploads/2018/02/HISTOPATHOLOGY.jpg.

Moreover, this focus on integrating cellular pathology with molecular identification marks an enormous leap over the conventional past of histopathology. While initial histopathological studies were primarily concerned with morphological assessments, a realization of the need for an integrated morphomolecular pathology model—a model that reconciles the cell and molecular aspects of disease—is present today. As noted in recent reviews, multidisciplinary approaches that integrate cellular pathology and genomics are increasingly relevant to cancer treatment. The introduction of programs to upskill pathologists in genomic environments emphasizes this groundbreaking transformation. This convergence is not only relevant to improving diagnosis but also to forcing precision medicine programs that tailor treatments against the patient's tumor biology. By encouraging the dialogue of old histopathology with fresh molecular findings, the science can remain in its mid-point role within cancer treatment while providing improved understanding of disease mechanisms (Cheng et al., 2017; Jones et al., 2018) (Figure 14.3).

14.1.2. Key Figures in Tissue Morphology

The evolution of tissue morphology, particularly in the context of pathology, has been influenced by its pioneers, whose work laid the foundation for current comprehension. It is one field that has emphasized the way cellular structure is associated with disease expression. The early tissue morphologists employed histological techniques to identify and classify various pathologies and, ultimately, further our understanding of the role of structural abnormalities in disease diagnosis and treatment. One such use is the application of these techniques to coral pathology, highlighting the need for the establishment of proper diagnostic criteria that include both gross observation and microscopy. This trend underscores the essential contribution of diagnostic histopathology to uncover the subtleties of disease processes, as encouraged by retrospective workshops for distinguishing and clarifying nomenclature within the examination of coral diseases (Bochsler et al., 2007). Moreover, advances in imaging technologies enabled an investigation into tissue morphology at hitherto unprecedented resolution. Research by scientists who have deployed scanning electron microscopy and transmission electron microscopy has been important to understand microarchitectural differences in diseased tissues. For instance, studies of calcified heart valves have unraveled the complex spatial arrangements between bioapatite crystals and their local microenvironments through such multiscale examinations. It has been identified that pathological crystallization processes can be differentiated to gain insights into the mechanisms of heart valve disease. By understanding such relationships, scientists are better positioned to effectively design interventions and improve clinical outcomes. This intersection of innovative imaging techniques with morphological studies presents a model for investigating other processes of disease, towards an enhanced appreciation of tissue health and disease (Cavarretta et al., 2015). Finally, the integration of traditional histological techniques with modern techniques remains crucial to further advance tissue morphology in pathology. Such interaction between pathologists and biomedical scientists has provided an environment where critical knowledge transfer occurs, bridging descriptive and mechanistic science. It is out of these interactions that critical advances are formulated for overcoming the new challenges of diagnosis and treatment of different diseases. As the need for detailed tissue characterization grows, the roles of these key players in tissue morphology will shift, affecting teaching and interdisciplinary research. Continuous exploration of microscopic tissue anatomy enables clinicians and researchers to be prepared to address the challenges of pathological processes, ultimately enhancing patient care through better diagnostic and therapeutic interventions (Bochsler et al., 2007).

14.1.3. Evolution of Techniques and Technologies

Pathological tissue morphology evolution has been greatly assisted by advancements in diagnostic methods and technologies. Traditional histopathology previously relied on manual visual inspection of stained tissue samples under a microscope. This is no longer the case with the advent of computer systems and digital imaging technologies. Digital pathology not only enhances the precision of morphologic assessments but also enables the storage and sharing of high-resolution images for collaborative diagnostic reasons. Later, pathologists can conduct remote consultations, greatly improving specialist opinion access in underserved regions. Moreover, such innovations enable the integration of robust data analytics, thereby promoting new paradigms in diagnostic precision and reproducibility that are central to patient care and research. The application of genomic information in cellular pathology has been noted over the last few years as a milestone in controlling complicated diseases such as cancer. The old dichotomy of morphological observation and molecular description is slowly being bridged to allow for a combined knowledge of disease pathology. Advances in the last few years have seen the uptake of the molecular description of tumors through next-generation sequencing as a standard procedure, enhancing the accuracy of diagnostics and treatment strategies enormously. This evolution constitutes a paradigm shift toward "morphomolecular pathology," a strategy that recognizes the requirement for the interpretation of morphological data alongside genomic profiles in order to gain an integrated view of pathology. Such convergence can be expected to further position cellular pathology at the center of oncology while expanding its reach in precision medicine approaches toward ultimately improving the outcomes of cancer therapy (Jones et al., 2018). With it, new therapeutic techniques such as microwave thermal ablation are a great reflection of how technology is revolutionizing treatment paradigms in pathology. This minimally invasive procedure has been increasing in clinical use due to the fact that it has a shorter recovery time and can be useful in treating patients who are not good candidates for surgery. Real-time monitoring of tissue response after treatment is key to optimizing outcomes. Current imaging techniques are lacking here, necessitating the development of new techniques like microwave tomography. The method quantifies dielectric tissue properties after ablation, facilitating easier monitoring of treatment response (Cavagnaro et al., 2018). The findings of recent *ex vivo* experiments suggest that microwave tomography can effectively image transitions between treated and untreated tissues, highlighting the potential to enhance therapeutic efficacy and patient care while further enriching pathological tissue morphology (Figure 14.4).

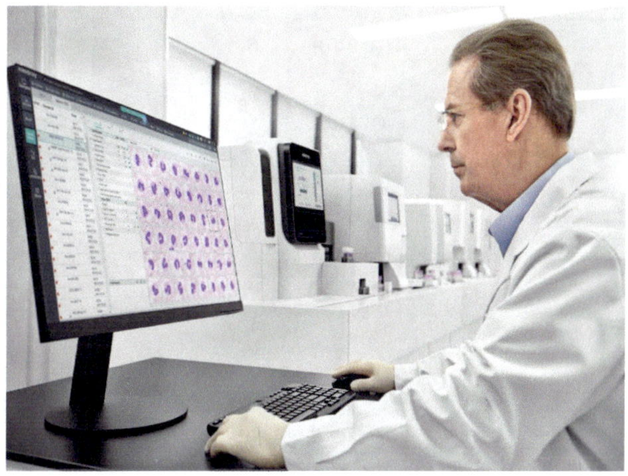

Figure 14.4. Evolution of techniques and technologies.

Source: https://www.mindray.com/content/dam/xpace/en/media-center/press-center/news/mindray-launches-new-mc-80-automated-digital-cell-morphology-analyzer-taking-morphology-analysis-to-the-next-level/mc-80-news-s2.jpg.

14.2. Types of Pathological Tissues

Knowledge of pathological tissues is crucial in the diagnosis and treatment of diseases, including cancer. Among the pathological tissues, neoplastic tissues are of specific interest as they are benign or malignant. Benign neoplasms, like lipomas or adenomas, are typically well-circumscribed with well-delineated borders and do not infiltrate into neighboring tissues. In contrast, neoplastic malignant tumors such as carcinomas and sarcomas exhibit uncontrolled growth with a propensity to invade adjacent tissues and metastasize to other sites. The morphologic attributes—size, shape, nuclear appearance, and growth pattern—of these neoplastic tissues are crucial for understanding tumor behavior and prognostication. Identification of these features in histopathological specimens is a valuable skill for pathologists with a substantial bearing on treatment and patient outcome. A second significant pathological tissue form is inflammatory tissue, which follows injury or infection. Inflammation involves the recruitment of immune cells to the site, such as neutrophils and macrophages, which contribute to the repair of the injured tissue.

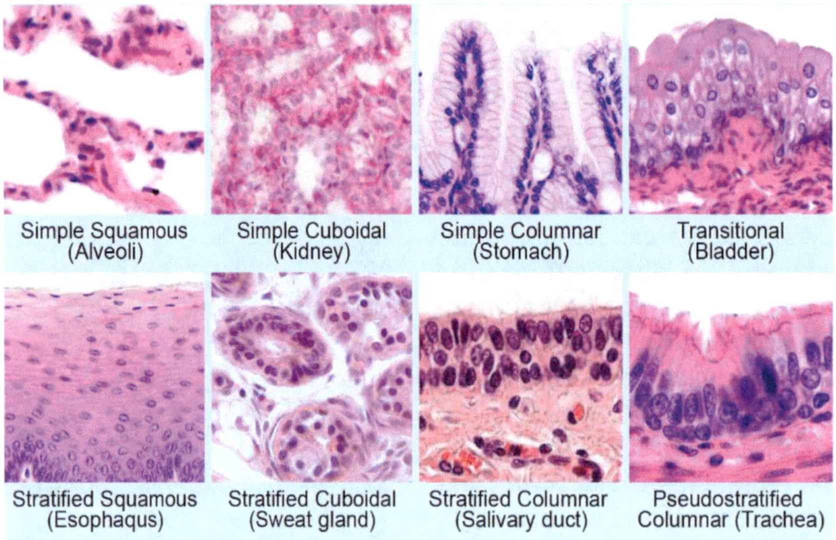

Figure 14.5. Key figures in tissue morphology.

Source: https://rsscience.com/wp-content/uploads/2022/04/epithelium-classification-types.jpg.

Acute inflammation is beneficial, but prolonged or chronic inflammation may lead to detrimental pathological changes, e.g., fibrosis or granuloma formation. In a number of diseases, including autoimmune diseases and persistent infections, inflammatory tissue persistence distorts the architecture and function of the normal tissue. Understanding the morphology of such tissues is crucial because it allows distinguishing between acute and chronic inflammation and recognizing the mechanisms of disease. Additionally, advances in imaging techniques and histopathological examination can also enhance our ability to investigate inflammatory tissues and their contribution to disease progression. Finally, the examination of connective tissue diseases reveals another facet of pathological tissues responsible for impairing human health. Fibrosis or scleroderma, for example, involves the deposition of extracellular matrix components in a way that is inappropriate, causing stiffness of the tissue and loss of function. Morphological studies of such tissues can reveal vital information regarding the degree and progression of such diseases. For example, fibrosis can be the result of a wide variety of etiologies, including chronic inflammation or direct tissue injury, and its morphologic assessment often shows alterations in collagen fibers and cellular components.

Understanding the pathological changes in connective tissues contributes to our knowledge of disease mechanisms and informs therapy. Thus, extensive studies of the morphology of many pathological tissues, including neoplastic, inflammatory, and connective tissue types, form the basis upon which modern diagnostic pathology is founded, with significant effects on treatment protocols and patient prognoses (Figure 14.5).

14.2.1. Neoplastic Tissues

Neoplastic tissues, which result from the uncontrolled growth of cells, exhibit certain morphological characteristics that describe their origin and mode of growth. Abnormal tissues can be benign or malignant; benign tumors typically grow slowly and tend to remain localized, whereas malignant tumors can invade surrounding tissues and metastasize to distant sites. The histological architecture of neoplasms reveals critical information regarding their nature, including cellular pleomorphism, abnormal mitotic images, and variable differentiation ranges. Their characterization is purely indispensable in diagnosing neoplastic disease because they greatly aid in the planning of treatment strategies and in the prediction of patient prognosis. Furthermore, technological advances in imaging techniques and molecular pathology have demystified the characterization of neoplastic tissues with greater levels of precision, allowing more personalized and optimal therapeutic practices. Particular attention must be paid to the neoplastic microenvironment, which in most cases is marked by a complex relationship between tumor cells and the extratumoral stroma. This stroma comprises immune cells, vasculature, and fibroblasts, all of which significantly contribute to the tumor growth and response to treatment. Pancreatic ductal adenocarcinoma (PDAC) is a good example of the role played by stellate cells in the process of neoplastic transformation. These cells not only contribute to the fibrotic character of the tumor but also confer drug resistance. YAP and its homolog TAZ have been recently implicated in stellate cell activation, thus revealing a pathway by which the stroma microenvironment can promote drug resistance and malignancy. These findings underscore the importance of determining the neoplastic microenvironment to develop targeted therapy protocols in cancer treatment (Dhall et al., 2015).

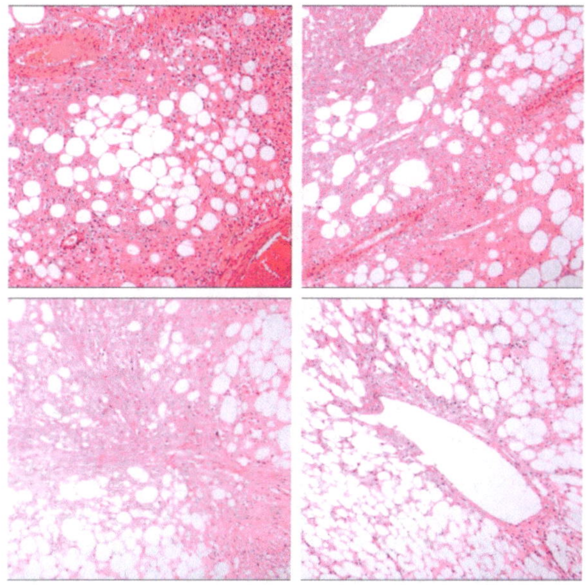

Figure 14.6. Neoplastic tissues.

Source: https://www.researchgate.net/publication/356641240/figure/fig1/AS:1102392229670913@1639842197145/Sections-show-neoplastic-tissue-composed-of-adipose-tissue-epithelioid-cells-and.jpg.

In addition, some of the neoplastic tissues, such as posttransplant lymphoproliferative disorders (PTLDs), underscore the central role of immunosuppression during tumor development. In solid organ or stem cell transplant recipients, the use of immunosuppressive therapy to prevent graft rejection has a seemingly contradictory effect of causing lymphoproliferative disorders from dampened T-cell activity. Studies have shown that such conditions, i.e., monomorphic PTLDs, are typically associated with viral pathogens such as macaca lymphocryptovirus and thus further complicate the clinical picture. The unique histopathological features of PTLD are noteworthy and provide insight into its pathogenesis, suggesting that intensive viral load monitoring could serve as an early diagnostic intervention, with timely therapeutic interventions to control disease progression (Badin et al., 2016). Understanding these morphologies of diseased tissues not only determines treatment but also stimulates further research into more effective therapeutic regimens (Figure 14.6).

14.2.2. Inflammatory Tissues

Inflammatory tissues characteristically show a feature of pathological changes that reflect chronic responses to injury, infection, or environmental insult. This alteration involves complex interactions among cellular and molecular activities that result in activation of inflammatory pathways. For instance, in chronic tendon lesions, the excessive production of matrix components is an example of an inability to effectively repair or remodel the extracellular matrix. Studies have shown that TGF-ß isoforms, particularly TGF-ß2, are implicated in the process and, hence, their potential participation in the pathogenesis of inflammatory tissues. Inasmuch as TGF-ß2 exists, a lack of TGF-ßRI may lead to nonproductive signaling, and that is why chronic tendon lesions do not heal appropriately (Curry et al., 2001). Hence, understanding these molecular pathways is significant in the construction of therapeutic therapies to enhance inflammatory tissue diseases. Apart from structural changes, inflammatory tissues have cellular composition changes that undermine homeostasis. Immune cell infiltration into the damaged site is an ordinary biological reaction to infection and injury. For example, periodontitis demonstrates how chronic inflammation may not only lead to tissue destruction at a local level but to systemic consequences. Certain oral pathogens, such as Porphyromonas gingivalis, have been shown to infect the central nervous system from the oral environment and to have adverse effects on the health of neurons. This highlights the bimodal character of inflammatory tissues, where local responses become amplified into systemic problems, a sign of an even greater implication for diseases such as Alzheimer's. This evidence supports the need to investigate the intricate interplay between inflammatory responses and their systemic implications for diseases that spread beyond the initially involved tissues (Chukkapalli et al., 2014).

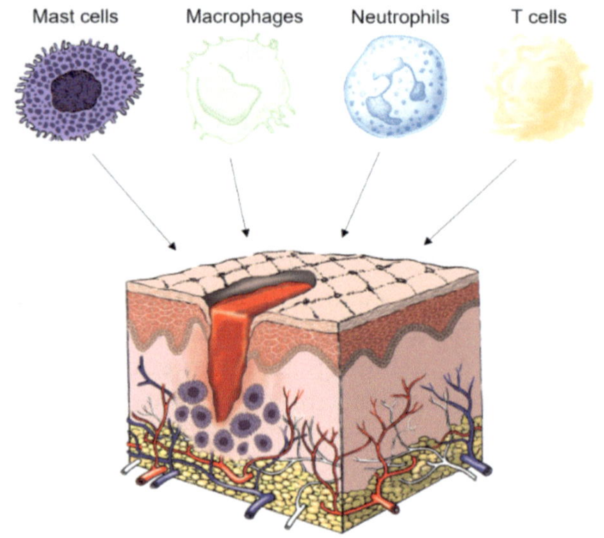

Figure 14.7. Inflammatory tissues.

Source: https://www.frontiersin.org/files/Articles/883239/fimmu-13-883239-HTML/image_m/fimmu-13-883239-g001.jpg.

The pathological morphology of the inflammatory tissue can provide important diagnostic and prognostic information. Through a detailed histopathological analysis, the scientists can pick up the characteristic alterations such as enhanced vascularity, altered cellularity, and the presence of immune cell aggregates. These alterations indicate an ongoing inflammatory process, and clinicians from here can assess the severity and potential course of conditions. Moreover, an awareness of the morphological background of inflammatory tissue also helps differentiate among types of immunity, whether acute or chronic. Repeated activation of pro-inflammatory signaling in chronic inflammatory diseases like tendinopathy or periodontitis may result in tissue remodeling that exposes individuals to further severe complications. Thus, characterization of the morphological features of inflammatory tissues not only aids the understanding of the pathological bases but also influences treatment modalities aimed at regaining tissue integrity and function (Figure 14.7).

14.2.3. Degenerative Tissues

Degenerative tissue analysis lies at the core of understanding pathological morphology of tissue, as it often develops as a manifestation of cellular loss of function in maintaining tissue homeostasis. For instance, degenerative tissues such as those found in tendinopathy are characterized by structural and functional loss, often due to repetitive micro-trauma that outstrips the capacity of extracellular matrix repair. This dynamic cycle of damage and repair depicts the failure of the biological response that cannot reconstruct tissue integrity. Recent advances in molecular and biochemical techniques have illuminated the complexity of these pathways to degeneration, revealing the highly evolved patterns of signaling that control tissue remodeling. It is worth noting these processes not only for the sake of proper diagnosis but also for the preparation of proper treatments for conditions that include degenerative changes in the tissues, caused by habitual activities or serious traumas. Tendons' conditions are such examples of the issues with degenerative tissues where healing is unresponsive or incomplete. The majority of tendons, particularly in athletes, undergo repeated strain or injury, resulting in a degenerative condition with pathological lesions. The chronic tendon lesions are significant as they reflect the failure to repair or remodel the extracellular matrix, causing dysfunction and pain. The molecular pathophysiology of these conditions is complex, where the involvement of multiple growth factors and cellular pathways plays an important role in directing the destiny of repair of tissues. Investigation of these variables is significant for understanding how degeneration establishes a cyclical pattern within the tissue microenvironment, in which deterioration can exacerbate rather than resolve, thereby perpetuating the disease process (Riley., 2004). Research seeking to clarify the role of transforming growth factor-beta (TGF-β) in tendon disease has provided useful insights into the mechanisms that regulate degenerative tissue. TGF-ß is critical for tissue repair but, when dysregulated, can lead to failed healing. It has been confirmed that while TGF-ß2 is uniformly expressed within normal and degenerative tendon tissue, TGF-ß receptor expression is dramatically disrupted. Specifically, the absence of TGF-ßRI from the fibrillar matrix suggests a block in the TGF-ß signaling pathway that is most probably responsible for the chronic nature of these lesions. Increased cellular signaling through overexpressed TGF-ß2 in the involved tissues versus ineffective receptor interaction is due to the preservation of degenerative alterations. Grasping this signaling dysregulation is pivotal in the design of therapeutic interventions directed against the causes of tissue degeneration, which may then promote a shift away from the chronic condition and toward a more rehabilitative status (Curry et al., 2001).

14.3. Techniques for Analyzing Tissue Morphology

Methods of tissue morphology analysis play crucial roles in the understanding of pathological conditions, particularly in cancer research. Traditional methods of histological section analysis rely on manual segmentation, a time-consuming and subjective process susceptible to human errors. Automated approaches have transformed this area, with greater accuracy in the identification of pathological features. Among these developments, unsupervised color clustering has become a successful technique for segmenting immunohistochemical images, enabling scientists to automatically delineate cancerous lesions from the stroma, thereby improving diagnostic reliability. In doing so, it enhances the visualisation of tumor heterogeneity, which is vital for effective treatment planning and prognosis. The accuracy of such machine-based methods relative to manual segmentation underscores their potential in day-to-day clinical practice and research facilities. Advances on the basis of automated approaches have also increased the accuracy of nuclear segmentation of tissue images using morphological methods. Accurate nuclear segmentation is not only essential for the quantification of some protein activity associated with cancer formation but is also necessary to help provide correct diagnoses and therapeutic interventions. A fully automated technique designed for nuclear segmentation addresses the challenges introduced by heterogeneous staining and inhomogeneous layers of tissues.

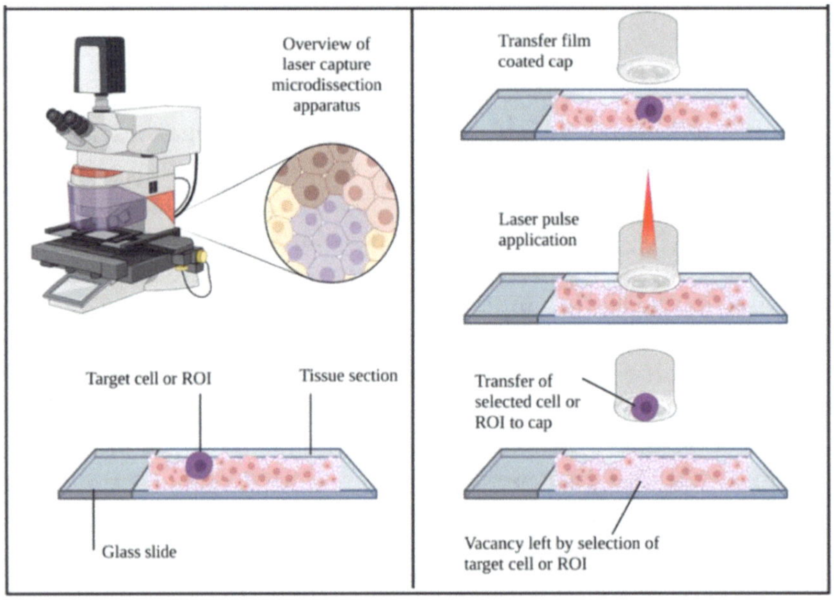

Figure 14.8. Techniques for analyzing tissue morphology.

Source: https://api.intechopen.com/media/chapter/78769/media/F3.png.

Through encouraging morphological segmentation of nuclear membranes, this approach surpasses traditional semi-automated active contour-based solutions that often fail in sophisticated tissue contexts. Considering the pressing need for precision in cancer diagnosis, the use of such new techniques is essential for the improvement of outcomes in cancer treatment and the determination of fundamental mechanisms of tumor biology (Acquaviva et al., 2010). Additional refinement in tissue morphology inspection techniques has been found to possess the potential for outperforming existing techniques in terms of speed and accuracy of performance. A comparative evaluation of computerized segmentation techniques with traditional methods, such as active contours, reveals considerable advantages in reliability and consistency. Active contours provide a point of departure for segmentation, but with shortcomings in involved immunohistochemical scenarios, providing evidence that there is a call for advanced methodologies that can dynamically shape themselves along evolving patterns of staining and tissue morphology. With the abundance of experimental evidence proving the superiority of more novel approaches, it is clear there is a significant imperative to integrate these automated techniques into research and clinical practice. Further refinement of these techniques not only enhances diagnostic accuracy but also facilitates a deeper understanding of pathological mechanisms at a molecular level, ultimately translating to more targeted therapies (Acquaviva et al., 2010) (Figure 14.8).

14.3.1. Histological Staining Methods

Histological staining techniques are central to the investigation of tissue morphology because they enhance the visibility of cellular and extracellular features in various tissue specimens. Histological staining refers to the treatment of tissues with dyes and other chemicals that selectively bind to specific constituents, thereby allowing pathologists to recognize cellular structures and to recognize changes that are suggestive of disease. Staining is not only critical in the case of microscopy but also for the identification of tissue architecture and cellular relations. Several staining methods, including hematoxylin and eosin (H&E), Masson's trichrome, and immunohistochemical stains, are employed to identify various features like cell nuclei, collagen fibers, and proteins. Thus, the overall effectiveness of such procedures is based on the nature of tissue and the pathological conditions under observation; that is, proper selection of staining methods is always required in any histopathological study. The emphasis on the requirement of staining methods, and the comparison of the histopathological features of tissues under different conditions is crucial. For example, in congenital bicuspid aortic valve (CBAV), research reveals clear pathological features in leaflet specimens of patients with AS. In one such study, it was found that the degree of calcification and inflammation was not significantly different in CBAV-AS patients compared with TAV-AS patients, while fibrosis of the valves appeared more evident in CBAV-AS patients. These findings indicate the value of reliable histological staining in accurately representing these alterations, facilitating a better understanding of disease processes and pathogenesis. The ability to effectively identify and assess these differential histological alterations plays a critical role in enhancing diagnostic and treatment methods in cardiovascular pathology (Mazzone et al., 2016). Moreover, the improvement of staining methods has spurred the development of completely automated systems that offer increased accuracy in nuclear segmentation in histological images, particularly in cancer tissue analysis. Traditional methods, such as active contours, have limitations regarding heterogeneous staining and the presence of multiple layers of tissues that could complicate the identification of nuclear morphology. New studies have demonstrated computerized techniques superior to conventional ones, which yield superior results in circumscribing nuclei and quantifying protein activity of utmost significance for cancer diagnosis and therapy. As histological staining's future unravels, the advances in technology bring greater diagnostic precision, better facilitating an in-depth analysis of pathological tissue morphology and its implications in patient treatment (Acquaviva et al., 2010).

14.3.2. Imaging Techniques (e.g., Microscopy)

Pathological tissue morphology investigation relies heavily on advanced imaging techniques, notably microscopy, that provide a high-resolution insight into tissue architecture at the cell level. Routine light microscopy can yield some results, but resolution constraints require more sophisticated methodologies to be utilized.

Fluorescence microscopy offers one such method, able to visualize individual proteins within cells and thus allowing close examination of their spatial arrangement and molecular interactions. More advanced techniques, such as confocal microscopy, enhance this capacity by eliminating light that is not in focus, resulting in higher-resolution three-dimensional images. These advances facilitate more accurate assessment of disease-specific tissue alterations, such as those in cancer, and aid in improved diagnosis and therapy planning. Automated techniques are emerging as the imaging technology continues to advance beyond manual observation with microscopy. Current research provides computer-based segmentation methods that are able to efficiently detect cancerous regions in immunohistochemical tissues. The first method utilizes unsupervised color clustering for separating target cancerous regions from nearby stroma, while the second method seeks computer-based segmentation of cancer cells' nuclear membranes based on color separation and morphological processing. More importantly, the methods are more accurate than traditional methods and far better than manual methods and common computerized methods. These developments not only facilitate interpretation of complex tissue images but also enhance the consistency and standardization of appraisals for specific proteins in specific pathological conditions (Acquaviva et al., 2010). The combination of polarized-light imaging methods, such as second-harmonic generation microscopy and polarization-sensitive optical coherence tomography, is a significant advance in the study of cartilage morphology, particularly in the understanding of diseases such as osteoarthritis. These light-imaging techniques are extremely informative regarding cartilage architecture and composition, and offer a non-invasive means of evaluating structural changes. With these imaging modalities, researchers can monitor the efficacy of tissue engineering strategies to heal articular cartilage, an extension of ongoing research since conventional treatments have failed. The key observations are that not only do these methods enhance our understanding of cartilage pathology, but also make it possible to create pathogenetic therapies that may halt cartilage deterioration as part of degenerative joint disorders (Matcher, 2009) (Figure 14.9).

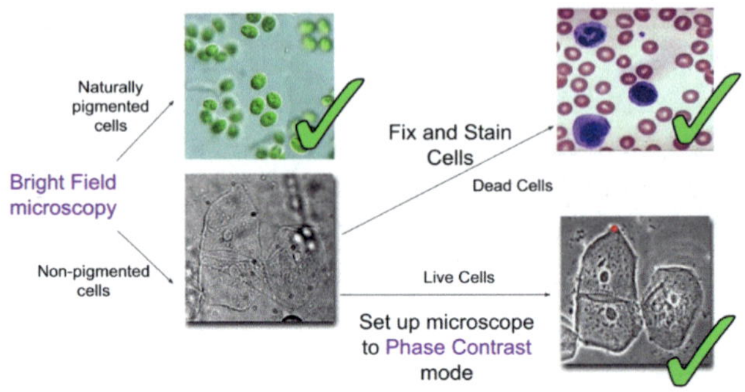

Figure 14.9. Imaging techniques (e.g., microscopy).

Source: https://i.ytimg.com/vi/doxGqBOp5MM/maxresdefault.jpg.

14.3.3. Molecular Techniques (e.g., PCR, FISH)

The use of molecular techniques in the examination of pathological tissue has drastically altered the landscape of diagnosis and treatment. Of the most glaring of these techniques, Polymerase Chain Reaction (PCR) enables the amplification of sequences of DNA, which assists in the identification of genetic content in various samples. The technique is of tremendous importance to identify mutations, pathogens, and also tumor-associated gene expressions. The specificity of PCR enhances the ability to delineate the molecular characteristics of tumor tissue, thereby guiding clinical practice. In addition, PCR's quick turnaround time makes it an important tool in time-sensitive diagnostic contexts, such as infections or tumors. By correlating molecular data with histological findings, doctors can design personalized treatment regimens that are better suited to the unique molecular microenvironment of each tumor type, with improved patient outcomes. Fluorescence In Situ Hybridization (FISH) is another important molecular pathology technology that allows imaging of specific DNA sequences in the tissue cellular context of clinical samples. FISH employs fluorescent probes to attach to target regions of chromosomes, allowing one to identify chromosomal abnormalities and gene amplifications, which are often pivotal in cancer biology. As is clear from recent advances, FISH could yield critical data regarding the spatial architecture of genetic material and its relevance to comprehending tumor heterogeneity and formation. Its use in evaluating cervical cytology specimens, particularly to determine the role of human papillomavirus (HPV) in neoplastic lesions, exemplifies its diagnostic utility (Filho L et al., 2008). Moreover, FISH enables the association of molecular change with morphological characteristics and thereby improves the diagnostic platform of pathological tissue morphology. The innovative application of single-cell sequencing technologies, such as Topographic Single Cell Sequencing (TSCS), indicates the evolving role of molecular methods in pathology. This technique, preserving the spatial organization of single cells in tissues, provides an integrated perspective of clonal evolution in tumors, as observed in the studies of synchronous Ductal Carcinoma *in situ* and Invasive Ductal Carcinoma (DCIS-IDC) (Casasent, 2018). Through enabling genomic heterogeneity at the individual-cell level, TSCS reveals how single subclones of cancer cells engage with their environment, providing a more complete picture of tumor growth and metastasis. These insights enable the personalization of targeted therapies in consideration of not only the total composition of the tumor but also the intricate subclonal interactions. Altogether, these molecular techniques are reshaping our approach toward handling pathology in a more specific way, enhancing the link between morphology and molecular biology for the treatment of diseases.

14.4. Role of Pathological Tissue Morphology in Disease

The intricate interplay of pathological tissue morphology and disease mechanisms is exemplified in amyotrophic lateral sclerosis (ALS), a neurodegenerative illness characterized by motor neuron loss. Pathological features of ALS, including the prevalence of mutant superoxide dismutase (SOD1) in familial ALS, demonstrate the way in which some modifications of neuronal tissue morphology promote disease progression. In ALS, changes in glial cells and the muscle microenvironment create a non-cell autonomous condition that promotes motor neuron degeneration. Evidence has emerged that microglia, the resident immune cells of the central nervous system, are morphologically changed to create an inflammatory microenvironment that is detrimental to motor neuron survival. This brings forward the importance of tissue morphology study since the adaptive changes in cell architecture play crucial roles in triggering disease processes and may signify targets for therapeutic strategies (Cocozza et al., 2019). Other than neurodegenerative diseases, pathological cardiac tissue morphology has also become a central force behind cardiovascular disorders. Advances in imaging, such as cardiac magnetic resonance and computed tomography, facilitate the identification of ectopic cardiac fatty images, which may be indicative of various pathological processes. These images may reflect a process ranging from normal physiological presence of adipose tissue to frank diseases such as arrhythmogenic right ventricular dysplasia and post-myocardial infarction lipomatous metaplasia. Identification of these morphological variations is essential because they influence diagnostic considerations and therapeutic intervention. While not all fatty images will be of clinical significance, some may reflect underlying disease processes for which there is evidence to substantiate that morphological assessment is a fundamental component in understanding and managing cardiovascular disease (Cannavale et al., 2018). Examining pathological tissue morphology is not only important in the understanding of disease pathology but also in improving patient outcomes with personalized therapies. Through tissue structural changes research, scientists can identify new biomarkers indicative of disease progression and treatment outcome. As an example, research on the activation of microglial cells within ALS has triggered studies attempting to modulate the inflammatory response, and it is interesting to observe the direct correlation between morphological alteration and therapeutics. Similarly, fluctuations in cardiac adipose tissue predict the likelihood of pathological significance, enabling clinicians to distinguish benign from malignant processes. By integrating pathological tissue morphology into medical practice, medical practitioners can enhance diagnostic accuracy and tailor interventions to target the morphology-based aspects of diseases, ultimately leading to enhanced patient care and outcomes (Cannavale et al., 2018; Cocozza et al., 2019) (Figure 14.10).

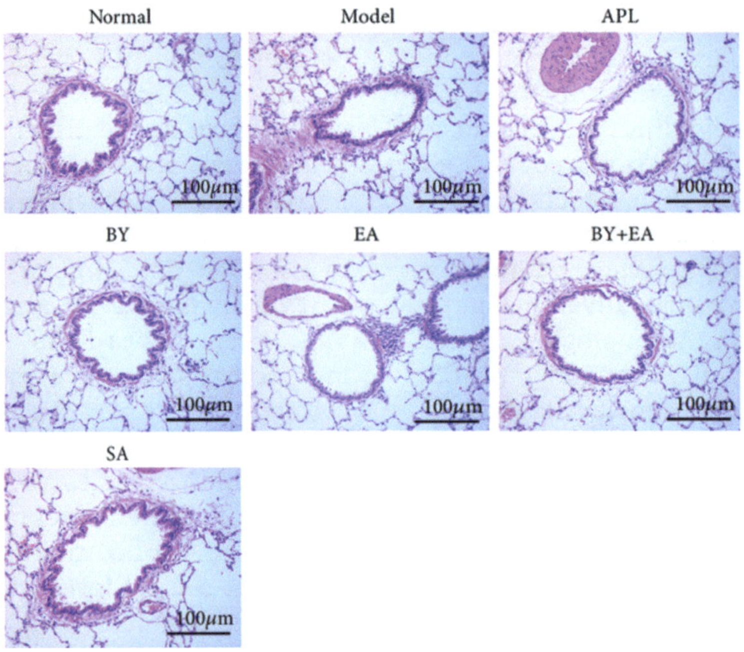

Figure 14.10. Role of pathological tissue morphology in disease.

Source: https://www.researchgate.net/publication/333472097/figure/fig4/AS:1086065611931654@1635949628100/Changes-in-the-lung-tissue-morphology-in-all-groups-a-Pathological-changes-in-the-lung.jpg.

14.4.1. Cancer Diagnosis and Staging

The role of imaging modalities in cancer diagnosis is increasingly important, particularly in the context of accurate identification and staging of disease progression. Magnetic Resonance Imaging (MRI) and Magnetic Resonance Cholangiopancreatography (MRCP) have become indispensable tools in the evaluation of pancreatic cancer. Their high specificity and sensitivity make them indispensible to clinicians evaluating tumor behavior and resectability. Curiously, MRI and MRCP were found to demonstrate good performance in differentiating the character of pancreatic lesions in one research, with a sensitivity of 88% and specificity of 95% (Turowska et al., 2009). Moreover, the accuracy of these imaging techniques for assessing tumor resectability was up to 95%, underscoring their vital role in clinical treatment planning and management. Since staging of cancer is of utmost significance in planning for appropriate treatment modalities, the incorporation of newer diagnostic technologies is of utmost significance. Histopathological evaluation remains the gold standard for the diagnosis of cancer, but digital pathology has transformed the field. Pathologists can interpret large volumes of digital histopathological images using machine learning algorithms, thereby improving diagnostic yield and clinical outcomes. However, the technique has some limitations, such as the need for high-resolution image acquisition and standardized protocols to prevent variability in analysis. These complications need to be addressed for computer-aided diagnosis systems to thrive in clinical settings, thereby optimizing cancer staging and treatment planning (Ishikawa, S., & Komura, D., 2017). Ultimately, proper diagnosis and cancer staging depend on a multifaceted approach that combines advanced imaging modalities and sound histopathological analysis. The interaction between these modalities extends clinicians' ability to make educated decisions, tailor treatments, and evaluate patient prognoses. As science advances, the integration of newer technologies, e.g., digital imaging and machine learning, will further refine cancer diagnosis and staging procedures. This continuous advancement also guides timely intervention strategies while fostering improved understanding of tumor biology, which is critical for the development of novel therapeutic modalities in the future. Emphasizing innovation in pathological tissue morphology is thus critical for maximizing outcomes in cancer treatment and care.

14.4.2. Infectious Diseases and Tissue Response

The interaction between infections and body tissue response is one that is extremely complex and central to the comprehension of pathological tissue morphology. When pathogens infect the body, they initiate an immune response that can cause radical alterations in tissue structure. A component of this response is inflammation, in which invading immune cells migrate into infected tissue, thereby increasing blood flow and the secretion of signaling molecules. As pathogenic microbes increase, as in the case of oral pathogens like *Porphyromonas gingivalis*, they can penetrate the blood-brain barrier, which leads to a cascade of immune responses resulting in neuronal damage and tissue architecture disturbance. Results indicate that chronic infections can develop as pathological changes, proving the widespread impact infectious pathogens have on tissue structure and well-being. Pathological tissue structure that is associated with infectious illnesses may be very dissimilar depending on the nature of the pathogen as well as the tissue involved. For instance, in systemic infection, the accompanying inflammatory response may lead to changes such as fibrosis, necrosis, or even tumor growth in the infected tissue. Immune cell infiltration can result in local tissue damage, which, as periodontal disease research has shown, can have far-reaching consequences, even with potential neurological manifestations. The chronic inflammation stemming from polymicrobial infection could not only compromise local structural integrity but also create a fertile soil for other diseases to take root, as studies indicating the link between oral pathogens and neurodegenerative diseases have shown. Hence, it becomes essential to identify the characteristic pathological changes due to various infectious agents so that therapeutic strategies can be effectively designed. Moreover, persistent surveillance of pathological changes in infection-prone tissues is crucial for early diagnosis and treatment. As evidenced by research on elephant foot pathologies, where the pathologies are often multifactorial in nature, an early assessment can reveal the underlying causes prior to their becoming severe. The development of osteoarthritis or infective osteoarthritis may mirror the complex responses caused by infective disease in other mammals, including man. Using advanced imaging techniques and diagnostic methods, researchers can better understand the impact of infections on tissue morphology. These data not only contribute to veterinary practice but also underscore the need for active response in human medicine, particularly the detection of early pathological changes to prevent long-term effects of infectious diseases on the morphology and health of tissues (Figure 14.11).

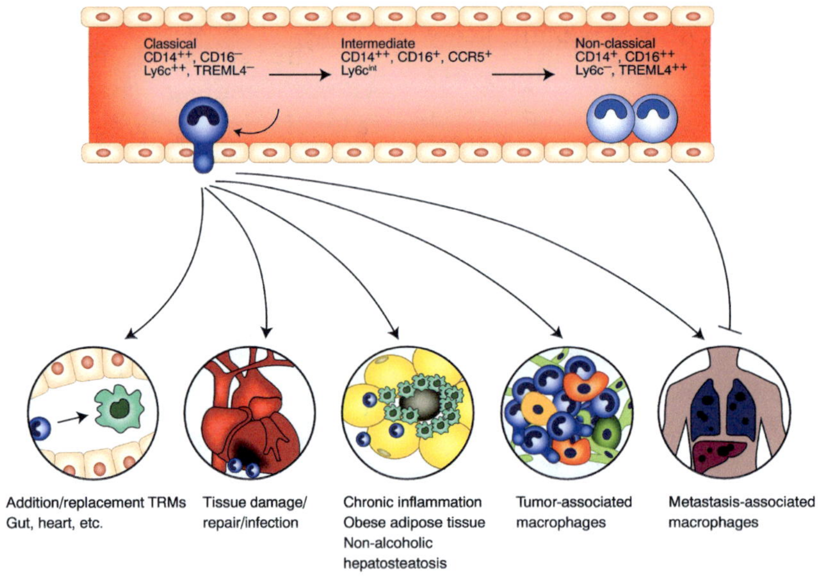

Figure 14.11. Infectious diseases and tissue response.

Source: https://els-jbs-prod-cdn.jbs.elsevierhealth.com/cms/attachment/d08cd273-e928-4f60-84e0-caf845b3b405/gr1_lrg.jpg.

14.4.3. Autoimmune Disorders and Tissue Changes

The complex association between tissue alterations and autoimmune diseases is critical to understanding pathological tissue morphology. Autoimmune diseases, such as multiple sclerosis (MS) and Menieres disease, produce characteristic changes in tissue architecture, mainly resulting from the action of immune-mediated damage and repair mechanisms. In MS, the pathologic alterations are closely associated with demyelination and inflammation, followed by subsequent degeneration of neural tissues. This inflammatory response not only damages myelin-producing oligodendrocytes but may also result in axonal integrity disruption, which classically manifests in radiologically apparent lesions on magnetic resonance imaging (MRI). The inflammatory milieu is responsible for a cyclical pattern of tissue injury and healing, further compounding the morphological terrain of compromised tissue. Moreover, the integrity of the blood-brain barrier (BBB) and the microvasculature plays a key role in autoimmune disease. In Meniere's disease patients, meticulous ultrastructural analysis illustrates relevant changes in the blood-labyrinthine barrier (BLB). Capillary structure research reveals signs of vascular degeneration, including increased vesicular transport and basement membrane thickening, consistent with clinical symptomatology and disease severity. These structural abnormalities detail how immune processes can disrupt vascular integrity, with the potential for severe systemic and neurological impact. Since tissues are continuously subjected to inflammatory attack, the morphologic alterations that ensue emphasize the need for further investigation on the mechanisms controlling these pathological alterations in autoimmune diseases. The mechanisms of coagulation, as well as thrombotic occurrences, also contribute significantly to morphologic degradation of tissue in autoimmune disorders. Findings from observations on MS indicate that perivascular fibrin(ogen) deposition is associated with early inflammatory processes, which suggests that hemostatic factors enhance tissue injury. The availability of thrombin not only initiates inflammation but may also have neurotoxic actions on glial cells under certain circumstances. Thus, alterations in the normal physiology of microglia and astrocytes following perturbation of the coagulation cascade are responsible for the rapid progression of these diseases. Thus, the interplay of immune dysregulation and coagulation factors provides a complex model for investigating tissue remodeling in autoimmune disorders, with promising lines of therapeutic attack aimed at inhibiting damage and promoting repair pathways in target tissues (Figure 14.12).

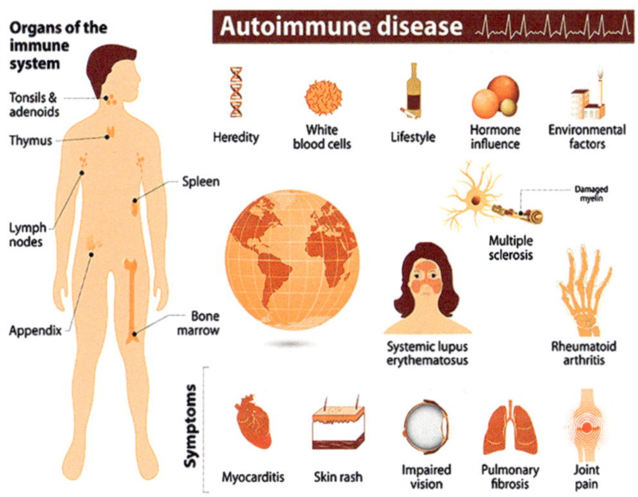

Figure 14.12. Autoimmune disorders and tissue changes.

Source: https://www.niehs.nih.gov/sites/default/files/health/assets/images/autoimmune_disease.jpg.

14.5. Case Studies in Pathological Tissue Morphology

The examination of pathological tissue morphology through case studies provides useful information regarding the alterations that define various stages of illness. In particular, cardiovascular disease patient tissue sample analysis has identified strong morphometric changes linked to structure and function. By focusing on the aortic wall deposits, researchers have learned that thermal characteristics of biological apatite may be applied as a marker of pathological changes. For instance, it has been shown that the presence of sodium and magnesium can influence mineral properties, suggesting their non-chance involvement in calcified tissues, which reflects pathological processes at play. Delineation of such conversions enables a finer strategy for diagnosing and treating cardiovascular diseases and ultimately opens up new possibilities for therapeutic intervention, attesting to the clinical importance of studying tissue morphology in these diseases. The most recent advancements in imaging techniques and computational analysis have greatly enhanced the research of pathological tissue morphology, particularly in cancer biology. By applying sophisticated segmentation algorithms to immunohistochemical tissue images, researchers can accurately detect and isolate cancer regions within complex biological samples. An example technique applies unsupervised color clustering in order to demarcate tumor areas independently of nearby stroma, which is critical to knowing about tumor growth patterns. Besides, a second computational approach stresses the color separation for attaining the precise nuclear membrane segmentation of cancer cells. These technologies exhibit higher accuracy compared to the traditional manual procedures and provide a uniform method to study the tissue morphology and the behavior of specific proteins involved in cancers and other pathologies. Thus, these methods possess high potential not just for research purposes but also for clinical diagnostics and therapy. The use of these novel techniques in clinical practice underlines the growing importance of case studies in revealing the complex interdependencies between tissue structure and disease onset. By thoroughly investigating pathological specimens through automated means, researchers can revolutionize the discipline of diagnosis from a qualitative assessment to a quantitative and objective process. This shift facilitates data reproducibility and enables the examination of larger datasets, providing a strong foundation for understanding disease mechanisms at the tissue level. As demonstrated by current studies, including work performed on the alteration of bioapatite in atherosclerotic plaques, this technology can identify novel biomarkers for disease development. By improving such methods further, pathological tissue morphology can have a major impact on personalized medicine, delivering information that is tailored to the unique needs of individual patients.

14.5.1. Breast Cancer Histopathology

The histopathological complexity of breast cancer hugely dictates diagnosis and, consequently, therapy. Pathologists depend heavily on morphologic features of tumor cells in evaluating malignancy and in making patient management decisions. Moreover, assessment of cellular arrangement, size, and form is of utmost importance for accurate breast cancer diagnosis. In some instances, small tumors are not always detectable, and this may lead to misdiagnosis if one only relies on visual observation. This negatively affects the outcomes of patients. Recent advancements involving label-free multiphoton microscopy (MPM) have shown the ability to overcome these limitations by quantitatively examining breast tissues in more dimensions. The novel approach allows for an enhanced examination of tumor characteristics, and thus the precision of breast cancer diagnoses and treatment protocols attuned to meet individual patient needs, resulting in improved prognostic outcomes (Zhong et al., 2025). In the histopathology of breast cancer, precise nuclear morphology analysis has emerged as a significant aspect in malignancy identification. Segmentation of nuclei provides critical information regarding cell growth and malignancy of tumors, which determines the choice of treatment strategy. Standard segmentation, however, proves to be inefficient in the delicacy of nuclear composition, especially with overlapping nuclei or changing size and shape. To address these issues, the advent of advanced multi-scale context-aware approaches, such as the M3-Net model, is a milestone in computerized histopathological analysis. By integrating global and local tissue features, M3-Net improves the accuracy of nuclei segmentation and enables pathologists to derive critical information from the histological terrain. This technological development is not a refinement of imaging techniques; it transforms the diagnostic model fundamentally by making possible a more advanced assessment of tumor histopathology (Sufyan et al., 2025). With the evolution of breast cancer histopathology, integration of machine learning and advanced imaging techniques is at the forefront of diagnostic breakthroughs. With tools such as MPM and sophisticated segmentation algorithms, physicians can make more informed decisions regarding the care of patients. Not only do these technologies enhance diagnostic sensitivity but also permit measurement of response to treatment, providing a data-driven basis for making therapy adjustments. Additionally, prediction of the efficacy of treatment based on characteristics measured pathologically may transform personalized medicine in oncology with therapeutic approaches customized to the patient's pathology. With constant progress in research in this area, there is a hope that such progress will enhance the survival and quality of life in patients with breast cancer, thereby emphasizing the vital importance of histopathological assessment in contemporary clinical practice (Figure 14.13).

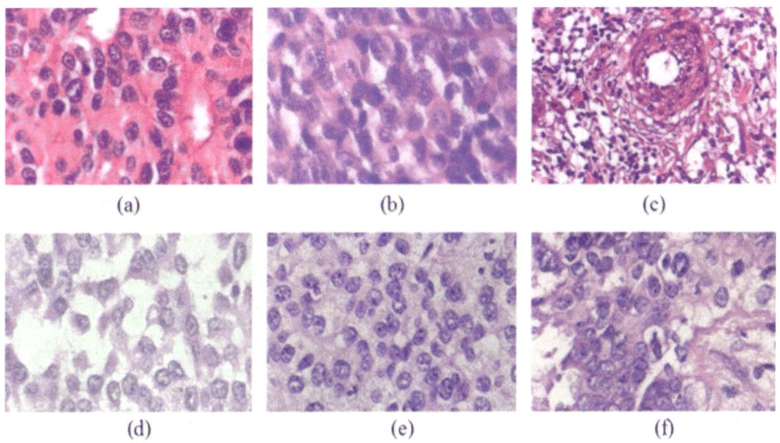

Figure 14.13. Breast cancer histopathology.

Source: https://www.researchgate.net/profile/Xipeng-Pan-2/publication/329486028/figure/fig1/AS:941760410824734@1601544587790/Breast-cancer-histopathology-images-samples-a-e-are-ductal-carcinomaDC-sample-f-is.png.

14.5.2. Chronic Inflammation in Autoimmune Diseases

Chronic inflammation is a feature of many autoimmune disorders and has profound impacts on tissue morphology and organ function. In autoimmune disease, the immune system targets normal tissue, leading to chronic inflammatory reactions that may lead to tissue damage and architectural alterations. For instance, in rheumatoid arthritis and systemic lupus erythematosus, inflammatory cells penetrate joint tissue and other organs, resulting in a pattern of injury and repair, ultimately ending in pathologic changes. The interaction between tissue cells and immune mediators is usually multifaceted and culminates in the formation of granulomas and fibrosis, destroying the normal tissue architecture of the involved tissue. This dysregulated inflammatory reaction not only underlies clinical presentation but also poses stringent challenges to therapy, since avoiding inflammation while ensuring immune defense remains a tenuous balance in the therapy of such diseases. In a specific instance of a pediatric patient with chronic inflammation presenting atypical features, the diagnostic process mirrored the complexity of issues involved with autoimmune diseases. The child had chronic fever, arthralgia, and neuroinflammation, and skin biopsies showed nodular vasculitis, possibly secondary to diseases such as childhood-onset polyarteritis nodosa (c-PAN). This case illustrates how chronic inflammation may manifest differently across individuals, complicating diagnosis and management. Significantly, the inflammatory process became apparent not just in the joints but also in systemic manifestations like uveitis and skin lesions. While the therapy with corticosteroids demonstrated the initial disappearance of symptoms, their tapering resulted in relapse and left a trace on the persistence of the inflammation following changes in tissue morphology. These characteristics emphasize the necessity of careful clinical and immunologic investigation to reveal the pathways of these inflammatory conditions and make a significant contribution to the morbidity of patients. New therapies targeting chronic inflammation in autoimmune disease are giving promise to modify the disease process and reduce tissue injury. For instance, therapy with siponimod and other sphingosine 1-phosphate receptor modulators is promising in managing autoimmune diseases by inhibiting lymphocyte migration and dampening neuroinflammatory cascades. In the preclinical models, such as *Theiler's murine encephalomyelitis virus model, their actions on microglial activation and tissue integrity have been studied and demonstrated to result in* some attenuation of disease in some cases. While initial reports describe suppression of inflammation, more work is necessary to characterize their actions on long-term neurodegeneration and lesion formation. The nuanced understanding of the way chronic inflammation distorts tissue morphology and the development of targeted therapies will provide worthwhile perspectives into maximizing care approaches for autoimmune disorders, emphasizing the significance of comprehensive approaches to care in such complex diseases.

14.5.3. Tissue Changes in Infectious Diseases

When considering pathological tissue morphology under consideration, it is clear that infectious diseases trigger a range of tissue alterations that play a major role in shaping overall health outcomes. When pathogens infect host tissues, they tend to activate inflammatory reactions, triggering a cascade of cellular and molecular changes. These alterations include cellular necrosis, apoptosis, and hyperplasia, which indicate the body's efforts to control the infection. For instance, periodontal infection demonstrates the way in which microbial invasion can transcend local tissue to affect remote structures, for example, the central nervous system. The oral pathogen *Porphyromonas gingivalis* has been reported to invade brain tissues via complement activation, thereby causing bystander neuronal injury, as suggested by ApoE-/- mouse studies. This highlights the interconnectedness of tissue response and systemic manifestations of infectious disease pathology, and thus, it becomes important to understand such mechanisms holistically in order to come up with appropriate therapeutic interventions (Chukkapalli et al., 2014). Pathological changes resulting from infectious diseases are not confined to a single organ system. A clear example is in research conducted using elephants, where foot diseases illustrate the magnitude of pathological alterations. Research employing post-mortem computer tomography has revealed a marked prevalence of bone remodeling, osteoarthritis, and enthesopathy in the African and Asian elephant feet. These pathologies are indicative of chronic stress and inflammation, enhanced by weight-bearing locomotor mechanisms. Furthermore, the study revealed differences between the incidence of these pathologies with respect to sex and age, pointing out the multifaceted nature of tissue response to infectious diseases. These findings underscore the necessity of ongoing monitoring and active care of the elephant's foot condition, which signifies the value of tissue change surveillance in disease-prone species (Benjamin et al., 2017). Finally, tissue changes in infectious diseases involve a multi-disciplinary approach to appreciate their meaning. It is essential that pathologists, immunologists, and clinicians collaborate to investigate the wide variety of ways in which pathogens influence host tissues at the molecular and histological levels. Using advanced imaging and molecular technologies can provide a wealth of information on the degree of change in the tissue, as well as pathway-specific processes responsible for disease. For instance, in infection-induced neuropathology, detection of pathogen-derived DNA in brain tissues via polymerase chain reaction provides new avenues for therapeutic targets. Unraveling these intricate interactions between infection and tissue pathology will not only drive improvement in treatment modalities but also enhance preventive practices in many fields of medicine and veterinary practice. With the continued interplay between tissues and pathogens, the necessity to learn pathological tissue morphology among infectious diseases is made all the more apparent (Figure 14.14).

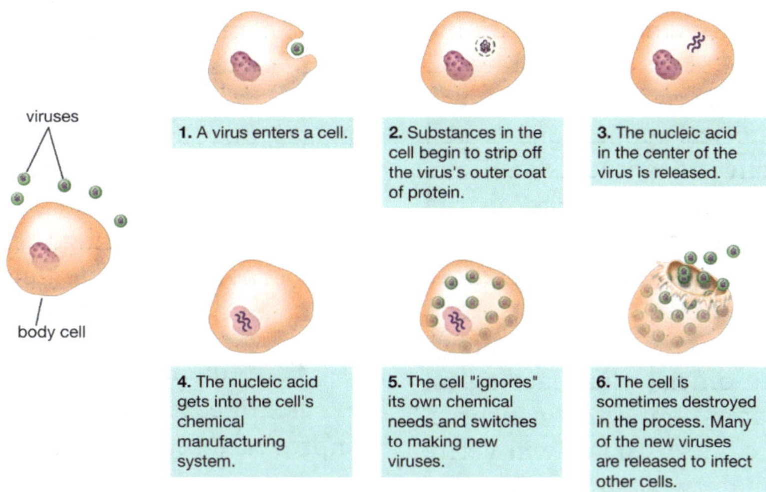

Figure 14.14. Tissue changes in infectious diseases.

Source: https://cdn.britannica.com/17/95417-050-D08C7F24/process-virus-cell.jpg.

14.6. Current Research Trends

The study of pathological tissue morphology has documented impressive advances in recent years, with the advances observed being in concordance with current trends in research directed at the issues in cell aging and related neurodegenerative diseases. With the world's aging population, conditions such as Alzheimer's disease and Parkinson's disease are significant health issues confronting the world, which need novel therapeutic approaches. Experiments probing the mechanism of brain aging reveal the critical roles of oxidative stress, chronic inflammation, and mitochondrial injury, and studies have shifted toward therapy with cellular components instead of whole cells. Of these, mesenchymal stem cells (MSCs) have been the focus of significant attention due to their regenerative capacities, and MSC-derived extracellular vesicles have been established as a consequence. These vesicles, or MSC-Exo, present a hopeful solution, retaining the biological benefits of MSCs but avoiding safety concerns, such as immune rejection and tumor formation, paramount in the new age of neurodegenerative disease treatment (Quan et al., 2025). Furthermore, a study on botanical compounds within the realm of pathological tissue morphology presents yet another modern research avenue. The research on L. (black seed), with its dense medicinal potential, is a good example of how traditional knowledge is able to integrate itself with contemporary scientific research. This research seeks to elaborate on the chemical and botanical composition of black seed, exploring its historical applications as well as the impact of its active constituents on tissue wellness. Trends now depict a focus on the extraction processes and formulation strategies that maximize the therapeutic efficacy of these plant materials, in alignment with the trend towards plant-based therapeutics in pathology. Their integration into official pharmacological systems raises regulatory and safety concerns, but the forthcoming clinical studies will verify their efficacy in treating various diseases, illustrating the extensive overlap between traditional medicine and modern biochemistry in shaping future research directions (Usmani et al., 2024). Ongoing research sees the most significant trend being quality control and standardization for stem cell therapy and for the use of botany. The necessity of rigorous regulatory oversight is evident in that the health care system relies on trustworthy information regarding the efficacy and safety of such therapy. Such rigorous quality assurance not only ensures quality to the therapeutic products derived from MSC-Exo and plant sources like black seed but also inspires trust among the consumers. Current research bridges the commercialization gaps to enable the integration of state-of-the-art therapeutic modalities into clinical practice. Hence, there needs to be an interface of quality research, regulatory compliance, and innovative therapeutic strategy for advancing the science of pathological tissue morphology to improve health outcomes and therapeutic interventions in neurodegenerative disorders and beyond.

14.6.1. Advances in Digital Pathology

The integration of digital pathology into pathological tissue morphology practice is a histopathological examination revolution. The advent of whole-slide scanning technology has enabled the digitization of tissue samples, transforming the pathologists' processes of disease diagnosis and research. The method enables the archiving and sharing of high-quality images, thereby greatly enhancing collaborative research across institutions and geographies. Besides, it encourages the application of computer-aided diagnosis (CAD) systems that provide complementary pathologists' interpretations with robust data-driven results.

Consequently, digital pathology innovation has greatly eased disease diagnosis processes and improved disease detection precision, thereby maintaining the capabilities of pathologists in formulating highly informed decisions in patient treatments and care plans (Boucheron et al., 2009). Utilization of machine learning techniques in digital pathology has greatly increased the analytical potential of digitized histopathological images. By leveraging large datasets, algorithms can detect patterns and abnormalities in tissue morphology that may be undetectable to the naked eye. This capability addresses increasing demands for precise diagnostic tools capable of navigating the complexities of modern pathology.

Assertively, the continuous innovations in CAD technology for histopathology have exhibited efficacy in enhancing the accuracy of diagnosis, particularly in detecting cancer and other areas. Still, challenges remain, including demanding standardized protocols and minimizing algorithm training biases. Overcoming them is essential in maximizing the utility of machine learning, therefore paving the way for more accurate diagnostic outputs (Ishikawa, S., & Komura, D., 2017). In addition to technical advancement, the adoption of digital pathology requires rethinking teaching practices in the field. As pathology education continues to progress, skill development in digital technology and data analysis is necessary for the next generation of practitioners.

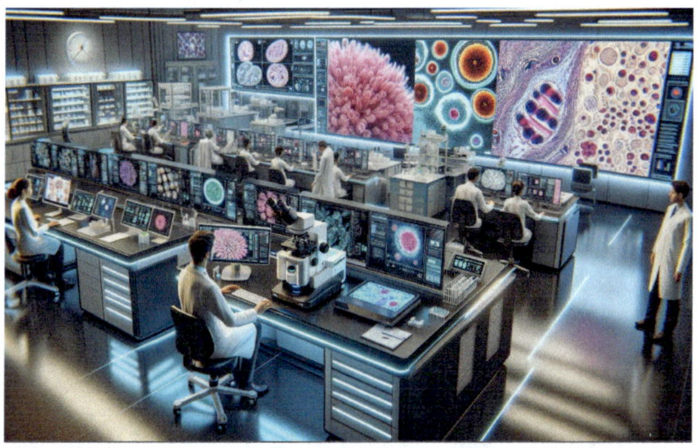

Figure 14.15. Advances in digital pathology.

Source: https://digestley.com/wp-content/uploads/2024/02/Digital-Pathology.webp.

Those programs that integrate digital imaging and machine learning into their curricula can better prepare the students for the evolving landscape of pathology. Additionally, continuous professional development activities related to digital technologies can empower pathologists to adapt to the rapid pace of the discipline's evolution. The intersection between machine learning and digital pathology is most likely to revolutionize the professional roles in clinical labs, concentrating on the demand for intersectoral competencies that bridge traditional histopathology and modern technology, thus creating an adaptable workforce (Boucheron et al., 2009; Ishikawa, S., & Komura, D., 2017) (Figure 14.15).

14.6.2. Integration of Artificial Intelligence

The application of artificial intelligence (AI) in pathological tissue morphology within the global arena is revolutionizing diagnostic potential in oncology. Pathologists employed traditional manual observations of tissue samples, which were subject to human error and time-consuming, in the past. AI technology is, however, being increasingly utilized to examine complex patterns of tissue morphology with better accuracy and speed. For instance, sophisticated algorithms assist in the identification of microcalcifications in mammography images, an essential indicator of breast cancer, according to recent literature on the use of fractals and wavelets in cancer diagnosis (Fuente et al., 2008). This technology not only improves the diagnostic accuracy but also assists in early identification of malignancies, improving patient outcomes. In the application of AI in pathological inspection, potential for bias and ethical issues should be addressed. Also, the rapidity of advancements in AI in cancer diagnosis and imaging raises questions about how machine learning models will be used in clinical routines. The issues include the need for transparency in AI systems, as algorithms must be understandable to practitioners to ensure accurate interpretation of results. Besides, regulatory settings that manage the ethical use of AI in healthcare are the current imperative. From recent analysis, investigating the impact of AI on cancer pathology diagnosis shows the benefit of enhanced efficiency as well as challenges that may emanate from implementation (Alsup et al., 2023). It is critical that healthcare stakeholders sail through such intricacies to harness the actual potential of

AI to meet the needs of patient welfare. The ongoing development of AI applications in pathological tissue morphology reaffirms the revolutionary potential of the technology in cancer management and prevention. With the use of sophisticated machine learning algorithms, clinical professionals and researchers are able to perform such critical activities as regression, classification, segmentation, generation, and compression of cancerous tissue data. As an illustration, segmentation methods have the capacity to precisely isolate cancerous from non-cancerous tissue, a characteristic that can impact the choice of treatment enormously. With an increasing amount of research, future experiments will be building upon these fundamentals, driving innovation towards personalized treatment and targeted therapies (Alsup et al., 2023). Not only is the implementation of AI enhancing diagnostics, but it is also ushering in a finer understanding of cancer pathology, a significant step forward for the discipline.

14.6.3. Future Directions in Tissue Morphology Studies

The history of tissue morphology studies is intertwined with the evolution of imaging devices that enable improved visualization of pathological and normal tissues at various resolution levels. New techniques, such as high-resolution computed tomography (HRCT), have enabled investigators to distinguish morphological patterns of disease, such as fibrotic interstitial lung diseases. Imaging modalities combined with advanced algorithms for texture analysis hold considerable promise for improving diagnostic accuracy. For example, an experiment established that topological texture features outperformed traditional texture analysis methods in automatic tissue characterization, registering significant classification accuracy rates. Greater knowledge of tissue morphology through these means can lead to earlier diagnosis and personalized treatment protocols, thereby revolutionizing clinical pathology practice (Huber et al., 2010). Upcoming research needs to focus on enhancing such technologies and integrating more data-intensive approaches to quantify tissue change complexity over time. In addition to imaging advances, the interface of computational models with machine learning techniques is reshaping the tissue morphology research field. By using large datasets, researchers can explore complex interactions between cellular structure and disease state to support predictive modeling. For instance, the application of machine learning algorithms to pathology has the potential to quantify histological parameters linked with specific morphological alterations. Such data-driven studies, in addition to enabling identification and classification, illuminate more about the associated biological processes. Additionally, studies of cellular behavior, like those illustrated in studies of ovarian cyclicity, highlight the dynamic nature of tissue morphology across various physiological and pathological states. These studies underscore the importance of synchronizing molecular and biological data in morphological assessments to achieve a holistic understanding of tissue integrity and pathology (Chatdarong, 2003). The future of research in tissue morphology also lies in the translational route, wherein findings of basic science can be successfully translated into clinical application. With emerging new technologies and techniques, it is essential that interdisciplinary cooperation among biologists, pathologists, and engineers is established to evolve innovation in this field. Interdisciplinary studies can offer the development of new diagnostic devices and therapeutic interventions tailored to the specific needs of an individual patient. Moreover, as more information becomes available on tissue morphology, the possibility of studying rare diseases and those diseases with no effective diagnostic methods expands. By targeting unexplored areas, the field can make significant strides in improving patient outcomes. Lastly, the convergence of advanced imaging, computational modeling, and translational research will definitely redefine the fate of tissue morphology research and further elucidate the understanding of pathological processes of human disease (Chatdarong, 2003; Huber et al., 2010) (Figure 14.16).

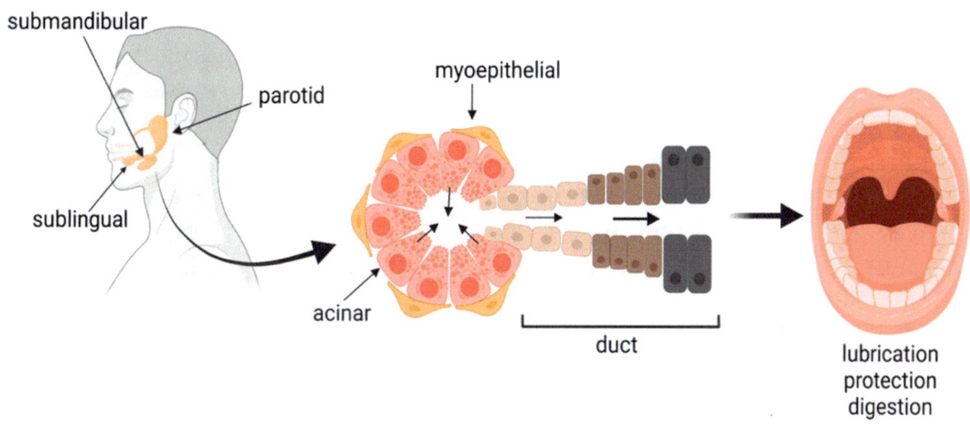

Figure 14.16. Future directions in tissue morphology studies.

Source: https://pub.mdpi-res.com/cells/cells-10-01723/article_deploy/html/images/cells-10-01723-g001.png?1626156112.

SUMMARY

In summarizing the major findings on pathological tissue morphology, it is evident that sophisticated analytical approaches significantly enhance our understanding of disease mechanisms. Advances such as spatial transcriptomics provide significant insights into cellular and molecular heterogeneity, which will untangle the complexities of such pathologies. The building of models like UPSST demonstrates the capability to choose pathological regions with precision and correlate them to specific morphological characteristics. By achieving high performance metrics, as in recent studies, researchers can obtain significant biological findings that augment our knowledge of tissue morphology in disease (Chen et al., 2025). Such progress not only directs diagnostic workup but also opens the way for the development of targeted therapies to oppose the underlying cause of tissue anomalies. Furthermore, the clinicopathological characteristics of rare tumors, such as alveolar soft part sarcoma (ASPS), demonstrate the dynamic interaction involved between morphology and clinical conduct. The pathological features of ASPS allow differential immunohistochemical profiling, thus facilitating more accurate diagnosis and prognostication. Retrospective studies emphasize the importance of morphological assessment, which may help clinicians in decision-making regarding management strategies for affected individuals. Surprisingly, factors such as tumor size and metastasis have been potent prognostic indicators, illustrating that pathological morphology is not only a descriptive parameter but a crucial determinant of patient outcome. These findings highlight the significance of combined strategies employing clinical history and histological examination to maximize patient care and survival (Zhang et al., 2024). Overall, the examination of pathological tissue structure is a basis in basic science as well as clinical investigation. The concert between modern techniques and traditional histopathological methods provides the avenue for an unequivocal comprehension of disease formation and therapeutic sensitivity. As illustrated by procedures like UPSST and tumor studies like ASPS, the vigorous scrutiny of tissue morphology transcends mere observation to yield vital information on the pathobiology of disease. Such an active landscape highlights the need for continued study and refinement in the field, ultimately resulting in greater diagnostic capability and therapeutic intervention. As scientists build on these initial discoveries, the development of more sophisticated methods will further elucidate the complex interplay between pathology and tissue morphology, ultimately enabling more precise and personalized medicine.

Pathological tissue morphology should be known in order to diagnose and treat a number of diseases correctly. This implies a proper knowledge of tissue structural alterations due to disease processes. Such examples include solitary pterygoid sinus lesions, which are puzzling to clinicians due to their uncommon clinical presentations and complex anatomical structures. Systematic retrospective analysis also revealed great variation in clinical symptoms, including headaches, ocular symptoms, and nasal symptoms, among patients presenting with such lesions. By correlating imaging with clinical findings, clinicians can more accurately diagnose, thus reducing rates of misdiagnosis as well as enhancing patient outcomes. Thus, ensuring that clinicians have a good understanding of such tissue morphologies is imperative in advancing medical practice and the efficiency of treatments (Yu et al., 2025). At the same time, research on conditions such as thin endometrium highlights the intricate interdependence of morphology and function of tissue. Dysfunction of the lining in the endometrium may hinder fertility, illustrating how pathological changes may establish significant clinical implications. Studies have shown that ischemic conditions adversely affect the endometrium, causing alterations in cytoskeletal proteins and cell junctions of epithelial cells. Using advanced imaging and investigative methods, researchers found that morphological changes constitute an adaptation to poor blood supply and insufficient oxygen, ultimately leading to increased cell death and apoptosis. Understanding these mechanisms will not only facilitate enhanced diagnosis but also assist in the development of targeted therapies to restore endometrial function and promote reproductive health (Peng et al., 2024). Hence, a summary of key points in pathological tissue morphology should emphasize the classification and functional assessments of various types of tissue under physiological and pathological conditions. Marriage of clinical statistics with a deep understanding of morphological changes allows for more advanced diagnostic criteria and treatment protocols based on individual conditions. The findings of the above experiments clearly show the need for urgent exploration of pathological tissue morphology, as application of this topic extends beyond the field of diagnostics into that of therapy. Enabling health practitioners to understand tissue changes enhances patient care and guides public health policies toward limiting the impact of diverse diseases through early intervention and detection (Peng et al., 2024; Yu et al., 2025).

A LOOK TO THE FUTURE:

BIOCHEMICAL TECHNIQUES:

Biochemical techniques form the foundation of experimental investigation in the life sciences, allowing scientists to observe, measure, and manipulate the molecular machinery of living organisms. These techniques encompass a wide range of laboratory methods used to analyze biomolecules such as proteins, nucleic acids, lipids, and carbohydrates, and to understand their structure, function, and interactions within biological systems. By enabling precise experimentation and quantitative analysis, biochemical techniques have become indispensable in research, medicine, biotechnology, agriculture, and environmental science. At their core, biochemical techniques are designed to isolate, separate, quantify, and characterize biological molecules and processes. Fundamental approaches such as centrifugation and electrophoresis allow researchers to fractionate complex mixtures, separating cellular components or biomolecules based on size, density, or electrical charge. For example, differential centrifugation can isolate organelles from cell homogenates, while electrophoresis separates proteins or nucleic acids by charge and size, revealing important information about molecular composition or identifying specific variants.

Other methods, such as chromatography techniques, exploit differences in molecular properties to purify and analyze mixtures. Techniques like high-performance liquid chromatography (HPLC) and ion-exchange chromatography enable detailed separation of compounds, making it possible to study individual biomolecules in isolation and monitor their behavior under controlled conditions.

Spectrophotometry plays a crucial role in many biochemical assays by measuring how molecules absorb or transmit light, which can indicate concentration, purity, or chemical changes during reactions. This non-destructive analytical tool, often paired with colorimetric assays, is widely used to quantify proteins, nucleic acids, and enzyme activities. Modern biochemical laboratories also employ advanced techniques such as isothermal titration calorimetry, which measures the thermodynamics of molecular interactions, adding depth to understanding binding events and reaction energetics. Methods like the Western blot extend these capabilities by allowing the specific detection of proteins and their modifications, critical for both basic research and clinical diagnostics.

The importance of biochemical techniques goes far beyond the laboratory bench. In medicine, they underpin disease diagnosis, the development of targeted therapies, and the monitoring of treatment efficacy. In biotechnology, these methods drive innovations in drug discovery, genetic engineering, and biomaterial development. In environmental science and agriculture, they help unravel metabolic pathways and assess biological responses to external stresses. This work aims to provide readers with a comprehensive introduction to the principles, applications, and significance of key biochemical techniques. By integrating theoretical foundations with practical insights, it seeks to cultivate a deeper appreciation for how these methods enable the exploration of life at the molecular level and contribute to the advancement of scientific knowledge and societal well-being.

REFERENCES

1. Di Cataldo, S., Ficarra, E., Acquaviva, A., & Macii, E. (2010). Automated segmentation of tissue images for computerized IHC analysis. *Computer Methods and Programs in Biomedicine, 100*(1), 1–15. https://doi.org/10.1016/j.cmpb.2010.02.002Acquaviva, A., Bresson, X., Caselles, V., Chan, T., Chang, S. K., Chen, Y., Chen, S., et al. (2010). Achieving the way for automated segmentation of nuclei in cancer tissue images through morphology-based approach: A quantitative evaluation. *https://core.ac.uk/download/pdf/11412919.pdf* (accessed on 6th August 2025).
2. Adams, R. A., Akassoglou, K., Akenami, F. O., Albright, A. V., et al. (2018). A perspective of coagulation dysfunction in multiple sclerosis and in experimental allergic encephalomyelitis. *https://core.ac.uk/download/195777098.pdf* (accessed on 6th August 2025).
3. Alyaldin, E., & Bale, P. (2024). OA26 Atypical multisystem inflammation related to infection or just plain old polyarteritis nodosa? *Rheumatology Advances in Practice, 8. https://www.semanticscholar.org/paper/390e0c2e9f5c4ace11f4e579235e1c797b9b407b* (accessed on 6th August 2025).
4. Arbab Sufyan, M., Ahmad Fauzi, M. F., & Wong, L. K. (2025). M3-Net: A multi-scale nuclei segmentation model for breast cancer histopathology using contextual patches and attention mechanism. In *2025 IEEE 22nd International Symposium on Biomedical Imaging (ISBI). https://www.semanticscholar.org/paper/b2c75585f9cefa6cf2777e31890f347bbe45c612* (accessed on 6th August 2025).
5. Badin, R. A., Cavicchioli, L., Cozzi, E., Crossan, C., et al. (2016). Posttransplant lymphoproliferative disorders in neuronal xenotransplanted macaques. *https://core.ac.uk/download/293883125.pdf* (accessed on 6th August 2025).
6. Benjamin, M., Carciofi, A., Carlson, M., Choudhury, B., Craig, J., Csuti, B., Dyson, S., et al. (2017). Skeletal pathology and variable anatomy in elephant feet assessed using computed tomography. *https://core.ac.uk/download/76981012.pdf* (accessed on 6th August 2025).
7. Bochsler, V. S., Galloway, S. B., Harley, R. A., Kramarsky-Winters, E., et al. (2007). *Coral Disease and Health Workshop: Coral Histopathology II. https://core.ac.uk/download/11017972.pdf* (accessed on 6th August 2025).
8. Boucheron, L. E., Can, A., Gurcan, M. N., Madabhushi, A., et al. (2009). Histopathological image analysis: A review. *https://core.ac.uk/download/46378.pdf* (accessed on 6th August 2025).
9. Buckley, C. D., Curnow, S. J., Denniston, A. K. O., Fairclough, M., et al. (2010). Distinct types of fibrocyte can differentiate from mononuclear cells in the presence and absence of serum. *https://core.ac.uk/download/pdf/19179.pdf* (accessed on 6th August 2025).
10. Cannavale, G., Carbone, I., Catalano, C., Francone, M., et al. (2018). Fatty images of the heart: Spectrum of normal and pathological findings at computed tomography and cardiac magnetic resonance imaging. *https://core.ac.uk/download/141696736.pdf* (accessed on 6th August 2025).
11. Casasent, A. (2018). *Investigating invasion in ductal carcinoma in situ with topographical single cell genome sequencing. https://core.ac.uk/download/212897087.pdf* (accessed on 6th August 2025).
12. Cavagnaro, M., Crocco, L., Lopresto, V., Pinto, R., et al. (2018). Monitoring thermal ablation via microwave tomography: An *ex vivo* experimental assessment. *https://core.ac.uk/download/195776752.pdf* (accessed on 6th August 2025).

13. Cavarretta, E., Cottignoli, V., Familiari, G., Giovanna, S., et al. (2015). Biological niches within human calcified aortic valves: Towards understanding of the pathological biomineralization process. *https://core.ac.uk/download/54521879.pdf* (accessed on 6th August 2025).

14. Chen, G., Hong, X., Zhang, L., Ding, L., Li, L., Jiang, C., Ni, J., et al. (2025). UPSST: Unsupervised pathology domain identification by integrating tissue morphology, imputing and clustering of spatial transcriptomics with GAT. *IEEE Transactions on Computational Biology and Bioinformatics, 22*, 298–309. *https://www.semanticscholar.org/paper/36721beccfb24318269f022b1b0498b2868b149b* (accessed on 6th August 2025).

15. Huber, M. B., Leinsinger, G., Nagarajan, M., Ray, S., et al. (2010). Classification of interstitial lung disease patterns with topological texture features. *http://arxiv.org/abs/1005.5086* (accessed on 6th August 2025).

16. Ishikawa, S., & Komura, D. (2017). Machine learning methods for histopathological image analysis. *http://arxiv.org/abs/1709.00786* (accessed on 6th August 2025).

17. Peng, T., Yang, S., Lian, W., Liu, X., Zheng, P., Qin, X., Liao, B., et al. (2024). Cytoskeletal and inter-cellular junction remodelling in endometrial organoids under oxygen-glucose deprivation: A new potential pathological mechanism for thin endometria. *Human Reproduction. https://www.semanticscholar.org/paper/f3b6c47b86781c1b671b8fd23fbac7b2b97083c7* (accessed on 6th August 2025).

18. Yu, Z., Yu, Y., Chen, X., Wang, Y., Cheng, P. (2025). Clinical diagnosis and treatment experience of 21 case report of isolated sphenoid sinus lesions. *Medicine, 104. https://www.semanticscholar.org/paper/1a7a034b0b48a15daa8024235e5d8bab934f71a3* (accessed on 6th August 2025).

19. Zhang, Y., Huang, Y., Qin, Y., Yang, N., Yang, P., Li, N., Feng, Z. (2024). Alveolar soft part sarcoma: A clinicopathological and immunohistochemical analysis of 26 cases emphasizing risk factors and prognosis. *Diagnostic Pathology, 19. https://www.semanticscholar.org/paper/50bcae6834bcedf08fc12f22500a8a7d18d83053* (accessed on 6th August 2025).

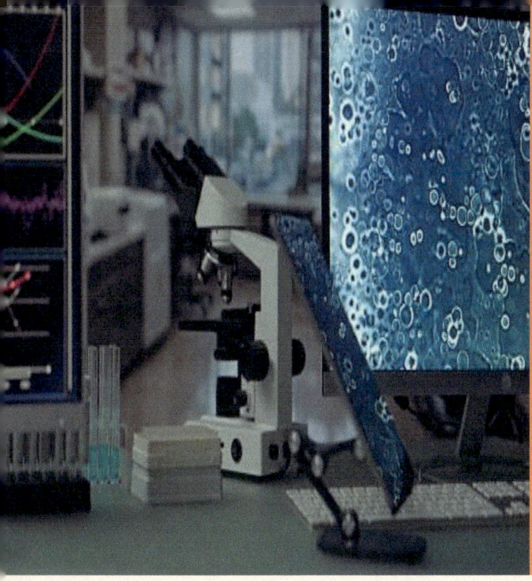

Chapter 15

DIGITAL PATHOLOGY AND AI IN MORPHOLOGICAL ANALYSIS

Contents

Introduction

Artificial intelligence (AI) application in digital pathology is a paradigm shift method of conducting morphological analysis that drives medical diagnostics to an entirely new level of practice. Pathologists have been using their skill and hand-eye coordination to examine tissue samples before, an effort with numerous drawbacks such as subjectivity and time-wastage. Digital pathology offers avenues for enhanced visualization and analysis, leading to enhanced efficiency and accuracy in the detection of diseases. Through the use of advanced image analysis techniques, digital pathology readily digitizes the pathology slides into high-resolution digital images, offering a window for AI algorithms to assist in quantifying histological features and detecting anomalies that would otherwise go unnoticed. This development not only serves to streamline workflows but also increases diagnostic consistency, eventually contributing to better patient outcomes. An integral aspect of this technological adoption is that neural networks are being designed to enable more user-friendly, productive analysis of whole-slide images (WSIs). Research indicated the power of neural networks to provide robust, quantitative opinions in medical contexts but was limited by training difficulties and the need for expert knowledge. Groundbreaking alternatives such as intuitive interfaces have met this deficiency, allowing pathologists to use neural network forecasts instantly within familiar digital workplaces. For instance, through a human-in-the-loop approach, pathologists are able to minimize the workload associated with WSIs annotation by quite a large extent, enhancing the experience and efficiency of employing AI in pathological diagnosis.

These innovations represent one way in which AI can support human expertise in pathology, enabling substantial improvements in diagnostic accuracy and efficiency (Ginley et al., 2018). Moreover, the work on automatic tissue segmentation techniques demonstrates the great mileage that can be achieved through integrating AI in morphological analysis. It has been shown that automated segmentation approaches work better than the traditional methods, including manual annotation and existing computerized systems, particularly in complex tasks like immunohistochemical tissue image recognition. With the application of unsupervised color clustering technology and advanced morphological processing, researchers have developed methods able to precisely delineate cancer areas with minimal false positives in surrounding tissue. In addition to enhancing diagnostic validity, these developments provide standardized and reliable measures for assessing the biological activity of individual proteins involved in multifactorial genetic diseases. This transition to these automated approaches is a significant step towards more reproducible and objective analyses, signaling a new era in pathology that relies heavily on the synergy between novel computational methodologies and essential medical knowledge (Acquaviva et al., 2010) (Figure 15.1).

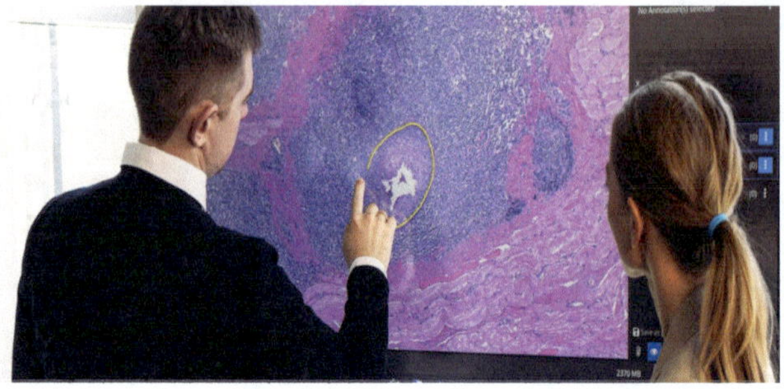

Figure 15.1. Digital pathology and AI in morphological analysis.

Source: https://websites.fraunhofer.de/smart-sensing-insights/wp-content/uploads/2023/09/digital-pathology-software_MICAIA-1500x500.jpg.

Definition of Digital Pathology

Digital pathology is a revolutionary medical diagnostic tool that combines traditional histopathology with advanced digital technology. It involves the capture, management, and examination of pathology data generated through digitized glass slides. Digital pathology is not merely the digitalization of samples but the enhancement of pathologists' workflow through electronic slide storage, retrieval, and review. This advancement facilitates the seamless sharing of high-resolution images across networks to facilitate remote consultations and collaborative research, effectively bridging geographical distance. Such advancements point to the capacity of digital pathology to deliver timely and accurate diagnoses and to streamline traditional practices associated with tissue examination. By integrating technology throughout the pathology workflow, digital pathology is a change agent for patient outcomes and healthcare delivery. Also, integrating artificial intelligence (AI) into digital pathology is a watershed moment for morphological analysis. AI algorithms enable sophisticated computational techniques that maximize image analysis and allow automatic tissue pattern recognition and classification. These advancements have demonstrated significant potential to supplement pathologists' expertise, enabling them to process and analyze enormous volumes of data successfully. For example, learning deep models can assist segmentation processes—dissolving complex tissue architectures into fragments that are easier to examine, thereby improving diagnostic accuracy. By leveraging AI technologies, digital pathology not only addresses the quintessential need for precision in diagnostics but also reduces the workload on pathologists significantly by allowing them to concentrate on more complex cases. The complementarity between digital pathology and AI exemplifies the move towards contemporary medical practice, where efficiency and precision have both been appreciated. Finally, the language of digital pathology coincides with the broader implications of health informatics and telemedicine's usage. As healthcare increasingly adopts digital tools, the applications of digital pathology extend beyond image digitization to encompass robust data analytics. Advances in technologies such as cloud computing and machine learning offer the functionality to handle enormous data sets, thus driving diagnostic protocols and patient care methodologies. This shift not only enhances diagnostic accuracy but also allows for continuous professional development of pathologists through access to advanced tools and materials. Moreover, research into open-source software tools in digital pathology promotes an open culture for innovation that enables clinicians and scientists to adapt and implement these technologies for use in various clinical environments (Adams et al., 2003; Cabibi et al., 2024). Overall, the definition of digital pathology serves to indicate a shift in paradigm to an integrated, efficient, and technologically advanced health system.

Overview of AI in Healthcare

The use of artificial intelligence (AI) in medicine, particularly that of digital pathology, is a paradigm shift in the capability for diagnosing and treating diseases. With complex algorithms and machine learning techniques, AI has the potential to speed up and automate much of morphological analysis, ranging from tissue segmentation to classification. Such advances facilitate greater diagnostic precision and speed, allowing clinicians to make more accurate decisions. As Alsup et al. (2023) observe, the application of AI on cancer tissue imaging has ushered in immense advancements with models that are tailored to perform vital functions such as regression and classification. This increased reliance on AI not only streamlines workflow processes but also enhances a broader insight into pathological data and improves, in turn, patient outcomes. Further, computer pathology systems have transformed the area of disease classification and diagnosis at its fundamental level. By supporting distant consultation and multi-specialist collaboration, the systems enhance the accuracy and efficiency of diagnostics. Molecular profiling, guided by AI software, provides invaluable data in relation to the genetic etiology of diseases, thus maximizing the treatment modalities. According to Hussain (2023), the intersection of molecular, histological, and clinical data allows for dynamic classification schemes that significantly improve prognostication and disease stratification. This integration of technology and medicine drives a paradigm shift toward precision medicine, where individualized treatment protocols can be formulated according to the patient's unique genetic profile and disease characteristics. However, the accelerated development of AI in healthcare is accompanied by ethical concerns and challenges that must be addressed to enable effective implementation on a widespread scale. Data privacy, algorithmic bias, and the requirement for rigorous validation of AI systems are a few of the serious concerns that require exhaustive frameworks and guidelines. As cited in Alsup et al. (2023), with the potential of AI to transform cancer pathology, concerns regarding its ethical application within existing healthcare frameworks arise. To overcome these challenges, solutions that integrate cooperation among medical professionals, data scientists, and ethicists must be pursued. By generating discourses around such complexities, stakeholders can collaborate in establishing standards that achieve maximum advantages of AI while curbing risks, thus optimizing the integration of this technology into health care practice (Figure 15.2).

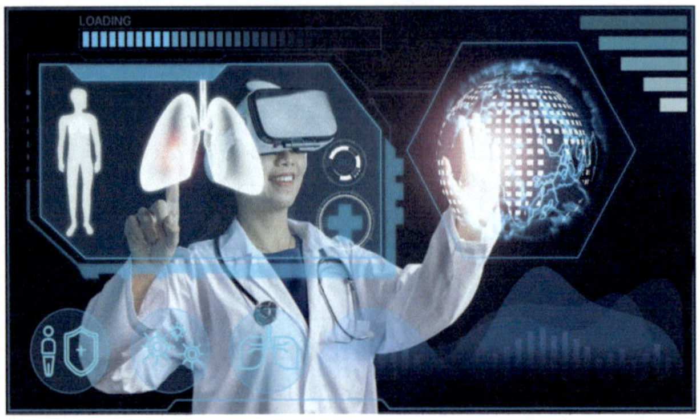

Figure 15.2. Overview of AI in healthcare.

Source: https://d3l9a8mvoa6cl8.cloudfront.net/wp-content/uploads/sites/3/2023/08/21165645/Banner-%E2%80%93-2.jpg.

Importance of Morphological Analysis

The importance of morphological examination in digital pathology lies in its ability to enhance diagnostic precision and reproducibility. Traditional microscopic examination, which relies on pathologists' judgment, typically has limitations like inter-pathologist discordance and intra-observer variation in diagnosis. This discordance is particularly observed in dermatopathology, where high biopsy rates necessitate efficient diagnostic processes. Use of artificial intelligence (AI) in morphological analysis overcomes these issues by regular assessment of histopathology images. An example is the development of a deep learning algorithm that classifies digitized dermatopathology slides into four classes with high accuracy, improving skin cancer diagnoses and enabling identification of those requiring specialist analysis, thereby streamlining the diagnostic process (Ayyagari et al., 2020). Moreover, applying neural networks to facilitate morphological analysis yields robust and quantitative evaluations, which are essential in the medical community. The ubiquity of user-friendly interfaces, such as the Aperio ImageScope, allows pathologists to benefit from these advanced AI tools without technical training. Such ease is crucial as it bridges the gap between medical scientists and advanced neural network algorithms, opening doors for the broader use of AI in pathology. Human-in-the-loop methods substantially reduce the workload of whole-slide image (WSI) annotation and decrease the time required for diagnosis, while improving the accuracy of knowledge derived from morphological information (Ginley et al., 2018). Therefore, these innovations reflect the evolving character of pathology, such that morphological examination is inextricably bound to improving outcomes for patients. The utility of morphological examination is more than a matter of mere classification; it is the gritty comprehension of tissue architecture and cellular morphology that informs clinical decision-making. With AI-based algorithms, pathologists can perform multi-class segmentation of various histological observations and further augment their diagnostic abilities. This is particularly critical in the case of complex tissues like renal and prostate tissues, where precise segmentation has important implications for treatment planning. AI's capability to deliver quantitative measures regarding tissue composition can result in more individualized approaches to medicine that enable clinicians to personalize therapies for unique patient profiles. With morphological analysis in progress to advance the frontiers via the newest digital pathology techniques, its contribution towards shaping the destiny of diagnosis and treatment planning cannot be overestimated, with a revolutionary era unfolding in patient care outcomes.

15.1. Historical Context of Pathology

The historical context of pathology is intricately tied to the evolution of diagnostic practices that have shaped contemporary medicine. From its inception in the early 19th century, pathology emerged as a scientific discipline focused on understanding disease through the examination of tissue and cellular structures. Pioneers such as *Rudolf Virchow* advanced the field by establishing cellular pathology, which emphasizes the significance of cellular alterations in disease processes. This initial work paved the way for modern diagnostic techniques, where histopathology was the standard for disease diagnosis. As microscopy technology advanced over the 20th century, the ability to observe tissue samples under the microscope revolutionized disease diagnosis and significantly enhanced diagnostic accuracy. This trajectory through time emphasizes the great importance of technological innovation in streamlining techniques applied in pathology, paving the way for the contemporary trends toward digital pathology and artificial intelligence. The past years witnessed the convergence of pathology and digital technology initiate a spectacular transformation within the field.

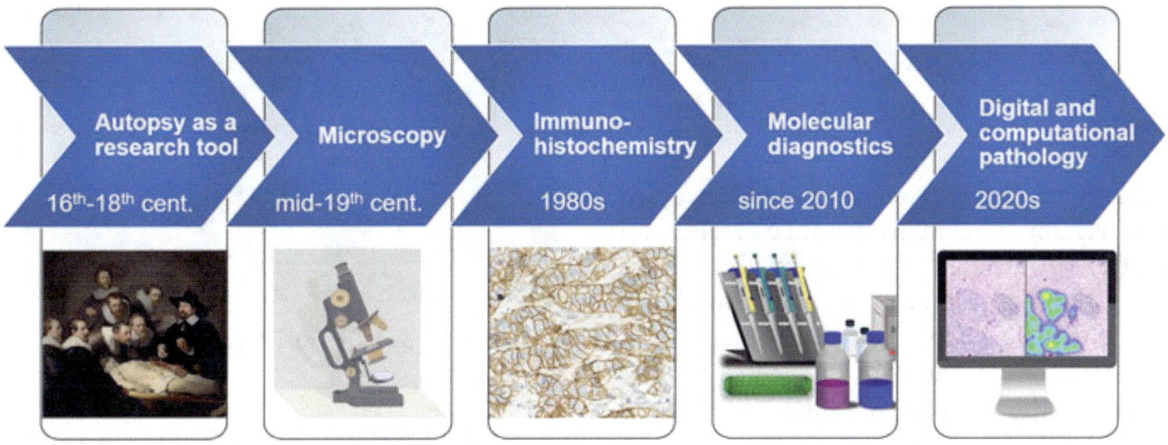

Figure 15.3. A history of transformations in pathology.

Source: https://www.researchgate.net/publication/364257292/figure/fig1/AS:11431281119583909@1676125400468/A-history-of-transformations-in-pathology-The-specialty-is-again-on-the-verge-of-major.ppm.

The use of digital imaging techniques enables the creation of high-quality, digitized slides that are accessible for remote examination by pathologists, improving accessibility and efficiency. Digitization not only streamlines the workflow but also addresses some of the inherent limitations of traditional pathology, such as inter-pathologist discordance and biopsy rates, which call for better reproducibility of diagnosis. To demonstrate the impact of such advances, researchers have developed deep learning algorithms to classify digitized dermatopathology slides with very high accuracy. These models draw on large databases of images to train algorithms, resulting in a deep learning model that is as much as 98% accurate in routine use, demonstrating the power of computational technology to influence diagnostic practice in pathology (Ayyagari et al., 2020). While digital pathology keeps evolving, it is important to think about the broader implications and potentialities of artificial intelligence. Computational pathology has hastened clinical diagnosis, enabling the identification of new morphological biomarkers, the prediction of patients' outcomes, and the personalization of therapeutic strategies. While certain AI-based diagnosis systems have received regulatory approval for clinical assistance, there are still significant technical barriers that prevent them from widespread implementation into practice. The transition from historical pathology principles to current AI-based use is a paradigm shift in disease diagnosis and management. Additionally, as the field continues to expand further, the future provides a much more intricate relationship between digital technology and pathological examination, possibly revolutionizing research and clinical practice (Jaume et al., 2023) (Figure 15.3).

15.1.1. Evolution of Pathological Techniques

The history of pathological methods has been characterized by the shift away from conventional histopathology to digital pathology, drastically changing the field of morphological analysis. Pathologists have traditionally used glass slides and optical microscopes to analyze tissue samples, but the process was also susceptible to human fallibility and subjective inaccuracies. Increased slide digitization has also enabled the growth of full whole slide imaging (WSI), yielding high-resolution, accessible images that may be remotely reviewed. This is a breakthrough for the industry because digital pathology not only accelerates and enhances diagnostic accuracy but also increases opportunities for collaboration among medical specialists, reducing geographic barriers to expert consultations and second opinions. With evolving technology, artificial intelligence (AI) also has a growing part to play in the creation of pathological techniques. Implementation of AI, and particularly neural networks, offers quantitative evaluation not previously possible by any other methodology in traditional settings. For instance, using a human-in-the-loop technique maximizes the annotation effectiveness of WSIs by providing tools for pathologists that complement their abilities rather than replacing them. Current methods observe the improvements in the performance of neural networks, presenting their efficiency in segmenting complex histological outcomes, for instance, renal microcompartments. The iterative learning process not only streamlines the accuracy of classification in renal tissue characterization but also broadens the scope of these advanced techniques in various medical imaging fields, revealing the adaptability and dependability of AI applications in pathology (Ginley et al., 2018).

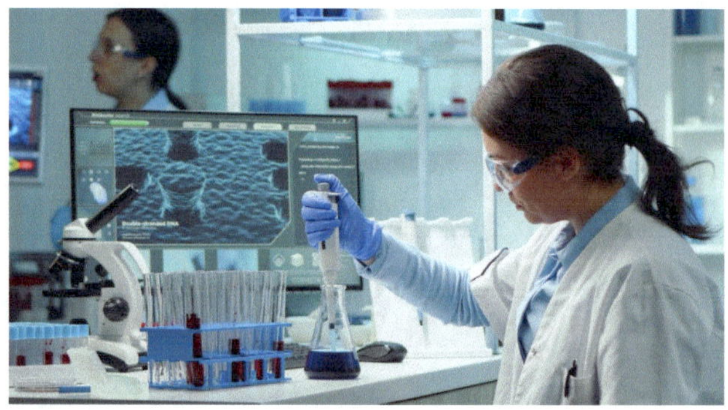

Figure 15.4. Evolution of pathological techniques.

Source: https://external-content.duckduckgo.com/iu/?u=https%3A%2F%2Fmiro.medium.com%2Fv2%2Fresize%3Afit%3A1200%2F1*gfsHgY-6KZZcvDGwcvlVdA.jpeg&f=1&nofb=1&ipt=35b692e5994c8bce3936c22150865b6eae0c6f570c1cd320c9b31dc705df58b7.

The pathological study of ear structure in various animals likewise illustrates how enhanced pathological techniques can be applied beyond their conventional histological applications. For example, familiarity with the correlation between mammals' ear morphology, such as that of red foxes, domestic dogs, and cats, is significant for the prediction of hearing sensitivities from anatomical observations. Although ear morphology is similar, slight differences can make significant contributions to hearing capacity, making a nuanced methodology for morphological analysis crucial. Significantly, previous models predicting hearing parameters from ear measurements do not always agree with functional data, revealing a complicated interdependence of structure and auditory function. The establishment of pathological techniques thus not only increases our understanding of anatomy but also increases the complexities that are involved in biological systems and thus the potential for future research and fields of application across disciplines (Burda et al., 2020) (Figure 15.4).

15.1.2. Introduction of Digital Technologies

The use of information technologies in pathology is a breakthrough in disease diagnostics and analysis. Pathologists previously relied on conventional techniques such as glass slides and manual examination, which were slow and laborious in terms of precision and speed. With the emergence of digital pathology, whole-slide imaging (WSI) has become a groundbreaking tool that enables specimens to be scanned and pathologists to read and interpret them on high-quality screens. Besides the improvement in the recording of fine morphological detail, this shift also permits remote consultation, thus expanding access to pathological services. Moreover, the incorporation of advanced software platforms to analyze and annotate images has optimized workflows while promoting collaborative opportunities among medical practitioners, ultimately with the aim of optimizing diagnostic accuracy and patient care. With ongoing advances in AI, the application of AI in digital pathology is increasingly evident. The employment of neural networks transforms the process through which pathologists interpret complicated data sets since the machines are capable of handling images with high precision and speed. The challenge of training neural networks, however, has prompted the development of interfaces that are user-friendly as well as compatible with existing digital pathology systems such as Aperio ImageScope. By applying a human-in-the-loop strategy, researchers are confronting the difficulties of WSI annotation, thereby enabling AI algorithms to continue being optimized. This iterative process not only improves morphological analysis accuracy but also expands these features to other medical imaging domains, demonstrating the flexibility and efficacy of AI in enhancing diagnostic practice (Ginley et al., 2018). Besides, the use of digital technology is not just applicable to image analysis but spreads throughout the laboratory process, including verifying for pre-analytical errors that may compromise diagnostic integrity. Developments such as barcoding systems have transformed laboratory processes, ensuring accurate sample identification and tracing from diagnosis. This matters most in hematology and oncology, where diagnostic precision can greatly determine treatment plans. The integration of digital imaging methods and genomic analysis broadens the diagnostic scope even more by allowing for end-to-end analyses that marry morphological data with molecular data. The combined impact of this synergy underscores the adoption of digital methods in pathology as it portends enhanced clinical practice and patient-focused care (Hospital et al., 2021).

15.1.3. Impact of Technology on Diagnostic Accuracy

The inclusion of technology in diagnosis has dramatically changed the accuracy of pathology assessments, especially in digital pathology and AI. Diagnostic techniques are often characterized by substantial inter-pathologist variation and subjective interpretation error, which affect the reliability of diagnostic results. Digital pathology helps in scanning histological slides to digitize slides so that pathology specimens can be viewed under improved imaging techniques. The rise of deep learning networks aims to address such limitations by classifying digitized tissue slides into distinct categories to improve diagnostic accuracy. In research that utilized a deep learning platform on a dataset of 5,070 images, a 98% accuracy rate was demonstrated using confidence scoring, showing the power of revolution that AI can bring in increasing diagnostic reproducibility and efficiency (Ayyagari et al., 2020). This innovation is quintessential of the shift towards better diagnostic criteria in the era of technology-enabled medicine. Additionally, the application of neural networks in medical diagnosis has huge potential for efficiency and the grade of morphological inspection. The principal barriers to implementation are the complexities of training and incorporating such systems within existing healthcare systems. To combat such hurdles, novel interfaces like the Aperio ImageScope allow seamless interchange between medical professionals and neural network responses. Through human-in-the-loop processes, the load of WSIs' annotation can be minimized, enhancing the workflow in general. Pilot experiments on renal histologic findings, for instance, demonstrate substantial improvements in segmentation performance with such methods. This adaptability of neural networks across various medical image modalities signifies their central function in enabling increased diagnostic accuracy along with process ease within clinical procedures (Ginley et al., 2018). As such technologies advance, they are likely to bridge the gap between current procedures and future diagnostic modalities. Lastly, the role of technology in diagnostic accuracy is an ever-changing story because continuous developments in digital pathology and AI redefine the game of morphological examination. The emphasis on quantitative assessment in pathology drastically enhances the accuracy of diagnosis conclusions, particularly when combined with difficult specimens and clearly interpretable cases. Not only do they accelerate the identification of malignancies, but they also facilitate targeted workflows, allowing experts to sequence cases with increased priority. Furthermore, the capacity for iterative learning in these systems fosters a culture of progressive improvement, in which diagnostic models become increasingly precise over time through real-world data and feedback cycles. As these technologies continue to grow within clinical settings, the potential for achieving diagnostic results with increased accuracy and reduced human error becomes more feasible, in the long term transforming medical diagnostics and patient care (Figure 15.5).

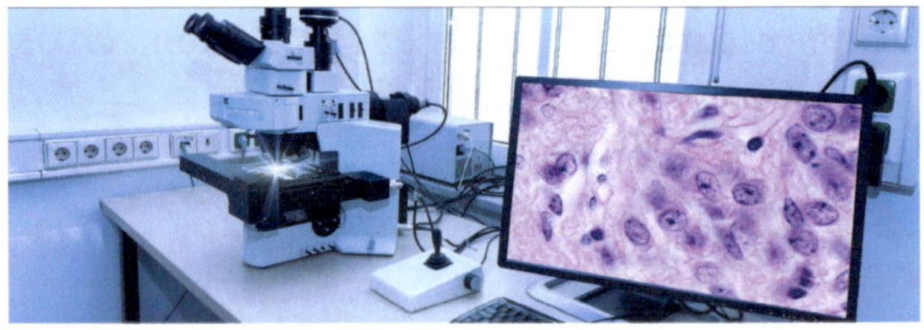

Figure 15.5. Impact of technology on diagnostic accuracy in pathology.

Source: https://external-content.duckduckgo.com/iu/?u=https%3A%2F%2Fwww.hospitaltimes.co.uk%2Fwp-content%2Fuploads%2F2022%2F01%2Fshutterstock_1926391706-scaled.jpg&f=1&nofb=1&ipt=cbd908adbbe7765d197d008287d564bde668ccf8898fb329dfb680916bc44354.

15.2. Fundamentals of Digital Pathology

At its foundation is the evolution of digital pathology in the transition from traditional microscopy to whole slide imaging (WSI). This platform enables the scanning of entire glass slides at high magnification, generating digital images that can be analyzed with sophisticated software tools. The integration of machine learning algorithms within this platform has significantly enhanced diagnostic ability by increasing accuracy, efficiency, and reproducibility for morphological analysis. Tools such as QuPath and HistomicsTK offer pathologists user-friendly platforms with support for WSI analysis, facilitating a better workflow and reduced manual effort. As digital pathology evolves, attention to automation and reduction of inter-observer variability underscores the demand for a technology revolution in the practices of pathology. This advancement is due to the growing computer science-clinical medicine intersection, putting digital pathology at the forefront of diagnostic innovation (Castagnola et al., 2024). In addition to enhancing diagnosis processes, digital pathology encourages more study of intricate biological traits. Computer vision image analysis with AI enables cellular and tissue morphology recognition with unprecedented precision, enabling disease characterization at the molecular level. For instance, digital imaging techniques in the analysis of blood samples allow for the measurement of important parameters such as cell size, shape, and composition, essential for effective medical assessments. Microfluidics and machine learning image analysis provide new avenues for research in blood test applications. The ability to isolate and categorize features with digital image processing not only accelerates the examination of blood cell morphology but also enhances the value of diagnostic tests. Such innovations underscore the paramount role of integrated technologies in advancing medical diagnostics (Amarasinghe et al., 2021). However, the adoption of AI technology and digital pathology is not without its own set of challenges. Critical considerations related to data quality and machine learning model interpretability underscore the limitations inherent in digital pathology practice. While open-source software and machine learning platforms hold considerable potential for simplifying analyses and enhancing diagnostic accuracy, their effective application requires a solid appreciation for data quality and also for the nuances of model interpretations. While investors in the practice strive to close these gaps, continued research seeks to build incrementally on machine learning algorithms and training data sets. That progress will seek to bring digital pathology technology to a point where it can be relied upon to provide accurate, actionable clinical knowledge. Equilibrium between scientific validity and technological innovation remains essential for the practice's transition to more efficient and reliable diagnostic tools (Castagnola et al., 2024) (Figure 15.6).

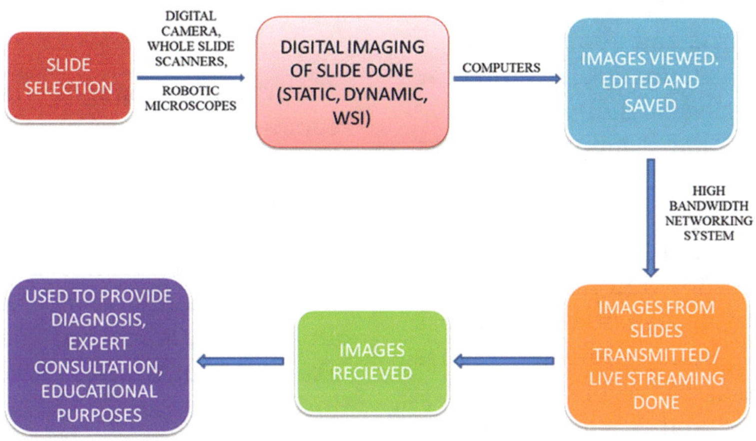

Figure 15.6. Process of digital pathology.

Source: https://external-content.duckduckgo.com/iu/?u=https%3A%2F%2Fwww.researchgate.net%2Fpublication%2F315972481%2Ffigure%2Ffig1%2FAS%3A621697606635522%401525235668747%2FProcess-of-digital-pathology.png&f=1&nofb=1&ipt=eb6bc87f4d4ac2ef0f653e8bf05fc88de8f31ad2d0ffa28d4747f1b90f1ce7f7.

15.2.1. Components of Digital Pathology Systems

The use of digital pathology systems has revolutionized traditional techniques used in histopathology by integrating advanced technologies to optimize diagnostic accuracy and efficacy. The core of these systems are whole slide imaging (WSI) technologies, which acquire high-quality digital images of tissue samples. These images enable detailed inspection and allow pathologists to examine entire slides, no longer limited by the physical confines of the microscope. Besides WSI, digital pathology systems also encompass sophisticated software that enables image analysis, quantitative measurement, and even the detection of subtle morphological variations. Such technical refinement enables pathologists to perform morphological analysis with enhanced accuracy and rapidity, further leading to improved patient outcomes through more timely and informed clinical decisions. Digital pathology platforms are a fundamental component of computerized image analysis software, using artificial intelligence (AI) to optimize diagnostic accuracy and workflow. The software can be trained to detect patterns and abnormalities in histological images, consequently alleviating the burden of subjective analysis otherwise inherent in traditional methods. For example, AI-driven automated scoring of the Human epidermal growth factor receptor 2 (Her2) in breast cancer showed how AI can complement pathologists' judgment. In a recent study, automated grading not only improved the assessment process but also provided a strict, objective score that minimized inter-observer variability, a typical issue in visual grading systems (Berseth et al., 2017). These developments in computer-aided analysis demonstrate the enormous potential of harnessing AI in combination with digital pathology to provide higher diagnostic consistency and reliability. Beyond image acquisition and analysis, digital pathology system architecture also includes data management and collaboration tools that significantly enhance its utility in the clinical setting. Digital systems contain comprehensive patient data, such as imaging and clinical histories, within secure, accessible repositories. This infrastructure facilitates interdisciplinary discussions between pathologists, oncologists, and researchers through mutual information and experience, hence facilitating diagnostic concordance and research opportunities. Moreover, clinical application of digital pathology systems offers the possibility for systematic pooling of large datasets, which can be utilized for machine learning applications aimed at enhancing diagnostic algorithms. The use of advanced methodologies, such as biphasic hydrogel techniques for tissue analysis, attests to the increasing complexity of digital pathology systems, which form core solutions to the challenges posed by diverse pathological contexts (Arda et al., 2017). Through such advanced integration, the functions of such components put digital pathology at the forefront of paradigmatic healthcare solutions.

15.2.2. Image Acquisition and Storage

The process of imaging in digital pathology is responsible for the efficacy of morphological assessment. Whole Slide Imaging (WSI) is now the norm, enabling high-resolution scanning of entire histological tissue sections to be made feasible. This technology not only facilitates extensive examination of cellular architecture but also enables digital images to be integrated into computational pathology workflows. However, tissue digitization involves a range of artifacts and variations influencing the accuracy of subsequent analyses considerably. It is therefore necessary to employ advanced preprocessing techniques to mitigate these effects, including artifact detection and color normalization. By providing access to high-quality images for examination, practitioners can increase the reliability of diagnostic results and facilitate more accurate interpretations of underlying biological processes (Engan et al., 2022). Storage and management methodologies of images are just as crucial in the digital pathology landscape, with ever-increasing volumes of data. Patients' tissue samples, when digitized into WSIs, produce large amounts of data that need to be stored using robust solutions. Efficient storage systems must be able to store the various formats of image data such that images are retrieved rapidly for clinical or research purposes. These storage systems must also provide user-friendly interfaces to enable pathologists to access and analyze images efficiently. Advanced data management technologies are needed, not only to automate clinical workflows but also to enhance collaboration among researchers. As digital pathology increasingly relies on artificial intelligence to interpret images, a systematic image storage strategy will enable the incorporation of AI-based technologies into morphological assessment (Jaume et al., 2023). Advancements in new image acquisition and storage technology portend the potential of more sophisticated artificial intelligence applications in pathology. Recent advances in computational pathology suggest a , when AI has the capability to automate clinical diagnosis and even derive new biomarkers from tissue images. Such potential is, however, contingent upon the quality of the digital images and the stability of the storage devices involved. If the underlying data is tainted due to inadequate acquisition or storage practices, the effectiveness of AI algorithms will inevitably be compromised. Therefore, a clear understanding of these considerations is required to implement AI successfully in clinical environments. With ongoing research, the integration of new image capture technologies with better data management systems will be crucial in realizing the full potential of AI in augmenting diagnostic accuracy and patient outcomes in digital pathology (Jaume et al., 2023) (Figure 15.7).

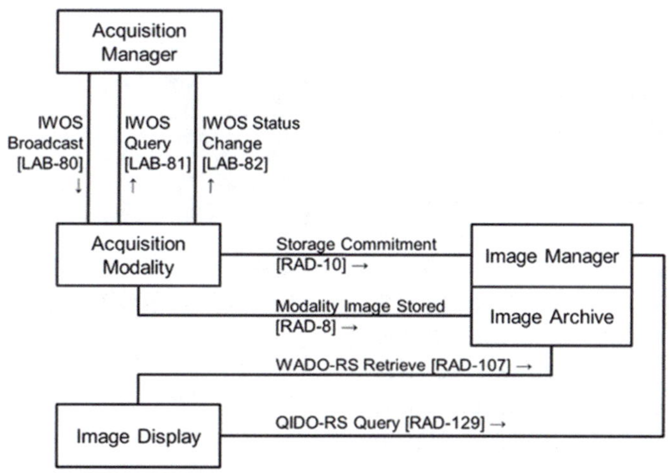

Figure 15.7. Digital pathology image acquisition.

Source: https://www.researchgate.net/publication/350345855/figure/fig4/AS:11431281152837688@1682183826959/Digital-pathology-image-acquisition-profile-Transactions-to-acquire-store-and-display.ppm.

15.2.3. Software Tools for Analysis

The integration of software solutions in digital pathology significantly enhances morphological analysis in terms of better data handling and interpretation capability. The software tools facilitate the interpretation of complex histological data into significant information, allowing pathologists to navigate enormous biological information with ease. Complex software programs employ artificial intelligence algorithms to examine tissue structures, identify patterns, and categorize conditions, enhancing the accuracy of diagnosis. For instance, the transition from traditional histological methods to computer platforms enables quantitative tissue structure measurement, translating qualitative data into measurable parameters. This change not only streamlines workflow processes but also facilitates better collaboration between clinicians, enabling multi-disciplinary teams to interact with digital data from various perspectives, thus improving the overall diagnostic approach. Recent advances highlight that computer programs with three-dimensional imaging capabilities address limitations inherent in conventional thin-section histology. Conventional methods often cannot represent the spatial arrangements of tissues properly, and it is challenging for us to comprehend physiological and pathological states. The establishment of biphasic hydrogel methodologies is only one case of the need for novel solutions in this field. These strategies facilitate high-throughput volumetric interrogation of asymmetrical and delicate tissue structures that are resistant to effective examination by traditional techniques. Facilitating automated analysis within these software platforms not only enhances the precision of morphological measurements but also evidences their utility in both research environments and clinical environments. Validation of such tools is required since they have quantitative advantages that carry profound implications for ongoing research on diseased tissues, like the critical examination of pancreatic innervation and development (Arda et al., 2017). The field of digital pathology is poised for a revolution through the development of software tools that leverage natural language processing (NLP). Such technologies are focused on optimizing data retrieval speed and interaction in the health sector and, therefore, critically influence the result of diagnostics and research. By using NLP in medical databases and online libraries, clinicians can retrieve relevant studies, reports, and analyses at high speed and thus make better-informed decisions. The integration of NLP with picture analysis software allows for an enhanced comprehension of concepts and pathology terminology, further enhancing education tools and resources in the medical environment. Such integration can enhance both the functional capabilities of medical interventions and the resulting quality of patient treatment and control, and therefore, NLP will be a key component in the future of digital pathology and morphology analysis enhanced by artificial intelligence (Adams et al., 2003) (Figure 15.8).

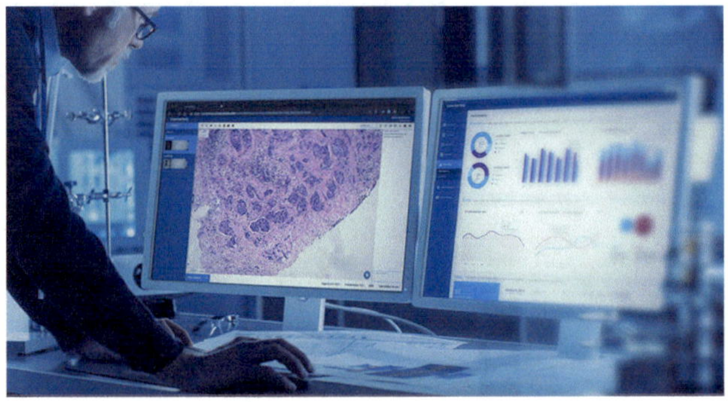

Figure 15.8. The integration of software tools into digital pathology.

Source: https://proscia.com/wp-content/uploads/2019/12/proscia-img-where-is-it-headed.jpg.

15.3. Role of AI in Morphological Analysis

The advent of artificial intelligence (AI) has radically transformed the application of morphological analysis in the general case, and particularly in digital pathology. AI can now analyze extensive sets of histological data far more quickly and with greater precision than earlier methods with the help of advanced algorithms and machine learning software. This results in a higher diagnostic capability than the traditional approach. The capability of AI to identify and classify intricate tissue structures gives pathologists access to highly effective decision-making tools, enhancing both the accuracy and effectiveness of diagnoses. For example, AI models can be designed to identify subtle morphometric differences that may escape the human eye, thereby enabling earlier and more accurate detection of pathological conditions. As the integration of AI advances further, it can potentially enhance our understanding of disease onset and care of individual patients in practice. Furthermore, morphological analysis by AI is not only beneficial for diagnosis but also assists in the quantified evaluation of tissue structures. The requirement for extensive analysis most often occurs because of the complexities found within soft and irregular tissues, which may prove challenging for standard histological methods to measure with high precision.

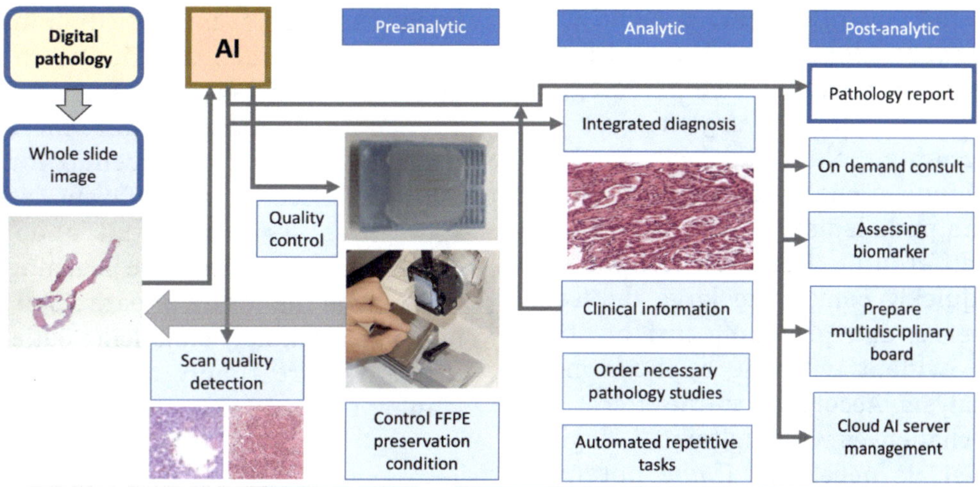

Figure 15.9. Role of AI in morphological analysis.

Source: https://pub.mdpi-res.com/diagnostics/diagnostics-12-02794/article_deploy/html/images/diagnostics-12-02794-g001.png?1668503302.

Recent breakthroughs have introduced new techniques, such as the biphasic hydrogel method, that facilitate high-throughput volumetric studies of these recalcitrant specimens. By employing the method in combination with computer-based AI analyses, researchers are able to generate enhanced knowledge of normal and pathological tissue dynamics. Such techniques have recently been highlighted to have demonstrated quantitative advantages over conventional thin-section histology in various aspects, making them enhance the possibility of wide applications both in research and clinical environments (Arda et al., 2017). Such a level of integration marks an important step towards even more comprehensive data-based patient care. Beyond patient care, advances in AI morphological analysis also have implications for other research areas in regenerative medicine. Understanding tissue regeneration is derived from intricate knowledge of cellular actions and resultant morphological change. AI technology, for example, has been responsible for investigating the Tendon-derived Stem/Progenitor cells (hTSPCs) after therapies like extracorporeal shock wave therapy (ESWT). By monitoring differentiation processes, AI systems can classify and count responses of the stem cells effectively relative to morphological changes and thereby gain insight into injury repair mechanisms. Hence, AI not only enables analysis but also enriches our understanding of biological processes, allowing clinicians to refine treatments and optimize recovery regimens for conditions like tendinopathies (Ferretti et al., 2016). This holistic view corroborates the indispensable role played by AI in morphological analysis as well as the overall advancement of healthcare (Figure 15.9).

15.3.1. Machine Learning Algorithms

The application of machine learning algorithms to digital pathology represents a significant step toward morphological analysis. With the incredible growth in digital histopathological images, there has been an urgent need for quick and accurate tools for analysis. Machine learning techniques enable computer-assisted diagnosis, and pathologists' work is now being conducted differently. These algorithms are capable of quickly computing large datasets, finding patterns, and providing insights that may not be evident with the application of standard analysis. According to the literature, meeting the challenges with digital pathological image analysis is necessary if the potential of machine learning applications in the field is to be achieved (Ishikawa, S., & Komura, D. , 2017). This integration of AI and digital pathology has a more interactive process of diagnosis with more precise and efficient testing of cancer and other morphological studies. But naturally, the intersection of machine learning algorithms in digital pathology is not without issues. Training neural networks, for example, requires gargantuan amounts of annotated data in order to perform efficiently. One of the critical aspects of this work is the construction of usable interfaces for medical researchers to train and refine these networks. A case in point is the use of software such as Aperio ImageScope, which can significantly ease the process of annotation. If done using a human-in-the-loop methodology, iterative refinement towards network enhancement is achievable, which ultimately results in improved segmentation of complex renal histologic features (Ginley et al., 2018). Overcoming these technological barriers is indispensable to realizing the potential of machine learning for accurate pathologic image interpretation. As digital pathology advances, the versatility of machine learning algorithms in becoming acceptable across various fields of medical imaging is noteworthy. The approaches developed in renal histologic evaluation provide the foundation for applying them in oncology and radiology as well. The ability to automatically divide such organs as human prostate glands from radiologic images demonstrates the versatility of such algorithms in addressing diversified morphological issues. Additionally, as scientists continually optimize these techniques, there is a promising avenue for improving diagnostic accuracy and efficiency across various specialties. This potential underscores the crucial role that machine learning algorithms will play in the future of pathology and medical imaging, ultimately enhancing patient outcomes through more timely and precise diagnoses (Ginley et al., 2018).

15.3.2. Image Recognition Techniques

In computerized pathology, image recognition techniques play a central role in maximizing the effectiveness and accuracy of morphological examination. By simplifying complex algorithms for processing histopathological images, scientists have developed automated approaches that can identify cancerous tissues and distinguish them from non-cancerous backgrounds. One particular promising technique involves using unsupervised color clustering for efficient segmentation of target cancerous tissue and removal of extraneous tissue elements. Such a method not only reduces the complexity of analysis but also standardizes the process of evaluating individual tissue characteristics to a much greater extent, significantly reducing variability associated with manual assessment.

The use of such image recognition algorithms is a revolutionary step towards the search for reliable, reproducible diagnostic procedures in pathology, as it serves to overcome the constraints present in traditional methods based largely on subjective interpretation. In addition, the application of advanced image recognition techniques to digital pathology calls for movement towards more accurate and automatic diagnosis. For instance, techniques that focus on color separation and morphological processing have established their capability to segregate nuclear membranes in cancer cells automatically. This particularly holds in immunohistochemical image analysis, where accurate determination of specific cellular structures is paramount for proper diagnosis and subsequent treatment planning. Experimental observations indicate that such automated approaches outperform traditional accepted approaches like supervised learning and active contours, with improved accuracy and efficiency in morphological assessment. These developments are significant, especially considering mounting digital histopathological image numbers, presenting challenges to human interpretation and calling for reliable, scalable tools that can tap computational capacities to improve diagnostic performance (Acquaviva et al., 2010). Despite the tremendous potential of the developments, there are serious challenges to digital pathological image analysis that must be addressed with care. Challenges such as variability in imaging quality, the need for high-quality training datasets, and the difficulty of developing stable machine learning algorithms can prevent the effective utilization of image recognition techniques in pathology. These must be addressed as they directly impact the effectiveness of computer-aided diagnostic systems in pathology. There are options to address these challenges, such as improving imaging protocols, applying data augmentation, and refining algorithmic strategies, to maximize the use of machine learning in digital pathology. Working ahead of these challenges, researchers open up new possibilities for image recognition techniques to revolutionize morphological assessment, yielding more accurate and trustworthy results that contribute to better patient care overall (Ishikawa, S., & Komura, D., 2017) (Figure 15.10).

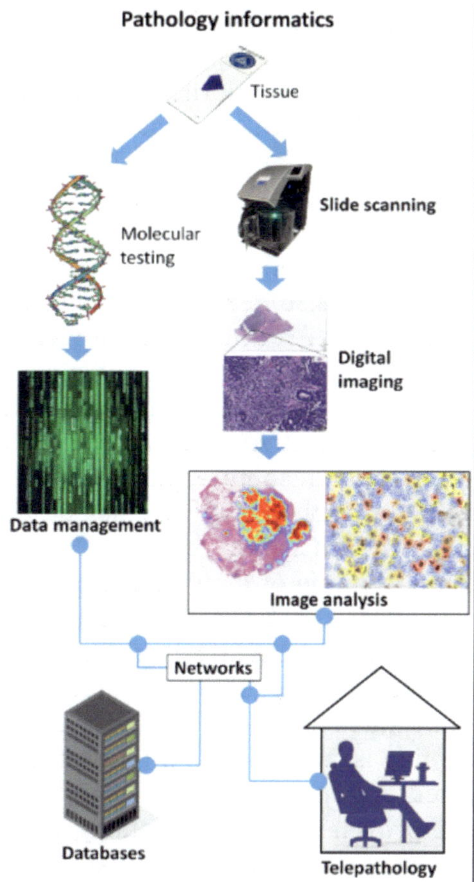

Figure 15.10. Image recognition techniques of digital pathology.

Source: https://upload.wikimedia.org/wikipedia/commons/d/d0/Major_topics_of_pathology_informatics.png.

15.3.3. Data Interpretation and Decision Support

In digital pathology, the union of data interpretation and decision support systems is paramount to enhance the precision and efficiency of diagnosis. With digital histopathological images being accumulated at great speed, applying machine learning approaches for their examination has turned out to be imperative. Such developments are anticipated to provide computer-aided diagnosis instruments that can efficiently analyze large datasets, identifying patterns that may lie outside human perception. But even with advancements, challenges such as data heterogeneity and the requirement of robust algorithms still persist, necessitating additional research and innovation to further optimize these technologies. Addressing these challenges is crucial in ensuring that digital pathology not only enhances the capabilities of pathologists but also becomes organically part of existing clinical routines, hence facilitating a culture of enhanced diagnostic efficiency and accuracy (Ishikawa, S., & Komura, D., 2017). The need for objective data interpretation is also emphasized in some applications, such as cancer diagnostic biomarker assessment. Human epidermal growth factor receptor 2, or Her2, is a prime example of a significant prognostic factor in invasive breast cancer. Classical visual immunohistochemical scoring of HER2 is not objective and generates inter-observer variation, influencing the reliability of diagnosis. To solve this issue, artificial intelligence-based automated scoring tools have been designed and have proven to be valid. Notably, there has been a competition that evaluated AI algorithms for Her2 scoring and established that such automated scoring tended to outperform scores given by pathology experts, opening the way towards more objective diagnostic methods. Such advancements highlight the paradigmatic potential of AI in providing standardized and precise interpretation of information in the digital pathology field (Berseth et al., 2017). Ultimately, the convergence of data interpretation and decision support technologies gives rise to a new era in diagnostic medicine. The use of AI algorithms for image interpretation enables better decision-making, enabling pathologists to focus on complicated case assessments rather than redundant testing. Not only does this enhance the quality of diagnostic procedures, but it also optimizes treatment options for patients through better biomarker analysis. As digital pathology continues to evolve, the implementation of standardized benchmarking criteria will become a requirement in order to evaluate the performance of automated systems. With more coordination among researchers, clinicians, and technology developers, the field can unlock its full potential with AI and lead to improved patient outcomes and an empowered health system (Berseth et al., 2017; Ishikawa, S., & Komura, D., 2017).

15.4. Benefits of Integrating AI in Digital Pathology

The use of artificial intelligence (AI) in digital pathology provides groundbreaking benefits in diagnostic accuracy as well as efficiency. With advanced image analysis algorithms, AI can scan histological images to identify patterns that may be missed by the human eye. Not only does this increase the pace of diagnosis, but it also eliminates human error, allowing pathologists to focus on more complicated cases requiring nuanced judgment. As recent studies have shown, the integration of AI programs into digital pathology systems significantly improves diagnostic precision, particularly for diseases with atypical features. This results in more precise treatment protocols tailored to each patient individually, a huge advancement for personalized medicine. The combined impact of AI and digital platforms ultimately enhances the overall level of care, promoting better patient outcomes in the field of pathological diagnostics (Hussain 2023). Beyond improving the diagnostic function, AI integration in digital pathology optimizes workflow efficiency in laboratories. AI programs have the potential to automate routine tasks, such as image segmentation and quantification, freeing pathologists to focus on interpretation and decision-making. Such automation is particularly pertinent in the context of increasing case loads along with the pressing requirements of rapid diagnosis.

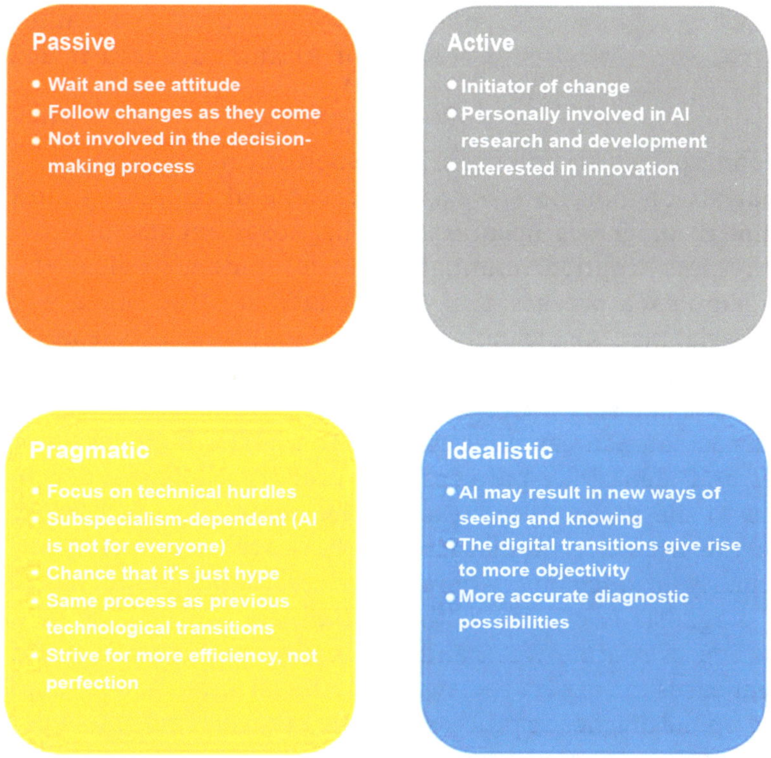
Passive
• Wait and see attitude
• Follow changes as they come
• Not involved in the decision-making process
Active
• Initiator of change
• Personally involved in AI research and development
• Interested in innovation
Pragmatic
• Focus on technical hurdles
• Subspecialism-dependent (AI is not for everyone)
• Chance that it's just hype
• Same process as previous technological transitions
• Strive for more efficiency, not perfection
Idealistic
• AI may result in new ways of seeing and knowing
• The digital transitions give rise to more objectivity
• More accurate diagnostic possibilities

Figure 15.11. Integrating artificial intelligence in pathology.

Source: https://media.springernature.com/full/springer-static/image/art%3A10.1038%2Fs41379-022-01123-6/MediaObjects/41379_2022_1123_Fig1_HTML.png.

The innovations in digital pathology in recent times are a reflection of the necessity for meticulous deployment of technological advances, where planning is a component equal in importance to reap maximum dividends. With the help of AI, laboratories not only ease operations but also facilitate coordination among experts, leading to interdisciplinary solutions to complex cases. The increase in productivity that comes from the integration of AI puts digital pathology at the forefront of innovation, sooner or later resulting in a more responsive healthcare system (Dawson., 2022). In addition, the integration of AI has an effect that transcends the efficiency gains solely; it provides pathologists with the ability to extend the boundaries of research and clinical practice. The intersection of molecular characterization and computer systems driven by AI offers the entire landscape of disease mechanisms, initiating therapy strategy development. By enabling the review of big data, AI is accountable for finding novel biomarkers and disease types, enhancing the quality of patient care. The interdisciplinary nature highlighted in ongoing investigations underscores the need to integrate knowledge from various domains, including genomics and computational pathology. This combined strategy not only improves disease understanding but also prognostication, thereby complementing the aims of precision medicine. Therefore, the addition of AI to digital pathology is not a technological upgrade but a key move towards advancing the entire field of medical diagnostics (Hussain , 2023) (Figure 15.11).

15.4.1. Enhanced Diagnostic Accuracy

The use of artificial intelligence (AI) and digital pathology in the analysis of morphology has greatly enhanced clinical diagnosis accuracy. In the past, pathologists applied manual inspection to tissue samples, a process prone to human error and variability. AI technology has introduced machine learning algorithms that can process enormous datasets with speed and accuracy that surpass human capabilities. By examining images and identifying patterns that may be invisible to the naked eye, these AI systems enhance the accuracy of disease identification, particularly in oncology, where accurate and timely diagnosis is crucial. With the ability of automation of routine work and notification of unusual cases for expert review, not only does AI speed up the diagnostic process, but it also guarantees the accuracy of results, enhancing patient outcomes in a timely way (Alsup et al., 2023). Naturally, trends in three-dimensional (3D) tissue-structural relationships have overhauled traditional practices in histology, significantly relying on thin-section imaging methods. These conventional methods usually cannot capture the complexity of tissue structure and thus lead to compromised pathological examination. Recent advances in intact-tissue imaging techniques, as realized by new hydrogel methodologies, have now overcome such limitations. By enabling high-throughput volumetric interrogation of spatially heterogeneous tissues, this approach significantly improves the evaluation of normal as well as disease states. Applying these methods to clinic samples facilitates improved comprehension of the disease dynamics of conditions such as pancreatic cancer, highlighting the advantages of embracing inclusive imaging methods for diagnostic improvement (Arda et al., 2017). Extensionally, the union of 3D imaging and AI analysis is extremely promising in redefining diagnostic perfection in pathology. With the progress of digital pathology, the integration of AI and advanced imaging techniques holds the potential to fuel growth in diagnostic methods. Utilizing big data analysis and sophisticated algorithms, doctors are not only capable of improving the validity of individual diagnoses but also of providing input to larger-scale epidemiological studies, improving the foundation of evidence required to gain a greater understanding of disease patterns and outcomes. The potential of AI to assist in risk stratification and personalized treatment planning is its role as a transformational agent in modern medicine. Future research and development will also have the potential to further extend the application of AI across a variety of areas in pathology, necessitating meticulous validation studies to maintain the validity of diagnostic processes. Lastly, the integration of digital pathology and artificial intelligence is going to revolutionize the branch of morphological analysis and cancer diagnosis so that patients receive the optimal standard of care (Arda et al., 2017; Alsup et al., 2023) (Figure 15.12).

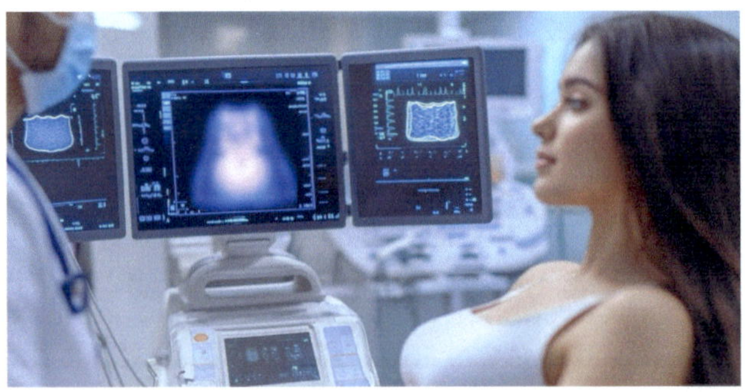

Figure 15.12. AI-powered diagnostics in healthcare.

Source: https://tateeda.com/wp-content/uploads/2024/11/ultrasound-diagnostics-with-AI-1.jpg.

15.4.2. Increased Efficiency in Workflow

The use of artificial intelligence (AI) and digital pathology has transformed workflow efficiency in the environment of morphological analysis. Traditional pathological processes are time-consuming, with pathologists manually examining samples under microscopes and thereby introducing variation in diagnoses through subjective interpretation. The use of digital pathology replaces traditional procedures by digitizing slides and employing advanced algorithms to observe images, which enhances diagnosis and minimizes human error. For instance, one deep learning model designed to diagnose dermatopathology slides attained a high accuracy rate of up to 98% when coupled with confidence scoring, demonstrating the potential of technology to enhance diagnostic accuracy and efficiency exponentially (Ayyagari et al., 2020). Such advances not only reduce the time for analysis but also enhance the reproducibility of test results, leaving pathologists to focus more on tricky cases that need specialist review. Moreover, the capability of AI systems to review large sets of data is crucial to improving workflow efficiency. By their capacity for handling vast quantities of images at top speed, genetic information can be analyzed, comparing morphological features to potential diagnoses, and all of this with accuracy. Computer systems can sort and prioritize cases based on established criteria, significantly reducing the workload for pathologists. Such an algorithmic structure is particularly critical in high-throughput labs, where the need for timely and reliable assessments becomes essential. Utilizing methods like barcoding, as seen in contemporary lab processes, pre-analytical errors can be minimized to a significant extent, thereby facilitating effective tracking and handling of samples throughout the assessment process (Hospital set al., 2021). The union of digital pathology and AI enhances both individual diagnostic performance as well as aiding in a more streamlined overall lab process. Beyond accelerating diagnostics, the use of AI in digital pathology facilitates a culture of ongoing learning and growth. Because such AI systems operate on heterogeneous data from multiple institution settings, they are increasingly refined through machine learning processes and thereby become versatile across a range of pathological situations. Such versatility is particularly valuable in arriving at areas of discordance between pathologists, where diagnostic confidence can vary based on individual interpretations. The application of deep learning technology helps not just with the harmonization of interpretations across various laboratories but also allows for the quick identification of cases that need to be reviewed again. With more accurate and efficient diagnosis, AI-augmented digital pathology ultimately means improved outcomes for the patient, marking a dramatic shift in the manner by which diagnostic services can be made efficiently and reliably accessible within the current medical setting (Ayyagari et al., 2020).

15.4.3. Reduction of Human Error

The advent of digital pathology is a revolutionary intersection of technology and histological analysis that has significantly reduced human error. Traditional approaches subject pathologists to fatigue and subjective judgment, leading to incorrect diagnoses. Digital platforms, on the other hand, provide a better process of analysis that is less susceptible to such vulnerabilities. For example, machine learning techniques improve diagnostic uniformity by examining large volumes of imaging data with precision. As Arda et al. (2017) suggest, the blending of computer-assisted diagnosis allows for more uniform analyses, thereby reducing discrepancies caused by subjective perceptions. This initial reformulation not only optimizes diagnostic efficiency but also ultimately enhances patient outcomes by yielding more reliable findings. Further enhancement in imaging methods, such as the biphasic hydrogel technique described in current literature, further validates pathological diagnoses. With the capability to execute high-throughput quantitative volumetric interrogation of complex tissues, the technique serves as a substitute for the limits of conventional thin-section histology, which is unable to adequately document the involved three-dimensional architecture characteristic of most biological samples. The technique's demonstrated validity makes it a strong candidate for clinical use, where accuracy is paramount. As noted in Arda et al. (2017), the quantitative advantages of intact-tissue techniques can greatly reduce human error related to misinterpretation or incomplete analysis of samples. These advancements highlight the criticality of integrating advanced tools in routine use, allowing for a more objective and reliable platform for diagnostic examinations. Moreover, the utilization of artificial intelligence in digital pathology extends beyond the mere image analysis to provide a system for continuous improvement and error reduction. The employment of sophisticated algorithms can identify patterns and abnormalities that may go unnoticed by even the most experienced pathologists, thus acting as an important support system. By addressing specific challenges inherent in computerized pathological image analysis, as discussed in Ishikawa, S., & Komura, D. (2017), AI can learn and adapt processes to enhance diagnostic accuracy with time. This adaptive capability not only serves to neutralize the cognitive biases inherent in humans, but it also better arms pathologists with the tools for making decisions. In a profession in which precision is paramount, combined synergy between human expertise and AI is a valuable method in the quest to minimize diagnostic errors and enhance the quality of care in medical pathology (Figure 15.13).

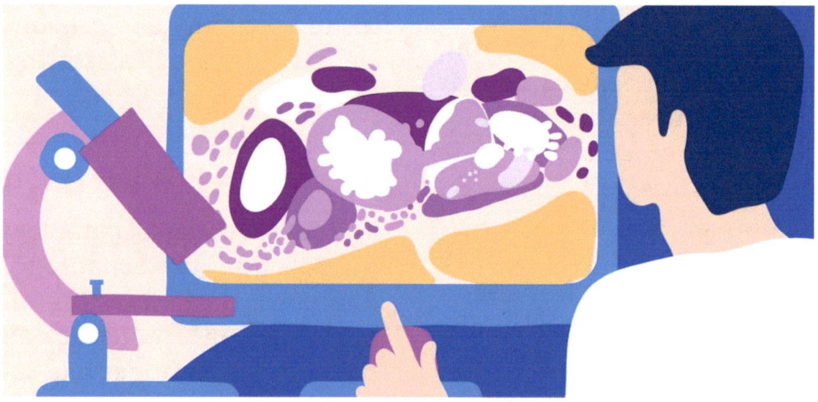

Figure 15.13. Reduction of human error in digital pathology.

Source: https://roche.scene7.com/is/image/RocheDiaProd/hero-computation-digital-pathology-impacting-patient-care?wid=1440&hei=702&fit=crop,1.

15.5. Challenges and Limitations

One of the main issues in combining digital pathology with artificial intelligence (AI) for morphological analysis is tissue sample heterogeneity. Heterogeneity can be caused by a wide range of factors, including fixation variability, staining protocols, and natural biological variability between samples. This heterogeneity is a dominant factor in the performance of automated segmentation algorithms, often leading to nonsensical or flawed outcomes. Whereas traditional manual examination allows pathologists to make up for these differences, AI programs must be trained on a broad range of data sets to generalize. Automated methods must thus be robust to such variation to be consistent and accurate across samples. The need for extensive training datasets is yet another complicating factor, given that preparation of representative samples is time- and resource-intensive, making it further challenging for computer-based techniques in morphological analysis (Acquaviva et al., 2010). Another significant limitation is explainability in AI systems, particularly deep learning methods used in digital pathology.

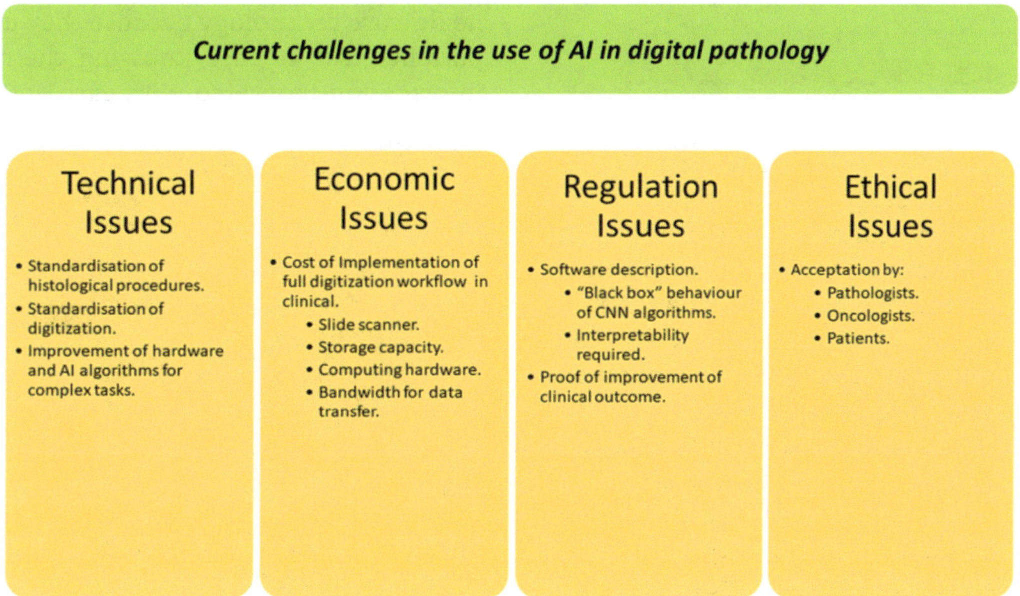

Figure 15.14. Current challenges in the use of AI in digital pathology.

Source: https://www.researchgate.net/publication/353430826/figure/fig16/AS:11431281250091352@1717770704282/Current-challenges-in-the-use-of-AI-in-digital-pathology.png.

AI algorithms are inherently black boxes, and it is challenging for clinicians to identify the decision-making processes. Difficulty opening the black box makes it harder for pathologists to trust and adopt AI-driven results, as they are reluctant to accept AI-driven results without clear explanations. For the integration of AI into clinical workflows, there is a need not just for accuracy but also for explainability in order to facilitate co-working between human experts and machine learning. As a response to this issue, scientists have begun crafting natural interfaces that reconcile AI predictions with user-friendly tools, evident from the work of developing a human-in-the-loop methodology to optimize annotation operations while enhancing network performance (Ginley et al., 2018). This approach emphasizes the necessity of interpretability for broader acceptability and seamless integration into clinical workflow. Second, the technological advancement required for AI model training is a major barrier to broad implementation across digital pathology. Consistent algorithm training demands a wealth of tagged data, which is incredibly expensive and labor-intensive to obtain. Moreover, computational resources for processing WSI are substantial in most instances, limiting use to high-end infrastructure available in only some institutions. This kind of technological disparity not only constrains the broader use of AI for pathological analysis but also presents concerns about equity in healthcare. Disparities in access to advanced tools may exacerbate existing inequities within the medical community, affecting patient outcomes across groups. As artificial intelligence moves forward into digital pathology, the resolution of these technical challenges will be essential to enabling equitable and effective healthcare solutions (Acquaviva et al., 2010) (Figure 15.14).

15.5.1. Data Privacy and Security Concerns

The rapid adoption of artificial intelligence (AI) in digital pathology brings significant data privacy and security concerns, particularly given the sensitive nature of patient information on morphological examination. With conventional histopathology becoming increasingly digitized, extensive amounts of data, such as patient scans and diagnostic images, are being generated, stored, and processed. This switch demands rigorous defense against unlawful access and loss of data, which could betray patient confidentiality and the integrity of medical records. Recent literature suggests that the effective application of AI tools hinges not only on their mathematical prowess but also on the rigorous practice of data management so that it is privacy standard-compliant. In addition, regulatory frameworks such as HIPAA must be adapted to deal with such new challenges in the time of virtual space, where information could be relocated and potentially misused, and therefore, new security measures must be rethought constantly in healthcare facilities. For AI-assisted morphologic analysis, the algorithms will be prone to requiring huge datasets to train effectively. However, the necessity raises ethical issues regarding data ownership and consent. Patients may be oblivious to the fact that their medical data can be utilized for training AI, and therefore, their rights can be infringed upon if proper consent processes are not followed. The use of higher-level imaging techniques and machine learning algorithms, while promising for more precise cancer diagnosis, needs to protect patient autonomy and confidence as the topmost priority. The thin line between applying these technologies to deliver improved results and behaving ethically in the use of data cannot be overstated. As highlighted by the latest studies, implementing open data usage policies and informed consent are significant steps towards achieving trust in AI-based healthcare technology because they ensure that patients feel at ease knowing their sensitive information is treated with care and integrity.

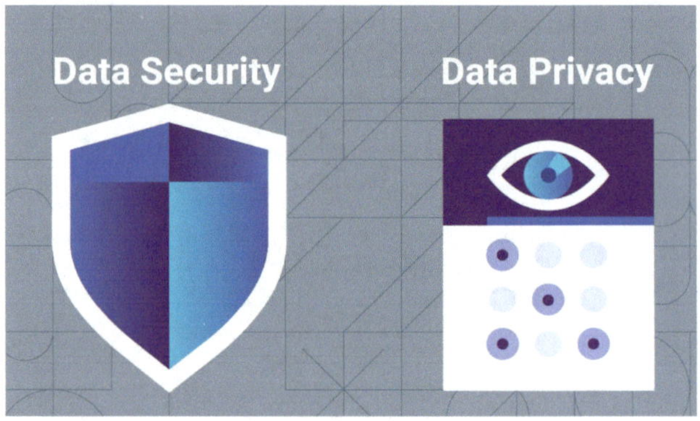

Figure 15.15. Data privacy and security concerns of digital pathology.

Source: https://static.endpointprotector.com/blog/2023/04/tofu-data-security-security-vs-policy.jpg.

The threat of data misuse is a constant problem in the digital pathology environment. Because of the complexity of cybersecurity threats, both external hacking and inherent negligence present a threat, the clinical effectiveness of AI applications and patient data is put at risk. According to current studies, the issue is beyond mere technological obsessions; healthcare units need to cultivate a culture of technological security among their staff and invest in ongoing training programs to implement protections against data-handling threats. With the deployment of advanced encryption techniques and multi-factor authentication processes, organizations are able to protect their online platforms from potential invasions. At last, maintaining a strong framework with both its technological and human aspects is most essential in an effort to have strong data security in the aftermath of greater application of AI in morphological analysis, aligned with principles of patient safety and quality of care for this emerging digital era of healthcare (Naser et al., 2024; Firuzpour et al., 2025) (Figure 15.15).

15.5.2. Need for Standardization in Technology

The rapid evolution of digital pathology, combined with breakthroughs in artificial intelligence (AI), brings monumental challenges to bear on the necessity of standardizing technology at once. As more hospitals and research institutions rely on digital histopathological images, consistency is the most pressing need in data handling and processing. Variability in image capture, storage, and analysis would lead to inconsistencies and, in turn, undermine the accuracy of computer-aided diagnosis systems using machine learning approaches. There needs to be standardized protocols and guidelines in place for integrating AI into morphological analysis to be effective. Standardization not only ensures consistency among diverse systems but also permits collaboration among the scientific community, paving the way for innovations in research and clinical applications that leverage reliable data transfer and reproducibility (Ishikawa, S., & Komura, D., 2017). Additionally, heterogeneity of digital imaging technology and its applications further exacerbates the issues implicit in the science of digital pathology. Different institutes might utilize different imaging modalities, which results in non-comparability and verification between studies. Utilizing commonly accepted standards is crucial in limiting such differences to attain comparability in data interpretation and enhance the collective knowledge of pathological results through AI-based algorithms. This approach would potentially enable a more conducive framework to train and test machine learning models that are the core of the diagnostic system of the future. By regulating these platforms, stakeholders are able to optimize the performance of AI tools to make them not only become trusted but also effective and precise in morphological analysis (Hospital et al., 2021). Besides that, the adoption of standardized protocols can significantly reduce pre-analytical errors within digital pathology labs that participate in clinical labs. These errors commonly stem from differences in sample handling, imaging protocols, and data processing algorithms, which contribute to adverse effects on diagnostic accuracy. Quality control culture programs can promote a culture of quality control, whereby standardized protocols ensure that digital images are captured and processed under the same parameters. This is particularly important in light of the considerable volume of histopathological images generated for processing by machine learning. By increasing efficiency and adhering to standardized processes, the field can accelerate the development and deployment of AI tools, leading to improved patient outcomes and more reliable diagnostic methods (Ishikawa, S., & Komura, D., 2017).

15.5.3. Resistance to Change in Clinical Settings

Resistance to change in clinical settings typically stems from strong habits and entrenched routines that healthcare professionals have worked out over years of practice. Adjusting to novel technology, such as digital pathology and morphological analysis using artificial intelligence, entails technical adjustment but also a culture shift among medical staff. Most clinicians will be resistant to innovation since they fear that new systems may disrupt current workflows or diminish their roles. This leads to low adoption of advanced technologies, ultimately eroding the potential gains associated with enhanced diagnostic accuracy and efficiency. Hence, these issues have to be addressed to facilitate a culture for change and innovation in clinical practice. Besides, insufficient training and education in new equipment can perpetuate resistance to change in health environments. With the rapidity of advances in healthcare, the use of advanced digital systems necessitates a perpetual process of learning and adaptation by health professionals. Doubt concerning digital tools typically creates fear and apprehension concerning their use in day-to-day practices. For instance, its use in AI algorithms for morphological data processing may be perceived as a threat to clinicians' professional expertise. When professionals themselves cannot grasp the operational details of new technology, they become vulnerable to myths about their effectiveness and reliability. Hence, involving practitioners in the design and implementation phases of these technologies, as well as investment in adequate training, is the key to overcoming resistance and achieving successful adoption of digital pathology. Moreover, the relationship between organizational structure and resistance to change should not be overlooked. Clinical settings have hierarchical models that can dampen the spread of innovative ideas and collaboration. If leadership is not committed to adopting digital tools, it fosters an environment in which resistance thrives. Not only is management support critical to the introduction of new technology initially, but it is also critical to long-term investment and support. The promotion of a feedback- and participation-based culture can assist in breaking down resistance from the staff by creating a sense of collective ownership of the process of change. For instance, successful digital pathology implementation often depends on the development of interdisciplinary groups focused on inclusion to ensure that the voices and opinions of all are heard and valued during the transition to AI-enabled morphological examination. With ongoing medical progress, managing resistance to change effectively will be very challenging in order to fully enjoy the benefits of these revolutionary technologies (Figure 15.16).

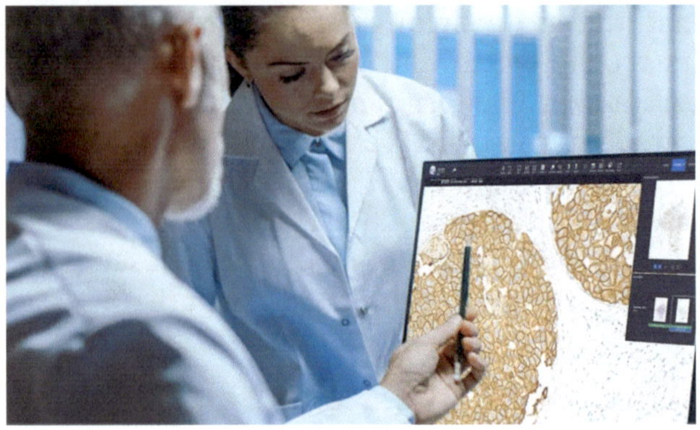

Figure 15.16. Resistance to change in clinical settings of digital pathology.

Source: https://img.mlo-online.com/files/base/ebm/mlo/image/2024/02/65de3f9cdfdaab001e0f2be5-ventana_0001_rgb_figure_4.png?auto=format,compress&fit=max&q=45&w=950&width=950.

15.6. Future Directions in Digital Pathology

The future of digital pathology is significantly influenced by the evolution of artificial intelligence (AI) technologies, which have the potential to revolutionize morphological analysis. AI in digital pathology not only aims to enhance diagnostic accuracy but also optimizes workflow efficiency. The prime strategy is utilizing neural networks to automate tissue sample segmentation and classification. For instance, recently introduced efforts have presented more user-friendly interfaces that enable the annotation of whole slide images (WSIs), thereby maximizing the training of neural networks. The human-in-the-loop technique reduces the enormous amount of labor usually consumed in annotating WSI and greatly improves the performance of such networks on subsequent rounds of training. Such confluence is a step toward an increasingly collaborative framework that synergizes human expertise with machine abilities, creating an integrated diagnostic system that promises to revolutionize patient care in pathology. In addition to maximizing efficiency, the future of digital pathology will also see more focus on the robustness and flexibility of algorithms across various domains of medical imaging. Current literature draws attention to the universality of neural networks beyond conventional histology, as can be seen from their use in segmenting renal microcompartments from renal tissue slides and other image modalities such as radiology. The universality presents a promising avenue for AI-based analysis to shatter many facets of the medical imaging paradigm. Following up on the research into multi-class segmentation algorithms serves to enhance the precision of diagnoses like renal dysfunction, as well as provide the promise of standardizing interpretation across various types of cancer and tissues. Development of these cutting-edge analytical tools in this regard continues to be essential to the creation of universal frameworks for morphological analysis. Moreover, the inclusion of texture features in AI algorithms emphasizes a vital aspect of future breakthroughs in digital pathology. Recent research has shown that the use of advanced statistical tools, such as the Gray-Level Co-occurrence Matrix (GLCM), improves the classification of certain granulomatous disorders. The method illustrates that texture features can prove to be even superior to usual morphological features like size and shape for diagnostic accuracy. The precise accuracy achieved with the application of algorithms like Scaled Conjugate Gradient Back-Propagation Neural Networks (SCG-BPNN) demonstrates the degree to which texture analysis, in conjunction with sophisticated machine learning techniques, may automate diagnostic processes. With continued developments in AI technology, the integration of these sophisticated analysis techniques will be critical to advancing the efficacy of digital pathology and advancing the development of personalized medicine approaches in treatment and diagnosis (Figure 15.17).

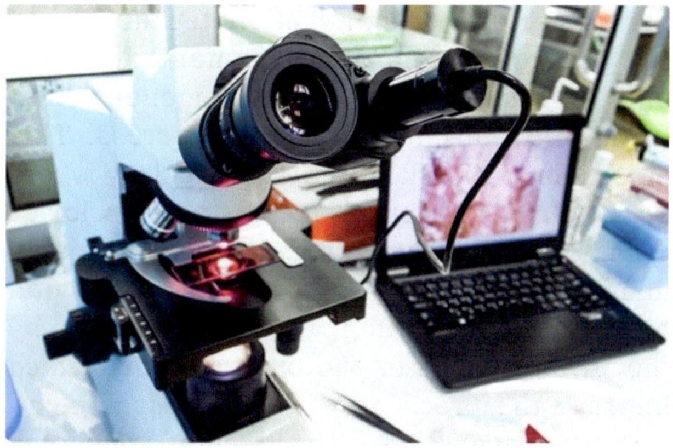

Figure 15.17. Future of digital pathology.

Source: https://www.news-medical.net/image-handler/picture/2020/5/shutterstock_554423998-1.jpg.

15.6.1. Advancements in AI Technologies

The rapid development of artificial intelligence (AI) technologies has profoundly redefined the digital pathology scene, particularly in morphological examination. AI systems, powered by machine learning software, are now capable of processing large collections of histological images at unprecedented speed and accuracy. Through deep learning techniques, these systems can identify minute patterns that are often outside human reach. For example, image recognition technology enables various cell types in a sample to be identified, thereby increasing diagnostic throughput and accuracy. As such, pathologists can rely on AI-supported analyses to aid their diagnosis, reducing human error and improving laboratory throughput, which is critical to the efficient management of clinical workflows and the timely care of patients. In addition, the use of AI in the analysis of histopathological images has opened up new realms of research and application, particularly in insight into multifactorial diseases. The use of AI algorithms to manage diverse morphological features makes it easier to delve deeper into the pathogenesis of diseases such as cancer.

For instance, the ability of AI technology to analyze tumor microenvironments enables one to research tumor heterogeneity and its implications for treatment success. This innovation is especially critical in oncology, where personalized medicine is increasingly a priority. Techniques such as feature extraction and digital image processing are capable of extracting vital biological information, as demonstrated by the advancements in photomicrography, which improve the precision of cellular assessment. With the development of AI technologies, they continue to prove themselves as invaluable tools towards pushing the frontiers of medical research (Hospital et al., 2021).

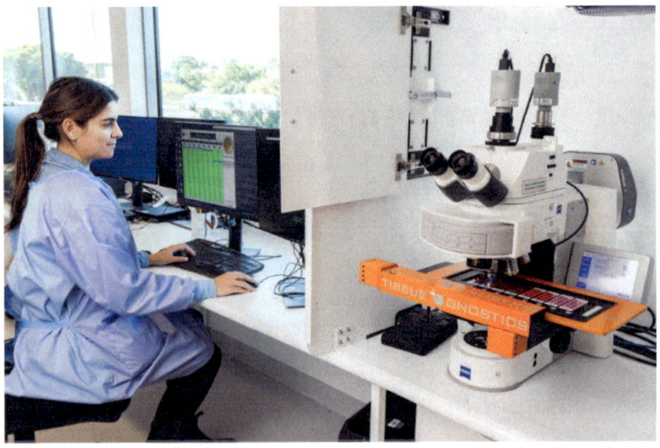

Figure 15.18. Advancements in AI technologies in digital pathology.

Source: https://assets.rbl.ms/34709844/origin.jpg.

In addition, ongoing innovations in AI are transforming the procedures used in routine laboratory practice, particularly in blood work and overall hematopathological diagnosis. Computer-image-based imaging combined with classification software empowered by AI is revolutionizing basic tests such as the full blood count (FBC) to allow for rapid analysis of cellular morphology and functionality of patient samples. Advanced imaging technologies and integration of AI enable precise identification and counting of various blood cell types, finally providing complete information regarding a patient's health status. This is not only crucial for the diagnosis of current conditions but also for the early identification of potential health complications, hence allowing proactive health care management. The ongoing development of smart AI systems continues to hold immense promise for enhancing the quality of laboratory testing and advancing innovations in the care of patients (Amarasinghe et al., 2021) (Figure 15.18).

15.6.2. Potential for Personalized Medicine

The combination of digital pathology and artificial intelligence (AI) holds revolutionary potential in personalized medicine. With the aid of advanced imaging techniques and machine learning algorithms, physicians are able to achieve a more precise picture of individual patient profiles, particularly with regard to morphological analysis. The specificity opens the doors for the identification of disease-specific characteristics on a cellular level, paving the way for personalized therapeutic approaches. Integration of digital pathology and AI enhances diagnosis accuracy and enables therapeutic response monitoring, optimizing treatment approaches with real-time data analysis. Patients thereby gain from treatment strategies optimized to their unique biological and pathological profiles, illustrating the great potential of personalized medicine in modern healthcare strategies. Personalized medicine is based on the assumption that genetic, environmental, and lifestyle factors individually predict health outcomes. The integration of AI in digital pathology allows clinicians to better interpret complex datasets of genomic and morphologic assessments. By leveraging big data analytics, AI systems can detect patterns and relationships that are not readily observable with traditional methods. This is entirely in alignment with the trend towards precision medicine, which recognizes individualized treatment plans over a one-size-fits-all ideal. As researchers continue to explore how AI-driven intelligence can be incorporated into pathology processes, personalized therapies become increasingly within grasp, thus enhancing patient care outcomes and healthcare system efficiency. The efforts towards bridging this technology-clinical practice gap demonstrate the vital role that AI will play in the future of healthcare. To yet more fully advance a vision for the future of personalized medicine, the promise of integrating non-conventional treatments such as Qigong with advanced medical technology is compelling. Such an integrative approach considers the many-sided aspects of patient health that are often overlooked by standard therapies. Evidence indicates that AI-Medicine training databases can enable synergy between Eastern and Western technologies to further the personalization of care. Through the identification of unique breathing patterns with machine learning, clinicians may be able to learn about how to tailor interventions for specific patients. Such novel mashups might lead to developing a vitality score index (VSI) and thereby allow treatment outcome prediction and lifestyle adaptation. This depiction of interdisciplinary collaboration for personalized medicine highlights the promise of new technologies to optimize patient care, with treatments aligned as closely as possible with the patients themselves (Dethlefs et al., 2019).

15.6.3. Integration with Other Healthcare Technologies

The integration of digital pathology with other health technologies has transformative value for morphological examination, a highly efficient and accurate diagnostic process. With the use of digital pathology platforms that enable the digitization of slides, healthcare providers are able to integrate histopathological information with sophisticated imaging devices to produce a better picture of a patient's condition. This team-oriented approach not only facilitates remote consultation between expert teams but also enables a more nuanced understanding of complex cases. With various healthcare technology systems integrated, pathologists are able to see molecular profiling data and AI-driven analysis tools simultaneously, enhancing robust diagnostic procedures with the fusion of multiple data streams. This convergence showcases the virtue of interdisciplinary collaboration, enabling customized treatment plans that are sensitive to individual patient needs. The integration of artificial intelligence (AI) with digital pathology is another significant aspect of health technology integration. AI is capable of processing large datasets of histopathological images, enabling automated image analysis with enhanced diagnostic accuracy. The incorporation of techniques such as machine learning allows for the detection of subtle abnormalities invisible to the naked eye, therefore improving early disease diagnosis for conditions such as cancer. The incorporation is part of the greater trend of precision medicine, in which AI-driven insights support individualized treatment protocols, refining interventions based on individual characteristics of patients' disease. The synergistic effect of AI technologies embedded in digital pathology platforms not only enhances workflow but also enables the reliability of morphological assessment, and thus enhances clinical outcomes. Moreover, the integration of advanced molecular techniques into digital pathology platforms offers the promise of novel diagnostic modalities. Next-generation sequencing, for example, can be paired with histological assessment to give further information on the genetic etiology of disease. This intersection of molecular profiling and digital pathology highlights improved categorization and prognostication of disease, ultimately directing therapy. Moreover, as demonstrated by recent advances in dermatopathology, the intersection of multidisciplinary wisdom from genetics, pathology, and clinical medicine encourages an integrated understanding of patient care.

By the integration of these diverse fields, healthcare practitioners are well placed to navigate the challenges of disease management, as exemplified by recent developments that emphasize technology as a catalyst for innovation in disease understanding and treatment pathways (Hussain, 2023; Firuzpour et al., 2025) (Figure 15.19).

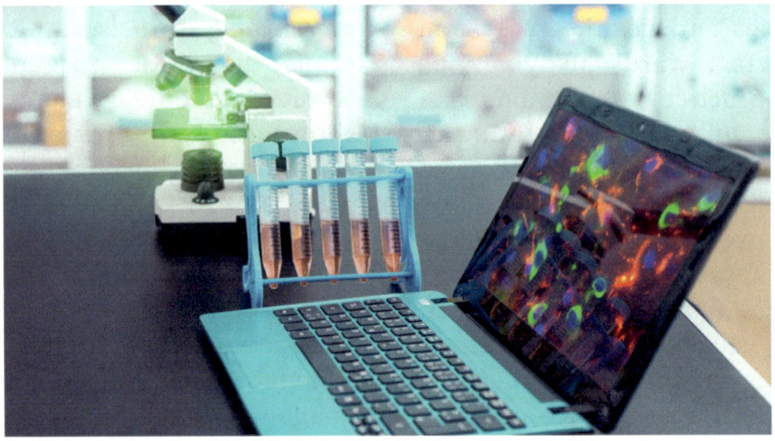

Figure 15.19. The integration of digital pathology with other healthcare technologies.

Source: https://cdn.sigma.software/wp-content/uploads/2024/01/blog-digital-pathology.jpg.

SUMMARY

Lastly, the integration of artificial intelligence (AI) and digital pathology in morphological analysis holds significant potential for the medical field. Synergizing diagnostic confidence, accelerating workflows, and assisting in the nuanced interpretation of complex biological systems, this pairing is poised to make a lasting impact. With the ability to rapidly and accurately analyze vast datasets, AI-facilitated tools are capable of identifying patterns and abnormalities that are not visible to the human eye. These technologies not only advantage patients by being able to diagnose early and accurately, but also allow for research studies that apply these technologies to examine complex disease processes. The convergence of these fields is a transformative shift for the practice of pathology, towards one that is more analytical and data-based, on the horizon to establish new standards of care. As the technologies evolve, ethical and pragmatic considerations must be addressed. Application of AI in diagnosis raises the issue of transparency of algorithms and explainability of results. Physicians should exercise caution in understanding the limits of AI technologies and effectively utilize them in practice. Providing equal access to these technologies to different healthcare centers is also imperative in avoiding inconsistencies in patient treatment. As has been highlighted in the recent debate regarding digital pathology, the implementation of successful AI solutions needs a collaborative approach between healthcare professionals, technologists, and policymakers. It is necessary to ensure collaboration in order to facilitate a robust base that can not only be utilized to build AI systems but also to integrate them into existing healthcare workflows. Finally, the future of AI within morphological analysis and digital pathology holds exciting potential, warranting additional research and investment. Innovations such as machine learning and deep learning stand to unlock new capacities for analytical applications, enabling more insightful appreciation of disease processes and tailored treatment plans. As the technology continues to mature, having standardized guidelines and prudent assessment measures will become essential to the assurance of the consistency of AI tools in practice. Additionally, collaborative research among multiple disciplines will broaden our understanding of how to maximize the usage of these technologies across different pathological conditions. In the future, harnessing the complementarity between artificial intelligence and digital pathology can open the way for groundbreaking new advances in medical diagnosis and patient care, ultimately resulting in a smarter and more responsive healthcare system.

The integration of digital pathology and artificial intelligence (AI) into morphologic analysis has revolutionized the practice of diagnostic medicine, with particular focus on the evaluation of biomarkers such as human epidermal growth factor receptor 2 (Her2) in invasive breast cancer. Traditionally, Her2 IHC scoring relied on subjective visual interpretation, which led to interobserver variation that compromised diagnostic accuracy. A paper presented in recent computerized scoring competitions demonstrated how AI-enabled algorithms might offer more precise and unbiased scores through an astounding reduction of human bias in Her2 scoring. Significantly, it was demonstrated that the algorithms outperformed pathology experts in scoring contests and could be used to assist pathologists and enhance cancer diagnostic accuracy (Berseth et al., 2017). Moreover, the accumulation of digital histopathological images has generated a demand for sophisticated analysis techniques, particularly involving machine learning algorithms. The utilization of digital images makes it possible for computer-aided diagnosis, which can ease the diagnostic process and make it more efficient. Nevertheless, image analysis presents special challenges, including variations in image quality and the need for standard evaluation protocols. Resolution of these issues is necessary for the efficient implementation of AI solutions in pathology. Machine learning approaches, while promising, must evolve to prevent such barriers since clinical results are based on image analysis accuracy. Recent literature suggests that research into solutions to such inherent problems is crucial to advancing the validity of digital pathology (Ishikawa, S., & Komura, D., 2017). Ultimately, the convergence of digital pathology and AI is a giant leap towards enhancing diagnostic capacity in healthcare. The potential for machine systems to deliver objective findings not only surpasses the limitations of traditional methods but also shatters new ground for enhanced patient management by way of individualized treatment regimens. With technological advancements, continued interaction between developers of artificial intelligence and pathologists will be essential to idealize algorithms and ensure they are acceptable with clinical requirements. Emphasis on the use of AI in morphological analysis directs attention toward a transition toward an improved, more efficient, accurate, and objective system for diagnosis of disease, thus transforming diagnostic pathology practice for the better (Berseth et al., 2017; Ishikawa, S., & Komura, D., 2017).

A LOOK TO THE FUTURE:

BLOOD CELL MORPHOLOGY:

Blood cell morphology is a foundational concept in clinical hematology and laboratory medicine, involving the examination and interpretation of the shapes, sizes, structures, and physical characteristics of blood cells under a microscope. It focuses particularly on cells observed in peripheral blood smears, including red blood cells (erythrocytes), white blood cells (leukocytes), and platelets. This morphological analysis plays a crucial role in diagnosing, monitoring, and understanding a wide range of physiological and pathological conditions that affect the blood and the body as a whole. The discipline of blood cell morphology traces its roots to the development of blood smear techniques and staining methods that made cellular details visible under light microscopy — a practice that remains vital despite the advent of automated hematology analyzers. While modern instruments provide rapid quantitative data such as cell counts and indices, visual assessment of a stained smear reveals qualitative information that machines cannot fully capture. For example, subtle changes in cell shape, color, or arrangement often provide early clues to underlying disorders, making manual morphology evaluation indispensable in many clinical settings.

Normal erythrocytes typically appear as biconcave discs with central pallor and uniform size and shape. Deviations from this typical morphology — such as variations in size (anisocytosis), altered shapes (poikilocytosis), or abnormal aggregations like rouleaux — can signal diverse clinical conditions such as anemia, nutritional deficiencies, chronic inflammation, or hematologic malignancies. Similarly, white blood cells exhibit morphological features that reflect their development and functional status: changes may indicate infection, immune response alterations, or bone marrow disorders. Platelet morphology and distribution also yield key diagnostic insights, particularly in bleeding and clotting disorders.

Blood cell morphology is not merely descriptive; it provides interpretable evidence that guides clinical decisions. By integrating morphological findings with clinical history, laboratory data, and other diagnostic tests, healthcare professionals can differentiate between disease etiologies, evaluate disease progression, and select appropriate therapeutic strategies. In cases of anemia or suspected hematologic disease, a carefully examined blood smear may even point directly to specific diagnoses or suggest targeted follow-up tests.

This work aims to introduce readers to the principles, methodology, and clinical significance of blood cell morphology. By combining foundational concepts with practical insights, it seeks to enhance understanding and appreciation of how detailed morphological analysis continues to support better patient care, enrich hematologic education, and inform ongoing research in blood disorders and related fields.

REFERENCES

1. Di Cataldo, S., Ficarra, E., Acquaviva, A., & Macii, E. (2010). Automated segmentation of tissue images for computerized IHC analysis. *Computer Methods and Programs in Biomedicine, 100*(1), 1–15. https://doi.org/10.1016/j.cmpb.2010.02.002Adams, R., Amsler, M., Bangalore, S., Barker, A., Benoît, J., Bian, X., Bondale, P., et al. (2003). Natural language processing. https://core.ac.uk/download/9015693.pdf (accessed on 6th August 2025).
2. Aga Khan University Hospital, Karachi. (2021). *LABRAD: Vol 46, Issue 4 – October 2021*. https://core.ac.uk/download/482026963.pdf (accessed on 6th August 2025).
3. Alsup, A. M., Fowlds, K., Hajighasemi, A., Koomey, C., et al. (2023). The state of applying artificial intelligence to tissue imaging for cancer research and early detection. http://arxiv.org/abs/2306.16989 (accessed on 6th August 2025).
4. Amarasinghe, R., Basnayake, B. A. D. J. C. K., Hettiarachchi, S. P., Melroy, R., et al. (2021). Review on photomicrography based full blood count (FBC) testing and recent advancements. https://core.ac.uk/download/577886377.pdf (accessed on 6th August 2025).
5. Arda, H. E., Burns, V. M., Chakravarthy, H., Charville, G., et al. (2017). Pathways to clinical CLARITY: Volumetric analysis of irregular, soft, and heterogeneous tissues in development and disease. https://core.ac.uk/download/129069108.pdf (accessed on 6th August 2025).
6. Ayyagari, D., Bonham, M. J., Chamarthi, R. V., Cockerell, C. J., et al. (2020). Tailored for real-world: A whole slide image classification system validated on uncurated multi-site data emulating the prospective pathology workload. https://core.ac.uk/download/288847206.pdf (accessed on 6th August 2025).
7. Berseth, M., Bhalerao, A., Bueno, G., Denzler, J., et al. (2017). Her2 challenge contest: A detailed assessment of automated HER2 scoring algorithms in whole slide images of breast cancer tissues. https://core.ac.uk/download/96620936.pdf (accessed on 6th August 2025).
8. Cabibi, D., Comelli, A., D'Aprile, S., Denaro, S., Giannone, A. G., Parenti, R., Pavone, A. M., et al. (2024). Digital pathology: A comprehensive review of open-source histological segmentation software. https://core.ac.uk/download/638996026.pdf (accessed on 6th August 2025).
9. Castagnola, M., Coghe, F., Didaci, L., Faa, G., et al. (2024). The quest for the application of artificial intelligence to whole slide imaging: Unique prospective from new advanced tools. https://core.ac.uk/download/614060218.pdf (accessed on 6th August 2025).
10. Chen, G., Chen, Y., Dey, N., Sherratt, R. S., et al. (2019). Texture features based microscopic image classification of liver cellular granuloma using artificial neural networks. https://core.ac.uk/download/323052639.pdf (accessed on 6th August 2025).
11. Dawson, H. (2022). Digital pathology – Rising to the challenge. https://core.ac.uk/download/541129482.pdf (accessed on 6th August 2025).
12. Dethlefs, B. A., Lee, K. L., Li, S. C., Loudon, T. L., et al. (2019). Breathing signature as vitality score index created by exercises of Qigong: Implications of artificial intelligence tools used in traditional Chinese medicine. https://core.ac.uk/download/323075335.pdf (accessed on 6th August 2025).
13. Engan, K., Kanwal, N., Molina, R., Pérez-Bueno, M. C., et al. (2022). The devil is in the details: Whole slide image acquisition and processing for artifacts detection, color variation, and data augmentation: A review. https://core.ac.uk/download/527689265.pdf (accessed on 6th August 2025).

14. Ferretti, A., Leone, L., Malisan, F., Raffa, S., et al. (2016). Extracorporeal shock wave treatment (ESWT) enhances the in vitro-induced differentiation of human tendon-derived stem/progenitor cells (hTSPCs). https://core.ac.uk/download/54530853.pdf (accessed on 6th August 2025).
15. Firuzpour, F., Kozak, M., Majd, H. S., Saeidnia, S., et al. (2025). Advancing cancer diagnosis and treatment: Integrating image analysis and AI algorithms for enhanced clinical practice. https://core.ac.uk/download/637013191.pdf (accessed on 6th August 2025).
16. Ginley, B., Govind, D., Jain, S., Jen, K. Y., et al. (2018). Iterative annotation to ease neural network training: Specialized machine learning in medical image analysis. https://core.ac.uk/download/573411151.pdf (accessed on 6th August 2025).
17. Hussain, A., et al. (2023). Updates in dermatopathology: Emerging trends in diagnosis and classification. https://core.ac.uk/download/596247500.pdf (accessed on 6th August 2025).
18. Ishikawa, S., & Komura, D. (2017). Machine learning methods for histopathological image analysis. http://arxiv.org/abs/1709.00786 (accessed on 6th August 2025).
19. Jaume, G., Lu, M. Y., Mahmood, F., Miller, J. B., et al. (2023). Artificial intelligence for digital and computational pathology. http://arxiv.org/abs/2401.06148 (accessed on 6th August 2025).
20. Naser, M., Nasr, M. M., & Shehata, L. H. (2024). Advances of AI in cancer breast: Review. https://core.ac.uk/download/636457352.pdf (accessed on 6th August 2025).

INDEX

D

E

F

G